Domestic Animal Behavior for Veterinarians and Animal Scientists

Fifth Edition

Domestic Animal Behavior for Veterinarians and Animal Scientists

Fifth Edition

Katherine Albro Houpt, VMD, PhD

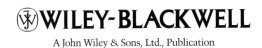

A John Wiley & Sons, Ltd., Publication

Edition first published 2011
© 2011 John Wiley & Sons, Inc.

Blackwell Publishing was acquired by John Wiley & Sons in February 2007. Blackwell's publishing program has been merged with Wiley's global Scientific, Technical, and Medical business to form Wiley-Blackwell.

Editorial Office
2121 State Avenue, Ames, Iowa 50014-8300, USA

For details of our global editorial offices, for customer services, and for information about how to apply for permission to reuse the copyright material in this book, please see our Website at www.wiley.com/wiley-blackwell.

Library of Congress Cataloging-in-Publication Data

Houpt, Katherine A.
  Domestic animal behavior for veterinarians and animal scientists / Katherine Albro Houpt. – 5th ed.
    p. ; cm.
  Includes bibliographical references and index.
    ISBN 978-0-8138-1676-0 (hardback : alk. paper)   1. Domestic animals–Behavior.   2. Animal behavior.
I. Title. [DNLM: 1. Animals, Domestic.   2. Behavior, Animal.
SF 756.7 H839d 2011]
    SF756.7.H68 2011
    636.089–dc22

                                                                                                2010020442

A catalog record for this book is available from the U.S. Library of Congress.

Set in 10/12 pt Times by Aptara® Inc., New Delhi, India
Printed and bound in Singapore by Ho Printing Singapore Pte Ltd

4   2013

To my friend of fifty years for bringing me joy

Contents

About the author

Katherine Albro Houpt, VMD, PhD, is emeritus professor of Animal Behavior at Cornell University College of Veterinary Medicine. She is a diplomate of the American College of Veterinary Behaviorists. She is director of Animal Behavior Consultants of Northern Michigan.

Preface

The fifth edition of Domestic Animal Behavior reflects the genomic age. A new chapter on the genetics of behavior has been added. Although the search for *the* gene for a specific behavior or behavior problem is still all too often fruitless, the field is moving so quickly, the techniques improving, and the costs of genetic analysis falling that it will not be long. Demethylation of genes explains why a cloned bull or cat may not have behavior as the original animal did. Another—not unrelated—field that has received a lot of attention in the past decade is laterality or handedness in animals. There are interesting sex differences in laterality and, in some cases, behavior problems are associated with lack of laterality.

The field of domestic animal cognition has continued to expand and there have been several studies on horses in addition to the growing number of studies on dogs. Episodic memory in pigs, observational learning in horses, and inferential learning by exclusion in dogs are a few of the new topics.

The most interesting development in maternal behavior is the stimulation of maternal behavior in mares using hormones and a dopamine blocker to induce lactation and cervical stimulation to induce specific maternal behavior to a foal.

Acknowledgment

Thanks to Charles E. Houpt for the cover photo and for solving many other problems concerning this book.

1 Communication

The position of the ears and tail, and the overall posture, are most indicative of the animal's immediate intentions. Flehmen (tonguing and gaping in carnivores) and the vomeronasal organ function in sexual behavior are discussed. Visual communication is an aid to understanding animals, but both vocal and olfactory communication can be problems.

INTRODUCTION

Communicating with animals, in particular, learning to understand the messages the animal is sending, is the most important part of diagnosis. Communication is a vital part of animal husbandry and the art of veterinary medicine, and a very useful adjunct to the science of veterinary medicine. Before ordering a complete blood count and liver function tests, the astute clinician will already know that a dog is suffering from abdominal pain because it assumes an abnormal posture with rump high and head low, or that a horse that paces in its stall and kicks at its belly is suffering from colic.

Another important aspect of communication between veterinarian and patient or between handler and stock is assessment of an animal's emotional state or temperament. Adequate restraint or, preferably, a quiet, tractable patient is necessary for thorough examination and diagnosis. Most practitioners learn eventually to recognize animals that will be aggressive or fearful and, therefore, require tranquilization, muzzling, or more stringent methods. It would be helpful for agriculture and veterinary students to learn in advance how to recognize animals' moods. Learning by experience to recognize behavior problems may occur at the expense of a badly bitten hand or kicked leg. For their own safety, as well as for acuity of diagnosis, clinicians should learn to listen to and watch for the messages their patients are transmitting both to them and to each other. Farmers can prevent injury to themselves and to their stock if they can interpret the animals' messages.

Communication between animals and humans occurs frequently, especially between dogs and their owners and cats and their owners. Dogs can respond to pointing by choosing the correct container, and it is not surprising that trained working gun dogs are better than pet gun dogs. Horses are more limited in their ability to interpret human gestures. Of the four horses tested, three could respond to touching the correct bucket out of two; in one test, only one horse responded to pointing by approaching the correct bucket.[1285] In another test, horses did respond to pointing by approaching one of two buckets, if the pointer was close to the bucket or the pointing gesture was longer than a second but only if the pointing gesture was sustained (dynamic).[1221] Goats rival dogs in their ability to follow human pointing and gazing.[977]

Domestic Animal Behavior for Veterinarians and Animal Scientists, Fifth Edition by Katherine Albro Houpt
© 2011 John Wiley & Sons, Inc.

Dogs and cats can determine where hidden food is when a person indicates the hiding place by pointing to it momentarily or dynamically from as far away as 80 cm. When the animals knew where the food was, but could not reach it, dogs were more likely to look at the owners sooner and for a longer time than cats.[1322] Dogs owned by blind people apparently do not realize that the owner is blind because they also look at unobtainable food, then at the owner, then at food, but they add a sound, noisy mouth licking (licking their chops).[675] Dogs will watch a human (owner or stranger) searching for, manipulating, and eating a hidden treat longer than they watch familiar dogs. They spend the least time observing feeding behavior.[1580] A single dog has been trained to use arbitrary signs to communicate. She would press a striped symbol for a walk, a toy, or water. Best of all, she would touch a sheet of newsprint to signal that she wanted access to her urination area.[1641] Despite their ability to communicate with humans, dogs do not seek help for their owners in an emergency situation such as when the owner has a heart attack or when the owner is pinned under a bookcase.[1201]

Animals communicate not only by auditory signals, as humans do, but also by visual and olfactory signals. Many olfactory messages cannot be detected by humans, although male pheromones, such as those contained in the urine of tomcats and the very flesh of boars and billy goats, are quite discernible to humans. We are all aware of vocal communication by animals, but many of these calls remain to be decoded. It is the visual signals made by ear, tail, mouth, and general posture that are of most benefit in gauging the temperament and the health of the patient.

PERCEPTION

Vision

Acuity

Communication in animals depends on their ability to perceive messages. The sensory abilities of domestic animals, with the exception of dogs and cats, have not been studied systematically. The perception of animals is almost always compared with that of humans. Dogs and cats have a higher critical flicker fusion (point at which a flickering light appears to be fused, or a steady light) than humans, which means that dogs and cats can see television, but in some cases the image may appear jerky to them.[368] Cats respond to television especially rapidly moving animate (mice, birds) or inanimate objects (balls) and will spend 6% of their time watching the screen.[536] Cats can discriminate illumination at one-fifth the threshold of humans, but their resolving power is only one-tenth that of humans.[558] Cross-eyed Siamese cats do not have stereoscopic vision; other cats do.[1463] Environmental conditions affect visual acuity. Free-ranging cats have been shown to be hypermetropic, whereas caged cats are myopic.[203] The visual acuity of cattle, measured by using a closed or partially opened circle at various distances from the cow, is inferior to that of humans.[539] Bulls have fairly poor vision; they are able to discriminate a 36-cm solid black disc from a similar disk with a white center if the center was 1 cm or larger and the bull was within 1.5 m.[1590] This indicates a visual acuity of only 23°, similar to the horse (23°) or the dog (10°).[1328] In some studies, pigs have been found to have poorer visual acuity than cattle—a hundredth or a thousandth of a humans.[2085] In the Snellen system, humans have 20/20 acuity whereas horses have 20/30, dogs have 20/85, and cattle or pigs 20/200 acuity.[1876] This means that what a person could see from 200 feet would have to be within 20 feet for a bull to see. Cattle can discriminate objects at 2 lux of illumination. Cattle are also poorer in brightness discrimination than are humans. They have a brightness discrimination threshold of 66 lux in bright light and 4.8 lux in dim light, whereas humans have discrimination thresholds of 105 and 4.2 lux.[1511] Horses can see in dimmer conditions than humans, they can make visual discrimination at a level of light equivalent to the illumination in a dense forest on a moonless night.[753]

An important question is, "Do all people look the same to animals, that is, can an animal tell the difference between people?" The answer is definitely yes. Pigs can tell people apart, even if olfactory cues are masked, on the basis of visual cues such as height and facial appearance. They can even distinguish humans apart in dim (20 lux) light.[1042] Cattle recognize people by their faces or the color of their coveralls, and use height to discriminate between people.[1383,1671] Sheep can recognize faces of other sheep and differentiate them on the basis of photographs. They can remember at least 25 different sheep faces for more than a year. In addition, they are able to recognize human faces, even faces of those they have not seen for many months.[999] Dogs associate their owners, voice with their face and when a strange voice is played while the owners picture is displayed the dogs gaze longer indicating that their expectations had been violated.[4] All people do not look the same to sheep, cattle, dogs or pigs, and probably this is true of most domestic animals. Therefore, the animals can remember who has treated them well or painfully.[1382]

Color vision

A question often put to a behaviorist is whether animals have color vision. All species of domestic animals have been shown to possess color vision in that they will make discriminations based on color, but color probably is not as relevant to these animals as it is to birds, fish, and primates. For example, teaching cats to discriminate between colors is very difficult, although they learn other visual discriminations with ease and have two types of cones that absorb green and blue. Nevertheless, cats,[1721] dogs,[1406] horses,[723] cattle,[419,688] pigs,[1036,1406,1407] goats,[298] and sheep[1381] can all make discriminations based on color alone. Color vision in domestic animals is not identical to that in humans. In the most carefully conducted studies, dogs appear to see the world not in shades of gray but rather in shades of violet, blue, and yellow. Their vision is similar to that of color-blind or dichromat humans, who see the green light as pale yellow, the yellow as yellow, and the red as dark yellow.

Ruminants can discriminate medium and long wavelengths (yellow, orange, and red) better than they can short wavelengths (violet, blue, and green). Cattle can discriminate red from blue and green but have difficulty discriminating green from blue. Animals can not only perceive colors but also be influenced behaviorally by color. For example, calves are more active in red light and less startled by loud noises in green light.[1508] Bulls, indeed, can perceive the matador's red cape.[1607] Horses can discriminate red from blue but some horses have difficulty distinguishing green or blue green (wavelength 480 nm) from gray.[327,389,1202,1513,1782] It may be easier to teach horses to discriminate colors if the stimuli are presented on the ground rather than at nose level. Color may be a more important feature of the equine environment than previously thought because horses do not habituate to objects of different colors and shapes, but do habituate if all the objects are the same color. Apparently, one blue blob is similar enough to another blob that the horse realizes it is not a threat.[353] Some colors—blue, black, white and yellow—cause more reaction when the horse encounters them on the ground than others—brown, green, red, and gray.[745]

Monocular and binocular vision

Eye placement in the skull also affects vision. Horses have eyes set quite laterally and can, therefore, see to the side and far to the rear. They cannot see well right in front of their heads. Lateral vision is necessarily monocular, and horses see binocularly only in the 70° directly in

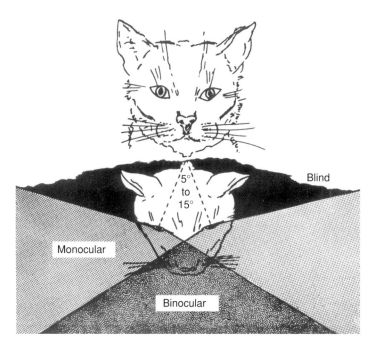

Fig. 1.1   Fields of vision of the cat, showing a large binocular area resulting from the forward position of the eyes. (J.H. Prince, reprinted from M.J. Swenson, ed. Duke's Physiology of Domestic Animals. Copyright 1970, 1977 by Cornell University. Used with permission of Cornell University Press.[1553])

front of the head. Contrary to many popular and scientific sources, horses do not have a ramped or slanted retina;[1773] the retina is similar to that of other animals. Figures 1.1 and 1.2 illustrate the fields of vision of the cat and horse, respectively. The binocular overlap (areas where the horse is viewing objects with both eyes simultaneously) is down the nose and not straight ahead.

Horses can see clearly with their heads lowered, contrary to popular belief.[160] They do so by adjusting their eyeball to a horizontal position.

When the horse lowers its head, the binocular field is directed toward the ground for grazing and the monocular fields are in position to scan the lateral horizon. When the head is raised with the nose pointing forward, the horse uses the binocular field (both eyes) to scan the horizon, and the monocular (single eye) lateral vision becomes limited.[763]

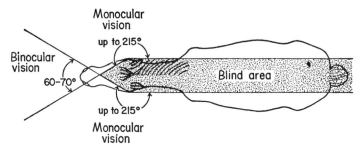

Fig. 1.2   Fields of vision of the horse. Note that there is only a small area of binocular vision but a very wide field of monocular vision.[1974] (Copyright 1975, with permission of Bailliere Tindall and W.B. Saunders Co.)

Audition

Acuity

In hearing, as in vision, cats and dogs appear to perceive more than humans. Humans can hear 8.5 octaves; cats can hear 10. Cats have 40,000 cochlear fibers and humans have 30,000, although the range of hearing in cats is only 1.5 octaves greater than that of humans because higher frequency detection requires a disproportionate increase in cochlear nerve fibers; the number of fibers needed per octave is not constant but, rather, rises with the rise in frequency.[1627] Cats, despite their mobile pinnae, can discriminate between sounds 5° apart, whereas humans can discriminate sounds 0.5° apart. The pinnae significantly lower the auditory threshold in the cat. The absolute upper limit of hearing in cats is 60–65 kHz (kilohertz = kilocycles per second) and 45 kHz in dogs.[802] Dogs and cats can discriminate one-eighth to one-tenth tones.[558,1403] Sheep also appear to perceive higher frequencies than do humans.[48] Dogs and adult cats are not known to produce ultrasonic calls, but rodents do make ultrasonic noises[45] that the carnivores use to locate them.

Practical application

The importance of hearing to cattle is indicated by the fact that they will avoid the side of a maze where milking facility noises are played.[88] Dogs are quieter when classical music is played but more reactive when heavy metal is played.[1998] The auditory acuity of dogs has been used in silent dog whistles and ultrasonic (but not to the dog) distracting devices.[317]

Olfaction

Acuity

Olfaction is to animals what writing is to humans—a message that can be transmitted in the absence of the sender. The sender must be present for auditory or visual signals to be sent, but an odor persists for minutes (or days) after the sender has gone. Olfactory acuity is probably the most important sense of domestic animal species because individual odor recognition and pheromonal release are an important part of their communication. Dogs probably have the greatest olfactory acuity, and this macrosmatic species is the one most investigated. Dogs can detect aliphatic acids at one-hundredth the concentration detectable by humans;[1374] The lowest concentration of amyl acetate that dogs can detect is two parts per thousand.[1963] They can distinguish between the odors of identical twins[974] and detect the odors of fingerprints 6 weeks after the fingerprints were placed on glass.[1027] Dogs frequently are trained to sniff out drugs and natural gas leaks, and bloodhounds have been used for centuries to track people; apparently, no modern invention is as reliable as the canine olfactory mucosa. However, when thermally stressed or physically tired, their rate of detecting explosives falls from 91% to 81%.[677]

When administering drugs to odor-detecting dogs or those used in tracking, care must be taken by the veterinarian because a combination of corticosteroids can interfere with olfactory discrimination.[559]

Considerable controversy exists about the ability of dogs to match a human scent from one part of the body, for example, the hands, with another part, such as the elbows. Although dogs can be trained to do so, it appears to be a difficult concept for them to grasp. This is probably because they can easily discriminate odors from different body parts.[284,1736] The same dog can learn to detect at least 10 different odors.[2030] Dogs can be trained to detect cadavers and live scent. Dogs trained to do both are less accurate—more distracted by cadaver odor when commanded to find a live human scent.[1170]

Pheromones and the vomeronasal organ have been identified in the intermammary area of lactating sows, bitches, mares, and doe goats as well as the cheek glands of cats,[1464] and these may be of value in reducing aggression and fear and encouraging feeding. The use of synthetic versions of these pheromones and that of the feline cheek glands are discussed under the appropriate species.

The vomeronasal organ lies between the hard palate and the nasal cavity in all species except humans. It is a paired tubular organ into which nonvolatile material can be aspirated. Receptor neurons in the lining of the organ detect pheromones and send information more directly to the hypothalamus than neurons in the main olfactory system. In ruminants and horses, flehmen or lip curl accomplishes this by closing the nostril while the animal breathes deeply. Cats gape and dogs tongue using their tongue to move material into the opening of the incisive ducts that open into the vomeronasal organ. Each neuron expresses only one pheromonal receptor gene. In mice, the vomeronasal organ allows recognition of sex and individuals are recognized by combinatoral activation of neurons.[797] Domestic animals are not as dependent on the vomeronasal organ for reproduction as rodents, but it still plays a role as will be discussed for each species.

HORSES

Vocalizations

Neigh

The neigh (or whinny) is a greeting or separation call that appears to be important in maintaining herd cohesion. It is most often heard when adult horses or a mare and foal are separated. A separated mare and foal will neigh repeatedly. These appear to be nonspecific distress calls, which the mare, but not the foal, may recognize individually.[2055] Some horses will call to their owners, but usually only when they are in their line of sight.

Nicker

The soft nicker is a care-giving (epimeletic) or care-soliciting (et-epimeletic) call. It is given by a mare to her foal upon reunion and probably is recognized specifically by each.[1909] A horse may also nicker to its caretaker and a stallion to a mare in estrus.

Snorts, squeals, and roars

Nickers or neighs usually elicit a reply; other equine vocalizations, such as snorts, squeals, and roars, do not. The roar is a high-amplitude vocalization of a stallion and is usually directed to a mare. A sharp snort is an alarm call. More prolonged snorting or sneezing snorts appear to be a frustration call given when horses are restrained from galloping or forced to work. Snorts and nickers are sounds from the nostrils. The mouth is closed. Other calls are given with the mouth open.

When two strange horses meet, or when horses have been separated for some time, they greet each other by putting their muzzles together nostril to nostril (Fig. 1.3). The nostrils are flared, but if any vocal signals are given, they are inaudible to humans. Usually one, the other,

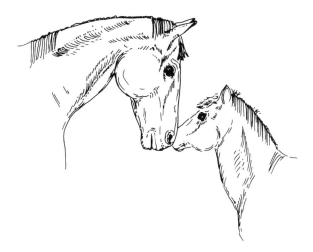

Fig. 1.3   Greeting. Nostril-to-nostril investigation, in this case by a horse and a pony.

or occasionally both of the horses will squeal and strike or jump back although neither has been bitten or threatened. The squeal is, therefore, a defensive greeting. It is heard frequently when horses are forming a dominance hierarchy and many bites are being exchanged. Mares that are not in estrus squeal and strike when a stallion approaches too closely. A squeal may also be a response to pain.

Visual signals

Expression

The horse's ears are probably the best indicator of its emotions. The alert horse looks directly at the object of interest and holds its ears forward. Ears pointed back indicate aggression, and the flatter the ears are against the head, the more aggressive the horse[1902] (Fig. 1.4). Frequently, veterinarians are called upon to examine a horse for soundness for a prospective buyer. If the horse reacts to examination, or even saddling, by swiveling its ears back, it may not be a desirable purchase, even if it is perfectly sound physically.

Other facial expressions of the horse are more subtle; nevertheless, they can be used profitably to understand a horse's mood. A submissive horse turns its ears outward. Young horses (less than

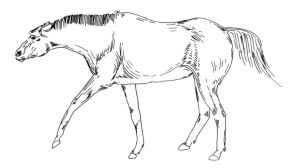

Fig. 1.4   The aggressive posture of a horse. The ears are back, and the horse is striking out with its front leg and lashing its tail.[867]

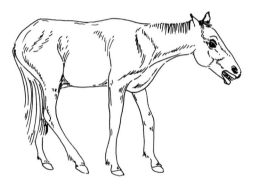

Fig. 1.5 The submissive posture of a horse. The tail is tucked in and the ears are turned outward. The horse is also snapping (opening and closing its mouth while retracting the lips).[867]

3 years old) have a more dramatic display, snapping, also called champing or tooth-clapping, in which the lips are retracted, exposing the teeth that are sometimes clicked together (Fig. 1.5). This expression is shown by a yearling colt to an approaching stallion or toward an adult who is threatening him. The sexually receptive mare shows a unique expression, the mating face, in which her ears are swiveled back and her lips hang loose (Fig. 1.6). She may also exhibit snapping. The flehmen response, or curled upper lip, of the courting stallion is discussed in the next section. A horse that sees but cannot reach food, or is anticipating food, makes chewing movements and sticks out its tongue (Fig. 1.7). This may be a submissive signal. More difficult to identify is the horse in pain. A horse that is exhausted and in pain will show loose lips but clenched masseter or cheek muscles. Before a horse is in such pain with colic that it kicks at its belly, it will repeatedly swivel its ears back as if attending to its abdomen. The various facial and postural expressions of horses have been illustrated by McDonnell.[1255] Horses tend to position their ears in the same direction in which they are looking. Thus, when the horse's ears are pointed straight ahead, it is looking straight ahead. This can be a clue that the horse is

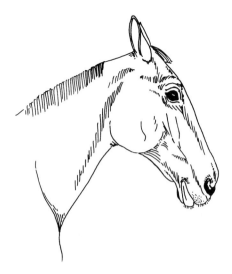

Fig. 1.6 The mating expression of the mare.[867]

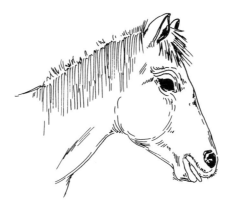

Fig. 1.7 The food-anticipating expression of the horse.[879] (Copyright 1978, with permission of Elsevier Scientific Publishing.)

about to shy at an object. Usually, the rider can identify the frightening object by looking where the horse's ears are pointing. The horse can then be coaxed to investigate and conquer its fear of the object. When the horse turns its ears to the side and back, it is looking to the side.

Posture

The posture and bodily actions of the horse are also useful in interpreting its moods. The relaxed horse stands quietly, whereas its nervous counterpart prances and chafes at the least restraint. The aggressive horse, when threatening to kick, lashes its tail and may even lift one of its hind legs. The frightened horse tucks its tail tightly against its rump and stands with its feet close together. Muscle guarding is seen, especially if the animal anticipates pain. A few mares will urinate and lash their tails, splattering urine, as they are being chased, and it should not be confused with the frequent urination but with deviated tail seen in estrous mares. The stallion moving his mares assumes a unique posture, called herding, driving, or snaking, with head down, nearly touching the ground, and ears flattened (Fig. 1.8).

Horses paw the ground not in aggression but rather in frustration when they are eager to gallop or, more commonly, when they want to graze and are restrained by rope or reins. Pawing to eat may be a behavior derived from pawing through snow for grass and might be considered a form of displacement behavior. Tail lashing and pawing can be signs of discomfort.[987]

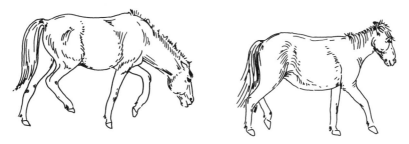

Fig. 1.8 Driving posture of the horse. The stallion, left, drives a mare. This behavior is also called snaking, herding, or driving (rounding).[867]

Tactile sense

Horses can detect a fly on their skin and respond either by moving their skin or swishing their tails. Riders make use of the horse's ability to perceive a slight pressure on his flank in order to signal dressage movements. Very light pressure on the skin is used to calm a horse.[1859] Another use of the horse's tactile sense or more likely pain receptors is the twitch. When the horse's upper lip is twisted with a chain or rope, endorphins are released and analgesia is produced.[1084]

Olfactory signals

Scent marking

Olfactory communication plays an important part in the sexual behavior of horses. Stallions curl their upper lip in the flehmen position or "horse laugh" when they smell the urine of a mare (Fig. 1.9). Estrous urine alone does not stimulate more episodes of flehmen by stallions than does nonestrous urine,[1220,1801] but the frequency of flehmen by a stallion toward a particular mare in his herd increases as she approaches estrus, perhaps because the mare urinates more frequently. After the stallion investigates urine by putting his lip in it, the flehmen position carries the urine into the nasal cavity. When his lips are raised in the flehmen position, the nostril opening is partially blocked and the horse, by breathing deeply, carries the urine into the vomeronasal organ. Although stallions flehmen most frequently, geldings and mares also exhibit the behavior in response to olfactory or gustatory stimuli. Cough medicine or a new bit often causes the horse laugh or flehmen—obviously, not a sign of amusement. Stallions usually urinate on the urine (scent mark) as they are exhibiting flehmen.

Horses also use olfactory cues, especially from their own or other horses' manure, to find their way home. Wild stallions use manure piles, or stud piles, along well-used pathways, possibly to scent mark.[573] These piles may separate bands of horses both spatially and temporally. Even in a pasture, stallions select one place to defecate and then back into the pile to eliminate, so the pile does not grow much wider. On the other hand, mares and geldings face outward, gradually increasing the diameter of the pile. Because horses do not eat grass contaminated with feces, a pasture containing mares and geldings rapidly becomes "horsed out" or inedible.[1442] Despite the discrimination of older horses against feces, foals show coprophagia, as discussed in more detail in Chapter 6, "Development of Behavior." Horses respond to predator odor by

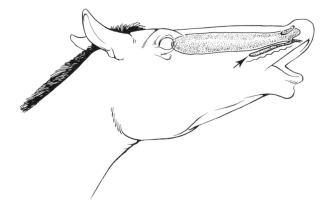

Fig. 1.9   The flehmen response or lip curl. The location of the vomeronasal organ is indicated by the arrow.

increased sniffing, but only seem frightened (refuse to eat and increase heart rate) when the odor is combined with the sound of a plastic bag being dragged over the ground[352] Horses have individual sensitivities. Some are more reactive to odors, others to tactile or auditory stimuli, but there is no general sensitivity. A horse that responds strongly to a sound is not necessarily going to respond strongly to a spicy taste.[1095]

Artificial pheromones

The equine appeasing pheromone, from the intramammary sulcus of the lactating mare can reduce the signs of fear and the elevation of heart rate in response to a novel stimulus—a bridge.[563]

DOGS

Vocalizations

The common vocal communications of dogs are the bark, whine, howl, and growl.

Bark

Barking is a territorial call of dogs. It is used to defend a territory and to demarcate its boundaries. Stray dogs, whose resting places may be quite temporary, rarely bark.[192] As a stray dog passes the yards of owned dogs, however, it precipitates territorial barking. The observant owner can recognize various types of barks. The bark to be let in the house differs from that directed at human intruders, which may differ from that directed at canine intruders. Barking occurs in wild canids; a wolf in a semi-naturalistic pen will bark at an intruder, but barking has been a trait selected for in domesticated dogs. People obtain dogs because they bark and can serve to warn their owners of the approach of intruders. Unfortunately, dogs are much more likely to bark in response to another dog's bark than to the sound of a human intruder.[11] The barking trait can become a problem in a highly urbanized environment. Two thousand two hundred complaints about barking are filed in Los Angeles per year.[1729] For this reason, a dog's barking can be a problem for the owner. A more acute problem is the barking of kenneled or caged dogs in a veterinary clinic. The noise level generated by barking can exceed the 90-decibel limit of the Occupational Safety and Health Act.[15] Animal hospitals must, therefore, be constructed with very good sound insulation.

Excessive barking can be punished with a collar that sprays citronella on the dog's chin[972,1997] or an electric shock collar could be used to teach the dog to keep barking to a minimum. The only type of electronic collar that is humane is that which is activated by the animal's bark rather than by the human. A final resort is vocal cordectomy (debarking), which may save the life of a dog that has been a barking problem. Various procedures are described for vocal cordectomy.[71] Dogs are not rendered silent, but the strength and pitch of their voices are lowered.

Whine and howl

Whining is an et-epimeletic or care-soliciting call of the dog. It is first used by puppies to communicate with the mother, who provides warmth and nourishment. Mature dogs whine when they want relief from pain or are in even a mildly frustrating situation, such as when they want to escape outdoors or reach a rabbit for which they are digging.

Howling is a canine call that has not been deciphered well. It occurs more frequently in wild canids, coyotes, and wolves and in some breeds of dogs, such as huskies, malamutes, and to a lesser extent hounds. Harrington and Mech[765] found that the incidence of howling in wolves increased 10-fold during the home-site season. As the year's pups mature, the pack becomes more dispersed and the howling apparently takes the place of scent marking in coordinating pack member spacing and activity.

Harrington[764] also has found that wolves can discriminate strange adult from strange pup howls and answer only the former. A different component, lower in frequency, occurs in the answering howls of wolves approaching the source of a strange howl. Whether this is true in dogs as well remains to be determined.

Growl

Growling is an aggressive or distance-increasing call in dogs.

Visual signals

A dog's emotional state can be determined by observation of its ears, mouth, facial expression, tail, hair on its shoulders and rump, and overall body position and posture (Fig. 1.10). The calm dog stands with ears and tail hanging down. When it becomes alert, its tail and ears are pointed upward. The dog may point with one front foot. As the dog becomes more aggressive, the hair on the shoulders (hackles) and the rump rises and the lips are drawn back. The ears remain forward and the tail may be slowly wagged. With increasing aggression, the lips are retracted and the teeth exposed in a snarl. The dog stands straight. As the dog becomes frightened, the ears go back until they are flattened against the head and the tail descends until it is between the legs.

Posture

The posture of the fear-biting dog, the one most likely to injure a veterinarian, is that of the frightened dog with tail and ears down and the body leaning away from the source of fear. It will have raised hackles and lips retracted in a snarl, which may expose the molars as well as the canines. Care must be taken when approaching a dog to notice any lifting of the lip, because this may be the only prediction of defensive aggression or fear biting. The fear biter will escape if possible; but if it is approached within its critical distance, which may be a yard (approximately a meter or less) from it, it will attack.

More common, fortunately, is a dog in which fear is not mixed with aggression. The fearful dog crouches with its tail between its legs and its ears flattened down. If the dog is abjectly submissive, it will lie on its side and lift its hind leg, displaying the inguinal area. It may also make licking intention movements, that is, sticking its tongue out but not contacting anything. Finally, it may urinate. This behavior probably represents a reversion to puppy habits in which the puppy lies down on its side and presents the inguinal area to the mother (who is, of course, dominant over the puppy) and allows her to lick and clean it.

General posture is also a good indication of the dog's mood. A lowered body posture with depressed tail is associated with fear and fear-based aggression[787] and a tall, especially a rigid,

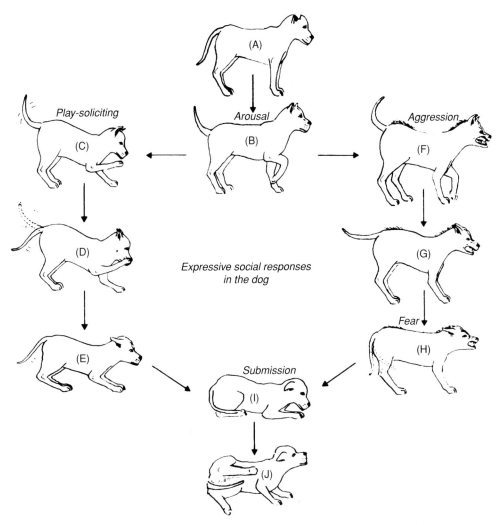

Fig. 1.10 Body postures of the dog. (A, B) Neutral to alert attentive positions; (C) play bow; (D, E) active and passive submissive greeting—note tail wag and shift in ear position and in distribution of weight on fore and hind limbs; (F–H) gradual shift from aggressive display to ambivalent fear-defensive aggressive posture; (I) passive submission; and (J) rolling over and presentation of inguinal-genital region.[616] (Copyright 1975, with permission of W.B. Saunders Co.)

posture with tail raised and stiff is associated with offensive aggression. Dogs wag their tails to the right of center when encountering their owner or a stranger, but to left when encountering a strange dominant dog.[1564]

During a submissive approach, dogs curve their bodies, wiggling toward the superior, whereas a dominant dog stands straight and walks stiffly with tail and ears erect. This stiffening of posture can be used to predict when an initially friendly greeting is about to become an attack.

Dogs greet their owners as they did their mothers: by licking their faces. As puppies, dogs lick their mothers' faces to beg for regurgitated feed. Although wild canids frequently regurgitate food for their pups, not all domestic dogs do so; nevertheless, the begging behavior is shown by domestic puppies. The behavior persists in the adult dog who either licks the owner, or, if prevented by discipline or its small stature, makes licking intention movements. Licking their own lips, yawning, or even falling asleep sitting up are all signs of ambivalence in dogs. A few dogs will "grin" as a submissive greeting. They show their teeth with flattened ears.

Dogs have a play signal; it is necessary to signal that the action that follows is play because, otherwise, the recipient of the playful act will consider it genuine aggression or sexual activity and respond in kind. A bowing with the forequarters lowered and the hindquarters elevated and topped by a rapidly wagging tail is the signal for canine play.[200] Often, one paw is waved or rubbed at the dog's own muzzle. Interspecific communication is important, too. People use various motions and vocalizations to signal that they want to play with a dog. The most successful are lunging or bowing toward the dog while whispering or speaking in a high-pitched voice.[1624]

Genetic and surgical alteration

Ears, tail, and hair position are all important in visual communication between dogs, but communication tends to break down in breeds that have been modified either genetically or surgically. Dogs with dependent ears, such as hounds, can only hint at attentiveness or fear. It is hard to detect piloerection on a long-haired dog. Can an Afghan raise its hackles? Hair also prevents many breeds from seeing the signals of other dogs. The Old English sheepdog is a good example because it has hair across its face and cannot see, and because of coccygeal amputation, its tail position must be left to the imagination. Merely cutting the hair that obstructs a dog's vision can improve its temperament. Dogs with docked tails learn to wag their whole hindquarters so that pleasure, if not fear, can still be expressed.

Olfactory signals

The legendary olfactory acuity of dogs has already been mentioned. Because dogs can smell so well, it is not surprising that dogs use odors as a means of communication.

There are applied uses of canine olfactory abilities too. Although olfactory repellents are seldom effective in dogs, odors can have a positive effect. Wells[1995] has found that lavender oil reduces canine vocalization and locomotion during car travel. A chemical has been synthesized from the epithelial cells of the bitch's mammary sulcus and is available commercially as Dog Appeasing Pheromone®. It has calming effects on newly weaned puppies, dogs afraid of fireworks, and in the veterinary clinic and reduces barking amplitude and increases resting behavior in shelter dogs.[673,674,1124,1335,1745,1856,1881]

The importance of olfactory communication to dogs is exemplified by the diligence with which male dogs scent mark vertical objects by urinating. Dogs are believed to be capable of identifying species, sex, and even individuals from the odor of the urine. Dogs scent mark much more frequently in areas where other dogs have marked. The record may be that observed by Sprague and Anisko[1797] of 80 markings by one dog in 40 hours. Even though male dogs rarely empty their bladders completely, such efforts exhausted this dog's supply; the last urinations were dry.

Elimination postures

It is appropriate at this point to discuss elimination postures in male and female dogs. Owners are often concerned because their young male does not lift his hind leg but, rather, still squats.

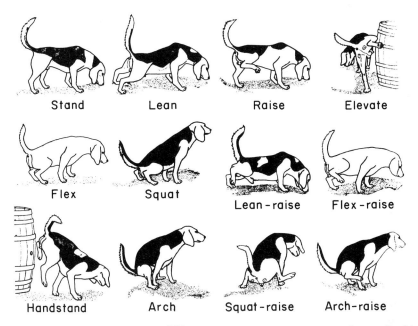

Fig. 1.11   Elimination postures of the dog.[1797] (Copyright 1973, with permission of E.J. Brill Publishers.)

Although standing and lifting the hind leg are typical innate male behaviors mediated by testosterone,[212] 3% of the time males urinate in other positions. Bitches assume not only the squatting position (68% of the occasions that they urinate) but also lift their hind legs (2%) and use various combinations of the two postures.

Urine marking is the most common form of scent marking in dogs, but vertical objects may also be marked with feces, as any kennel cleaner has observed. Again, males are more likely than females to mark with feces[1797] (Fig. 1.11). Hart[769] found that castration reduces scent marking in male dogs. Dogs that cannot smell (anosmic) and that, therefore, cannot identify other dogs' urine, mark less frequently and, in contrast to intact dogs, do not urinate on the urine of other dogs. When dogs scratch after eliminating, they are not making rudimentary burying movements but are spreading the scent and possibly adding the odor of secretions from interdigital sebaceous glands. Intact male dogs mark more during the breeding season; lactating bitches mark around their nest area.[1469]

Urine

The most powerful means of olfactory communication in the canine species is the urine of an estrous bitch. Doty and Dunbar[481] have shown that male dogs are more strongly attracted to the urine of an estrous bitch than to vaginal or anal sac secretions, although Goodwin et al.[702] present strong evidence that the vaginal secretion methyl p-hydroxy-benzoate is what induces the actual mating behavior sequence in the male (see Chapter 4, "Sexual Behavior"). Dogs "tongue," that is, flick their tongues against the palate just behind their incisor teeth, introducing estrous urine into the vomeronasal organ. This is the canine equivalent of flehmen.

Dunbar[496] also demonstrated the marked preference by an estrous bitch for male urine as compared with either estrous or nonestrous urine. The urine contains pheromones, substances secreted by one animal that affect the behavior of another animal. In estrous urine, these compounds are probably estrogen metabolites. The urine of a bitch in heat can attract males from great distances. The attractant effect of the bitch's pheromone is usually considered a nuisance, but it has practical applications. For instance, the pheromone could be used to attract stray dogs that could then be easily captured. One might expect that male dogs would inevitably be attracted to the urine of a receptive female, but Beach and Gilmore[174] noted that a dog without mating experience did not investigate estrous urine in preference to anestrous urine, whereas sexually experienced dogs did.

Anal and aural secretions

Urine is not the only olfactory means by which dogs communicate. The anal gland secretions normally are eliminated with the feces and, no doubt, give them a unique odor.[481] Dogs, on meeting, usually sniff under each other's tails. This behavior is probably one of identifying the individual by its smell. A very excited dog can express its anal sacs forcefully; the resulting odor is pungent enough to be smelled by humans and may function as a fear pheromone.[475] The secretions of the ears are also believed to function in individual identification,[616] and investigation of one another's ears is a common greeting behavior of dogs.

Submissive urination

Submissive urination is a frequent behavioral problem. It occurs more often in young dogs and small dogs. Living with a dog that is dominant over its owner may be difficult, but living with a dog that urinates submissively is messy. Punishing the dog for urinating in fear or excitement aggravates the problem. The dog is already afraid of its owner, and punishment only confirms and reinforces that fear. The wisest course is to avoid overexciting the dog.

Overenthusiastic greetings and overly harsh punishments should be avoided. If the person in the household who most often elicits the submissive behavior generally ignores the animal, the problem may be minimized. Submissive urination often declines as the dog matures.

Urine marking

Another type of communication by pet animals that is not appreciated by humans is urine marking. The stimulus for urine marking in the house is a vertical object, but the motivation of the dog may be elimination, marking, or even separation anxiety. Elimination problems are addressed in the "House breaking" section of Chapter 7, "Learning". The marking of every vertical object in a city block is another source of pollution that may not only kill the trees sprayed but also spread such urine-borne diseases as leptospirosis. Urine marking may increase the level of aggression in male dogs. Smelling the urine of other dogs does, no doubt, excite a dog regardless of whether it might lead to aggression directed toward humans. For a number of reasons, therefore, dogs should be encouraged to urinate on their own territories only.

CATS

Vocalizations and audition

Many more feline vocalizations exist than those described in Table 1.1; some of these vocalizations may not be recognized by every cat owner.[274] The wild ancestor of cats *Felis sylvestris lybica* is less vocal and meows in fewer contexts; its call is longer and lower in frequency and deemed less pleasant by humans.[1413] Apparently, we have selected cats to communicate with us in "pleasant" voices. Humans can distinguish positive and negative affect in feline

Table 1.1 The vocalizations of cats.

Murmur	A soft, rhythmically pulsed vocalization given on exhalation. Murmurs are the request, or greeting call, which can vary from a coax to a command, and the acknowledgment, or confirmation call, which is a short, single murmur with a rapidly falling intonation.
Purr	A soft, buzzing vocalization that is easy to recognize. It occurs only in social situations and may indicate submission or a kitten-like state. Remmers and Gautier[1596] have shown that purring is associated with rapid contraction of the muscles of the larynx. The laryngeal muscles are driven by a central pattern generator with a cycle of contraction every 30–40 ms.[640]
Growl	A harsh, low-pitched vocalization,[309] usually of long duration and given in agonistic encounters.
Squeak	A high-pitched, raspy cry given in play, in anticipation of feeding, and by the female after copulation.
Shriek	A loud, harsh, high-pitched vocalization given in intensely aggressive situations or during painful procedures.
Hiss	An agonistic vocalization produced while the mouth is open and teeth exposed. This vocalization is probably defensive and can be used to gauge whether a cat is defensively or offensively aggressing.
Spit	A short, explosive sound given before or after a hiss in agonistic situations. Saliva is expelled.
Chatter	A teeth-chattering sound made by some cats while hunting or more commonly when restrained from hunting by confinement.
Estrus call	A call of variable pitch, lasting a half-second to 1 second. The mouth is opened and then gradually closed. It is given repeatedly by queens in estrus, which is termed calling because the vocalization is so characteristic.
Howl and yowl of an aggressive cat	These are loud, harsh calls.
Mowl, or caterwaul, of the male cat	A variable-pitch call, usually given in a sexual context.
Mew	A high-pitched, medium-amplitude vocalization. Phonetically it sounds like a long "e." It occurs in mother–kitten interactions and in the same situations as the squeak.
Moan	This is a call of low frequency and long duration. The sound is "o" or "u." It is given before regurgitating a hair ball or in epimeletic situations, such as begging to be released to hunt.
Meow	This characteristic feline call, "ee-ah-oo," is given in a variety of greeting or epimeletic situations just as the mew and squeak are. Anyone who has tried to restrict a cat's food will not be surprised to know that cats can be trained to meow twice a minute for 2 hours when the reward is food.[564]

vocalizations.[1414] Agonistic calls are longer in duration and lower in frequency than affiliative calls. Because cats can hear ultrasound it has been used to deter cats from entering an area and, although the technique is only moderately effective, the efficacy increases with time.[1409]

Visual signals

Posture

The postures and facial expressions of the cat are shown in Figs. 1.12a and b. A cat carries its tail high when greeting, investigating, or is frustrated. The tail is depressed and the tip is wagged during stalking. When walking or trotting, the tail is held out at a 40° angle to the back, but as the cat's pace increases, the tail is held lower.[1015] A relaxed cat, as does a relaxed dog, usually stands with tail hanging, but the cat's ears are usually forward. When the cat's attention is attracted, the tail is raised and both ears are pointed forward and held erect. The aggressive cat walks on tiptoe with head down. Because the cat's hind legs are longer than its front legs, it appears to be slanting downward from rump to head. Its tail is held down but arched away

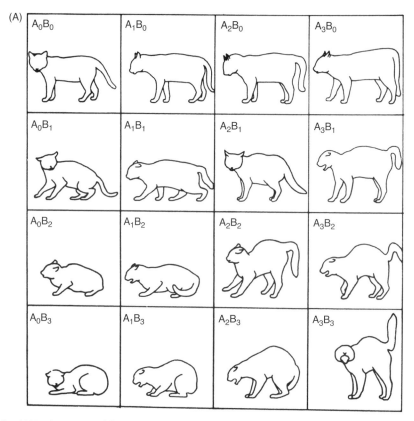

Fig. 1.12   (A) Body postures of the cat. Aggressiveness is increasing from A_0 to A_3, fearfulness from B_0 to B_3. A_3B_0 is the most aggressive cat, A_0B_3 the most fearful, and A_3B_3 the defensively aggressive cat.[1134] (English ed.; *Katzen–Eine Verhaltensstudien*, copyright 1975, with permission of Paul Parey, Berlin and Hamburg.) (B) Facial expressions of the cat.[1134] (English ed., *Katzen–Eine Verhaltensstudien*, copyright 1975, with permission of Paul Parey, Berlin and Hamburg.) A_2B_0 is offensively aggressive; A_0B_2 is defensively aggressive.

(B)

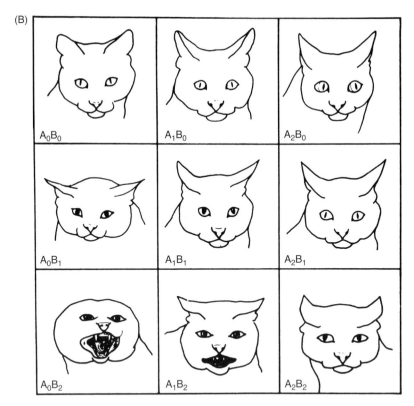

A_0B_0 A_1B_0 A_2B_0

A_0B_1 A_1B_1 A_2B_1

A_0B_2 A_1B_2 A_2B_2

Fig. 1.12   (Continued)

from the hocks; it is partially piloerected. Its ears are held erect and swiveled, so the openings point to the side. Its whiskers are rotated forward and its claws are protruded. Subordinate cats crouch in the presence of a dominant cat.

The frightened cat crouches with ears flattened to its head and it salivates and spits. The pupils of the aggressive cat are constricted; as the animal becomes more defensive, the pupils dilate. The light-colored iris of the cat's eye makes an especially prominent signal of the cat's mood; it is probably an important intraspecific signal and should be used also to advantage by the veterinarian. The eyes of an excited cat appear red because the retinal vessels can be seen through the dilated pupils. Contrary to popular belief, the "Halloween cat" is not the most aggressive one; this cat, with arched back, erect tail, and ears flattened, which is piloerected and hissing, corresponds to the fear-biting dog. The cat is fearful but will become aggressive if its critical distance is invaded. One clue to the cat's emotions is that the hind feet appear to be advancing while the front feet retreat; the paws are gathered close together under the cat.

Cats roll on their backs, but sex differences appear in this behavior. Most female rolling occurs during estrus and is directed toward males, whereas most rolling exhibited by young males is toward adult males and is presumably a sign of submission.[575]

The gape is a response to a strange smell. This expression is most commonly seen when the cat smells a strange cat's urine, and may be the feline equivalent of the flehmen response of the ungulates. The mouth is opened and the tongue is flicked behind the upper incisors where an opening in the hard palate communicates with the vomeronasal organ[1045] (Fig. 1.13). At the

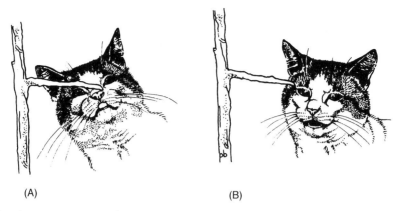

(A)   (B)

Fig. 1.13   The gape expression of a cat. (A) The cat touches the investigated object with its nose and may lick its nose; (B) then opens its mouth while gazing in a preoccupied fashion. (Drawing by Priscilla Barrett, Cambridge, UK.)

same time, an autonomic response to the odor is occurring whereby the urine brought to the hard palate is aspirated into the vomeronasal organ during parasympathetic stimulation. Fluid is flushed from the vomeronasal organ during sympathetic stimulation.[521]

Olfactory signals

Scent marking

Male cats scent mark, that is, spray urine, more than females, but both sexes do it. They spray trees along their most frequently traveled path. Spraying is also done by cats that are subjects of aggression.[1400] Free-ranging tomcats spray a dozen times per hour.[1907] Queens spray once an hour and are more likely to spray when they are in heat. Cats probably also use scent marking to arrange their activity temporally with other cats. Much of the signal value of urine is lost within 24 hours, as evidenced by a comparison of interest in fresh and older urine marks by male cats.[441] Cats can apparently distinguish the urine of familiar cats from that of strange cats.[1399] The smell of male cat urine is quite detectable by humans and usually objectionable to them. The smell of tomcat urine is probably caused by the sulfur-containing amino acid, felinine, which is present in highest quantity in tomcat urine and may be an important olfactory component in territorial spraying.[827]

Anal secretions

Cats are well known for their fastidious covering of their feces, but in some situations, such as outside their core living area, cats may leave their feces uncovered. Cats probably use fecal and anal sac odor for communication; two strange cats spend considerable time circling one another attempting to sniff in the perianal area. If the cats are not too antagonistic, they will eventually permit each other to sniff.

Rubbing

Cheek rubbing (bunting) behavior may also be a form of olfactory communication in that glandular secretion from the cat's face is deposited on the object bunted. Cats bunt the objects to which they respond with a gape. Urine up to 3 days old can elicit these responses.[1940] Cats also rub each other. In general, the subordinate cat rubs the dominant one. This behavior serves to exchange odors among all the cats in a group, that is, they all smell the same.

Inter-specific communication

Dogs and cats appear to interpret each other signals correctly even when the behaviors have opposite meanings in the two species, for example tail wagging which signals annoyance in cats and pleasure in dogs.[582]

BEHAVIOR PROBLEMS

House soiling or inappropriate elimination is the most frequent behavior problem of cats.[259,775]

Any animal with a behavior problem should be examined and treated for any concurrent medical problem. This is particularly true of feline house-soiling problems because of the association of urological problems with failure to urinate in the litter box.

The majority of cats prefer clumping litter[252] because it is made of fine particles similar to sand. More than one litter box per cat and daily cleaning solve many soiling problems.

Spraying by intact males or females in estrus should be treated by neutering. Spraying nearly always ceases if the tomcat is castrated before he is 4 months old.[1791] The result in mature males is more variable, but 87% of older males also abandon the habit after castration.[772] Spraying occurs in 5% of spayed female cats but usually is reduced by the same management techniques that improve nonspraying elimination—strict hygiene and a number of litter boxes.[1557]

Spraying synthetic cheek gland secretion in the area in which the cat sprays or using a plug-in defuser also is effective. If cats within the household are fighting, the pheromone is less likely to be effective.[624,1448] A long-term follow-up indicates that the cats do not habituate to it and spraying remains reduced or eliminated.[1337]

Clawing and scratching

Clawing or scratching behavior may be considered grooming behavior because the cat is loosening old layers of the claw, but seems to be primarily a form of marking behavior. The best teacher of a kitten is its mother, so kittens should be obtained from queens that use a scratching post.[768]

If all else fails, the cat should be declawed rather than euthanized or sent to a shelter for eventual euthanization. Without question, the cat will experience some pain at the time of declawing, so every effort should be made to improve analgesia, but there do not appear to be any long-lasting behavior sequelae to onychectomy.[211,1362,2071]

PIGS

Vocalizations

Vocal signals are probably the most important means of communication in pigs. Twenty calls have been identified,[738] and half a dozen are easily recognizable to humans. Kiley[1013] has analyzed the vocalizations of ungulates in depth.

Grunt, bark, and squeal

The common grunt is 0.25–0.4 seconds long and is given in response to familiar sounds or while a pig is rooting. The staccato grunt or short grunt is, as the name implies, shorter (0.1–0.2 seconds) and is given by an excited or investigating pig and may precede a squeal. A crescendo of staccato grunts is given, for example, by a threatening sow and may precede an attack on anyone who disturbs her litter. In a milder form, it can be a greeting. The bark is given by a startled pig. The long grunt (0.4–1.2 seconds) may be a contact call and is associated with pleasurable stimuli, especially tactile ones.[1216] The squeal is a more intense vocalization indicating arousal, and a pig that is hurt will scream.

The various grunts and combinations do not appear to have specific meanings, but the intensity of the vocalization varies with the intensity of the situation. A common sequence is to proceed from common grunts to staccato grunts to repeated grunts without interruption to grunt squeals to screams as the animal is approached, chased, picked up, and injected. Staccato greeting grunts are given by pigs that are reunited after a separation, and a series of 20 grunts with no pause may be given by the hungry pig. Nursing calls are described in Chapter 5, "Maternal Behavior." Changes in the frequency and length of calls can indicate need. When separated from the sow, hungrier piglets call more frequently and at a higher frequency than do satiated ones.[1981]

Isolation in a strange place causes pigs to vocalize. Short grunts are followed by screams. At the same time, the rate of defecation increases.[637] Mature pigs often react to restraint by tantrum behavior accompanied by very loud calls, but with no increase in heart rate.[1218] When disciplining a subordinate pig, a dominant pig will give a sharp bark as it feints with its snout. The pig in chronic pain grinds its teeth.

Visual signals

Posture

Possibly because the vocabulary of swine is so large, visual signals do not appear to be as important. One can learn something about pig thermoregulatory problems, if not about their moods, by observing their posture. Newborn pigs are relatively deficient in fur or fatty insulation and their surface volume ratio is large; therefore, maintaining body temperature is difficult. Pigs have compensated for their poor physiological abilities with several behavioral strategies to reduce heat loss. A warm piglet lies sprawled out, but a cold one crouches with its legs folded against the body. The surface area is thus reduced, and contact with a cold floor is minimized.

Tail position

The tail, particularly in piglets, is a good index of general well-being in most breeds. Although Vietnamese mini pigs do not curl their tails, a tightly curled tail indicates a healthy pig in most breeds, and a straight one indicates some sort of distress. The pig's tail is elevated and curled when greeting, when competing for food or chasing other pigs, and during courting, mounting, and intromission. The tail straightens when the pig is asleep or dozing, but curls again when the pig rouses unless the animal is isolated, ill, or frightened. The tail will twitch when the skin is being irritated. Amputation of pigs' tails removes a valuable, if crude, diagnostic aid.

Group behavior

Group behavior is even more important. Pigs, especially newborn pigs, huddle when they are cold. They thereby convert several small bodies into one large one, both decreasing their surface area and using one another for insulation. Pigs can select an optimal temperature when a gradient is present, both in the laboratory and on the farm. Therefore, heat lamps are provided, and newborn pigs, except those brain damaged by anoxia at birth, stay under the lamp at a comfortable 29°C (85°F). Adult pigs still huddle when they are cold, but their thermoregulatory problem is more apt to be one of hyperthermia. Pigs do not sweat, and although they pant, it is not sufficient for cooling. Again, behavioral thermoregulation takes over and pigs wallow in mud, which is more effective than plain water for evaporative heat loss.[1376]

Olfactory signals

Boars may use behavioral signs more than pheromones to determine the sexual receptivity of the sow. Boars are the only male ungulates that do not exhibit flehmen. Instead, they gape as a cat does when they encounter sow urine. Females can identify intact males, probably by the strong boar odor produced by the androgen metabolites present in both the saliva and preputial secretions of boars.[1768] Sex differences exist in the ability to detect androstenone.[480] Boars may habituate to this odor because it is present in their saliva. Females can detect the pheromone at one-fifth the concentration that intact boars do.[479]

  Olfactory stimuli serve to identify pigs individually, for pigs can distinguish conspecifics by means of odor,[1293] including urine odor.[1307] When visual, auditory, and olfactory stimuli were available separately and together olfaction appeared to be the most important sense in individual recognition.[1288] Pigs investigate any newcomer or any pig that has been temporarily removed by nosing it. The ventral body surface is a preferred site for sniffing. The ability of pigs to form a dominance hierarchy while blindfolded indicates that olfactory and auditory, rather than visual, signals are important to pigs.[556]

CATTLE, SHEEP, AND GOATS

Cattle posture indicates alertness, aggression, and submission (see Chapter 2). A subtle sign, the showing of the whites of the eyes, ($>15\%$ of the eye) can be elicited even by mild frustration such as visible but unreachable food or by social frustration such as removal of the cow's calf[1677,1679] or anticipation of food.[1678] Treatment with diazepam several hours before the frustrated experience decreases the percent of visible of eye white.[1680]

Vocalizations

Despite the intimate association of humans and ruminants for thousands of years, very little is known about communication in these species. Kiley[1013] has analyzed cattle vocalization phonetically and according to the motivation of the animal. The moo is low pitched. The other common vocalization—the call, hoot, or roar—is higher pitched and consists of repeated brief calls, usually by a distressed cow. A threatening bull gives a roar of high amplitude. A very hungry calf will give a high-intensity "menh" call. During copulation, grunting sounds are heard. Some humans can recognize cows by voice, so it would not be surprising if cattle were able to recognize one another. Cattle appear to respond to a vocalization with a vocalization of similar intensity. An excited call is answered by excited calls. Calves have a special moo, almost a baa, or play call.[294]

Vocal communication in a prey species such as cattle may be most important in transmitting information about general safety or danger. It may have been more important for cattle (and horses) to be alert and ready to flee than to communicate more precise information in their calls. If domestic animal communication is studied in as great a depth and with the same ingenuity as bird communication has been studied, vocal communication may be found to be more precise in domestic animals. Careful analysis of the situation in which a call is given, recording of the call, and playback of the call to conspecifics in a naturalistic setting may help to break the code of domestic animal languages.

Vocal communication in sheep consists of bleating in distress or to initiate contact. Ewes rumble to their newborn lambs (see Chapter 5) and rams make a similar call while courting. The snort is an aggressive communication in sheep.

Goats are frequently kept as pets and, like dogs, can annoy neighbors with their separation vocalizations. Analyzing the problem, as one would for a barking problem, may prevent de-bleating. Providing a companion goat often helps, as does ignoring the vocalization.

Visual signals

Submissive postures are the lowered neck and the headshake given mostly by small sheep in the presence of larger ones. Sheep have a visual signal for defensive aggression: they stamp. Threats in sheep are the foreleg kick, often repeated several times and sometimes actually contacting the opponent. The horn threat is movement of the head sharply downward. The twist and low stretch involves stretching the neck and twisting the head with accompanying tongue flicks. Some rams threaten by standing stiffly with their heads up, which causes their necks to bulge. Rams rub their horns on one another's face, probably spreading pre-orbital secretions. The other visual signals used in courting behavior are discussed in Chapter 4. Sheep rarely will huddle facing one another; head-to-head orientation is aggressive behavior in this species.

Adult sheep continue to use vocalizations as contact calls. Sheep also are able to distinguish conspecifics by means of olfaction.[136] Sheep can recognize photographs of familiar sheep and people, but a photograph of a familiar stock person is not as effective as the stock person himself in calming an isolated lamb.[1848]

The typical aggressive and submissive postures of cattle are described in Chapter 2, "Aggression and Social Structure."

Cattle can discriminate a photo of a cow from that of other ruminant species.[389] They are also capable of depth perception and have a fear of heights that can be demonstrated when they are first exposed to a milking pit.[89] Goats have pedal glands on only two feet and a tail gland. Aspiration of nonvolatile material into the vomeronasal organ has been demonstrated in goats.[1083] They stamp and produce a high-pitched sneeze when threatened. Kids have a distress call and an isolation bleat. The unique behaviors of courtship are discussed in Chapter 4.

Olfactory signals

Olfactory communication is very important for sexual activity in ruminants. Goats and cattle can distinguish conspecifics by means of urine. Male urine is more easily distinguished than is female urine.[126] The flehmen response is shown by all male ruminants in response to female urine.

Communication with humans

Sheep are aware of human visual activity. They look at a staring human more than a nonstaring human and they are more active and urinate more often.[186]

2 Aggression and Social Structure

The social structure of free-ranging domestic animals is that of groups of females with one or several resident males (horses and dogs), separate male and female groups (sheep and goats), groups of females and solitary males (swine and cattle), or groups of females that are flexible from solitary to matrilineal (cats). The determinants of dominance are age, weight, and sometimes sex. Methods of reducing aggression among newly mixed animals rely on environmental and management practices.

INTRODUCTION

Aggression is not a unitary phenomenon but serves a variety of functions in an animal's life. In some cases, aggression is used to obtain food; in others, it may facilitate access to a sexual partner or establish an animal's place in a social hierarchy. In some situations, aggression is highly desirable, as when fighting takes place to establish a dominance hierarchy. The importance of such fighting is that after the dominance hierarchy is formed, it provides the animals in the group a means by which additional serious combat may be minimized. For the animal practitioner, the problem is not to eliminate all aggression but to determine the type of aggression with which he or she is dealing; only then can the problem of control be dealt with, effectively. For example, castration may stop a tomcat from fighting with neighborhood cats, but it may have little influence on his hunting behavior.

CATEGORIES OF AGGRESSION

Social- or dominance-related aggression

Social aggression occurs when animals live in groups. It serves to establish the dominance hierarchy, i.e., who will be dominant over whom. When adult animals that previously have never been penned together are brought together for the first time, intense aggressive encounters may occur for several days until each animal has established its position in what generally turns out to be a hierarchy of dominant–submissive relationships. This type of social grouping contains an alpha animal, who is seldom challenged by subordinates; a beta, or second-ranked, animal, who is challenged only by the alpha animal, and so on. Within this organization, the type of aggressive encounter changes after the rank of each animal has been determined. No longer is an attack and subsequent fight needed for an alpha animal to establish its rights over a beta animal. Now, a direct stare, or the threat of a charge, usually serves to deter the beta animal

Domestic Animal Behavior for Veterinarians and Animal Scientists, Fifth Edition by Katherine Albro Houpt
© 2011 John Wiley & Sons, Inc.

from further confrontation. This assertion of dominance in the absence of a physical combat is called ritualized aggression. Although perception of an extensive hierarchy is questionable in domestic species, the relationship between any two animals certainly is recognized. The scarce resource over which social dominance is expressed can be food, a comfortable place to rest, a mate, or any action by one animal that is perceived as a threat or a challenge by the other. One of the best examples is of two horses sharing one bucket of food, with one horse displacing the other at the bucket and obtaining the scarce resource. Another example is of two dogs who usually coexist peacefully, but who fight when the owner tosses a ball.

Territorial aggression

Territorial aggression keeps others out of a particular geographical area. This is the type of aggression a domestic dog displays when it becomes a snarling menace to the delivery person. In essence, the dog is defending a territory that it considers its own and strangers—whether canine or human—simply are not welcome.

Pain-induced aggression

Pain-induced aggression develops directly out of induced pain or fear of pain. The function, of course, is to reduce the pain by eliminating the source. When an animal breaks a leg, it does not discriminate between the pain that comes from the break and the unavoidable pain induced by the veterinarian who tries to set the broken leg. A defense reaction of many species, including dogs and cats, is to attack the cause of pain.

   The veterinarian must expect to encounter pain-induced aggression frequently, for any animal will attempt to retaliate if it is suffering from acute pain. Therefore, a general discussion of this type of aggression is appropriate. Some species and some individual animals are more stoical than others, but most will bite or kick if the pain is severe. To judge when aggression may be induced by pain, we must consider the anatomical area involved. A wound on the face is more painful to the animal than a similar wound on the back because more receptors per unit surface are present on the face. Other areas that appear to be most sensitive are the ears, when afflicted with otitis, and the rectum, especially when the anal sacs are infected. Any animal will be in pain if a bone is fractured or the animal has been subjected to surgery.

   Injections usually cause pain, and the veterinarian must be prepared for the animal's reaction. Subcutaneous injections of a nonirritating liquid are virtually painless if placed in a loose-skinned area, but intramuscular injections of an irritating fluid such as tetracycline or ketamine are very painful even if no nerve is struck. Horses can become very "needle shy" and quite unmanageable. Equine practitioners are well advised to apply local or topical anesthetics before placing a large-gauge needle (>18) in the jugular vein of a horse and to reward the horse with a carrot immediately afterward. A horse that can be injected repeatedly is worth the few extra minutes and few extra cents involved in rendering the procedure painless. If they cannot escape, horses, dogs, and cats usually direct their aggression toward the veterinarian; cows, however, usually direct their aggression toward the painful area. A cow that can scratch her ear with a hind foot is quite capable of kicking someone standing at her shoulder, so one would do well to take advantage of the cow's pain-directed aggression. If possible, injections should be given on the side opposite that on which the injector is standing. The teats are probably the most sensitive area of the cow, with the possible exception of the muzzle, and should be handled from the opposite side of the udder if the procedure is to be painful or the cow is nervous.

An example of pain-induced aggression involves a cat with no previous history of behavioral problems that became markedly aggressive when admitted for treatment of a retro-orbital abscess. The cat was aggressive not only toward the hospital personnel but also toward his owner. The aggressive behavior, amounting almost to fury, did not subside until the cat had been in his home environment for several days. The fact that pain increases aggression should help to explain why corporal punishment of an aggressive dog may exacerbate, rather than attenuate its undesirable behavior.

Fear-induced aggression

Fear-induced aggression can be related to pain, but in some cases it is motivated by neophobia (fear of the unknown) or fear of a particular person or animal for no apparent cause. This type of aggression is usually accompanied by more physiological and visceral signs than those seen in pain-induced aggression, for example, crouching, spitting, and dilated pupils in a fearful cat or retreating with tail down and ears back in a dog.

Maternal aggression

Maternal aggression is directly related to the protection of the young. Although the male is generally considered the more aggressive of the two sexes, maternal aggression can equal the ferocity of any male attack.

Predatory aggression

Predatory aggression is usually directed toward another species and its purpose is to obtain food. Cats that are fully satiated will often hunt and not eat the catch indicating that predatory aggression is not entirely governed by hunger. During predatory aggression, the predator adopts an inconspicuous posture and usually does not vocalize.

THE BIOLOGICAL BASIS OF AGGRESSION

With this classification scheme in mind, we now can analyze aggression species by species. In subsequent sections, the major forms of aggression in domesticated species are discussed. Some species, such as the canids, show a much wider spectrum of aggression than others, or perhaps we observe a wider spectrum because of our close association with the species. We omit pain-induced aggression because it occurs in all species.

Genetic factors: breed differences

These are discussed in Chapter 10.

Environmental control of aggression

Various environmental factors can increase aggression. Hunger and crowding are the primary ones. Almost every study has found that decreasing enclosure size increases the rate of aggression. This is true of dairy cattle,[1315] beef cattle,[1860] and pigs.[951] Most aggressive interactions occur at the time of feeding. Unpredictability of feeding time also increases the rate of aggression.[323]

Hormonal control of aggression

In many species, the male is more aggressive than the female, both at the interspecies and intraspecies levels. Some notable exceptions exist, however, such as the female with the young. At other times, female aggression is generally limited to discouraging male suitors when the female is not sexually receptive and to maintaining the female's place in a female hierarchy if she lives in a group, such as a dairy herd. Female dogs do show territorial defense, but usually not with the gusto that males do.

Testicular hormones

Testicular hormones appear to play two distinct roles in the control of aggression. During very early development, the presence of testicular hormones establishes a heightened potential for aggression. This is one of the organizational effects of androgens on the brain. In the absence of testicular hormones, this aggression fails to develop. Hence, in the male, the presence of androgens during sexual differentiation enhances the potential for aggression, whereas the female escapes this influence.

Cats show sex differences in aggressiveness that are dependent on the neonatal hormonal environment.[931] Female puppies treated with testosterone in utero and after birth are, as adult dogs, more successful in competing for a bone than are normal females, but they still are less successful than males.[173] An organizational effect of testosterone can occur in female puppies of a predominantly male litter; these females are more apt to be aggressive after spaying.[256] Testosterone administration increases dominance rank in cows[263,266] and aggression in sheep.[1478] Castration has been practiced for centuries to improve tractability as well as to prevent breeding. Bulls, for example, are more aggressive than steers; the difference increases with age. Bulls also mount one another, which may be an expression of dominance rather than homosexuality.[1032]

In addition to their developmental effects, androgens have well-known activational effects upon aggression. Exposure to androgens during adulthood increases the probability that the male will show various forms of aggression (territorial, sexual, social, or dominance); androgens, however, have little to do with predatory aggression.

CATTLE

Free-ranging cattle

In contrast to most other domestic species, cattle are not often found in the feral state. Their large size and nutritional requirements may account for this. One group of cattle has remained relatively unmanaged on an estate in England for more than 500 years. These animals, the Chillingham or White Park cattle, form cow and calf herds, but the bulls live separately, either alone or in groups of two or three. They join the cow herds during the breeding season.[1104] Their home ranges are stable, but different areas may be used in different seasons. More aggression occurs among the cows than among the bulls or between cows and bulls when they are artificially fed.[746] The bulls maintain a hierarchy through displays with little overt aggression, but bulls from different home ranges rarely breed the same group of cows.

Confined cattle

Social behavior

Although cattle cannot choose their social group, they do form bonds with the cattle with which they associate. If released in a communal pasture, they remain close to and groom with cows from their own farm.[1842] They can learn to distinguish between cattle[739] and are less stressed in a frightening situation when familiar cattle are present, even if each cow has been placed in an individual stall.

Social aggression

The dominance hierarchy in cattle is known as the bunt order in polled cattle and the hook order in horned cattle. Dominance can be determined by observing the stances of the two cows involved. The dominant cow, when threatening the submissive one, will stand with her feet drawn well under and with her head down, but perpendicular to the ground. The ears will be turned back with the inner surface pointing down and back. The submissive cow also stands with lowered head, but her head is parallel to the ground and her ears are turned so that the inner surface points to the side. In the absence of horns, cattle use their heads as battering rams, pummeling each other's heads and shoulders until one can reach the more vulnerable flanks or simply inflict overpowering punishment on the other. Equally matched cows may fight for long periods, interrupting active aggression to rest in clinches; one cow will put its muzzle between the hindquarters and the udder of the other, effectively immobilizing her (see Fig. 2.1).

Aggressive bulls turn perpendicular to the opponent and display their full height and length. Some may paw and drop to their knees to horn the ground. Aggression is expressed, in the absence of horns by bunting or striking the opponent with the head.

Determinants of dominance. The determinants of dominance in cattle appear to be height, weight, age, sex, presence or absence of horns, and territoriality, with horns, age, and weight being the most important. The cow with horns dominates a polled animal. In general, the heavier animal is dominant over the lighter one,[264, 265] but in one study,[374] height was found to be negatively correlated with dominance. In an established herd, the older cows tend to be dominant, probably because initially the older cows are larger than the younger ones; after the hierarchy is formed, it remains stable.[1696] If strange cattle are added to the herd, they tend to be subordinate even if they are older and heavier. The reason is, presumably, that the cattle on their own territory have an advantage over those just introduced.[1696] Bulls were dominant over cows in a study of Holstein cattle.[1785]

The same cow does not "win" every interaction. To be dominant, a cow must win most of the interactions with the other cow.[2023] Dominance hierarchies can be observed simply by noting all agonistic interactions between cattle. However, this can be a slow process. Clutton-Brock et al.[364] noted only 0.1 agonistic encounters per hour in free-ranging Highland cattle, whereas they found that ponies engaged in agonistic behavior 1.9 times per hour. Provision of food to hungry cattle almost always provokes aggressive behavior and can be a technique for determining food-related dominance quickly. Cattle of the same rank feed within 2 m (6.6 ft) of one another at a trough, but the greater the difference in their rank, the farther apart they will be. Presumably, the lower ranked cow is the one responsible for the separation.[1214] The cow that delivers the most blows and spends the most time controlling the food is dominant. Physical contact is necessary for dominance to be determined, but vision is not. When two cows are in separate pens with the bucket anchored between the pens, both attempt to eat from it; neither retreats. If the cows are in the same pen, one defers to the other, with or without a struggle. The

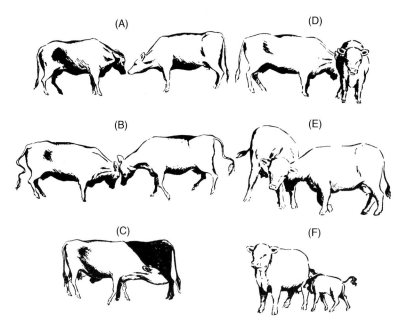

Fig. 2.1 Patterns of agonistic interactions in cattle. (A) Cows meeting after an active approach. The one on the left is threatening, whereas the one on the right has assumed a submissive posture. Note the head and leg positions of each cow. (B) Physical combat: a fight. The cows bunt or push against each other head to head, each striving for a flank position. (C) The clinch. One contestant of an evenly matched pair slips alongside the other; the head of the former is pushed between the legs and udder of the latter. In unusually prolonged contests, the cows rest briefly in the clinch between bouts of bunting. (D) Flank attack. The animal that gains a flank position is at a decided advantage over the other. The flanked animal either submits and flees or strives to regain the head-to-head position. (E) The butt. A dominant animal directs an attack against the neck, shoulders, flank, or rump of a subordinate, which in turn submits and avoids the aggressor. (F) Play fighting. The calf butts the mother.[735]

same process occurs even if the cows are blindfolded.[264] A unique way to determine dominance is to put the animals facing one another in a passage that is too narrow for them to turn around. The animal that is forced to back out of the passage is the submissive one.[1823]

Dominance hierarchies are similar, whether determined by aggressive interactions in many situations or just in feeding situations. Free-stall housing contains many areas where cattle compete: narrow passageways, drinkers, feeders, and cubicles. Entry into the milking parlor is not directly related to rank, although middle-ranking cattle tend to come first, with dominant cows in the middle- and low-ranking cattle last.[656,1020] In most cases, no correlation exists between milk production and dominance,[463] but in at least one study,[277] high-ranking cattle tended to be good producers. Herds in which the average behavior in the milking parlor is better (that is, less restless and aggressive) have higher milk production than herds with poor behavior.[1560]

The trend to automated milking results in interesting effects on cow behavior. Dominant cows spend more time chewing when entrance to feeding stations in an automated milking system is limited, although intake is similar in high- and low-ranking animals.[1301] High-ranking cows spend less time in the waiting area before automatic milking than low-ranking ones.[1300] Large herds have many triangular relationships because the number of cows is so much larger than that of a natural herd of cattle, which consists of a dozen cows.[744,1507] Furthermore, hierarchies fluctuate because dairy herds have so many changes in composition because of culling of poor producers, addition of replacement heifers, and movement of dry and calving cows to separate facilities. Cattle apparently remember one another, so when a cow leaves her herd and then returns within a few weeks, she will assume the same rank.[375] Sick cows and heavily pregnant ones will withdraw from the herd and, therefore, show a change in status—a fact that the stockperson and the veterinarian should note.[199]

When cattle are driven, the least dominant animals are first in the herd and the dominant animals are in the middle of the herd,[198] although when grazing freely, the dominant animals are the farthest from an observer.[197] During undisturbed grazing, the dominant cattle tend to be the leaders, but the individual cow that leads is variable.[1686] When feed is available from a stall in which only one animal can eat at a time, animals that are dominant in other situations do not supplant subordinate animals.[1822] Perhaps having protection on three sides allows the subordinates to maintain their positions.

Problems can arise when crush gates are used to speed entry into milking parlors; subordinate cows that would enter last are pushed into dominant cows. Aggressive interactions may result. Nonpregnant cows precede pregnant ones in the crush order.[474] Most cattle that refuse to enter a crush do so consistently. More bulls than steers were very agitated and more steers (40%) than bulls (25%) were calm.[709]

The individual distance of grazing cattle is about 20 m (66 ft), and intrusion into this area may be met with threats or bunts.[364] Cattle high in the hierarchy have an interanimal distance smaller than that of cattle that are low in the hierarchy; that is, they are not reluctant to approach another animal. Bulls tend to have greater interanimal distance than steers.[844] Interanimal preferences may also be related to dominance because animals found close to one another in a field are also close in rank.[1840]

The dominant cow is not the first into the milking parlor but is the first to a feeding area. Having arrived at a feeding area, the dominant cow spends more time eating[1289] and less time moving from place to place than does a low-ranking cow.[19] This is true both in the feedlot and on pasture. There are several interactions of reproductive status and dominance. Dominance increases with estrus and decreases with pregnancy.[197,1696] These physiological changes may be the reason that 25% of cows change rank in the course of a year in a stable herd.[1507] Prolactin levels are negatively correlated with dominance.[68]

Stage of lactation and adaptation to a challenging environment can have a destabilizing effect on dominance hierarchies. For example, when pastured in the Alps, Holsteins were subordinate to the native Swiss breeds[1435] although one would have expected the larger Holsteins to be dominant.

When formed, dominance hierarchies reduce overt aggression; only the lowest ranking animals may suffer deprivation of food when supplies are scarce or feeding space is limited. The importance of this can be seen when cows choose to eat a nonpreferred food alone than a preferred food next to a dominant cow.[1606]

Most aggression is seen during the initial stages of formation of a hierarchy. Stock managers should mix unfamiliar animals with care and avoid putting hungry animals together. When a previously unacquainted group of cattle is created, the hierarchy takes 24–28 hours to form. Four to forty days can elapse before nonphysical (that is, threats) replace physical interactions.[1046] In addition to physical injury, cattle may also suffer from lack of rest because of the general turmoil. The normal pattern of standing and lying as a group does not emerge for at least 48 hours after the group is formed. The stress resulting from lack of rest as well as rumination is added to the stress of transportation that usually precedes the formation of a new group.[2017] These considerations may explain why cattle are more susceptible to such diseases as the shipping fever complex when new groups are formed. Regrouping heifers up to 16 times does not decrease their aggressiveness nor hasten the time to form new hierarchies.[1584]

Aggression in bulls. In cattle, the greatest problem is the notorious and unpredictable aggressive behavior of bulls. Dairy bulls are generally more aggressive, as well as larger, than beef-breed bulls. One reason that artificial insemination of cows has been so enthusiastically accepted, despite its resulting lowered fertility, is that keeping bulls on the farm is no longer necessary. A teaser bull with a deviated penis or a vasectomy can detect cows in estrus but cannot impregnate them and is as dangerous as a fertile bull. The same hormones that motivate him to mount the cow also induce the bull to charge his owner. Elimination of those hormones reduces both mounting and charging. Now, most bulls are at artificial insemination centers where every precaution is taken to provide escape routes for the handlers.

Bulls are sometimes kept in groups; their behavior in this situation is described by Dalton et al.[425] and Kilgour and Campin.[1019] Bulls mount other males, and these animals retaliate by butting.[1345] Mounting in this case is probably motivated by dominance, not sex. Keeping bulls together can result not only in injury to the animals but also damage to the substrate, because the bulls paw and horn the ground.[938] Aggression can be reduced if the bulls are kept in the group with which they were raised; not only are they less aggressive, they are also less fearful at slaughter.[1375] Bulls who were hand-reared individually were more aggressive toward other bulls than were group-reared bulls.[1551]

Maternal aggression. Cows will attempt to protect their young, and caution always is warranted when a mother is with her offspring. Angus cows may be especially protective.

Grooming

Mutual grooming (licking) occurs, but this occupies only a few minutes per day. Cattle groom their age mates, their kin, and the cows closest to them. When one cow solicits grooming from another, the licking is of the head and neck.[636, 1687, 1688] In a free housing situation, most grooming takes place at feeding time. If feeding space per cow is reduced from 0.6 m/cow to 0.3 m/cow, grooming decreases and agonistic encounters increase.[1917] Older and larger cattle receive and give more grooming than younger cattle do. Milk production and milking order (order of entrance into the milking parlor) are also correlated with the amount of grooming received.[2056]

Environmental enrichment is often decreed to improve the welfare of confined animals. "Toys" do not seem to be used by many animals over the age of 2 months, but devices that, when manipulated, provide food or devices on which a cow can rub or scratch and groom itself are used.[2034]

Clinical cases of aggression

Aggression toward people, including butting, kicking, and crushing, is most apt to be a problem in dairy cattle that are handled several times a day. Dangerous animals are usually culled, but a high-producing cow may be kept. She will pose most danger to those unfamiliar with her temperament, that is, the veterinarians. Some cows can be handled only from one side so the astute clinician should try to work from the side of the cow where she is milked.

Veterinarians can be the victims of bovine aggression when their treatment is most successful. A cow recumbent with hypocalcemia may, when treated with calcium intravenously, leap to her feet and attack because, whereas severe hypocalcemia results in muscular weakness, mild hypocalcemia can cause irritability.

An unusual case of bovine aggression demonstrated the importance of visual cues to cattle. A herd of Hereford cattle and one Holstein were bred to a shorthorn bull. The Hereford shorthorn calves were red with a little white, but the Holstein shorthorn calf was mostly white with a few red spots. When the calf and its mother were released into the pasture a few days after the calf's birth, all the other cows attacked the calf. Altering olfactory cues had no effect, but the problem was dealt with immediately by putting the calf and its dam in a corral where they could be seen but not injured; eventually, the problem was solved by adding more cows with white calves to the herd.

SHEEP

Free-ranging sheep

Feral sheep in a natural setting form separate ewe and ram flocks. The ewe flocks also include lambs and immature rams. A flock seldom has more than 20 adult ewes. Ram flocks are much smaller (about six animals) and less stable. This type of social organization is seen in Soay sheep, which are a primitive form of domestic sheep, and among mountain sheep.[679,722] Domestic as well as wild sheep "camp" in one particular area at night. These areas are theorized to be useful because information can be exchanged between animals even though energy must be expended in traveling from food sources to the night camp.[1437]

In a large pasture, sheep divide into flocks with individual, but overlapping, territories. Newly introduced sheep, even offspring separated since weaning, are not allowed to join the original flocks but are relegated to less productive parts of the pasture,[907] which may explain their tendency to wander. Lambs may follow their mothers for up to 2 years after weaning, varying with the population.[1100,1645,1713]

Flocking

The formation of large commercial herds of hundreds of sheep is usually accompanied by a cacophony of baaing as the small flocks are lost within the large one and the individual sheep give separation calls. The formation of smaller or larger groups of sheep in farm situations is somewhat unnatural. Three sheep do not readily form a flock, and they tend to disperse; therefore, three sheep are often used in sheepdog trials as a test of the dog's ability to control the sheep. Sheep tend to select sheep of the same breed as flock mates when randomly mixed.[85,2043] Familiarity is very important to sheep. They quickly form associations that are slow to break down.[2044]

The nearest neighbor distance on pasture is approximately 5 m.[1763] Sheep were closest while resting and farthest apart when their activity was not synchronized, that is, some sheep were resting and others active.[1317]

Confined sheep

Dominance

Within an established, related flock of sheep, the oldest ewe is dominant over other ewes and is usually the leader in movements. Dominance is not related to body weight in commercial flocks of sheep of similar age. Very little overt aggression is seen among sheep, but dominance can be determined by limiting feeding space. Dominant sheep push out subordinates.[83,1799] One can observe the dominance hierarchy by entering a pen of sheep. The farthest sheep will be the most dominant.[485] The subordinate sheep will lie down less than dominant ones when lying area is restricted. Displacements increase from 7 to almost 30/ewe/day when space is reduced.[244] Aggressive sheep shoulder push; then, after the dominant animal has established itself, it displays behaviors toward the subordinate that appear identical to those used in courtship, that is, nudging, with head low and nose up, while striking with the front limb.

Age and weight, but not sex, are also important in determining dominance.[1637, 1638, 1711, 1712] Appearance must be important because shearing may reduce the rank of a dominant ewe.

Sexual aggression

Sexual aggression in sheep can actually interfere with breeding. Among rams, the dominant ram will usually breed more ewes than his subordinates unless he is so aggressive that his battles distract him from the ewes' estrus.[1759] Two rams may breed fewer ewes than one alone if they are often engaged in the butting contests typical of ram aggression. If three rams are present in a flock, two may fight, while the third one, which may be less aggressive but evolutionarily more competent, impregnates the ewes.

GOATS

Free-ranging goats

Feral goat herds can range in size from one to one hundred goats, but the mean size is four.[1737] Goats form sexually segregated flocks, except in mild climates where breeding takes place throughout the year. As with sheep, goats tend to spend each night in a particular area, a night camp. Home ranges of male goats are larger than those of females and vary with the season. The total range is 10–40 ha (25–99 acres).[1438]

Because goats, as an introduced species, are a threat to native wildlife, capturing and removing goats is undertaken. Use of a "Judas" goat who will lead the captors to the feral goats or attract the males when she is in heat is a technique that takes advantage of caprine social structure.[314] Does live in small, stable groups (heft-groups); each group comprises three to four animals and occupies its own range. Goats continue growing with age. Horn size as well as body size increases and, therefore, older goats are dominant over younger ones and males, who are larger, are dominant over females. This applies until the goats are 5 or 6 years old. Thereafter, the bucks decline in dominance; despite larger horn size, they may not be as strong and have a high mortality rate. Females decline more slowly. Does dominate kids except for their own, who are as likely as their dam to win a contest. Goats compete for food and the rate of aggression increases as food availability and day length decreases in the fall. More contests are resolved without overt aggression. The initiator approaches and the subordinate leaves the feeding spot and moves 3 m away.[1747] Most aggressive interactions occur when the goats are eating heather or other small shrubs rather than grass which is distributed more continuously.

Confined goats

Dominance

Dominance is much more obvious in a flock of goats than in a flock of sheep. Despite their close relationship, the two species are very different in behavior. Goats are much more aggressive and exploratory than sheep. In goats, as with horned sheep, the presence of horns is an important determinant of dominance. Because horns confer dominance, most agonistic interactions are brief feints or rushes in which the dominant animal lowers its head and points its horns at the subordinate. Horns, size, and age determine dominance.[158] When the animals are of equal or undetermined rank, long fights occur in which horns and heads are clashed together repeatedly. The goats that act as leaders have been born in the area and have more kin in the flock than do the nonleaders. Escos [544] and Syme [1839] found that a novel food will increase the level of aggression within a goat herd. Not surprisingly, restricting feeding space increases aggression, but the effect depends on the type of forage; there is more aggression over hay than over silage.[971] Goats do bite, especially polled goats who are 3 years old or older.[1884]

Grooming

A goat grooms itself by scratching its head and neck with a hind hoof and by oral grooming of the rest of the body surface. The oral grooming consists of an upward scraping motion of the lower canine and incisor teeth, a behavior that is suppressed by testosterone. Intact male goats groom orally less than wethers or does do.[1358] More self-grooming occurs following aggressive interactions, possibly indicating anxiety. Affiliative contact, through muzzle to muzzle contact or allogrooming by the aggressor, appears to reduce the postconflict anxiety.[1698]

HORSES

Free-ranging horses

Horses live in small groups called bands, which are composed of a stallion, several mares, and their offspring. A number of bands living in the same area are referred to as a herd. Nineteen populations of feral horses have been studied. In a free-ranging horse band, each stallion is associated with 2 to 28 mares (mean, 6).[214,993,1165,1909,1972] Band size is optimal at 5–7 mares. An older or larger mare is apt to be the highest ranking female, and she leads the herd in flight and in daily journeys to rest or to a new grazing area. The stallion drives the herd from behind, going to the front only to confront another stallion. Nevertheless, the stallion is usually, but not always, dominant over his harem.[215,878,2000] Mares apparently choose the stallion and the band that they ultimately join. Fillies usually leave their natal band at puberty, possibly to avoid an incestuous breeding with their sires.[504] The mares may switch bands several times, but by 5 years they are usually in their permanent band, but remain in the same general area, often joining a band that shares the same home range.[1166] They join another band or a bachelor band. The small percentage that does remain in its natal band have very low foaling rates, indicating that inbreeding depression of reproduction does occur.[995] The dominant stallion within the bachelor band is the one to form a new harem band with the young mare.

The best studies of feral ponies are those on Assateague Island off the coast of Maryland. These are known as Chincoteague ponies. About 20% of mares on Assateague Island change bands. Mares may leave bands for reasons having to do with the stallions. They are less likely to leave larger bands with older stallions who have had a harem for several years.[1667] Mares who change bands have a lower foaling rate than those who remain. Although this could be due to many factors, the fact that contracepted mares (to control population of horses the zona pellucida vaccine is used on many island populations) like naturally foal-less mares change bands more often than fertile mares indicates that reproduction may play a role.[1433]

If a mare enters a new band, the resident mares are aggressive toward her, but the stallion will protect her. The larger the herd, the higher the aggression rate per mare. Dominant mares interrupt nursing bouts of subordinates. The highest rate of aggression occurs at water holes.[1668] Dominance is important not only for immediate access to scarce resources but also for the reproductive success of one's offspring. Stallions born to dominant mares sire more foals.[570] The dominance hierarchies remain stable in undisturbed feral herds,[997] and age appears to be the most important determinant of dominance.

Stallions defend their mares, not a fixed territory. Two herd stallions, upon meeting, usually prance toward each other. When they are close enough to do so, they investigate each other with their nostrils. They then defecate and sniff at the manure. Feist and McCullough[573] noted that within bachelor herds, the most dominant animals defecated last. These displays between stallions can lead to a fight, but aggression is much more likely to result in the absence of the displays when a bachelor stallion tries to abduct a mare.

Stallions may evaluate their rivals on the basis of vocalizations. Subordinate stallions have shorter squeals that also begin at a lower frequency than those of dominant stallions.[1649] Rival stallions may be more likely to challenge a subordinate after having heard him squeal.

Large bands may have more than one stallion.[214,1330] The dominant stallion in the herd does most of the breeding; the subordinate stallion engages in most of the fighting with any other stallions that approach the band. The subordinate stallion sires 25% of the foals.[569] Bands of horses compete for fresh water; the band drinking usually will not be ousted by an intruding band.[626] The order of drinking is stallion, mares, and then juveniles. Only juveniles will be displaced by an intruder. Large, multimale bands tend to supplant smaller bands at water sources.[1331] Multimale bands have an advantage in that fewer mares leave these bands during the winter when food is scarce.[626] Some disadvantages of being in a multimale band exist: The mares are in poorer body condition and carry a heavier parasite load; they have traveled more and rested less. Their foaling rate is lower and foal mortality higher in multistallion bands.[1167] The advantages of being a subordinate stallion are not clear.[920]

In interspecies relationships, horses dominate cattle.[1909] Infanticide is reported in the domestic horse, but has also been observed in free-ranging Przewalski horses living in zoos,[271] in semi-natural reserves[572] and reintroduced into the wild in China.[345] The stallion kills a new born foal usually a colt and usually not his own offspring.

Domestic horses

What is a band? One or two horses are more restless than a larger group. Judging by the decrease in walking and increase in grazing compared with those of smaller groups, three horses are a band.[1079] Although the strict order by sex and age just described may be observed in wild horses, quite a different picture emerges when herds of domestic horses are studied. Dominance hierarchies tend to be linear unless the group is large, in which case triangular and more complex relationships appear (Fig. 2.2A,B). Montgomery[1352] studied one herd of 11 horses and found that dominance, as determined from observation of interactions of the whole herd, was determined by weight, not length of residency, but Clutton-Brock et al.[364] did not find any correlation between size and dominance in Highland ponies. In a larger study of 11 herds of horses and ponies, Houpt et al.[879] found that age and weight were not statistically correlated with rank in dominance hierarchies. All possible pairings of the herd members were made in food dominance tests so that both lower and higher rankings could be determined. During an 18-month period, the hierarchies in domestic horses were stable. The most aggressive horse was the dominant one who displaced other horses from food. Horses under 3 years of age are never dominant over adult horses and, in fact, display little aggression toward one another even when

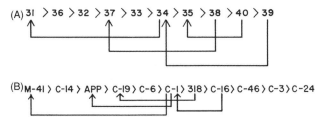

Fig. 2.2 Examples of dominance hierarchies in mares. (A) A herd of 10 thoroughbred mares. (B) A herd of 11 mares of various breeds. The greater than symbol (>) indicates that the horse on the right is submissive to the horse on the left. Arrows indicate direction of dominance in triangular relationships.[879]

vying for food, as Grzimek[724] had noted previously. Yearling fillies are more aggressive than yearling colts in a feeding situation.[1373] When yearling Icelandic fillies and geldings, maintained in separate herds were compared, both formed linear hierarchies, but the fillies showed more submission and less escalation or ignoring of aggression from another horse.[1941] The position of the stallion in the hierarchy is variable. In three herds of ponies of mixed size and age, geldings and mares were dominant over the stallions[877], but Arnold and Grassia[82] found that two stallions were dominant to the mares of their herds. Both studies used food competition as a measure of dominance. The advantage of high rank is most pronounced when environmental conditions are harsh. High-ranking Icelandic horses had more access to hay and used the bodies of the other horse as windbreaks. As a result, the higher ranking horse improved in condition over the Icelandic winter, whereas the lower ranking horses lost condition.[925]

Przewalski's horses have linear dominance hierarchies even on <30-ha (74-acre) pastures. The stallion is not always the highest ranking horse. Most aggressions consisted of displacements or threats rather than kicks or bites.[996]

Mothers are not necessarily dominant over their daughters. The daughters of dominant mares tend to be dominant within their own groups.[885] The hierarchy of foals is first related to birth order, but later, when size differences are not so great, the foal's rank is that of its dam.[67] Little change occurs in the rank of mares when they foal.[546]

Within a herd, the mares appear to have preferred associates—"friends," anthropomorphically—with whom they mutually groom, especially when their winter coats are shedding. Preferred associates share resources without competing. When the relationships of the mares are known, the preferred associates often are mother and daughter or siblings[1909] and are usually animals close in social rank.[364] When a member of a pair of preferred associates is allogrooming with another horse, the other partner may intervene either stopping the bout or replacing the nonpartner. The more subordinate animal of a pair is more likely to intervene. Subadult mares intervene in play bouts by males.[1929] Foals of high-ranking mares receive fewer aggression from other horses than those of low-ranking mares.[808]

Our modern manner of keeping horses in box stalls separated by bars prevents formation of relationships between adjacent horses despite olfactory and visual contact.[351] Apparently, horses must have direct contact to form a dominance relationship. Proximity does not cause horses to become preferred associates. In summary, the determinants of dominance in horses appear to be more closely related to the animal's temperament and the position of its mother in the band than to physical characteristics.

Types of aggression

Fighting can include a variety of responses in horses: running, chasing or fleeing, circling, neck wrestling, biting, and kicking.[1035] Horses neck wrestle and nip at one another even in play, but

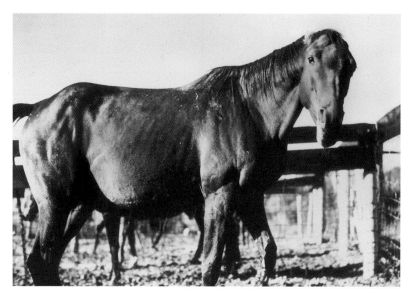

Fig. 2.3   An aggressive expression in a horse. A threat to bite.

biting or biting attempts with ears flattened to the head and lips retracted are signs of serious aggression (Fig. 2.3). Kicking is considered to be the horse's most aggressive act,[1909] and, although some have hypothesized that kicks are defensive—that is, directed up the dominance hierarchy[2000]—kicking more likely occurs when either the challenge or the danger is from the rear (Fig. 2.4).

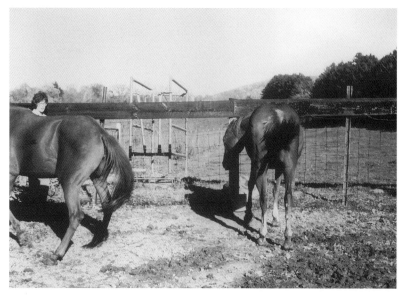

Fig. 2.4   Threat to kick. The horse on the right is threatening to kick the horse on the left. Note the lashing tail of the threatening horse and the tucked tail of the threatened horse.

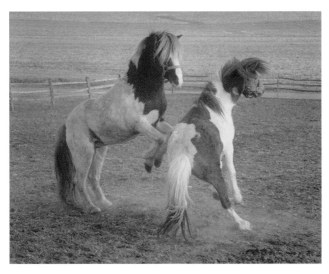

Fig. 2.5 Balking behavior by stallion on the right. (Photo courtesy of Dr. Sue McDonnell, University of Pennsylvania.)

Aggression between stallions can take many forms. Prefight behavior includes the arched neck threat, fecal pile display, head bowing, striking, threatening to bite, squealing, snorting, prancing in parallel, and pushing.[1255] The levade (rearing with deeply flexed hind limbs) is part of untrained stallions' interactions. This is probably the reason that Lippizaner stallions, rather than mares, are used by the Spanish Riding School. Stallions may rear and box with their forelegs or actually make contact with their forelegs. A horse may avoid the lunge of another horse by swinging its head in a dorsolateral direction away from an apparent threat while the hind legs remain stationary, a posture termed the balk[1261] (Fig. 2.5). A less intense version of this is seen when two horses share feed over which they might have been expected to fight. The horses turn away from each other. Avoiding eye contact as well as physical contact may be the goal of this behavior. Elements of sexual behavior such as resting the chin on the opponent's rump, rump presentation, and mounting also occur. These behaviors are seen in bachelor herds of stallions and may be play or determination of the hierarchy. The activities practiced in the bachelor herd are used to defeat a band stallion when a former bachelor acquires mares.

Horses can be severely injured in the process of forming a hierarchy, especially if they are so confined that the loser cannot escape. Horses that have been stalled separately for a few months may show much more aggression than when they have been together on a daily basis. Because neither age, weight, nor sex appears to be an important determinant of dominance, one should hesitate to predict a hierarchy in horses. It is safest to leave horses in the same group. Exercise on a treadmill does not change aggression level.[1117] A good management practice, therefore, is to introduce (or reintroduce) horses to one another across a fence. The horses can investigate and threaten each other but will be able to escape easily without being kicked, although the danger of injuring their limbs on the fence while striking or kicking is always present.

Grooming

Horses mutually groom one another. Licking of the foal is seen only in the short period after the foal's birth, but horses will stand shoulder to shoulder and nibble at each other's withers and back.

Horses tend to groom animals close to their own rank in the dominance hierarchy, which are also the horses nearest to them.[364] This behavior is more pronounced in the spring when the heavy winter coats are being shed. Horses that have been kept in individual stalls groom more when placed in a social situation, indicating a buildup of motivation for grooming.[351,874] Horse owners assume the role of grooming partner when they curry their horses. Grooming in the withers area reduces the horse's heart rate.[571] Rolling, which serves to scratch the horse's back, occurs more frequently in the spring. Horses rub their rumps and tails against fences. This appears to have erotic properties; males show penile erection. Rubbing can also be a sign of perianal pruritus caused by pinworm (Oxyuris spp.) infestation.

Summer weather brings horses irritating companions: flies, many of which are biting species. To escape flies, horses spend many of the daylight hours in the shade,[1909] in grassless areas, or, if available, in the snow or surf.[994] Some horses have a particularly effective way to deal with flies. They stand side by side, nose to tail, and keep the flies off one another's faces with their tails. Not all horses form pairs, despite the obvious advantages, but most will stand closer to one another during times of high fly density.[502]

Clinical problems

Treatment of equine aggression toward people

Aggression is an all-too-common behavior problem of horses. Aggression can be directed at people or other horses. Aggression toward people is seen most often in the stall, a small, easily defended space. Its appearance in the stall is probably a form of dominance and is influenced by the caretaker.[786]

A simple way to acquire dominance over a horse is to gain control over the animal on the ground. After rubbing the horse on the neck, placing the halter and lead, possibly with a chain, over the horse's nose, and backing it into a corner, one should pull down on the lead rope, releasing as soon as the horse lowers its head a little. Repeat until its head is close to the ground and then reward the horse by stroking. Some horses react violently to poll pressure, in which case an alternative technique should be used. Walk the horse around the stall clockwise so that it has to give in to the handler. Teach the horse to back away from a person on command, to never invade a person's space by touching, and to move to the side when touched. Free lunging, in which the person stops, starts, and turns the horse by moving in front of or behind or toward the horse's balance point, is another method of establishing control. A round pen is necessary to free lunge the horse easily. Another method to obtain dominance is to flex the horse's forelimb and strap it in that position for a few minutes. The horse is, in effect, three legged and should be urged to walk so that it is aware of its helpless situation. Of course, this exercise should be done only on a soft surface so that the horse will not injure itself if it should fall. When the horse has been restrained for 5 minutes, the limb should be freed and the horse walked again. This process is repeated several times until the horse has learned that the person can give him the use of his leg. This technique is most effective for a person with whom the horse has had no prior experience.

For simple cases of aggression (i.e., of a horse toward its owner), rewarding nonaggression is usually effective. A simple method of dealing with the horse that is stall guarding is to approach him and if he pins his ears stand still, backing away only when his ears come forward. This can be repeated gradually, approaching closer to the horse. The negative reinforcement is the presence of the unwanted person. The reward is removal of that person. Alternatively, aggression can be punished, but many owners of pleasure horses are unable or unwilling to inflict appropriate punishment. In addition, the punishment must follow the misbehavior within seconds. If a horse threatens its owner but the owner must run around the paddock to catch the horse before whipping it, the horse will not learn to stop threatening but only to avoid the owner. The same principle applies to punishing a horse for misbehaving in the show ring after it has left the ring.

Rewards must also be carefully timed, but the timing of rewards is not as crucial as that of disciplinary action. The best reward for horses is food, and grain fed in many small portions can be used to "shape" certain responses. For example, if the horse tends to swing its rump toward anyone who enters the stall, the following course of treatment should be used. On the first day, no grain should be poured into the horse's bucket until it turns 45° or more toward the front of the stall. By feeding grain in measurements of one cup or less, the owner gives the horse plenty of opportunities to learn that its movement toward the front of the stall will be rewarded. The next day, the criterion for reward should be raised to a 90° turn toward the front of the stall. This process can be continued until the horse learns that it must turn and face the front of the stall before it will receive its grain. The owner must be rigid about enforcing this, even if it means several days without grain for the horse. The process can be hastened using a secondary reinforcer such as a clicker (see Chapter 7, "Learning").

A similar method can be used for treating a horse that lays its ears back in a threatening manner. The horse should be fed only when it puts its ears forward. Eliciting the desired response may require whistling or throwing pebbles, and then the grain should be given only as long as the horse's ears remain forward. Each day a longer duration of this behavior should be demanded before the horse is fed. When the horse is responding well to this procedure, the owner can assume dominance by standing over the feed, starting with hay, and waving the horse off. This is the way that dominance is expressed between horses, but care must be taken to ensure that the owner is the "winner."

These simple behavior modification exercises should be performed by the owner because the horse must learn that it cannot threaten the owner. The horse must be rewarded and punished by each person affected by its behavior.

For severely aggressive horses, a more drastic treatment program must be used. The effectiveness of this treatment depends on three factors: (1) a stall or barn that is virtually lightproof, (2) the presence of only one source of food, and (3) the absence of other horses.

The horse should be put in the dark alone and handfed, receiving food and light only from people. Food should be withheld as long as the horse approaches aggressively. The animal should be given as many opportunities as possible to earn food and light, but initially the lights should be on for only a few minutes each day. If the horse refuses to eat for several days, hay may be provided, but grain should continue to be used as a reward for good behavior. The presence of another horse gives the aggressive horse companionship, and the appearance of a person, therefore, will not be as rewarding. Solitude is aversive to the herd-loving horse, and success is near when the horse nickers as people approach.

Treatment of equine aggression toward horses

Aggression between two or more horses can be treated by changes in management, such as separation of individuals. Horses that are stabled singly are more aggressive than those kept in groups.[351] In other cases, spacing feed buckets widely apart is the easiest way to prevent aggression between horses by reducing competition over resources; the resource is usually food. Holmes et al.[853] have shown how wire partitions along a feed trough allow a subordinate horse to eat in the presence of a dominant one. If aggression occurs in other circumstances, it is more difficult to treat, particularly if it occurs at pasture. Such behavior may be treated hormonally with progesterone (Depo-Provera) or medroxyprogesterone (Ova ban) 65–85 mg/day orally for a 300-kg horse. The pharmacological basis for the effectiveness of this treatment is not known. It is hypothesized that progestin administration inhibits those areas of the hypothalamus that induce aggression, especially sex-specific types of aggression. Regardless, the benefits achieved by such treatment must be balanced against the side effects. For example, long-term use may affect fertility in stallions. Tryptophan, as a feed additive or paste, should increase brain serotonin and reduce aggression. Alternatively, the serotonin reuptake inhibitor amitriptyline can be administered.

Aggression toward other horses that occurs under saddle or in harness is punished more easily, and most of these problems can be solved by a competent horse trainer.

Aggression in horses can be treated through a variety of ways. The method chosen should be determined by the type and severity of the aggression, as well as the circumstances under which it occurs. Owners should participate in treatment and should be urged not to breed vicious or unmanageable horses.

PIGS

Free-ranging pigs

Numerous populations of feral swine exist. They form groups of approximately eight, consisting most commonly of three sows and their offspring. The males are solitary for much of the year but may form all-male groups in the late winter.[711] The males travel farther than the females. Young pigs do not leave the sow until they weigh 27–32 kg (60–70 lb). The pigs have overlapping home ranges of 121–809 ha (300–2,000 acres).[1074]

Confined pigs

Social Aggression

Teat order. Pigs have the most intriguing of hierarchies because the ranks are formed soon after birth, not by uncoordinated pushing for a nipple as exhibited by puppies, but by vicious blows with the appropriately named needle teeth possessed by piglets at birth. To reduce the injury and infection from snout lacerations during the neonatal period, most swine producers clip the teeth to the gumline.[634] The resource over which the piglets are fighting is the pre-ferred pair of teats, usually the most anterior pair that produces the most milk and has the lowest incidence of mastitis. In addition, pigs sucking at these teats are much less likely to be kicked by the sow's hind legs. The hierarchy is formed within the first 2 days after birth; the heaviest and first-born pigs are usually dominant.[1239] Because the anterior teats produce the most milk, the pigs that suckle these teats grow fastest and remain dominant;[518,1240,1241] after its formation, the teat order of hierarchy remains stable, especially the top and bottom ranks.[554] By the sixth day after birth, the same teat is suckled by the same pig 90% of the time.[825]

Hierarchy formation. When unfamiliar weanling or older pigs are mixed, a hierarchy must be formed.[1240,1583] When young pigs (7–8 weeks old) are introduced, they spend a minute or two nosing one another, sniffing the face and anogenital regions—these investigations are longer between unfamiliar pigs[1790]—and then begin to butt the head and body and bite, especially the head and ears. Up to 80 bites may be inflicted before one turns away and retreats; the winner will continue biting.[955] Even week-old pigs will fight with strange piglets, although the fights are short. In older pigs, the process of hierarchy formation takes several days.[1294] Although most aggression is seen in the first 24 hours after mixing strange pigs, the food intake and weight gain of pigs is inhibited for more than 24 hours after mixing, and increased fighting continues for as long as 6 weeks.[529]

Mixing litters before weaning may be advantageous.[1521] "Socializing" piglets by letting two litters mingle from 10 to 30 days of age led to differences in their behavior when they were mixed with strange pigs at 51 days. The socialized piglets initiated aggression sooner, but formed hierarchies sooner, within 10 days, than unsocialized piglets.[447] The more pigs are regrouped, the more quickly they form hierarchies and the less serious the injuries, even when the pigs are always complete strangers to one another.[1926] Other consequences of regrouping occur as well: Pigs that have been regrouped are less likely to approach people than are pigs that have remained in a stable group; apparently, regrouping makes the pigs more fearful.[796]

Even simple physical factors such as a draft can cause pigs to be more aggressive.[1695] Pen size and shape can also affect aggression when strange pigs are mixed. Less aggression arises in a rectangular pen.[153]

When strange pigs are mixed, size disparity reduces the initial fighting; not surprisingly, however, the smaller pigs do not gain as well or remain as healthy as they do in groups of similar-size pigs.[1354] When pigs of disparate size must be mixed, however, smaller pigs fare better if the larger pigs are added to the pen so that the small pigs have the advantage of an established territory. The younger the pigs are when mixed—between 5 and 26 days—the shorter the time spent fighting.

Weight predicts success in encounters among newly mixed pigs, but aggressiveness predicts bullying behavior (one-sided aggression) and persistence of aggression.[448] Even at 4 weeks of age, intact piglets are more aggressive when mixed than castrated pigs.[1378] Females fight longer than castrated males.[1819] Boars are presumably dominant over sows, but when barrows (castrated males) and sows are penned together, the males might not be dominant.

When pigs are removed for 25 days or sows for 6 weeks[73] from a group that has been together for months, they assume their original rank, but the 12-week-old pigs that were dominant in a group formed for only 5 days may not be dominant when reintroduced to that group 3 weeks later.[554,1457] Small pigs and newcomers to an established group are usually subordinate.[636] Littermates show less aggression to one another than to unfamiliar pigs except over food, when similar levels of aggression are seen.[1558] The reduced aggression among littermates relates to familiarity, not kin recognition, as indicated by the fact that littermates cross-fostered onto another sow are treated like strangers.[1818] After separation, the dominant pig lies down and lets its belly be nosed by the other pigs. This behavior, the function of which remains unknown, is seen most often when the dominant pig has returned to its group after a separation.[634]

Age affects dominance among sows; older sows are dominant, feed more often and gain more weight.[1048] The immune status of subordinate pigs is inferior to that of dominant pigs,[1903] but both dominant and subordinate pigs may be immunosuppressed in a hot environment.[1372]

Sows. Dominant sows give birth to more male piglets than do subordinate ones.[1298,1309] The biological significance of this is that the offspring of the dominant animal is more likely to grow large and strong and to be dominant itself. The male offspring of a dominant sow has a better chance to dominate other boars, to gain access to estrous sows and, therefore, to sire many piglets. If the sow is not dominant, a greater risk exists that her sons will not sire any piglets. A safer way to ensure that her genes are passed on is to produce daughters, all of whom will have at least some offspring. Dominant sows give birth to piglets that are more active, more vocal and faster to touch a novel object (a large red container) than piglets of low-ranking sows.[1057] The best predictor of the dominance rank of a sow is the rank of her mother.[488] Low-ranking sows will lose weight unless feed is provided ad libitum.[290] A subordinate sow may produce small litters or low-birth-weight piglets,[1308] not because she lacks the genetic potential, but because she cannot obtain adequate nourishment. Sows were exposed twice a week for 3 weeks to different dominant sows, and, although their salivary cortisol rose immediately after the first five defeats, by the sixth confrontation, cortisol did not rise. The subordinate sow avoided the dominant pig or remained passive rather than fighting back by the third confrontation.[1923]

As in other species, after the hierarchy is formed, fighting is replaced by threats; these consist of a sharp, loud grunt and a feint with the snout by the dominant pig. Aggressive behaviors include thrusting the head upward or sideways against the head or body of the opponent. These activities may be accompanied by biting. Levering, in which the snout is put under the body of the opponent, usually from behind, also occurs. The submissive gesture in pigs consists in twisting the head away from the opponent.[952] The subordinate pig quickly gives ground (see Fig. 2.6). Leadership on a novel pasture is not correlated with dominance.[1295]

Not surprisingly, the sows that received the most aggressive acts showed the least estrous behavior. They did not mount or nose other sows as much as did high-ranking sows.[1485] The level of aggressiveness is not correlated with age, weight, or, in the case of sows, parity.[1377] Pigs in their home pen have some advantage over intruders.[1850] The greater the number of unfamiliar, as opposed to familiar, pigs, the more the fighting will occur.[74] Aggression can be a problem in pregnant sows, but management practices can reduce the fighting. If sows are returned to the group a week after being left to be bred, there is much less aggression than if they were gone for 4 weeks.[1800] Newly added sows rest apart from the original residents in a less desirable area of the pen, the dunging area. Only after 3 weeks does integration of the new and resident sows occur.[1353] Vision is not necessary for dominance hierarchy formation in pigs,

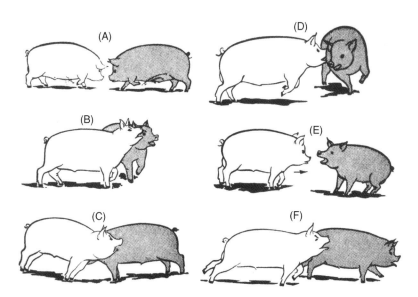

Fig. 2.6 Agonistic behavior in boars. (A) Pawing the ground during initial encounter. (B) Strutting. (C) Shoulder-to-shoulder contact and slashing. (D) Perpendicular biting attack. (E) Submission of pig on the right. (F) Pursuit of the loser.[738] (Copyright 1969, with permission of W.B. Saunders Co.)

as indicated by the fact that pigs that have been temporarily blinded with opaque contact lenses form a hierarchy, although overt aggression is reduced.[556] The lack of vision has advantages for a producer, resulting as it does in less aggression if strange pigs are mixed at night.[152] Producers routinely keep pigs in dim light to reduce aggression. Anosmic pigs are not as aggressive as normal pigs, perhaps because they have difficulty discriminating among pigs.[1291]

Most aggressive behavior appears in relation to food. If trough space is limited, the subordinate pigs are forced to eat at night, and they gain less weight.[1582] Average production may be acceptable, but the dominant pigs will gain too much weight and the subordinate ones too little.[681] Pigs may show aggression over entrance to an electronic feeder and form a queue in order of dominance.

The importance of confinement as a factor in dominance is that less aggression and milder consequences occur for subordinate pigs when they are housed outside.[1224] Crowding increases aggression in most species, and pigs show more aggression when the stocking rate is increased.[296]

Boars. A classic example of porcine sexual aggression is the confrontation of two boars. Pigs tend to use loud vocal communications in general, but two boars threatening one another are eerily quiet. They strut shoulder to shoulder, champing their jaws, from which fall clumps of thick, white saliva containing an androstenol pheromone (refer to Fig. 2.6). When they face each other, they often paw the ground, a sign of aggression in many artiodactyls. The animals meet in frontal assault. They slash at each others' shoulders with their well-developed tusks, inflicting severe lacerations. The stronger pig will achieve a flank attack and, consequently, victory. The winner of a conflict usually chases the loser. Aggression between sows and barrows is similar to that of boars, except that champing and strutting are restricted to intact males.

Preventing aggression among newly mixed pigs. Strange pigs typically are mixed in two types of circumstances: when pigs are grouped by sex or size after weaning or after sale to a feeder pig operation; and when sows are grouped for breeding and gestation.

Many methods are available for minimizing aggression among newly mixed pigs: tranquilization, provision of shelters, and boar pheromone. The aggression can be reduced by tranquilizers such as azaperone 2.2 mg/kg[1841] or amperozide 1 mg/kg,[228] but these are not readily available. McGlone and Curtis[1273] used hides, small recesses in the pen, into which a pig could put its head. The reason that hiding the head reduces aggression is not clear. Perhaps the sight of the head stimulates aggression in the more aggressive pig. A simpler explanation is that the pig's head is protected. Furthermore, his weapons are the teeth and snout, and if they are in the hides, they are not being used on other pigs. Provision of toys can reduce aggression.[230]

Simple masking odors have no effect on aggression.[154] Spraying or dabbing the boar pheromone 5-α-androstenol on the pigs reduces aggression among young pigs[1269–1271] but not older ones. Perhaps the explanation is that young pigs are always submissive to adult boars, whereas an older pig may challenge an adult male or a pig that smells like one. A more practical method of reducing aggression is to add the amino acid tryptophan and reduce the amount of other neutral amino acids because these compete with tryptophan for the carrier across the blood–brain barrier. Tryptophan will be converted into serotonin in the brain. When pigs are exposed to a dominant pig, those fed with tryptophan have lower levels of cortisol before and 2 hours after the confrontation although their behavior during the conflict is not affected.[1051] Little information exists about reducing aggression when sows are mixed, although more should be learned before gestation crates are no longer used. The presence of a boar does not reduce aggression among sows and actually increased their salivary cortisol level.[1723] Providing partitions longer than the body length of the sows and between which individual sows can eat reduces aggression. Feeding a diet diluted with water also helps.[49]

Tail biting

Another type of aggression that is seen mostly in penned pigs housed on artificial floors is tail biting.[549] Crowding encourages the outbreak of tail biting,[554,1709] but the main cause appears to be lack of opportunity for oral stimulation in a species that normally spends 7 hours a day rooting on pasture.[738] Quite possibly, bored pigs begin to nibble on each other's tails for lack of anything else to do. After a tail has been bitten severely enough to bleed and the bleeding has been aggravated as the victim swishes its injured tail, the pigs become much more aggressive and bite in earnest.[1925] The blood itself appears to be the stimulus for play to become true aggression.[630] Some pigs are killed outright, but more often losses occur as the result of infection of the wounded tails. If only one or two pigs are responsible for most of the biting, they should be removed. Often, simply giving the pigs corn on the cob to chew will stop an outbreak of tail biting that has not progressed to the cannibalistic stage. Tail biting can be reduced by providing a rooting source such as soil that is also a source of iron;[66] this soil is helpful because iron deficiency can be a cause of tail-biting.[631] The incidence of tail biting increases when pigs are housed without bedding on slatted floors and are fed automatically. Feeding by hand, providing straw bedding and manipulatable objects decreases the incidence.[273] Docking of the pigs' tails at birth is performed on many hog farms. This approach eliminates the target, but not the vice, and ear biting may arise instead.[1492]

Grooming

Subordinate pigs groom dominant ones. The dominant pig lies on its side while the subordinates nibble at its belly. The pig has areas that it cannot reach with its own snout or hind feet (Fig. 2.7). These areas, the flanks and back, are groomed by other pigs. Singly penned pigs scratch themselves on inanimate objects instead. If scratching seems particularly prolonged or intense, skin parasites may be present.

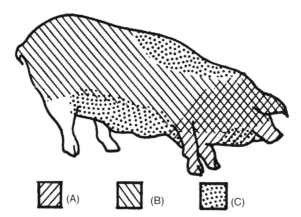

(A)   (B)   (C)

Fig. 2.7 Grooming behavior of the pig. (A) The area scratched by the hind legs. (B) The area rubbed on vertical objects. (C) The area licked and nosed by other pigs.[738] (Copyright 1969, with permission of W.B. Saunders Co.)

DOGS

Social behavior

Urban dogs are either solitary or form small groups, most often of two or three.[192,218,428,616,1118] Wolf packs contain 2–12 members.[1290] Perhaps we have selected dogs to be less social, or pack living, than their lupine ancestors. Another explanation is that dogs perceive their owners as part of their pack because the majority of the dogs in these studies were free-ranging pets, not strays. Large groups of urban dogs are seen only in association with estrous bitches.[429] Rural dogs form slightly larger packs that often contain two to five dogs.[1717] Dogs in packs are more dangerous to humans than solitary dogs. This kind of aggression is usually predatory; the pack, usually underfed, chases a person who is on foot or on a two-wheeled vehicle.[254]

Regardless of the size of a canine group, social relationships are formed. The importance of a companion of the same species is illustrated by in a study of dogs afraid of thunder. Their cortical rose over 200%, but rose less if there was another dog in the household.[486] There is considerable controversy about whether dogs or even wolves have strict dominance hierarchies.[276] Resource holding potential relies on the animal valuing the item more than it fears the other dog. For that reason, a dog might guard a bone, but not a bowl of dry dog food from another dog or from its owners. Dominance is a function of the relation between two individuals and in some pairs of dogs dominance is very apparent. A dominant dog typically assumes a T-position in relation to the submissive dog's shoulder (Fig. 2.8). The submissive dog turns its head away, avoiding the

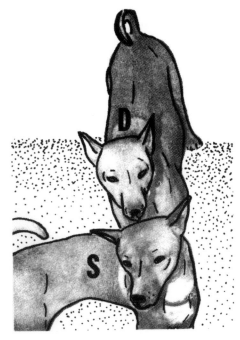

Fig. 2.8   Dominant and submissive postures in dogs. The dominant dog (D) forming an intimidating T-position relative to the position of the subordinate (S), who attempts to avoid a confrontation by turning away.[612] (Copyright 1972, with permission of Coward, McCann, and Geoghegan.)

eye contact that might elicit an attack. The submissive animal often remains stationary because running usually elicits an attack or chase.[612] Dogs seem to be able to identify their own breed and will choose their own littermates in a two-choice test.[829] There is not only preference for their own breed but also aversion to others. For instance, the attack of fox terriers will be more aggressive toward a dog of another breed.

Determinants of dominance

Territorial aggression

According to clinicians, this is the most commonly observed type of aggression. The examples of such aggression include dogs barking at one another from their respective territories and dogs threatening or actually attacking either dogs or people that encroach on their territory. The typical dog fight involves bites to the head and disproportionately to the eyes and the thoracic region.[146] This type of aggression between dogs is difficult to treat because the dog cannot be desensitized to all other dogs. Males are more likely than females to be the victims and the aggressors. It can be controlled, and the owner can defuse a potentially aggressive situation by not pulling on the collar and by speaking in a high-pitched cheerful voice.

Fear-induced aggression

Fear-induced aggression is the type of aggression that most often directly confronts the veterinarian. The fear-biting dog will be most apt to attack when its critical distance has been invaded, an invasion that is unavoidable for the clinician to examine the dog. Every effort should be made to reduce fear in this type of dog. The astute behaviorist should be able to judge which animal is the fear biter and should not be further frightened, and which is the generally aggressive dog that will be more easily handled when made submissive. Fear and aggression are sometimes ambiguous in that a dog may be guarding a scarce resource (dominance), but be afraid of a confrontation with a human who outweighs it (fear). It will still bite. This type of aggression is termed conflict or competitive aggression. The fact that the majority of dogs that have bitten their owners exhibit fear in other situation indicates that dominance is rarely the problem.[731]

Aggression and hormonal influences

See Chapter 5, "Maternal Behavior," for a description of pseudopregnancy in bitches that may be accompanied by aggression. There are nonmaternal forms of female aggression. Spayed females tend to be more aggressive than intact ones, possibly because the source of progesterone has been removed, especially if females were outnumbered by males in their litters.[257,1445] Lactating bitches may aggressively protect their puppies. Pronounced aggression by a lactating bitch with a large litter may be a sign of lactation tetany.

Predatory aggression

Predatory behavior by dogs is often a clinical problem. A solitary dog will attack sheep, but the latency to attack is shorter if another dog is chasing.[355] Dogs that kill chickens, deer, lambs, or cats are frequently presented for treatment. The easiest approach is proper restraint of the dog. A dog on a leash or in a pen is not only prevented from killing other animals but also is no longer at risk of automobile-induced trauma. One method is to "socialize" the dog to the prey animal by penning the dog and prey together. At first, however, the prey animal might have to be caged for protection. A more drastic treatment may also be used. Electric shock collars have been used successfully to inhibit dogs from attacking sheep.[354]

Guard Dogs for Predator Control. In the western United States, coyotes are the major predator of sheep; in the eastern United States, dogs are the primary predator. In both areas, guard dogs, not herding dogs, have been moderately successful. The breeds used are the Anatolian Shepherd, Maremma, Shar Planinetz, Spitz, Komodor, and Great Pyrenees. Sixty to seventy percent of sheep producers who use these dogs believed that they were economically beneficial. The major problem is that 25% of the guard dogs injure or kill the sheep themselves, but most dogs can be trained not to chase the sheep.[384,712] Bonding sheep or goats to cattle may be a better means of reducing losses from predation.[52,54,904] The bonding will succeed more often if only one heifer is added to a flock of sheep.[53] If two or more heifers are present, they may not stay with the sheep. Llamas and donkeys have also been used as sheep-guarding animals.

Clinical problems

There have been many studies of aggression in dogs.[253,257,774,865,1215,2065] All these studies concur that males are more likely to be presented for aggression than are females, and that certain breeds such as spaniels predominate in the dominance aggression category,[1523,1524] whereas the more typically aggressive dogs such as German shepherds or rottweilers present as territorially aggressive. Hart et al., Horwitz et al., Horwitz and Nielson, Landsberg et al, and Overall,[100,257,773,910,1459,1893,1894,1924] discuss treatment of aggression. There are several books on small animal behavior problems that give much more detailed discussions of the treatment of aggression and other behavior problems.[100,188,839,862,910,1088,1459]

Aggression toward strangers

Territorial aggression toward people is probably the greatest canine behavior problem,[577] as can be seen from the following statistics. Two hundred seventy-nine people were killed by dogs in the United States in the years 1979 through 1994. In 1995–1996, 25 people, including 4 infants, died as a result of dog attacks.[909] An estimated half-million people are bitten each year. These figures are similar to those of earlier years.[1357,1674,2045] In 1995–1996, of 20 people killed by pit bulls, 19 were owned by men, seven of whom had convictions for violent crimes.[1177] In 1997 and 1998, rottweilers were the most commonly reported breed involved in fatal attacks, but they were the second most popular breed.[1673]

Military dogs used for patrolling also bite, usually a handler.[1116] Dogs bite strangers who are coming into the house or yard. This is termed territorial aggression. Most bites occur on or near the dog owner's property, suggesting that the dogs are protecting their territories. Delivery persons and postal employees are well-known recipients of canine aggression. Stray dogs do not inflict many bites, presumably because they do not have a territory to protect. Dogs chase cats and strangers who are running past. This is termed predatory aggression. Children receive the most bite wounds (60%), some of which are fatal.[578] Children tend to run, whether in play or in fear of the dog; running triggers pursuit and attack by the dog. Joggers and bicyclists are also frequent targets of aggressive dogs for similar reasons.

Most aggression toward strangers involves territorial boundaries—the front door or the yard. Many owners encourage this type of aggression because they want a watchdog. Unfortunately, they are not teaching the dog to discriminate between people with legitimate business and burglars. Both by their owner's approval and by the flight of the victim, the dogs are being rewarded for barking and lunging at visitors. For example, many dogs have learned that if they bark at mail carriers, the latter will leave. Of course, they would leave anyway, but the dog has been operantly conditioned (see Chapter 7).

Prevention of aggression. The first step in preventing aggression is to obtain dogs of nonaggressive breeds, because there are both environmental and hereditary influences on aggressive, as on all, behavior. Mackenzie et al.[1198] have shown that traits necessary for good, that is, aggressive, guard dogs are heritable. Fearfulness also is heritable.[695,1714] In fact, it was possible to develop a fearful and a normal strain of pointers within a few generations.[1388] Although dogs of mixed breed and of nearly every pure breed can be diagnosed as aggressive, some breeds are more at risk than others. German shepherds and rottweilers are more likely to show territorial aggression and, because of their popularity as a breed, are at or near the top of lists of breeds presented to behavioral clinics.[190,253,774,865] Behavior clinics also report that cocker and springer spaniels are frequently presented, usually for aggression toward the owner, either dominance or guarding (possessive) types of aggression. If the public were to stop buying dogs of breeds that tend to be aggressive, breeders would select dogs for suitable pet temperament as well as for conformation and coat.

Preventing the development of aggression is much easier than curing it. Puppies rather than adult dogs should be obtained as pets. The owner can then establish the correct relationship with the dog when it is easy to do so. Puppies should be acquired during the socialization period, 6–12 weeks (see Chapter 6, "Development of Behavior"). The source is important: Dogs from pet shops and those ill as puppies are more apt to have problems.[1733] Both parents should be friendly and approachable. The puppy should be outgoing, but not so assertive that it bites at hands when held or at feet when following people.

To avoid aggression toward other dogs, try to socialize the puppy to other friendly dogs of the same general size as soon as it has been properly vaccinated. If the puppy has plenty of pleasant experiences with other dogs while it is at its most playful age, it will be less apt as an adult to be either aggressive or fearful toward other dogs. Veterinarians should offer puppy socialization classes, not only to educate owners about puppy behavior but also to minimize the dog's fear of the veterinary clinic. Unfortunately, playing with other puppies and being handled by other people ("socialization") in these classes will not change the dog's innate response to social stimuli such as strange dogs or people.[1726]

Diet. The diet may be modified to one containing lower protein.[471] There is a common carrier for neutral amino acids across the blood–brain barrier. When the concentration of competing amino acids is reduced when a low protein is fed, tryptophan can enter the brain in higher concentration. Tryptophan is the precursor of serotonin. Serotonin metabolite, is lower in the cerebrospinal fluid of aggressive dogs, and higher serotonin is associated with lower aggression.[1595] The most aggressive dogs are fed the highest protein diet, and combining a low protein diet with supplementary tryptophan reduces aggression.[339,455]

Surgical procedures. Castration should always be advised for aggressive male dogs.[854] The effect of castration is twofold: (1) aggression may be reduced, particularly aggression that is sexual in motivation, although territorial aggression may not be affected;[1404] and (2) the dog will not be able to pass on its aggressive tendencies. For the same reasons, ovariohysterectomy should also be advised for aggressive females, particularly in cases of maternal or pseudopregnancy-related aggression. Spaying does increase aggression in bitches that were already aggressive, particularly if they were from predominantly male litters,[256,1445] so perhaps hysterectomy rather than ovariohysterectomy should be recommended for aggressive bitches. But it is more important to prevent reproduction.

Filing and capping the canines and incisors removes the most formidable of the dog's weapons. A large dog can still bite with its premolars and molars, and all dogs can still bruise or crush with their small jaws. Nevertheless, this procedure should be considered if a family insists on keeping a dangerous dog.

CATS

Free-ranging cats

Feline social organization is very variable. Group size varies from fewer than 10 on most farms to more than 30 in some urban areas where an abundant food source is located in a confined area.[1907]

In a rural setting, cats have territories as large as 200 hectares per female cat and 600 hectares per male cat,[1196,1907,2054] or one cat per square kilometer, whereas in an urban setting the density varies from 1000 cats per square kilometer (or ~2000 cats/sq mi.).[435,1399] Cats were considered to be a nonsocial species because they do not live in groups as adults if they are living on natural prey,[1907] but cats have been able to modify their social organization and live in groups, even multimale groups. Cats can adapt to a concentrated food source such as that found in dumps, fishing villages, and farms by living in groups, but these groups are of matrilineal female kin. Females rarely transfer from group to group, although males can. In general, the dominant tom's territory encompasses the females' (Fig. 2.9). Although he will not hunt on the females' territories, he will repel any marauding male, and the females will repel any female intruder. The larger the male's home range, the more female territories he encompasses and the greater his reproductive success. The males may make excursions outside their home range to mate with additional females.[1689]

Crowell-Davis and her colleagues have studied several groups of free-living cats and found may signs of affiliative behavior, especially cheek and tail rubbing of other group members.[159,400,406]

Confined cats

Social aggression

When two cats approach each other aggressively, they walk on tiptoe, slowly lashing their tails about the hocks and turning their heads from side to side while making direct eye contact. This threat may intimidate a subordinate cat so that it slinks off; evenly matched rivals will continue to approach one another (Fig. 2.10). They will walk slightly past one another before one cat will spring, trying for a grip on the nape of the opponent's neck. The attacked cat throws itself on its back, thus protecting the nape. The two adversaries will both lie on the ground belly to belly while they claw, vocalize, and bite at each other. After a few moments, one cat, usually the original attacker, will jump free. The other cat may adopt a defensive posture, attack, or run away. The victor usually pursues the vanquished.[1133] Cats that are aggressive toward other cats are not necessarily aggressive toward people, and vice versa.[1908] These differences in personality appear to be inherited, because a paternal effect has been noted.[6,567]

When placed together in a home or a laboratory or on a farm, cats will form dominance hierarchies,[156,369,1098] but marked aggression may persist in this originally solitary species.

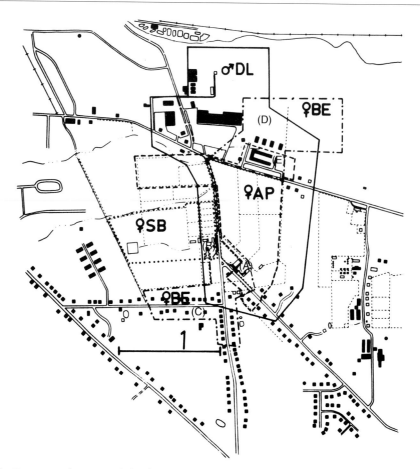

Fig. 2.9 Ranges used concurrently by three adult female (AP, BE, SB) and one adult male (DL) cats during 1979. AP and BE shared three of four barns at the home farm (A) and most of the yards and pastures immediately surrounding the barns. SB was the only female at her farm (B). BE used the southern section of her range (C) through most of 1978 and 1979 and started using the northern area (D) in the late summer of 1979 in a series of foraging excursions with that year's litter. One female kitten remained and eventually reproduced in this section of the range, whereas BE and a male kitten disappeared from this area in late 1979. The two section of BE's range were connected only by the road between SB's and AP's ranges; BE hunted frequently along the road shoulders, and SB and AP foraged only in the adjoining pastures. AP and BE shared the area around an apartment complex (E) but never were noted to contact one another here. DL's range included large areas of each female's range, and on most evenings DL visited each barn complex at least once. The enclosed line at the lower end of the map represents 500 m. Immediately above it, the north–south axis is indicated. Dark quadrangles represent homes, apartments and stores; open quadrangles barns and other out buildings. Narrow dotted lines indicated fence lines.[2054] (With permission of Veterinary Clinics of North America: Small Animal Practice.)

When feral cats, who voluntarily determine the group composition, are studied, a hierarchy emerges that varies with body size in females and age in males.[2066] More closely related cats are less aggressive.[274] The rank of cats for food may differ from their rank in social space in intact female laboratory cats,[505] but is the same in a large group of neutered cats of both sexes confined in one household and yard.[1041] Larger, older cats and male cats tend to be dominant over smaller younger female cats. Cats may divide up a house: one's territory may be the first floor; the other's the second floor. Roommates may find that the two cats belonging to one

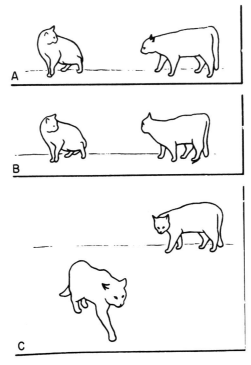

Fig. 2.10 Dominant and submissive postures in cats. The dominant cat is on the right. The submissive cat moves slowly away and avoids eye contact.[1134] (Katzen–Eine Verhaltensstudiend, copyright 1975, with permission of Paul Parey, Berlin and Hamburg.)

person will gang up on the single cat belonging to the other. Urination in the house, especially on beds or rugs, often occurs when strange cats are introduced.

Territorial behavior

Males maintain nonoverlapping territories in the nonbreeding season, but overlap considerably in the breeding season. Therefore, in both free-ranging and pet cats, intraspecies aggression among intact male cats is a very common problem. Many tomcats are presented repeatedly for treatment of bite wounds and abscesses resulting from fighting behavior. Castration is approximately 90% effective in eliminating roaming and fighting in adult male cats,[772] although the disappearance of one behavior may not be associated with a decline in the other.

In highly concentrated populations in which cats compete for food, males are dominant over females. The larger and older males are dominant over younger, smaller ones in competition for food or for females.[2066]

Cats can form harmonious social groups, but adding a new cat leads to fighting in 50% of households and there is a greater risk of fighting if the cats are allowed access to the outdoors. Ten percent of the cats are still aggressive a year after introduction.[1123]

Predatory behavior

The tall posture of the cat engaged in territorial or sexual aggression is to be contrasted with the stalking posture of predatory aggression. The predatory cat carries its body as closely as possible to the ground. It moves toward its quarry slowly, taking advantage of any natural cover. The closer the cat gets to its prey, the more slowly it advances. Almost inevitably, the cat will pause before leaping to attack. Only the tip of the tail will move as the cat lies in wait. There are usually two or three bounds from hiding to the prey. When attacking a large animal, cats try to make a nape bite to sever the spinal cord.[1133]

Predatory aggression is innate but has some learned aspects. Kittens raised with a mother who killed rats in their presence killed at their first opportunity; kittens raised alone seldom did, whereas those raised in a cage with a rat never did.[1073] Apparently, kittens learn to direct various innate predatory motor patterns to the prey (see Chapter 6) their mother brings to them. She does not simply let them eat the prey; she lets the prey go and catches it again. If the kittens attempt to catch or eat the mouse, the mother will compete with them for it. In this manner, the kittens are stimulated by the hunting game and, apparently, learn by observation. The types of prey brought to the kittens may influence the range of prey hunted by the kittens as adults. Although the mother can influence kittens' predatory skills by bringing prey and interacting with it, adult cats without such learning experience also become competent predators, so a kitten that is not a good hunter can acquire the skills as an adult.[1907]

Most cats will kill rats if fasted for two or more days, but they still prefer to eat commercial cat food rather than their prey.[6] Success of predatory attempts can be lowered by fitting the cat with a belled collar or a collar that emits beeps every 7 seconds.[1409]

One feline characteristic that is distasteful to some people is that cats sometimes play with their prey before and after it is dead. They will catch a mouse, let it go, and catch it again. After it is dead, they will throw it up with their paws and leap upon it. The function of this behavior is obscure, although it may be appetitive or, perhaps, displacement behavior, but it does indicate that the difference between predatory play and true predation is small. Truly hungry cats rarely play with prey; they eat it as soon as it is dead and they have recuperated from the predatory effort.

Grooming

Licking is a very important part of maternal behavior in cats, and self-grooming occupies a great deal of their time as adults. Cats sometimes lick one another; this is most likely to occur when a mother continues to groom her adult offspring, but long-term associates also allogroom and licking is part of courtship behavior. Feline grooming is an important part of daily activities. One of the simplest types of grooming is licking the nose and lips. These are two distinct motions that rarely overlap. Licking the nose occurs after gaping, for example, and the tongue goes dorsally on the midline and then is pulled immediately vertically and into the mouth. A common licking problem is an exaggeration of this behavior in which the nose is chronically irritated by the abrasive tongue. Licking the lips involves movement of the tongue along the edge of the upper lips to the corners of the mouth; this behavior is seen after eating or drinking.

Feline face washing is a stereotyped behavior. The cat is in a sitting position and applies saliva to the medial aspect of the front leg, which is held horizontally. The paw is rubbed from back to front over the nose with a circular upward motion. This motion is repeated a few times; each time, the paw reaches out a little farther until it reaches behind the ear (only after three rubs) and then travels downward over the backside of the ear, forehead, and eye. Other areas of the body are cleaned, but not in the stereotyped order in which the face is washed. The tongue is drawn over the coat in long strokes, mostly in the direction of the hair. If deprived of grooming by an Elizabethan collar, for example, cats will groom more, indicating the importance of the behavior. Grooming functions in external parasite control; we know this because when they are prevented from grooming, cats have more fleas.[524]

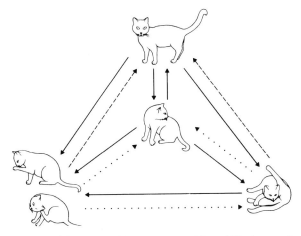

Fig. 2.11   Grooming postures of the cat. (*Top*) Nongrooming. (*Center*) Flank grooming. (*Clockwise*) Grooming of hindquarters; scratching ears; first step of face grooming, licking the front leg. Solid arrows indicate grooming sequences of normal cats. Dotted and dashed arrows indicate sequences in cats with tectal lesions.[1838] (Copyright 1977, with permission of *J. Comp. Physiol. Psychol.*)

During normal grooming, the saliva applied is licked up again, but in a hot environment the saliva is allowed to remain to aid in thermoregulation. The neck, chest, shoulders, and front paws receive the most grooming. The stomach, rear legs, back, croup, tail, and anal areas receive less attention. All the former regions are licked as the cat sits. The cat lies to lick the sides, stomach, rear legs, tail, and front paws[1133] (Fig. 2.11). A cat may sit like a bear on its haunches to lick the penis; this can be a sign of urethral obstruction. Grooming can also be a postconflict (cat–cat or cat–human) stress response.[1920] It is easy to understand how psychogenic overgrooming can result when a cat is stressed.

Allogrooming occurs among cats. Cats are more likely to groom relatives than nonrelatives and to groom cats they have known longer.[417]

Clinical problems

Pathological causes of aggression in cats are more common than in dogs.[1593] Meningiomas, feline ischemic syndrome,[450] and toxoplasmosis have all been associated with aggression. Although some meningiomas can be removed so that the cat's behavior returns to normal, the other conditions cause tissue damage in the limbic system that is diffuse and, therefore, untreatable. Sudden onset of severe aggression is a poor prognostic sign. Euthanasia should be recommended because the cats may climb up the owner and attack the face. The aggression is usually well directed. For example, a cat with toxoplasmosis attacked dogs, but only when she had been with her kittens. Beaver,[187] Borchelt and Voith,[257] Hart and Hart,[775] Hunthausen,[910] Landsberg,[1087, 1088] Overall,[1471] Askew,[100] Hetts,[839] and Horwitz[862] have addressed the problem of aggression in cats.

Aggression toward people

Predatory Aggression. Feline aggression toward people can be subdivided into predatory or playful, redirected, territorial, and dominance. The predatory type of aggression is preceded by stalking and pouncing and is usually directed toward the feet of a moving person. If the cat is young and has no other kitten to play with, the aggression is probably playful. In that case, the bite and scratches are usually inhibited; however, if the owners have not reprimanded the cat for biting too hard in play, it may not have learned to inhibit its bite. The progression of play to serious predation is a continuum and explains the behavior in which cats seem to tease or toy with their prey. Owners should be told not to encourage play directed toward their fingers or other body parts. Playful aggression should be redirected toward swinging toys. The owner may swing a toy from a string and praise the cat verbally for attacking the toy but punish the cat for biting at people's feet. The best way to punish a cat is to startle it. Water guns or aerosol sprays are very effective. Even a loud noise, such as a whistle, can be used. The best punishment is one that the cat does not associate with the owner. A similar strategy is used for true predatory aggression except that neither toys nor rewards are used, but the cat is sprayed for attacking.

Dominance. Dominant, status-related,[1459] or irritable aggression usually occurs when the cat is being stroked. The cat, particularly a male cat, may be giving the nape bite that it gives during copulation. The owner should pet the cat more gently and for less prolonged periods. Dominance over the cat can be attempted by getting up and thus forcing the cat to jump to the floor and by training; for example, it can be taught that it will receive a reward for sitting on command. The cat can be given a reward, a food treat, for allowing two strokes, then for allowing three, and so forth, to increase its tolerance for petting. Holding the cat down so that it cannot move for a few minutes a day may also help to eliminate the problem.

Redirected aggression. See section "Aggression Toward Other Cats." Cats may become aroused when they see a strange cat through a window, and they may attack their own owner. Owners should be advised not to pick up or pet an aroused, caterwauling cat.

Fear- or territory-related aggression. Attacks may be sudden and explosive, with or without vocalization (caterwauling), and may occur only once or recur. Common stimuli are the odors of other cats. Consequently, owners of cats that have become aggressive toward the owners after they have handled a strange cat should be careful to wash and change clothes before interacting with their own cat.

If no stimulus is identified, the cat may be exhibiting idiopathic aggression. If identified, the initiating stimulus should be removed. Severely aggressive cats should be isolated from the owner in a dark room for several days. Food and light are brought by the owner for brief periods several times daily until there is no indication of anxiety or aggression. Drug therapy with serotonin reuptake inhibitors may be indicated in cases of refractory or severe aggression. Benzodiazepines should be avoided because of the potential for disinhibition.

Aggression toward other cats

Aggression among cats in the same household is the most common feline aggressive problem, involving 10–50% of cats.[255,804] The reason for the wide variation is that owners are unaware of the subtle signs of aggression, such as staring, and may mistake the victim who is hissing with flattened ears for the aggressor whose upright posture is much more subtle. Male cats are more likely to initiate aggression than females. In contrast to dogs, male cats are aggressive toward females as well as males.[1156]

Territorial aggression. Introducing a new cat stimulates territorial aggression. The aggressor may be the newly introduced cat. The difference between territorial aggression and status-related aggression is that the aggressor seeks out the other cat rather than fight only when there is a scarce resource. Males are more likely to exhibit this behavior than females. The victim may be of either sex.[1156]

Redirected aggression. Redirected aggression occurs when a cat sees another cat outside a window and attacks its housemate. This type of aggression can be short lived, but may persist if the victim continues to flee whenever it encounters the aggressor. Apparently, the fearful behavior stimulates continued aggression by the other cat. If a new adult cat is introduced, aggression is to be expected, but aggression can also occur between cats that have lived peacefully together for years. In some cases, a physical change and/or a change in odor can precipitate the aggression. For example, if one cat is hospitalized, it may be attacked when it returns, either because it is weak or because it smells different. This could be termed nonrecognition aggression.

Treatment of aggression toward other cats. Separate the two cats for the entire day except at mealtimes, but rub each cat's cheeks and tail and then rub the other cat with the same towel. At mealtimes, feed the two cats in their separate environments for a few meals. Then gradually introduce them back into the same room, but feed them at opposite ends of the room, with the aggressor on a leash or in a cage so that it cannot reach the victim. Because the cats are together only at mealtimes, they will associate the reward of food with each other. If no hissing or fighting occurs at one meal, you may gradually bring the victim's dish closer to the aggressor at the next meal. Feed the cats three times a day instead of twice, because this will allow the cats to have more time in each other's presence. When the victim and aggressor can eat right next to each other with the aggressor confined, begin again to feed the cats at separate ends of the room but with the aggressor free (but with a leash and collar for easy catching). Gradually, day by day, move the bowls closer and closer, and increase the length of time in which they are together after mealtime. The synthetic cheek gland pheromone Feliway may also be applied to the feeding area to reduce tension and stimulate appetite.[716]

Interspecific aggression

Dogs and cats can exist amicably. The chances are best if the cat is less than 6 months old and the dog is less than 1 year.[582]

3 Biological Rhythms and Sleep

*Animals do appear to have a sense of time, which can explain the phenomenon of the dog who
wakes up and stands at the door shortly before the owner appears at the end of the working day.
They also realize when they have been confined for a longer or shorter period in identical cages
and will choose the place where confinement was shorter.*[1795]

The activity patterns of domestic animals vary considerably both between species and within
a species depending on the diet and environment. Horses spend the majority of their time
grazing on pasture, and ruminants spend the majority of their time grazing and ruminating; this
changes considerably in confined animals on high-concentrate diets. Cats and dogs rest or sleep
for a large percentage of the time. Pigs with free access to food also sleep many hours a day.
Circadian and other rhythms are important in determining activity and sexual cycles, as well as
physiological responses.

INTRODUCTION

One should be aware of the activity and sleep patterns of animals so that abnormality can be
detected. A horse that is lying down at night is probably sleeping; an adult horse that lies down
during the day (especially a cold, cloudy day) is abnormal and should be observed carefully
because this is an unusual time for a horse to be recumbent.

The patterns of behavior, especially those of activity and sleep, reflect internal rhythms.
There are several types of rhythms of differing duration. The circadian rhythms, occurring in
approximately 24-hour periods, are the best known and best studied. The activity cycles of
most animals are circadian in that the periods of activity and inactivity add up to approximately
24 hours. Other types of rhythms are high-frequency, ultradian, infradian, and annual cycles.
Biological cells are found in single cells. The various clocks appear to be linked in a hierarchal
organization that allows temporal coordination. The master clock appears to be located in the
suprachiasmatic nucleus.[1408]

HIGH-FREQUENCY RHYTHMS

High-frequency rhythms, for example, heart and respiration rates, occur in periods of less than
30 minutes. The heart rate varies inversely with body weight, so the heart rate of a cat (110–130

Domestic Animal Behavior for Veterinarians and Animal Scientists, *Fifth Edition* by Katherine Albro Houpt
© 2011 John Wiley & Sons, Inc.

beats per minute) is considerably higher than that of a horse (28–40 beats per minute). The respiratory rate does not vary linearly with body size, so the cow breathes 10–30 times per minute, and the pig, 8–18 times per minute. Respiratory cycles have an effect on the cardiac rate; it increases during inspiration. This effect, called sinus arrhythmia, is more marked in dogs than in other domestic species. The endogenous nature of biological rhythms can be best appreciated by a consideration of the contraction rate of the embryonic heart, especially that of a chick embryo, which does not have even the maternal heart rate to influence it.

ULTRADIAN RHYTHMS

Ultradian rhythms are more frequent than 24 hours; one example is the fluctuations of growth hormone output from the pituitary, which in cattle occur in cycles of 3.5 hours.[240] Body temperature also varies in ultradian cycles of approximately 1 hour in cats.[791] The physiological bases for, or influences upon, these short cycles are unknown but are believed to be the result of oscillations of cells in central pattern generators. The most interesting ultradian behavior rhythm is that of feeding. When food is available ad libitum, nearly all species eat 9–12 meals a day. This pattern is seen in dogs and cats,[978,1163] sheep,[341] horses,[1099] pigs,[221] and cattle.[1562]

CIRCADIAN RHYTHMS

A circadian rhythm is self-sustaining, maintained under conditions of constant light or dark, and has a cycle of approximately 24 hours.

Zeitgebers

Circadian rhythms are endogenous, that is, they persist under conditions of constant light or constant dark, but usually are influenced by, and entrained to, external factors, which set the biological clock. Some of these factors are temperature, barometric pressure, various drugs, hormones, and light. Of these factors, the most important is light. These factors are called zeitgebers (German for "time givers") because they set the rhythms just as one might set a clock.

Light

Circadian rhythms are entrained to light, that is, although under conditions of constant illumination a rhythm may have a period of approximately 24 hours, under naturally occurring light, the rhythm will be that of the light–dark cycle. The light must be present during a specific portion of the endogenous rhythm. Hamsters, for example, entrain to a 12-hour-light/12-hour-dark day and to a 6-hour-light/12-hour-dark day, but not to a 6-hour-light/30-hour-dark day.[535]

Considerable practical advantage has been taken of the entraining function of light to bring mares into estrus early, or conversely, to avoid injuries during hierarchy formation by keeping pigs in the dark. Even the simple act of putting a cover over a parrot's cage makes use of the effect of light on avian activity. The photoreceptors responsible for entraining circadian rhythms are not the same as those for vision, and some may even be extraocular.[314] Not all types of light are equally effective in entraining circadian rhythms. Green light is most effective and red light is least effective; therefore, red light may be used when visibility is desirable, but interference with an animal's circadian rhythms and dark activities is not.[1284] When zeitgebers are removed, the resulting desynchronization of internal rhythms may have deleterious results; for example, thermoregulation may be impaired.[651] When one travels, zeitgebers are removed or are not present at the proper period of time in the endogenous rhythm, causing jet lag because rhythms are not synchronized.

Barometric pressure

The influence of other factors on circadian rhythms has not been as well studied, but barometric pressure has been shown to influence activity patterns. Mice show higher activity levels when barometric pressure is increasing.[1798] Although the phenomenon has never been quantified, farm animals, such as horses and dogs, show high levels of activity before storms, and tail-biting episodes often occur in swine just before storms.

Drugs

Drugs can affect rhythms. Examples are caffeine and theophylline,[528] and lithium.[453,962,1266] The action of lithium on circadian rhythms of humans as well as of animals may be the basis for its amelioration of depression and aggression. The two compounds that may be useful for treatment of jet lag and sleep disturbances of shift workers are melatonin (see the following section, "Pineal gland") and benzodiazepines.[1724,1905]

More important from a clinical standpoint is that a given drug may have a greater effect and/or a lower toxicity at one time of day than at another. Hypoglycemic agents, if administered while liver glycogen and plasma glucose are low, are more apt to precipitate hypoglycemic convulsions than if administered at another point in the cycle.[963]

Pineal gland

The pineal gland is probably an important intermediary in the synchronization of circadian rhythms because it demonstrates marked rhythms of output of several hormones and neurotransmitters.[662] Melatonin is produced by the pineal, and is present in higher quantities in plasma and cerebral spinal fluid at night[801] (Fig. 3.1). Melatonin has an antigonadotropic effect in long-day breeders and a pro-gonadotropic effect in short-day breeders. It may be the means by which the hypothalamus is apprised of day length, the link between circadian rhythms and annual sexual cycles, for melatonin would increase as dark-period length increases, and the increased melatonin levels would depress gonadal activity. The practical application of this role of melatonin is that short-day breeders such as sheep may be brought into estrus earlier by oral administration of melatonin in the afternoon for several months.[72] Efficacy of melatonin for treatment of behavior problems remains to be investigated.

The peak level of the neurotransmitter serotonin is 180° out of phase with melatonin. Serotonin is a precursor of melatonin. The activities of the enzymes catalyzing the reaction (serotonin to melatonin) are influenced by light.[1267] Serotonin has been implicated as a sleep-inducing neurotransmitter. Day length will influence the relative amounts of serotonin and melatonin present in the pineal, thereby influencing the organism's sleep–wakefulness and reproductive condition. Aggressive behavior also may be influenced. Most owners are bitten by their dogs at night, when serotonin levels are low. Drugs that increase serotonin activity decrease aggression.

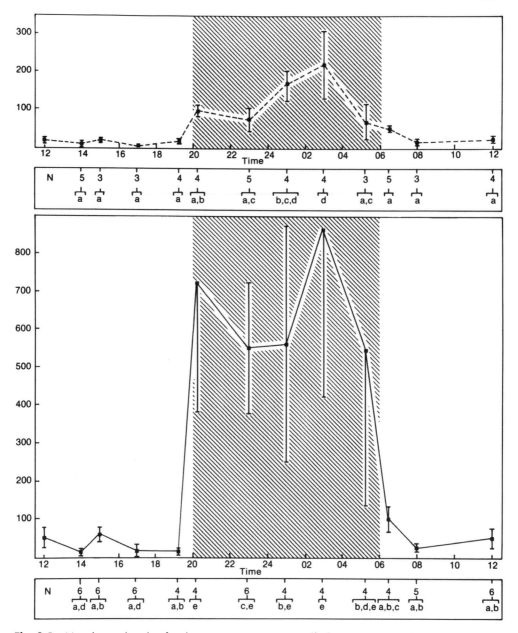

Fig. 3.1 Nyctohemeral cycle of melatonin concentration in calf plasma (upper) and cerebrospinal fluid (lower) at selected times of the day. The lights were on from 0600 to 2000 hours. Data points are means ± 1 standard error of samples from number (N) of calves. Letters indicate that when two means do not have any letter in common, they are significantly different.[801] (Copyright 1977, American Association for the Advancement of Science.)

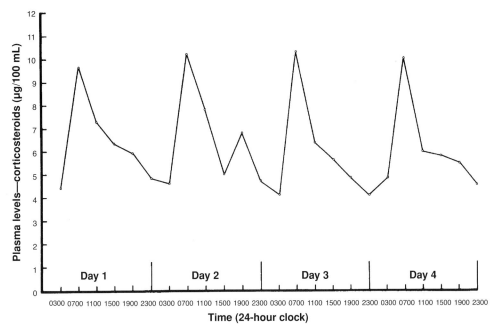

Fig. 3.2 Circadian rhythms of corticosteroid secretion in pigs. The graph is based on the mean results from six pigs. The peak of corticosteroid output occurs in late morning.[141] (Copyright 1973, with permission of Elsevier.)

Examples of circadian rhythms

In addition to gross activity, a number of cellular and endocrinological parameters vary in a circadian rhythm. Many hormones have been demonstrated to have circadian rhythms. Corticosteroids, including both cortisol and corticosterone, increase during the day in pigs and horses, with peak levels in late morning[262,2008] (Fig. 3.2). Both pigs and horses are diurnal (day-active animals) and show diurnal peaks in adrenocortical activity and adrenal responsiveness to ACTH during the day, whereas cats[1707] show increased adrenal activity at night. In stallions and boars, testosterone levels are highest during the day.[532,1029] Some hormones, such as vasopressin in the cat, show circadian rhythms in the cerebrospinal fluid but not in the blood.[1599]

There are age-related effects on the expression of circadian rhythms. For example, although there are circadian rhythms that occur in cortisol concentration in adult dogs, rhythms are not observed in either puppies or old dogs (>12 years of age).[1470] These age-dependent changes may be related to some of the problems of restlessness seen in older dogs (see Chapter 7, "Learning").

Not all hormones are secreted in greatest quantity during the day in diurnal animals; growth hormone, for example, decreases in output during the day in pigs.[1889] Circadian rhythms of heart rate, body temperature, white blood cell number, metabolic rate, liver glycogen and glucose, and glucose absorption from the gut have also been identified.[98,547] Dogs show circadian rhythms of body temperature having a period of 23.7 hours.[979] There is a circadian rhythm of body temperature in calves peaking in the afternoon and reaching nadir in early morning.[1195] Not all hormones exhibit a circadian rhythm. Insulin-like growth factor, unlike cortisol, has no circadian rhythm in horses.[1423] Lactate and urea show diurnal changes, but in opposite directions so that the postprandial efficiency of protein metabolism is greater, whereas efficient carbohydrate metabolism is decreased after an evening meal in comparison to a morning meal.[1051]

Feeding

Feeding is not only rhythmic, but also can entrain other rhythms. When an animal has meals imposed on it instead of freely feeding (the situation for most domestic animals), the animal anticipates the meal with an increase in activity. In order for this rhythm to be entrained, the meal must contain calories.[1343] Daily variations occur in activity and core body temperature of sheep, but these are entrained by feeding.[1512] And a period of activity occurs approximately 24 hours after a meal (when one meal a day is fed).[1346,2011] Rhythms of intestinal enzymes are also secondary to feeding.[589] Although animals usually drink prandially, that is, at the time they eat, evidence exists that drinking bouts may have a different rhythm than feeding. Goats drink mostly just before dawn and just after dark.[1642]

Parasitic rhythms

Still another facet of biological rhythms of importance to the clinician is the rhythm of parasites. Perhaps the best example is that of *Dirofilaria immitis*, canine heartworm. Microfilaria are most active and most likely to be found in the peripheral circulation in the evening.[790] The activity peak nicely coincides with that of the insect vectors, the mosquitoes that will carry the microfilaria to a new host. The clinician may have more success in making a positive diagnosis of the presence of the parasite by examining blood taken in the evening.

OTHER RHYTHMS

Infradian rhythms have cycle periods less frequent than 24 hours. Circatrigintan rhythms are rhythms of approximately 30 days. The sexual cycles of polyestrous domestic animals show periods of approximately three weeks. The sow and cow come into heat every 21 days. Examples of species that are seasonally polyestrous include the mare, which comes into heat every 17–24 days in the spring, and the ewe, which comes into heat, every 16–17 days in the fall.[566] These cycles may represent rhythms of hypothalamic, pituitary, or ovarian activity.

ANNUAL RHYTHMS

Annual or seasonal cycles are somewhat better understood. Horses and sheep are seasonal breeders. Horses are anestrous in the fall and winter and begin to show estrus as day length increases in late winter. Sheep show an opposite response in that they begin to be sexually active when days shorten in the fall. The evolutionary advantages to both species are obvious. The offspring of horses and sheep are born in the spring when food is abundant. Dogs now show sexual cycles of approximately six months' duration, but there is reason to believe that they, too, were once annual breeders. Basenjis, for example, still show an annual fall breeding season.[1714] Domestication, abundant food, and selective breeding also may have caused cattle and swine to become polyestrous throughout the year rather than during one season.

Not all annual cycles are reproductive. Cats show annual cycles of corticosteroids, thyroxine, and epinephrine levels. Peak levels of these three hormones occur during the winter.[1577] More familiar are the cyclic changes in hair coat. Hair-follicle activity in cats is highest in late summer and lowest in late winter, and as a result, fur is 0.5 mm (0.2 in.) longer in winter than in summer.[1672]

Adult ewes show a seasonal variation in heart rate, with a minimum in winter. In wethers, serum concentrations of prolactin, insulin, insulin-like growth factor, and thyroxine are all higher in the spring and summer than in the fall or winter; meal sizes are also larger when the days are longer.[1602]

Horses show seasonal rhythms in carbohydrate metabolism, but these may be related to training.[689] In a seminatural environment, horses also show a decrease in intake from 10 in late summer to 7 kg/day in late winter when the losses of body heat while foraging are greater than the gain from nutrient-poor winter forage.[1072]

Sleep occupies one-quarter (for ruminants) to one-half (for dogs) of the lifetime of animals, but the function of sleep remains unknown. One possible function is replenishing of neurotransmitters. A device to conserve energy, a means of remaining inconspicuous, a period for consolidation of memory, or simply a way to fill up time not needed for foraging are other hypothetical functions of sleep.[2081]

Types of sleep

Sleep can be classified into two types: the "sleep of the mind," slow wave sleep (SWS), or quiet sleep; and the "sleep of the body," paradoxical, active, or rapid eye movement (REM) sleep. The two types can best be differentiated from wakefulness and from one another by means of electroencephalography.

The electroencephalogram (EEG) of the alert animal is characterized by low-voltage, fast waves that are not synchronized. Slow wave sleep is characterized by synchronous waves of high-voltage, slow activity. During paradoxical sleep, the EEG shows low-voltage, fast activity similar to that seen in the wakeful state (Fig. 3.3), but very little muscular activity occurs; therefore, this type of sleep is called the sleep of the body. Although overall muscle tone is very low during paradoxical sleep, the muscles of the eyes frequently contract; hence, the term rapid eye movement. The low-voltage, fast activity of REM sleep does not result in many body movements because the medulla has an inhibitory area that, in effect, paralyzes the muscles of the body.[1367] Humans awakened from REM sleep report that they have been dreaming; the twitching of the face and legs (which are not completely inhibited) and whining during canine sleep indicate that dogs may also be dreaming. We can only speculate as to the presence or content of animal dreams. Total deprivation of either type of sleep is fatal. Deprivation of REM sleep results in behavioral abnormalities in all species tested, and rebound or extra REM sleep occurs during recovery from deprivation.[1652,1653,1914]

PATTERNS OF SLEEP AND ACTIVITY IN DOMESTIC ANIMALS

Sleep varies considerably among species.[316] The activity patterns of the various species described here are reported under specific environmental conditions. The behavior patterns may be different under different environmental conditions, and therefore, the numbers given should not be considered applicable to every animal under every condition. Allison and Cicchetti[46]

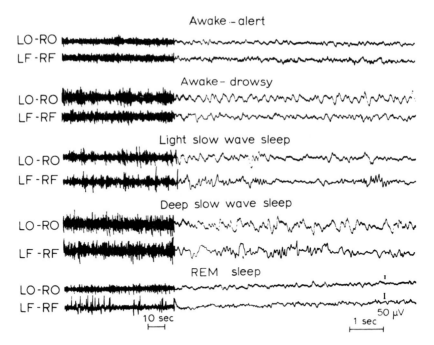

Fig. 3.3 The stages of vigilance and sleep in the cat. Polygraphic record at the speed of 30 mm per second showing the stages identified. LO-RO electroencephalographic record from the left and right occipital areas; LF-RF electroencephalographic record form the left and right frontal areas.[1913] (Copyright 1968, with permission of Pergamon Press.)

hypothesize that sleep time is inversely related to the danger of predation for a given species. Roughly speaking, predators sleep more than prey animals, and large animals more than small animals. See Fig. 3.4 for activity patterns of three species in the same pasture.

Dogs

Sleeping dogs often lie in a characteristic posture with their hind legs tucked up and their heads turned caudolaterally. Their eyes may be open or closed. Rapid eye movement (REM) sleep may be accompanied by leg movements, vocalizations, and by either polypnea or apnea. A dog awakened abruptly from REM sleep may bite, so it is best to let dreaming dogs, or at least sleeping dogs, lie, or to awaken them gently. Dogs show short periods of activity interspersed with periods of rest when free ranging,[192] when tethered outdoors,[454] and when caged.[790] Pet dogs appear to sleep at night, but their behavior may be entrained to that of their owner. Active (REM) sleep occupies only 6% of their time.[10,11] Dogs sleep in cycles of 16 minutes asleep and 5 minutes awake. House dogs and caged dogs sleep more than free-ranging dogs, but even the latter sleep 60% of the night.[12] Although sleeping dogs are relatively easily roused, owners who wish their dogs to guard property must be aware that dogs will sleep where they are most comfortable, that is, on soft surfaces, and not necessarily at the property line.[9] In the case of caged dogs, 30-minute to 2-hour periods of activity alternate with longer quiescent periods. Dogs in groups in kennels spend 7–24% of their time in active behavior (walking, trotting), 5–10% socializing with another dog, and the majority of the time inactive (sitting, standing, or

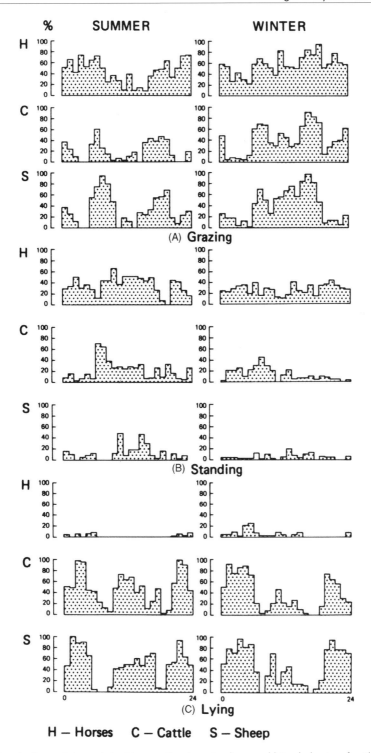

Fig. 3.4 Time budgets of domestic herbivores. Grazing, standing, and lying behavior of cattle, sheep, and horses living on the same pasture during two seasons.[78] (Copyright 1984, with permission of Elsevier Scientific Publishing and CSIRO.)

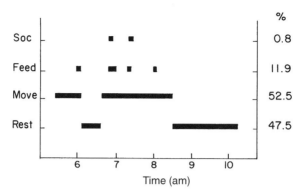

Fig. 3.5   Activity patterns of feral urban dogs. The activities of two dogs during a morning in the fall. Soc: social behavior with other dogs, including sniffing and chasing. Feed: feeding behavior, including rummaging through garbage and eating. Move: moving, walking, and running. Rest: resting or sleeping.[192] (Copyright 1973, with permission of York Press.)

resting), with 20% of inactive time in light slow wave sleep (LSWS), 25% in deep slow wave sleep (DSWS), and 10–12% in REM sleep.[840,846,896] Dogs position themselves so that they can see other dogs, but neither their activity level nor their barking rate changes when other dogs are visible.[1999] Free-ranging feral urban dogs are most active in early morning and in the evening. Foraging for food, usually garbage, socializing with other dogs, and traveling from alley to street to park are their major activities, and are usually interspersed with periods of rest (Fig. 3.5).[192] Similar periods of activity occur just after sunrise, and an hour or two before sunset in sled dogs tethered to their doghouses by 240-cm (8-ft.) leads. Under these conditions, dogs spend more than 80% of their time, night and day, lying down and sit only 2% of the time, mostly while observing another dog or a person.

Dogs exhibit similar behavior patterns whether in runs or on a tether; they are mostly lying down.[2071] Dogs with access to an outdoor run are more active, and are outside for over 2 hours per day in 100 trips per day.[1792] Dogs housed in group pens spend 40% of their time inactive, 12% moving around, 5% in maintenance behaviors such as eating and eliminating.[1428]

A pet dog's activity is controlled by its owner. Dogs are walked or let out early in the morning when their owners arise, and in early evening when their owners return from work.[218] A peak can also occur at noon in communities where people apparently return home for lunch.[1118] In mild climates, people often confine their dogs in their backyards rather than in the house. These dogs spend most of their time inactive, but do walk, run, chew, and explore. They spend a lot of time visiting the door into the house. Problems in these dogs such as barking and chewing are more likely to occur in untrained dogs.[1043]

The behavior of dogs in shelters is important because of concerns about long-term welfare of dogs that are not adopted in a no-kill (euthanasia only for medical problems or aggression). Interaction with a human for 15 minutes a week results in dogs that spend more time visible to the public and who wag their tails more often, which should increase adoptability.[1428]

Cats

General activity

In the laboratory, cats, like dogs, show short bursts of activity (1–2 hours of activity distributed throughout the day), and are 1.4 times more active during the day than at night.[1815] During the day, group-housed laboratory cats spend 36% of their time in maintenance behaviors such as resting, sitting, ingesting, or eliminating, and another 30% in comfort behaviors such as grooming and stretching. A quarter of their time is spent in motion.[1522] Caged cats in shelters spend 70% of their time in alert (easily disturbed) rest, 11% asleep, 14% sitting, and 6% active.[1068] Farm cats spend 40% of their time asleep, most of it at night. Although active at dusk and into the evening, cats are not really nocturnal. The rest of the farm cat's time is divided into 22% resting, 14% hunting (although this will vary from cat to cat), 15% grooming, 3% traveling, and 2% feeding.[1473] Urban cats are most frequently seen, and are presumably most active at night between dark and dawn.[218]

Sleep

Caged cats spend 10 hours per day sleeping. Slow wave sleep occupies 39% of the day and REM sleep, 8%. During REM sleep, the nictitating membrane covers the eye. SWS of cats, like that of dogs, can be subdivided into LSWS and DSWS, based on electroencephalographic characteristics and ease of arousal.[1912] The usual sequence of sleep stages in the cat is from wakefulness to LSWS to DSWS to REM to either LSWS again or to wakefulness. The two major sleep epochs occur at night. Drowsiness varies with feeding schedule. Cats fed three times a day drowse more than those fed once a day, and fasted cats drowse even less.[1655,1656] Older cats (>10 years of age) show less REM sleep and more SWS, as well as more brief episodes of wakefulness than do young cats.[267]

Elimination

Because house soiling is such a common behavior problem of cats, it is important to know how often they eliminate and the behaviors that surround the act of elimination. Cats eliminate 3–5 times a day. They spend 12 seconds digging before elimination, sniff the litter for 18 seconds, afterward especially if it is within their core area (where they spend 75% of their time), and cover for 12 seconds.[1830] House soiling cats dig less before eliminating, implicating litter qualities, such as odor or texture as factors discouraging cats from using the litter.[1830]

Pigs

Pigs, despite thousands of years of domestication, still forage optimally, that is, they obey the marginal value theorem and spend longer in each food patch when the cost of moving from patch to patch is higher.[729] Under the most modern conditions, pigs usually are kept in confinement so that the 7 hours of rooting (for example, food searching) noted on pasture[2060] fall to 2 hours per day of eating in a pen. If all oral, nasal, and facial activities are summed, sows housed outdoors spend 46 minutes of the 2-hour postfeeding period engaging in these behaviors in comparison to the 26 minutes spent in those ways by crated sows.[421] Sows living outdoors with access to shelters spend 25% of their time foraging and half their time outside, but newly farrowed sows spend 85% of their time in the shelters.[299]

The more hungry pigs are, the more time they spend rooting and the less time lying down. When kept in pens and supplied with peat in which to root, pigs still spend 10% of their time rooting, indicating that the behavior persists even when no food reward occurs.[1825] Hunger, too, may predispose to tail biting by increasing rooting time.[440] Increased time spent rooting results in decreased time spent manipulating penmates, a behavior that leads to aggression. The motivation for rooting can be hunger or curiosity (approaching novel stimuli) about the environment, which is the reciprocal of boredom (avoiding familiar stimuli). The ideal rooting material can be manipulated and destroyed like straw or peat.[1826] Frustration (that is, presence of inaccessible food) leads to changes in behavior. Oral activity is increased and the pigs are more likely to sit or lie on their sternums, and less likely to lie on their sides, which is the more relaxed position.[1131]

Pigs spend more time resting than do any other domestic animals.[783] They are recumbent 19 hours per day. They drowse 5 hours per day. Slow wave sleep occupies 6 hours per day; REM, 1.75 hours in 33 periods. Pigs are characterized by extreme muscle relaxation during sleep (see Fig. 3.6). Evaluating muscle tonus in a 400-pound sow is difficult, but when a sleeping piglet is picked up, it is as relaxed as a rag doll. Only 1–3 hours per day are spent in other activities, such as drinking, walking, playing, or fighting.[633] Domestic pigs are diurnal, and most activity takes place during the day.[1368] As do most diurnal species, pigs have higher melatonin levels during the scotopic, or dark phase, of the day; however, particularly bright light is necessary for entrainment.[717] Although motor activity and food intake increase during the day in pigs, these rhythms disappear in constant light, indicating that they are not circadian. Rhythms of body temperature depend on feeding, and do not occur in pigs fed ad libitum.[926] Pigs can entrain to 9 hours of light and 9 hours of dark, as well as to 12:12 cycles.[927]

Feral pigs and wild boars are more nocturnal in habit during the summer months, probably to avoid predation. Even wild pigs are not very active. Trapping and retrapping indicate that sows are usually found within 0.3 km (0.19 mi) of the point at which they are originally trapped; boars are within 2.0 km (1.24 mi).[1225] The sex difference may be in range rather than in activity.

Circadian rhythms are disrupted by changes in physical, social, or reproductive conditions. For example, putting a pig into a group after it has been housed individually, or tethering a pig, will disrupt circadian rhythms of cortisol for 1–4 days, as will surgery or estrus.[193]

Pigs defecate 4–7 times a day; the number decreases with body size. They urinate 3–5 times a day. When kept in partly slatted pens, pigs will lie on the slats when the temperature is warm and increase the number of defecations on the solid part, probably because there is little space on the slatted portion.[918]

To avoid stress and its detrimental effects on meat quality, animals are often placed in pens after transportation, and before slaughter. There are large differences among species in how rapidly they lie down. Swine lie down within an hour and cattle within 2 hours, although this will vary with the amount of space per animal and number of disturbances by people.[945,1025]

Horses

Horses may be able to drowse and even to engage in SWS while standing by means of the unique stay apparatus of the equine legs, but they lie down[740] when engaging in REM sleep. The horse in REM sleep lies either in lateral recumbency or in sternal recumbency with its muzzle touching the ground so that its head is supported during the atonia accompanying that phase. See Fig. 3.7 for lying and rising postures. A healthy horse seldom remains lying when it is approached, probably because a standing horse is better able to flee or to defend itself. A dominant stallion lies down first,[1651] that is, before subordinate horses lie down.

During the day, the horse is awake 88% of the time, and during most of this time, the animal is alert. Nighttime grazing also increases when days shorten. Both changes serve to keep grazing time, and therefore food intake, constant.[1168] Even at night, the horse is awake 71% of the time, but it drowses for 19% of the night.[1653] Stabled horses are recumbent 2 hours per day in 4–5 periods. Ponies are recumbent 5 hours per day, and donkeys even more.[1171] Slow wave

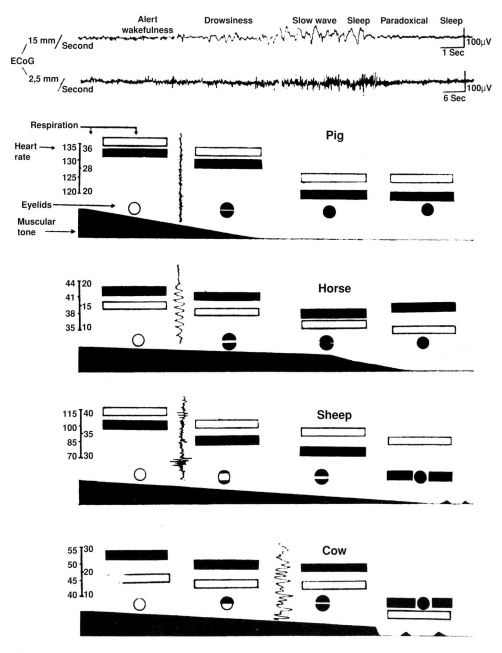

Fig. 3.6 (A) Physiological parameters of sleep in various species. The different electrocorticogram (EcoG) patterns for each species are shown at a speed of 15 mm per second: theta rhythm (horse), delta rhythm (ruminating cow), spincles (sheep), and alpha rhythm (pig).[1653]

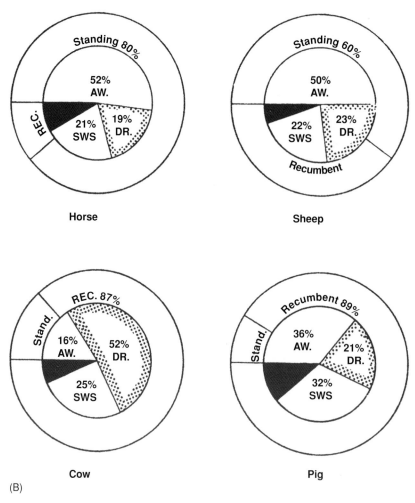

Fig. 3.6 (B) Mean comparative data of sleep and wakefulness states and of postures during nighttime. The inner circle shows the relative duration of the EcoG pattern (rapid eye movement, REM, in black) and the outer circle shows the relative duration of the postures. (Copyright 1972, with permission of Bailliere Tindall.)

sleep occupies 2 hours per day, and REM sleep occurs in nine 5-minute periods. Horses, in contrast to ruminants, show tachycardia, leg movements, and an increase in respiratory rate during REM sleep.[1653]

Management practices can affect equine sleep patterns. Previously stabled horses sleep less on pasture; they do not lie down during the first night, and total sleep time remains low for a month. Bedding affects how long horses lie; they lie longest on coconut husks, rarely on sawdust or coconut fiber and lie for an intermediate time on straw.[1419] Horse prefer bedding to no bedding.[907] Care must be taken not to deprive horses of sleep inadvertently. This is most apt to occur when horses are transported long distances or when they must be tied in straight stalls. If horses are tied short in a straight stall so that they cannot lie down, they may not have REM sleep. The horses compensate by sleeping while free during the day. Diet also affects the length of sleep in horses as it does in ruminants. An increase in lying occurs when the protein content

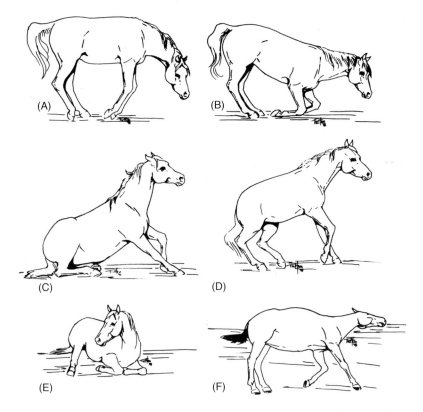

Fig. 3.7 The postures of the horse when lying down and getting up. (A,B) Lying down; (C,D) getting up; (E) sternal recumbency, the horse not lying symmetrically but with the lateral surface of one foreleg on the ground; (F) lateral recumbency, the upper foreleg anterior to the lower one. The horse exhibits rapid eye movement (REM) sleep in (F) or in (E) with the muzzle touching the ground.

of grasses increases in the spring;[500] a similar trend, an increase in lying, occurs when oats are substituted for hay. Fasting has the same effects.[422,423]

Ponies on pasture lie 7% of the night, 2% in lateral recumbency. Lying in lateral recumbency occurs almost always in the hours just after midnight. In stalls, the same ponies lie 12% of the time, probably in response to the drier stall environment. Horses can be seen lying in lateral recumbency during the day, usually after bad weather has kept them from lying down. Horses fitted with a urine collection harness lay down for only 0.5% of the time in contrast to control mares who lay down 3% of the time.[968] There has been controversy about the welfare of mares who must be tied while straddling a suspended urine collection devise, but the harness appears to affect the mares' behavior more.

Although horses lie, stand, and travel, their main activity is feeding. Feeding can be grazing or eating hay, if the hay is available free choice. Grazing time varies from 50% to 80% of the 24 hours taking place both day and night. The time of day when grazing takes place varies with the presence of biting insects. More time is spent grazing during the day in the winter when forage is scarcer (more steps between bites of food), and when biting insects do not drive the horses to refuge in snow, water, or barren areas.[502,994] Horses graze 15 minutes less for every extra hour of sunlight per day in the spring. Lactating mares graze more than barren or pregnant mares, reflecting the greater energy demands of milk production. Table 3.1 lists the

Table 3.1 Percentage time grazing by various populations of free-ranging feral horses.

Time of day (h)												Season	Population	Reference
0600	0800	1000	1200	1400	1600	1800	2000	2200	2400	0200	0400			
98	95	33	85	70	80	80	81	—	—	—	—	Winter	W. Alberta	2086
100	65	45	90	70	80	92	80	—	—	—	—	Summer	W. Alberta	2086
80	77	83	83	75	72	75	—	—	—	—	—	Summer	Assateague Is. MD-VA	993
—	—	—	—	—	—	—	63	53	53	40	70	Summer	Assateague Is. MD-VA	2087
					55–64[a]							Winter	Camargue, France	501
					51–60[a]							Summer	Camargue, France	501
					25–50[a]							Summer	Grand Canyon, CO	215
80	80	75	85	80	85	70	75	70	—	—	—	Winter	Shackleford Is. SC	2088
70	70	60	55	50	60	65	65	60	—	—	—	Summer	Shackleford Is. SC	2088

[a] Average percentage of time spent grazing over total time period.

percentage of time spent grazing by different populations of free-ranging or pastured horses and ponies. The circadian rhythms of most of our domestic animals are influenced by the provision of meals. This is especially true of herbivores, such as horses and ruminants, who normally would have access to grass at all times and whose hour-to-hour behavior would not depend on access to food. The large amount of time occupied by oral behavior indicates the reasons for the appearance of oral stereotypies, such as wood chewing and cribbing, in stalled horses on low-roughage diets (see Chapter 9).

Insects also affect equine time budgets and locations. They swish their tails 29 times an hour, skin twitch 11 times an hour, and shake their heads three times an hour. These behaviors are reduced on cool, windy, rainy days.[703]

The amount of traveling a horse does depends on two things: the availability of nutrients and the horse's social status. Young bachelor stallions travel more than harem stallions or mares, but otherwise, the distance that must be traveled to procure water or enough forage determines the amount of movement.[214] Isolated horses walk considerably more than those in sight of other horses. This type of walking, like that of the bachelor stallion, is presumably a search for companions. Camargue horses grazing on a large pasture walk 7–10% of the day, as do horses in a grassless corral.[501,872] Rapid traveling, that is, trotting and cantering, occupies a very small fraction, less than 1%, of the time budgets of adult horses studied in a variety of environments. Pasture or paddock design influences activity. Horses in rectangular paddocks make many more abrupt turns than those in square ones. The abrupt turns and stops can lead to leg injury.[1080] Horses do not spend as much time traveling at night as they do during the day. Ponies on lush pasture walk 3% of the night, whereas stalled horses and ponies walk less than 1% of the night.

Standing is the behavior that occurs when horses are not engaged in acquiring food, socializing, or sleeping deeply. Standing increases when feeding decreases (see Table 3.2 for time budgets of horses and ponies on a variety of diets, and Table 3.3 for time budgets of tethered horses) and when horses are satiated. Foraging in the bedding of the stall is a sign of hunger.[1421] Standing is also influenced by weather conditions in pastured horses. Horses stand rather than lie when it rains, and stand 20 minutes more per day for every Celsius degree drop in environmental temperature.[500]

Many riding horses are stalled most of the day and turned out in paddocks of varying sizes. The larger the paddock the more active the horse, but 45 minutes of exercise on an automatic walker decreases activity in all paddock sizes.[969] Horses turned out for only 2 hours per week trot, canter, and buck, but graze less than those turned out 12 hours per week.[343] Similarly, horses confined for 2 weeks are more active when released than those turned out daily.[874]

The time budget of a young horse depends on the housing. When first placed in individual stalls, 2-year-old horses eat less, are more often vigilant, but sleep more than pair housed horses. Although this difference in feeding and sleep disappears after two weeks in individual stalls, the individually housed horses continue to nibble walls and buckets, neigh, snort, and paw more than group housed horses.[1954]

Time budgets of Przewalski's horses have been recorded in various zoos, semireserves, and in the wild in Mongolia. At least three years after they were released into walking, which increased when the horses were released into the wild, and has persisted for the three years they have been living in the wild. The increased locomotion is most marked in the stallions.[270,271] The reason for this increase in walking may be increased vigilance. Seasonal differences appear, with horses grazing more at night in midsummer. Activity is lowest in the winter and highest in the late summer.[213] (see Table 3.4) In fact, during the Austrian winter, heart rate and body temperature of Przewalski horses drop, increasing again in May.[90]

Table 3.2 Time budgets of stabled horses and ponies.

| Time/Equid | Environment | Diet | Percentage of time | | | | | |
			Feeding	Standing	Moving	Drinking	Lying	Reference
Day/Horse	Metabolism cage	Limited Hay	50	45	0	1	4	2089
		Concentrates	32	62	0	1	5	2089
Day/Pony	Box stall	Ad libitum hay	76	19	3	2	1	1836
Day/Horse	Corral	Limited hay and grain	53	27	6	–	0	872
Night/Pony	Box stall	Limited hay and grain	15	17	1	–	13	907
Night/Horse	Box stall	Limited hay and grain	27	67	0.3	–	6	1740
24 h/Pony	Pen	Ad libitum grain	17	–	–	2	–	1099
24 h/Pony	Pen	Ad libitum pellets	31	–	–	–	–	2090

Table 3.3 Time budget of tethered horses.

Feeding	Standing	Stand resting	Lying	Drinking	Reference
50–58	19–22	20–24	1	2	2091
48	8	39	0	1	869
32	25		6.7		2092
36	58	19	6	1	2093

Table 3.4 Time budget of Przewalski horses.

Graze	Stand	Rest	Move	Environment	Reference
55	8	20	17	Free	271
54	12	24	8	Enclosure	271
51	20	13	13	Pasture	2094
48[a]	24	7	15	Yard	213
68[a]	18	0	12	Small pen	2095
44[a]	45	0	8.5	Large pen	2095

[a]Feeding.

Cattle

Cattle are essentially diurnal (day active). Their major activities are grazing, ruminating, and resting. Cattle lie down to sleep, to ruminate, or to drowse. Lying occupies nearly half the cow's day; when deprived of the opportunity to lie down, it will compensate by lying for longer periods when it is free to do so. This compensatory behavior indicates that rest is necessary. In fact, when both rest and food deprived, cattle lie down rather than eat when given the opportunity to do either.[1313] When limited in the time, they can spend feeding, lying, or in social interactions, cows prioritize lying, but may compensate for the decreased time spent feeding by eating more quickly so that caloric intake is not reduced in proportion to the decrease in time spent feeding.[1384] Many cattle are kept indoors now, and the amount of space can be limited. As space increases from 2.5 to 4 m²/animal, the time spent lying stretched out increases, and the number of times an animal steps on another decreases.[732]

Lying occupies 13 hours of a dairy cow's day in a loose housing environment, but this time will be reduced if the housing contains fewer cubicles than cows.[2023] Lying time is affected by the environment. Loose housed cattle spend less time lying than cattle in tie stalls, although their feeding times are similar.[1065] Stall design has a large influence on the ease with which the cow lies. If the number of free stalls is diminished, the cattle lie less and stand idle in the alley more, but still spend 5 hours per day eating.[842] Apparently, feeding is a protected behavior.

Milking frequency also affects resting patterns. Cattle milked three times a day have longer periods of lying and stand more easily than those milked twice a day, presumably because their udders are less engorged.[1455] Tethering reduces lying time and increases the time taken for cows to lie down in comparison with those that are box-stalled or pastured.[946] If dairy cows are confined in a small area, they lie less if the substrate is concrete or mud, and more if bedding is present. They compensate for the loss of recumbent time by lying when they next have access to pasture.

Space allowance or area affects activity patterns in calves. They eat and walk more in a larger pen, but ruminate and stand less.[1853]

Grazing

Most grazing takes place during the day.[101] Cattle on pasture spend anywhere from 5–8 hours grazing. Grazing time is inversely proportional to the quality of the pasture. Cattle on moderately good pasture spend 5 hours actually gathering food with their prehensile tongues and 2 hours walking.[964] As herbage is sparser, more walking between mouthfuls is necessary.

Grazing usually occurs in bouts, and is engaged in by the entire herd; social facilitation is strong in cattle. Two major grazing bouts take place, one just after sunrise and the other during late afternoon until sunset.[899] Midmorning and midafternoon are resting and idling times.[1964] Light may not affect grazing patterns immediately; a total solar eclipse shortens grazing times but does not affect rumination time.[1670]

By an hour after sunset, most cattle are lying down, although they will usually arise to graze during the night.[671] Night grazing may increase during warm weather, and may also increase as day length shortens. Both changes in behavior serve to keep grazing time, and therefore food intake, constant.[1720] Cattle drink 2–4 times a day during the summer on the range but only once a day or even every other day during the winter.[388] Grazing is covered in more detail in Chapter 8, "Ingestive Behavior: Food and Water Intake."

Distance traveled

The distance traveled by cattle or sheep can be measured by a rangemeter, a device that is similar to an odometer.[55,396] The distance covered by a grazing cow varies from 0.3–20 km/d (0.19–5.6 mi), depending on the size of the pasture or range and the abundance of forage. The longest distances are traveled by cattle foraging in a desert.[832] Beef cattle on range in Montana walk 3 km/d (1.9 mi) while spending 11–12 hours grazing per day at a bite rate of 50–60 per minute.[655] In rugged terrain, cattle create paths that involve the least effort—the shortest distance and the least hilly.[661] Dairy cows with free access to a pasture, a yard, and a barn travel 3 hours per day in summer but less than 1 hour per day in winter.[1066]

Housing conditions

Cattle live not only on the range but also in varying degrees of confinement. Dairy cattle are milked at least twice a day, and their grazing habits are organized around the milking schedule. The most intense grazing activity follows each milking. Two bouts occur after the afternoon milking, and one before the morning milking. A brief bout of rumination follows each grazing bout. A total of 5.5 hours during daylight are spent grazing, with an equal time being spent ruminating. In contrast, cattle in a loose-housing situation spend only half as much time eating and ruminating as do cattle on pasture. They spend 6–7 hours loafing, that is, standing while neither grazing nor ruminating, and they spend 12 hours resting. Time spent in walking decreases with the size of the idling area available to the cattle. Walking speed varies with the flooring type.

Cattle move more slowly on slatted concrete floors than on solid concrete or rubber floors and move most quickly with the longest stride on sand.[1858] When deprived of activity for as little as one day, cows will walk more when given the opportunity.[1936]

Cattle on feedlots are in a highly unnatural environment, as reflected in their activity patterns. Grazing bouts are replaced by 9–14 feeding periods, 70–80% of which occur during daylight hours. If hay and/or silage is fed, a total of 5 hours per day are spent eating, but the time decreases as the percentage of concentrates in the diet increases or if the roughage is ground.[1562]

Weather affects the time budget in that lying time decreases in cold wet weather.[588,698] This is particularly true for thin cows who are not as insulated by fat stores. Cows lie in different positions depending on the weather. They will fold their forelimbs under the body if the ground is cold or muddy and spend less time with their head touching the ground or their flank – the typical position for REM sleep.[1904] In hot climates, moving into the shade is another activity that appears to be a response to light rather than to temperature per se. Cattle should, of course, have access to shade, and shading behavior should be considered when management plans are made.

Elimination

Cattle defecate 7–15 times a day and urinate 5–13 times. The frequency of both excretory activities decreases in hot weather.[386] Rumination time also decreases under these conditions. When the environment is conducive, the cows are not confined; they will usually move away from their feces after deposition.[2009]

See Table 3.5 for activity patterns of cattle in different environments.

Sleep

The presence or absence of true sleep in ruminants has been controversial,[123,205,1310] but the extensive studies of Ruckebusch[1653,1654] indicate that cattle show both REM sleep and SWS. Rapid eye movement sleep occurs in 11 periods, so the total of 45 minutes of REM sleep and 3.5 hours of SWS are divided into many short naps. When cattle are in REM sleep, they usually are lying down with their heads resting on the ground and turned back into the flank. Cattle sniff the ground before lying down, and on arising, lick and scratch themselves. Cows in slings are sleep deprived, as are cows that have not yet adjusted to stanchioning or newly mixed groups of cattle. The stress of sleep deprivation should be considered by clinicians and stock managers. When kept in a corral at night, cattle, or Zebu cattle at least, tend to sleep in areas that remain constant for each individual from night to night. The resting places do not appear to depend on dominance.[1591] Most characteristic of ruminants are the extensive periods of drowsiness usually associated with rumination. Cattle are in a drowsy state 7.5 hours per day, divided into 25 periods that precede and follow sleep. Rumination and sleep are inversely related, so sleep time decreases with rumen development (see Chapter 6, "Development of Behavior") and decreases as the percentage of roughage in the diet increases.[123]

Environmental influences

Social changes can disrupt activity rhythms in ruminants as well as in pigs. For example, calves in a stable group show definite diurnal activity patterns; those in continually changing groups do not.[1047] Calves are affected by the lighting regime. They prefer a lighted area and spend more time lying there.[1988]

In summary, the normal bovine day depends on the diet , and on the housing conditions and in general, consists of alternating periods of eating and ruminating interspersed with resting or loafing and short periods of sleep (refer to Fig. 3.4). Activity patterns in cattle have been studied by other investigators in addition to those listed in Table 3.5.[599,751,760,1585,1744]

Table 3.5 Activity patterns of cattle in different environments.

Grazing (h)	Number of grazing bouts	Ruminating (h)	Lying (h)	Walking (h)	Standing (h)	Idling (h)	Type of cattle	Reference
								Cattle on pasture
5.5–7.5	6 (2 at night)	–	13	–	4	–	Dairy cows	101
5.5–10	–	–	–	–	–	–	Beef steers (Hereford)	2096
6.5	–	5.5	9.25	–	–	8.25	Dairy cows (shorthorn)	2097
8	5–7 (1 at night)	5.5	9.25	–	–	3.50	Dairy cows (shorthorn)	386
7–9	2	–	–	–	–	–	Beef cattle	2098*
7.25–7.5	4–5	4	–	–	–	2	Dairy calves	425
6	3	–	8.25	–	–	9	Beef cows (Charolais)	671
10–12	6 (1 at night)	8	–	–	–	4	Dairy cows	751
9	4 (1 at night)	8.5	9	–	15	6	Dairy cows (Holstein)	2099
7–8	–	4.5	5	0.25	3.25	–	Zebu cattle	760
9 (8–11)	2	–	–	–	2	–	Steers	2100
9–10	4	8	2	2–3	4	–	Beef cows (Hereford, Santa Gertrudis)	830
11.50	–	8.50	–	–	–	–	Dairy cows	2101
8	5	8	–	–	–	9	Beef steers (Hereford)	899
7–8	–	7	12	–	–	–	Beef cattle (Hereford)	964
11.50	5	7	–	1.25	–	5	Beef and dairy heifers	2102
7	2	7	–	–	–	–	Zebu and grade steers	2103
	4	–	–	–	–	–	Dairy cows (Brown Swiss)	2104

6–8	4–8	—	—	—	—	7–12	Steers	2105
10–10.5	—	—	9–11	—	2–3.5	—	Beef cattle (Hereford)	2106
9.5–12	3	—	10–14	—	1.25–4	—	Nonlactating cattle	2107
8–9.5	4	—	—	1.5	—	—	Dairy cows	1720
10	2	—	—	—	—	—	Beef cattle	2108[a]
—	3	6.25 (4.5–9.5)	—	1[a]	—	—	Beef cattle	1964
7 (5.5–8)	5	7	5	—	—	—	Dairy cows (Ayrshire)	2109
9	6	—	—	—	6	—	Beef steers (Hereford)	2110
							Cattle in confinement	
3–5	—	—	—	11	—	—	Dairy cows[b] (Holstein)	2111
4–5	—	—	—	8–11	—	—	Dairy cows[c] (Brown Swiss)	2112
3.5–5.25	9–12	7.5	9.5	6.5	14	1.25	Steers[d]	1562
3.5	4	—	—	12.25	—	6–7	Beef cows[d] (Hereford)	1693
3–4	—	—	10.5	—	8.5	—	Dairy cows[c] (Holstein)	2113
5	10	—	—	—	—	—	Dairy cows[d] (Ayrshire)	2114
6.25	18	—	—	—	—	—	Dairy cows[e] (Guernsey)	1985

[a]Daylight observation only.
[b]Free stall.
[c]Loose housing.
[d]Feedlot.
[e]Cowshed.

Table 3.6 Mean values of comparative data of sleep–wakefulness states and attitudes in four species of farm animals (three subjects of each species).

| Species and time period | Duration and Percentage | | | | | |
| | Wakefulness | | Sleep | | Attitude | |
	AW	DR	SWS	PS	Standing	Recumbent
Horse						
24-h period	19 h 13 min	1 h 55 min	2 h 05 min	47 min	22 h 01 min	1 h 59 min
	80.8%	8.0%	8.7%	3.3%	91.8%	8.2%
Nighttime (10 h)	5 h 14 min	1 h 54 min	2 h 05 min	47 min	8 h 01 min	1 h 59 min
	52.4%	19.0%	20.8%	7.8%	80.1%	19.9%
Cow						
24-h period	12 h 33 min	7 h 29 min	3 h 13 min	45 min	9 h 50 min	14 h 10 min
	52.3%	31.2%	13.3%	3.1%	40.9%	59.1%
Nighttime (12 h)	1 h 55 min	6 h 14 min	3 h 06 min	45 min	1 h 30 min	10 h 30 min
	16.0%	51.9%	25.8%	6.3%	12.5%	87.5%
Sheep						
24-h period	15 h 57 min	4 h 12 min	3 h 17 min	34 min	16 h 50 min	7 h 10 min
	66.5%	17.5%	13.6%	2.4%	70.1%	29.9%
Nighttime (12 h)	5 h 59 min	2 h 45 min	2 h 43 min	34 min	7 h 10 min	4 h 50 min
	49.8%	22.9%	22.5%	4.8%	59.7%	40.3%
Pig						
24-h period	11 h 07 min	5 h 04 min	6 h 04 min	1 h 45 min	5 h 10 min	18 h 50 min
	46.3%	21.1%	25.3%	7.3%	21.5%	78.5%
Nighttime (12 h)	4 h 23 min	2 h 30 min	3 h 52 min	1 h 15 min	1 h 20 min	10 h 40 min
	36.5%	20.8%	32.9%	10.5%	11.1%	88.9%

Source: [1653]

Sheep

Grazing and traveling

Until recently, sheep were seldom kept in confinement, so studies of their activities have dealt with range or pasture conditions (Table 3.6). Sheep on the range spend 50% of the daylight hours grazing,[388] of which 7 hours are spent grazing and 2 hours traveling.[477] On the range, sheep travel 6–14 km/d (4–9 mi), but they travel only 0.8 km/d (0.5 mi) on pasture.[395] Two factors determine how the range is used: familiarity with the area and social integration into the flock. Newly introduced animals may wander 14 km (9 mi), for example, when introduced to a new flock in an unfamiliar environment.[1976] On pasture, sheep spend 9–10 hours grazing in four periods, and they spend an equal amount of time ruminating in 15 bouts. Sheep allowed to graze only during daylight hours also spend 9 hours grazing,[216] similar to the time spent by sheep allowed 24 hours to graze. As has already been noted in the case of cattle, more time is spent grazing on a poor pasture (up to 12 hours per day), and twice as much distance traveled as on a good pasture. See Table 3.7 for sheep activity patterns.

Sheep, in particular, are synchronized in their behavior in that all or most of the sheep will be doing the same thing at the same time. Sheep may all begin to graze simultaneously, but much greater variation occurs in the end of a grazing bout. The satiety factors (discussed in Chapter 8) are more important in ending a meal, whereas the behavior of the other sheep is more important in starting it.[1622] Even on pasture, the type of feed can affect behavior patterns. For example,

Table 3.7   Activity patterns of sheep.

Grazing (h)	Number of grazing bouts	Ruminating (h)	Standing (h)	Lying (h)	Walking (h)	Reference
7	—	5.5[a]	—	—	2	477[b]
9–12	5	9–10.5	2.5	3.5	0.5	538
9	2	—	3.5	11.25	0.25	899
4–5.5	2	—	—	—	—	2115

[a]Includes idling and resting.
[b]Observed for 14.5 hours/day (daylight).

sheep grazing clover spend less time grazing and ruminating than do those grazing grass.[1491] Behavior is influenced by environmental temperature, and behavioral thermoregulation is, in turn, influenced by the animal's insulation. This is partially true in sheep who are sheared of their fleece rather than shedding gradually. This is reflected in their choice of substrate. Unshorn sheep in pens prefer expanded metal flooring, whereas newly shorn ones prefer solid floors.[755] Unsheared sheep spend 65% of their time lying, falling to 40% after shearing in winter, and only returning to preshearing levels after several weeks.[561]

Sleep

Sheep are awake for 16 hours per day. They drowse 4.5 hours per day, far less than cattle. Slow wave sleep occupies 3.5 hours per day, and REM sleep occurs in 7 periods for a total of 43 minutes.[1653] Sleep increases in sheep fed a low-roughage diet.[1359] While sleeping, sheep expend 10% less energy than while awake,[1897] so sleep deprivation would be expected to increase energy expenditure. Sheep will stand up 8–11 times during the night, usually to urinate or defecate.[538] Activity patterns in confined sheep have also been studied.[1969] In many colder climates, sheep must be confined during the winter. Because sheep choose to sleep against a natural or an artificial wall, it would seem logical that adding walls would increase testing time and encourage sheep to lie down in bedded area rather than on slatted floors, but a cross-shaped configuration increases aggression and cubicles increase time spent lying on the slats.[970]

The EEG, muscle relaxation, and other physiological parameters that accompany the various states of vigilance in farm animals are shown in Fig. 3.6A. The percentage of the night spent in sleep, wakefulness, and various sleep states and postures are shown in Fig. 3.6B. Comparative data for sleep and wakefulness in farm animals are given in Table 3.6.

Goats

Adults goats spend 41–47% of the time foraging, and kids spend 59–65%, depending on the stocking rate.[1555] Goats graze less and travel more when it is raining or when flies are abundant. These changes are more pronounced in shorn goats.[283] When food and water are available ad libitum, goats eat mostly at the beginning of the light phase, and at the beginning of the dark phase.[1642]

Feral goats on the Island of Rum spend their nights in caves. During the summer, there are two or three peaks in feeding interrupted by resting, but the percentage of time they spend feeding increases in the winter and their resting time decreases (See Fig. 3.8). Yearling spend more time feeding than adults or kids.[1748]

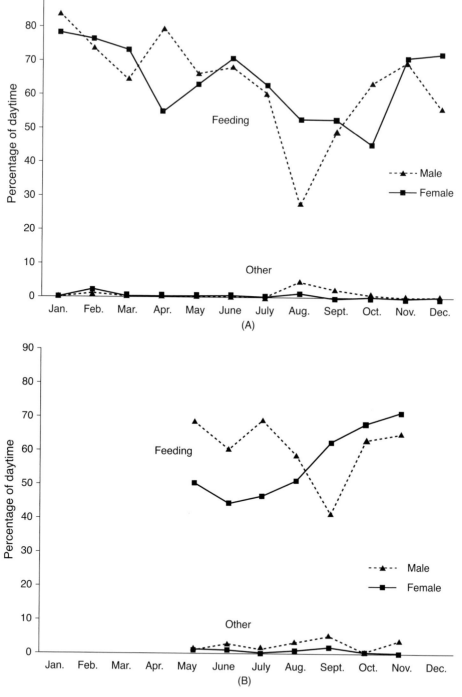

Fig. 3.8 Comparison of monthly variation in patterns of activity budgets of male and female adult goats on Rum in 1981 (A) and 2000 (B). Only the proportions of daytime spent feeding and in other activities are shown.[1748]

CLINICAL PROBLEMS

Human mental illness is often associated with disorganization of diurnal rhythms[1418], and with sleep disturbance.[1837] This has not been investigated in veterinary medicine, but owners of elderly dogs, in particular, complain that the animals are restless at night (see Chapter 6). The case of a cat that lacked the normal inhibition of movement during REM sleep, and was very active at that time has been reported.[826]

Hyperactivity

Hyperactivity is probably the behavior problem most frequently diagnosed by owners, and least frequently confirmed by the clinician. Most dogs that owners perceive as hyperactive are simply unruly. The owners usually have unconsciously rewarded the dog for hyperactivity by ignoring it when it is quiet and paying attention to it when it is rambunctious. For these dogs, even negative attention is preferable to no attention. The dogs usually are young dogs of working breeds. Although they actually may require more exercise than smaller breeds, they are more likely to cause more disruption when they are active than a little dog would. The running, jumping, and mouthing behavior may cause the owner to isolate the dog for long periods, which of course, leads it to be more excited when it sees people.

If the dog appears normal in the absence of the owner, then recommending more exercise, a canine companion (two or more owners could leave their dogs together so that extra dogs would not have to be acquired), and obedience training usually suffices to improve the dog's behavior. A specific behavioral exercise, "quiet training," is also recommended. The owner should pet and praise the dog or give a food reward whenever it is lying quietly. If it becomes hyperactive, the owner should either ignore or, if destruction of property is likely, isolate the dog, but only until the dog is heard to be resting quietly.

A few dogs are truly hyperactive. This condition can be diagnosed by measuring heart and respiratory rate, and activity of the dog, giving 0.5 mg/kg amphetamine, and then measuring the same parameters 30 and 60 minutes later.[1184] If the dog is truly hyperactive, the heart rate and respiratory rate will be lower after amphetamine. Dextroamphetamine 0.2–1.3 mg/kg or methylphenidate (Ritalin®) 5–20 mg per dog may be prescribed.

Narcolepsy

The number of clinical problems associated with sleep and circadian rhythm is small when compared with those associated with, for example, dominance and aggression. A syndrome involving sleep in dogs,[1344] cats,[1039] cattle,[1472,1820] and horses[609] is narcolepsy. Narcolepsy is characterized by attacks of inappropriate sleep. The affected dog will collapse and fall asleep for several seconds or minutes at a time. Play or food, especially very palatable food, often elicits the attacks. Interestingly, there are species and breed differences in the stimuli that elicit cataleptic attacks. Food is most apt to elicit catalepsy in dogs, but not in narcoleptic horses, which are most apt to collapse when petted or saddled. A familial occurrence of narcolepsy appears in miniature horses, in which the condition can be manifested at birth.[1186] Young dogs and Labradors are most apt to collapse when playing. Although Doberman pinschers are the breed most affected, Dachshunds and Labradors as well as poodles may also suffer from the syndrome. The best diagnostic test is to space small bits of food a foot or so apart, and time how long the dog takes to consume all the food and the number of times it collapses. The animal can be aroused with auditory stimuli. The drug imipramine reduces the severity and incidence of the attacks. In the Doberman pinscher breed, narcolepsy is inherited as an autosomal recessive gene[609] coding for the hypocretin receptor 2. Hypocretins are the major sleep-modulating neurotransmitters,[1153] and dogs lacking hypocretin are also narcoleptic.[1887]

Nocturnal wakefulness

Much more common than narcolepsy is the problem of dogs and cats that demand attention at night. In most cases, these are animals that are left alone during the day. The usual pattern is that the dog wakes the owner because it has a genuine need to eliminate. The dog learns after only a few nights that it can waken the owner and go for a walk or, at least, get some attention. Although sedation may be necessary in extreme cases, usually firmly enforcing a down stay command if the dog demands attention, combined with an increase in exercise and attention during the hours the owner is at home and awake, will solve the problem. Nighttime wakefulness usually accompanied by vocalization, and pacing is a common problem in old dogs (see Chapter 6).

The problem in cats occurs either in young cats that are seeking play or in cats subjected to a change in social or physical environment. More play in the evening will help to reduce nighttime, usually dawn, play periods in kittens. Free-choice food or a meal just before bedtime often is helpful, especially if the cat is crying for breakfast. Food in the bedroom is more effective because the cat may prefer to eat in the presence of the owner. Sometimes, punishing the cat with a water pistol suppresses the behavior, but cats often are able to avoid a stream of water, and still disturb the owner. Wrapping the cat in a blanket and restraining it for a moment is effective in some cases.

4 Sexual Behavior

Sexual behavior includes proceptive and receptive behavior by the female and courting and mate guarding by the male, as well as actual copulation. Tests have been developed to determine which bulls and rams will be successful breeders. A relationship exists between management practices, such as separation of the sexes at weaning, and later problems of homosexual or inadequate sexual behavior. Poor libido in breeding males and unwanted sexual behavior in castrated males are the most common behavior problems.

INTRODUCTION

Sexual behavior is important in all species of animals. The importance lies not only in maintaining adequate levels of libido in breeding animals but also in controlling the various aspects of sexual behavior that persist in neutered animals.

Mating systems have evolved within the framework of the morphological and physiological parameters of the individual species under continual ecological pressures. Although we have drastically reduced the nutritional, climatic, and health stresses to which domestic animals are exposed and have selected heavily for "good breeders," we still find remnants of this long-term evolutionary selection hindering our goal of high reproduction rates. Thus, we may continue to see problems that hinder breeding and production schedules, such as seasonal breeding in housed stock subjected to artificial control of photoperiodicity; poor libido in some of our artificial insemination (AI) programs, despite the absence of organic disease; and mate selection preferences that do not coincide with our ideas of desirable matings.

Physiological bases of sexual behavior

Adult male and female sexual behavior depends on a variety of factors for its expression: physiological, environmental, or psychological. These factors are (1) the genetic sex of the animal, (2) perinatal organizational action of hormones, (3) past social and sexual experience, (4) adult activational action of hormone and anatomical status, (5) the attractiveness of the potential mate, and (6) the external environment. Figure 4.1 illustrates the factors that affect sexual behavior, using the stallion as an example.

Domestic Animal Behavior for Veterinarians and Animal Scientists, *Fifth Edition* by Katherine Albro Houpt
© 2011 John Wiley & Sons, Inc.

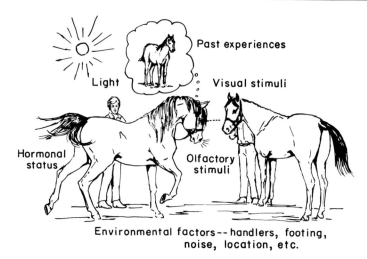

Fig. 4.1 Factors that affect sexual behavior.

Genetically determined sex

The sex of the animal is determined at the moment of conception, and the chromosomal sex will determine whether the indifferent fetal gonad develops into an ovary or a testis. Nevertheless, the potential for masculine and feminine behavior remains in both sexes. Studies on laboratory animals have revealed that the brain, and therefore, behavior is usually female unless the fetus is exposed to androgen during development. Similarly, without androgenic stimulation, the external genitalia will be female.

Organizational: perinatal hormonal influences

The role of sex hormones during ontogeny has been studied extensively in laboratory rodents and also in dogs. Male puppies have been castrated at birth and their behaviors are compared with that of intact dogs and dogs castrated as adults. Anatomically, these neonatally castrated dogs were altered in that their penes were very small. Despite this anatomical change, they still urinated in the masculine posture and were no different in their response to exogenous testosterone from dogs castrated as adults.[168] They were attracted to estrous females and mounted them; however, their underdeveloped external genitalia prohibited normal intromission. Both sexes have the genetic potential for male or female behavior, but neonatal androgens "defeminize" males, that is, make them less likely to show female sexual behavior. Therefore, as adults, when treated with estrogen, the neonatally castrated males show receptive behavior to other males.

Female puppies treated with androgens in utero and neonatally were markedly altered anatomically. They had no external vagina and did have small phalluses. They urinated in the masculine posture half the time. As adults, they were ovariectomized and treated with either female (estrogen and progesterone) or male (testosterone) hormones. The estrogen treatments revealed that the dogs had been defeminized; they would not stand or show any other signs of sexual receptivity. They were not even attracted to the male, as is a normal intact estrous female or an ovariectomized, estrogen-treated female. When treated with testosterone, the experimental dogs were obviously masculinized because they were attracted to, and would mount, other female dogs that were in heat. These studies indicate the powerful effects of perinatal androgens on the anatomy and behavior of animals of either genetic sex.[175–177]

Sheep and cattle are also defeminized by their neonatal androgens. The freemartin cow (born twin to a bull) is an example of a naturally occurring manipulation of the perinatal hormonal environment; as is described later in this chapter, these females exhibit masculinized behavior, although their external genitalia is not masculinized. Pigs appear to be unique in that they are defeminized not during the prenatal or neonatal period, but at puberty.[602]

Activational: adult hormonal status

The most important feature of the hormonal basis of sexual behavior is that hormones have a permissive role; that is, an animal requires a certain level of hormones for normal sexual behavior, but a higher level of hormones will not increase libido or receptivity. Hormonal treatment will not cure a deficiency of sexual behavior unless a deficiency of that hormone exists.

The complex relationships of the central nervous system, gonadal hormones, and behavior are discussed in more detail later in this chapter; in general, however, ovarian hormones result in an attraction to males and receptivity to male mounting. In some species (cats and pigs), the complete pattern of estrous behavior can be elicited by estrogen alone. In others (dogs and sheep),[179,219,1765] progesterone must also be administered. In ungulates, the behavioral action of estrogen is facilitated by a rapid preovulatory fall in progesterone, whereas in dogs, a rise in progesterone is important. Progesterone is administered before estrogen in the ewe and after estrogen in the bitch to induce estrous behavior.

Ovariectomy and castration. Ovariectomy (spaying) usually abolishes estrous behavior in females. Castration (orchiectomy) generally abolishes sexual behavior in males, but many exceptions exist. The more experienced the male, the longer sexual behavior, both arousal and copulation, will persist after castration. Prepubertal castration is, therefore, more effective than postpubertal castration in eliminating sexual behavior. Species differences appear in the effectiveness of prepubertal castration. Cats are affected more than dogs.[771,1105,1633,1634]

Anatomical factors. As mentioned previously, anatomical factors are important because a small penis precludes successful intromission. Intact afferent pathways from the penis are also necessary; experimental or traumatic neural damage to the penis results in misorientation in tomcats[92] and failure to ejaculate in bulls.[195] Similarly, desensitization of the vagina inhibits ovulation in the cat, an induced ovulator.[462]

The species differences in the structure of the penis are also important. For anatomical reasons, castration reduces the copulatory ability of male cats and horses more than it does for male ruminants and dogs. The muscular penis of the horse is more dependent on erection for successful intromission than is the fibroelastic penis of the ruminant. Similarly, the penile spines of the tomcat, which atrophy in the castrated male, are important for successful intromission and ejaculation as well as for induction of ovulation.

Social and sexual experience

It is much more common to observe animals that have been influenced by lack of adequate sexual experience than animals influenced by abnormal hormone levels. Male sexual behavior is affected by social influences. Having absolutely no social interactions, that is, being raised in isolation from weaning to adulthood, suppresses sexual behavior. The type of social interaction is important, but there are species differences. Rams raised in all-male groups from weaning to 1 year are less sexually active than those raised (or even given brief exposure) with females, whereas bulls, goats, and boars are independent of female exposure for normal behavior.[1544] Total lack of experience, homosexual experience only, too much sexual experience, or sexual experiences that are too unpleasant can all lead to sexual abnormalities.

Lack of socialization

The concept of critical or sensitive periods of development is discussed in Chapter 6, "Development of Behavior"; it should be emphasized here, however, that the most obvious effect of lack of socialization to conspecifics is on sexual behavior. Dogs raised without physical contact with other dogs from the age of 3 weeks showed normal libido toward estrous bitches but were very poor at orientation; they would mount improperly and seldom achieved intromission. This is probably an effect of lack of mounting experience because mounting forms a large part of male puppy play.[171] Similarly, boars raised in isolation from the time they were 3 weeks old showed very little sexual behavior.[820]

Within all-male groups, individuals may direct their sexual attentions to other males or be subordinate to other males. The dominant males may continue to mount males even in the presence of an estrous female; the subordinate animals often have little or no mounting experience. Some of these inappropriate responses will cease over time, but breeding efficiency is affected (at least temporarily).

Negative sexual experience

Unpleasant experiences during mating will have a deleterious effect on future sexual behavior, especially if the animal is young and has not had many (pleasant) experiences. The negative associations can be the result of overt aggression on the part of the sexual partner, rough handling by a stockperson, or an injury sustained during mating.

Effect on female sexual behavior

The effects of experience on sexual behavior have not been as thoroughly studied in females as in males. There may be less effect, in part because the female plays a less active role in mating in most management situations. Sows raised in isolation showed normal sexual behavior and were attracted to males when in heat.[1766] More research should be done on the effects of experience and age at weaning on female sexual behavior. Cats, in particular, may not be adequately socialized under normal rearing techniques and may reject toms, at least initially.

Attractiveness of potential mate

The element of attractiveness, or lack of it, of the sexual partner is not often considered, but higher mammals are influenced by this factor as well as by their hormonal levels. The attractivity of an estrous bitch's urine depends on her hormone state. If the donor of the urine is treated with estrogen, her urine becomes more attractive to males; if treated with testosterone, her urine is less attractive. Marking behavior of males is apparently an attempt to mask the attractiveness of bitch urine.[495,497]

Females may show individual preferences for one male over another. All females do not prefer the same male, indicating that the differences in attractiveness of males are based on the female's innate preferences and on past experience, rather than on some physiological characteristic of the male, such as pheromone release.

Male preferences can be based on physiological factors. For example, rams prefer ewes they have not bred before, as discussed later in this chapter. The action of ovarian hormones not only renders the female receptive but also increases her attractiveness, presumably by pheromonal release. Care must be taken when comparing the results of experiments on animals artificially brought into estrus with those involving females in natural estrus, because the latter may be more attractive than the former.

As do females, males also show individual mate preferences that are apparently psychological or idiosyncratic. An evolutionary basis may exist for some of these preferences. Males may prefer females that are similar, but not too similar, to themselves so that inbreeding will not occur and yet the same gene pool will be propagated.[164] Evidence for such behavior influencing sexual behavior of sheep,[794,1115] cats,[1137] and horses[995] has been found. The mechanisms and ramifications of mate selection are topics of considerable interest to researchers; extensive reviews of this work (primarily nondomestic species) may be found in Wilson[2032] as well as in Krebs and Davies.[1061]

External environment

The external environment is very important for optimal sexual behavior. Extremely inclement weather obviously will inhibit sexual behavior, but more subtle environmental factors, such as too many human spectators or a slippery floor, may also inhibit it. Not all additions to the environment are detrimental. In some cases, the presence of another male may stimulate sexual behavior. This has been well documented in cattle and goats.[238,1547] Males generally are more influenced by the environment than are females, so the female is usually brought to the male. Nevertheless, environmental factors in female sexual behavior deserve study. Time of day, for example, is important in cows, which show more signs of estrus at night. It is becoming clear that olfactory stimuli from the males, probably androgen-derived pheromones, affect sexual cycles in female ruminants.

The central nervous system and the control of sexual behavior

Females

Hypothalamic factors. In the female, gonadotropin releasing factor (GnRH) in the hypothalamus stimulates the release of follicle-stimulating hormone (FSH) and luteinizing hormone (LH) from the anterior pituitary. FSH induces follicular development, and FSH and LH together stimulate estrogen and progesterone production by the ovary. For most of the estrous cycle, estrogen and progesterone maintain low levels of LH and FSH through a negative feedback action on the hypothalamic–pituitary axis.

Near proestrus, however, the situation is reversed; rising estrogen levels have a positive feedback on LH secretion, resulting in the LH surge that causes ovulation. This preovulatory rise in estrogen is responsible for the hormonally based components of estrous behavior. The brain shows a refractory period during which biochemical changes presumably take place, which will result in estrous behavior.[1316]

Cyclical ovulation. In spontaneous ovulators (bitch, ewe, mare, and sow), the LH surge and, consequently, ovulation take place cyclically; but in induced ovulators, such as cats, external stimuli from the vagina either by natural coitus or artificial manipulation are necessary to trigger

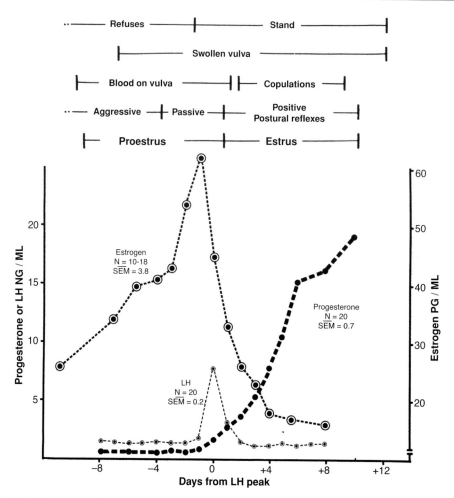

Fig. 4.2 Relationship of estrogen, progesterone, and LH levels to behavior in the bitch. Times of onset of behavior and physical signs represent means of a range of times.[377] (Copyright 1975, with permission of the Society for the Study of Reproduction.)

the LH surge. The relationship between hormone levels and sexual behavior in the bitch is shown in Fig. 4.2. The female's active solicitation of the male is called proceptive behavior.

The seasonal nature of reproductive behavior is also due to central neural variation in responsiveness to gonadal hormones. The same ewes had to be injected with a larger amount of estrogen to induce estrous behavior in the spring than was needed in the fall.

Olfactory influences and pheromones. Odors can have important effects on reproduction. This has been demonstrated in a variety of rodents, mice in particular.[287] In domestic animals, odor is probably not as important; nevertheless, the age at first puberty is lower in gilts exposed to a strange boar (continuous cohabitation with a boar will not produce the effect). Olfactory bulbectomy eliminates the effect, indicating that the odor is the important stimulus.[1030] Ewes show a similar response, called the ram effect, but odor may not be essential. Postpubertal cows show another response to odor; they will come into estrus sooner if exposed to the odor of estrous cow urine or mucus.[934] The best studied farm animal pheromone is the boar odor, which stimulates the estrous sow to assume the immobile, rigid posture that permits the boar to mount her and which can be used for estrus detection.

Males

Hypothalamic factors. The hypothalamic–pituitary axis is also involved in male sexual behavior. FSH is released in response to hypothalamic releasing factor. In the male, FSH stimulates spermatogenesis and LH testosterone release. Testosterone, in turn, acts upon the anterior hypothalamus–preoptic area in conjunction with appropriate stimuli from an estrous female to produce male sexual behavior. Inhibin, a testicular factor produced in the spermatic tubules, acts as a negative feedback on the hypothalamus.[1735]

Considerable evidence is accumulating that it is not testosterone itself, but rather a metabolite of testosterone, estradiol, that acts on the central nervous system to produce male sexual behavior. In general, estrogen and testosterone have similar actions in stimulating male sexual behavior in castrated animals, but an androgen that cannot be metabolized to estradiol, dihydrotestosterone, does not.[336,361] When freemartins are treated with estrogens and androgens, both hormones increase aggressiveness, mounting, and sniffing of the vulva of other cows, but only testosterone stimulates the flehmen response.[713] Testosterone itself, rather than a metabolite, may be responsible for this response (see Fig. 4.3). Dihydrotestosterone does stimulate

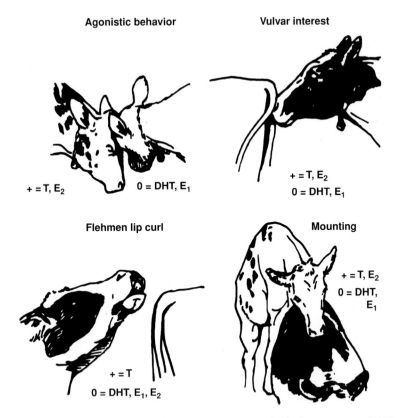

Fig. 4.3 Effects of testosterone (T), estradiol (E_2), estrone (E_1), and dihydrotestosterone (DHT) on agonistic behavior, vulvar interest, the flehmen response, and mounting.[713] (Copyright 1978, with permission of Academic Press.)

enlargement of the penis and of the sex glands, so when it is administered in combination with estradiol to castrated pigs, the full sequence of male sexual behavior, including intromission, occurs.[1479]

Stimulation of the brain by testosterone or its metabolites may facilitate appearance of male sexual behavior; it is the appearance of a female, however, that triggers the behavior. The stallion, for example, will exhibit the flehmen response and begin the courtship rituals of nibbling the crest and rump of the mare. At the same time, stimulation of the parasympathetic nervous system results in secretion of the accessory sex glands. The combination of penile stimulation after intromission and sympathetic stimulation leads to ejaculation.

Olfaction. Olfaction is, no doubt, important for identification of the estrous female; but elimination of the sense of smell by olfactory bulbectomy does not impair sexual performance of cats or rams, indicating that olfactory stimulation is not essential and that the male can identify the receptive female by visual or auditory means. The lack of resistance to his mounting attempts may be the most important information to the male.[93,776,1159]

Summary

In summary, hormones are important for normal sexual behavior, but the central nervous system can be relatively independent of them. This is indicated by the persistence of copulatory behavior in castrated male cats,[1633] dogs,[169] and rams[363] that had considerable precastration experience. Even prepubertal castration may not eliminate sexual behavior; one-third of prepubertally castrated bulls mounted cows.[597] A similar percentage of prepubertally castrated geldings showed sexual behavior.[1164] Apparently, after the brain is organized by androgens, external stimuli may be sufficient to trigger male sexual behavior.

CATTLE

The cow

The cow is a nonseasonal, continuously cycling breeder, but shows peak fertility from May to July and a low fertility from December to February. Puberty occurs anywhere from 4 to 24 months of age, usually at 6–18 months. The estrous cycle is 18–24 days long (mean, 21 days), although it is somewhat shorter in heifers and in the Bos taurus (Zebu) breeds.

Onset of estrus

Onset of estrus occurs more often in the evening and ceases in the morning. Actual sexual receptivity lasts 13–14 hours. The estrous cow shows a general increase in motor activity and a decrease in food intake[911] (Fig. 4.4). The more active a cow is, the higher her fertility.[2069] Investigative behavior such as flehmen, sniffing, rubbing, and licking increase as does premounting behavior such as standing behind the cow and resting the chin on the back of another, usually another estrous cow. She will bellow a great deal, switch her tail and raise or deviate it to one side, and urinate frequently. If a bull is available she will approach it.[1112] Estrogen levels peak when the cow stands to be mounted.[545,692] The cow that mounts is usually preovulatory. The mounting cows are also usually dominant over the mounted cows. This represents an interaction between hormonally mediated behavior and social influences.

Because visual cues are received over greater distances than olfactory cues, homosexual mounting may attract bulls who live apart from the cows (see Chapter 2, "Aggression and Social

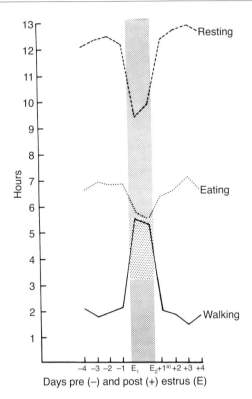

Fig. 4.4 Average composition of daily activities of cattle during estrous and nonestrous stages of the reproductive cycle.[911] (Copyright 1975, with permission of Department of Animal and Poultry Science, University of Guelph, Ontario, and Elsevier Science Publishers.)

Structure"). Furthermore, bulls choose cows who are mounting and being mounted in preference to those who are not.[678] Homosexual mounting in cows may have been selected for in dairy cattle because as long ago as medieval times, bulls were not routinely kept with cows, so only those cows that the owner noticed to be mounting were taken to a bull and bred.[121] Beef cows mount much less frequently than dairy cows, confirming this hypothesis.

The male effect, discussed in more detail later, is weaker in cattle than in sheep and goats. The presence of a bull hastens the onset of estrous cycles in postpartum beef cows but not in high-producing dairy cows.[1757] This is unfortunate because delay in return to estrous cyclicity means a delay in becoming pregnant, which in turn means a financial loss to the dairy farmer.

Aggressive behavior also increases markedly during estrus.[911] Cows mount cows both before and after the period in which bulls would mount[1021] (Fig. 4.5). Mounting behavior by cows may not occur if a bull is present.[1699] The intensity of estrus can be measured using frequency of sniffing the vulva of other cows, chin resting, and mounting of head or rear. The intensity of sexual behavior is not related to the dominance hierarchy.[1453] Severely lame cows display less intense estrus as well as lower progesterone levels, but the incidence of behavioral estrus is unaffected.[1965] Once a cow has been mated, she will no longer be receptive, but after an hour's rest she allows further copulation.[118]

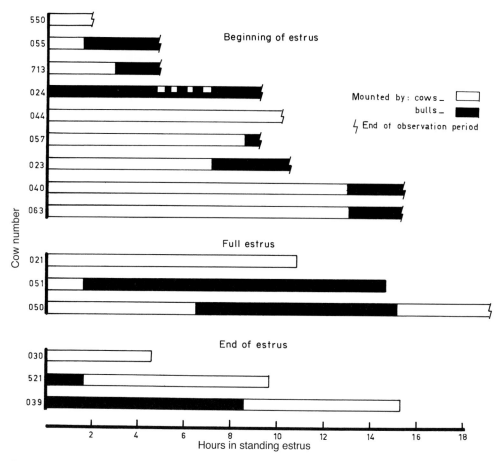

Fig. 4.5   Mounting of cows at different stages of estrus by cows and bulls.[1021]

Detection of estrus

Detection of estrus becomes more and more critical in the dairy industry as AI becomes more widespread (more than 90% of Holstein calves are conceived via AI). The physical signs of estrus, such as a copious vaginal secretion and vulvar relaxation, may be weak or absent. Estrous behavior may be less noticeable in housed cattle than in yarded or pastured ones.[1510] Footing can also affect a cow's willingness to mount.[1916] Traditionally, the bull is the best detector of estrus in the cow, with humans doing a poor to fair second. An estimated 19% of heats may be missed because behavioral signs are absent (silent heats) even though ovulation occurs, and an additional 15% are labeled as estrous periods even though ovulation does not occur (false heats). Some silent heats may have been behaviorally evident but were not observed by the herders. Pregnant cows—3–15%, depending on the criterion used to label a cow as estrous—may also show signs of estrus.[465,628]

Mounting behavior is used by the farmer to aid in heat detection, but it may not occur around the milking time or when the cows are usually observed. A commercial estrus detection device, which consists of a plastic vial containing a red dye, is glued to the dorsal tail base of a cow suspected to be in estrus. As she is mounted by other cows in the herd, the dye is gradually expressed into a viewing chamber; a full chamber supposedly is correlated with a sufficient number of mountings to indicate a full estrus.[2031] Several cows may be in heat simultaneously and one may not be mounted, so even the mechanical heat detector can give misleading false negatives.[1393] Pedometers are used to determine estrus because the cow is more active then (see Fig. 4.4), but the pedometers must be read several times a day to be accurate. Observation of chin resting and mounting are still the best indicators and correlate with estrogen levels.[1189]

A vasectomized bull or teaser bull with a surgically deviated penis may also be used to detect heat. The danger of keeping an unpredictably aggressive bull in close contact with people, however, has discouraged this practice. A freemartin heifer may be used satisfactorily. Fetal exposure to the androgens produced by the male fetus masculinizes the nervous system of freemartins; they are infertile and thus of little value as dairy animals. Freemartins are even more likely than the other cows in the herd to mount an estrous cow, and treatment with injectable androgens may heighten this behavior even further. Dogs have been trained to detect estrous cows, an interesting innovation presumably based on canine olfactory acuity.[1011] The dogs were 80–90% correct in detecting estrous cows.

Clinical problems of cows

Silent heats, a phenomenon to which heifers are especially subject, have already been discussed.

Nymphomania is more common in high-production dairy cows than in beef breeds. The cow shows intense estrous behavior either persistently or at frequent, irregular intervals. Herd milk production drops noticeably because these cows are often the best producers in the herd. Most commonly, the affected cow is 4–6 years old and has calved two to three times. Unlike a cow in normal estrus, however, the nymphomaniac does not stand for other cows. She actively seeks out other cows and mounts them. She paws and bellows like a bull and with time also becomes more male-like in voice and body conformation. Nymphomania is usually associated with follicular cysts, and treatment is sometimes successful using a source of LH, such as pituitary extract or chorionic gonadotropin.[1611]

The bull

In contrast to rams, bulls' sexual performance is not improved by raising them with females or exposing them to females at the time of puberty.[261,1551] Rearing bulls in individual pens does suppress sexual performance.[1552] Bulls can be trained to avoid a cow in estrus using electrical shock. Residual seasonality occurs in bulls as in cows. LH treatment results in higher testosterone levels if administered during the summer rather than during shorter days.[960] Bovine male courtship behavior is becoming an unobserved rarity in modern dairy farming with the advent and spread of AI. Bulls are now selected for (among other things) their willingness and ability to mount dummy cows, other bulls, or steers and to ejaculate into an artificial vagina. One might wonder how this willingness to leave behavioral interactions with the opposite sex up to random genetic drift eventually will affect the species. The courtship sequence is actually a series of reciprocal interactions between male and female. The female behavior has already been described.

Courtship behavior

Starting late in the cow's proestrus, the bull will begin to graze beside the cow, guarding her from any other cattle. His attempts to mount will be repulsed by the cow. During proestrus,

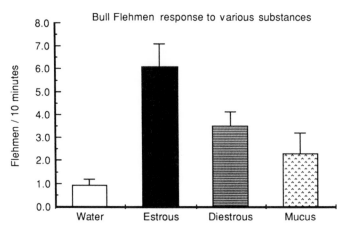

Fig. 4.6 The mean (±SEM) response of bulls to estrous and nonestrous urine, mucus, and water.[882] (Copyright 1989, with permission of Butterworth Publishers.)

most females are attractive to the male and attracted to him but not yet receptive. The bull may attempt to herd the cow away from rest of the herd.

Periodically, the bull will smell and lick the cow's vulva, often followed by the flehmen response (Fig. 4.6). Some, but not all, dairy bulls flehmen to estrous urine, and they do so more often than to mucus or to nonestrous urine.[882] Flehmen is followed by an increase in LH.[1187]

As estrus approaches, guarding becomes more marked as both other bulls and nonestrous cows are kept away. When the cow is in full estrus, the bull will have a partial erection while guarding her, and accessory gland fluid or precoital discharge will drip from the penis.[1006] The bull frequently nudges the female's flanks and either maintains head-to-head contact or, because of mutual genital sniffing and licking, stands in a reverse parallel (bigeminal) position with the cow. This position is common to the courtship sequence of all ungulates. The bull may rest his head across the cow's back while they stand in a T-position.[628] He makes several mounting attempts with a partial erection before the female will stand for him. When she is ready, the cow remains immobile and the bull mounts immediately. He fixes his forelegs just cranial to the pelvis of the female as he straddles her. Ejaculation occurs within seconds of intromission and is noted by a marked, generalized muscular contraction (Fig. 4.7). The bull's rear legs may be brought off the ground during this spasm. Dismounting and retraction of the penis follow rapidly. When bulls are used for hand breeding or for AI, lack of the stimulatory effects of the prolonged courtship may result in poor semen quality or poor reproductive behavior.

Sensory stimuli

Experimental manipulations have shown that a variety of sensory stimuli are needed to elicit male sexual behavior. Tape recordings of cows will sexually stimulate a bull,[446] but these sounds are probably of a nonspecific arousal nature. Bulls used for AI apparently become classically conditioned (see Chapter 7, "Learning") to the sounds in the collection arena, and these may help stimulate these animals. The stimulation of sexual behavior caused by a new female is called the Coolidge effect. The Coolidge effect occurs in bulls so that the mounts with intromission and decreased mounting intervals occur when a novel female is provided hourly. There is also more flehmen. Alternating two females has an intermediate effect.[118]

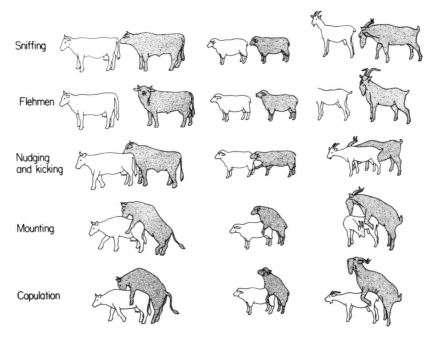

Fig. 4.7   Sexual patterns in cattle, sheep, and goats.[737] (Copyright 1974, with permission of Lea & Febiger.)

Olfactory cues seem to be used by the bull during early estrus to monitor the stage of the reproductive cycle of the cow; however, no studies have been able to show sexual excitation caused by olfactory stimuli alone. Although volatile compounds have been isolated from estrous urine, these compounds do not elicit interest from bulls. Urine from a bull used as a teaser did elicit flehmen and other signs of interest, but none of these olfactory stimuli affected sexual performance of dairy bulls in an AI center.[1538]

Visual deprivation seems to hinder sexual response generally, but most markedly when the blinded individual is presented with a female in a novel situation.[741] The inverted U-shape seems to be the visual stimulus most likely to stimulate sexual behavior, whether this be in the form of a standing cow, a dummy, or an unfortunate person bending over. Without special conditioning, a wild bovid will mount only an estrous conspecific female. One of the aims of domestication has been to obtain "easy" breeders, that is, bulls that respond to a less specific series of stimuli than those offered by a female and that do so with little sexual foreplay.

Sexual responsiveness is influenced by the range of stimuli to which the male is exposed during ontogeny. Free-ranging or wild bovids gradually restrict their sexual behavior to interactions with females. Bulls not exposed to females do not establish this more narrowed range of sexual stimuli; hence, the ability of some rather bizarre stimuli to instigate mounting and ejaculation. Dairy bulls are also rarely raised with females and so can be stimulated by other bulls.

Malnutrition rarely affects sexual performance, as evidenced by the continued reproductive success of starving cattle in parts of Asia and Africa. This phenomenon has been experimentally demonstrated by Wierzbowski,[2021] who found that underfed bulls actually were quicker to copulate than well-fed bulls.

Experiential factors

Individual bulls show marked differences in their levels of sexual behavior as measured by such parameters as mounts or ejaculation, the number of ejaculations per unit time, the latency to ejaculation, the number of ejaculations required for satiation, and the length of time to recover from postsatiation refractoriness. It seems unwise, therefore, to continue breeding a male that shows limited interest in mounting females, because doing so will only perpetuate the defect. Early experience and management, in addition to genetic factors, are important determinants of sexual behavior. For instance, Zebu bulls raised in small groups had a faster reaction time (time to the first mount) than did those raised on the range in large herds.[1197]

Serving-capacity tests

Blockey[237–239] has developed a procedure for testing serving capacity (libido and copulation competence) in potential beef cattle sires whereby several bulls are tested for 20 minutes with heifers restrained in stanchions. The relative performance in this short test is well correlated with sexual performance in a 19-day pasture breeding test. Because dominance hierarchies are not strong in bulls under 2 years of age, they do not fight in the group breeding situation, but they can interfere with one another.[664]

Hereford bulls will consistently mount females by 9 months of age, but are a year or older before they ejaculate. Therefore, Hereford bulls should not be given serving capacity tests before they are 18 months old, when their ejaculation frequency peaks.[1549] The sex ratio in serving-capacity tests should be 1:1, and breeds that differ in aggressivity (Hereford and Angus) should not be tested together.[1550]

Problems can arise with short-term tests of libido. A high environmental temperature can reduce libido, and the effect may not be the same in all the bulls, so one who normally has high libido may be more affected than one with low libido.[349] Other problems are that bulls are more responsive to preovulatory than to postovulatory cows,[664] so cows should be at that stage.

Clinical problems of bulls

Masturbation. Although commonly noted among bulls, masturbation causes no known reproductive problem. In general, masturbation is frowned upon on an anthropomorphic basis. Sperm quality or counts do not seem correlated with the frequency of this "vice." The bull performs pelvic thrusts, with his back arched, with a partially erect penis. Thus, the penis moves in and out of the preputial sheath until ejaculation occurs. All bulls masturbate, especially at times of inactivity.[884] As shown in the following sections, all domestic animals have been observed to masturbate, and so it would be difficult to label this an abnormal behavior. See Fig. 4.8 for patterns of masturbation in dairy bulls.

Impotence. Loss of libido must be approached as a clinical problem with a rather large differential diagnosis in mind. The problem may be secondary to almost any other organic disease. Bulls used for AI seem especially susceptible to musculoskeletal diseases, rendering them lame and unable or unwilling to mount. Obesity may be considered a pathological condition, and it caused many problems in the early development of the AI program. Obese bulls were difficult or impossible to arouse. Now the diets of bulls are more closely controlled; however, obesity should still be considered in assessing a case of loss of libido. Balanoposthitis or injury to the penis are specific conditions of the genital urinary tract that might be confused with a libido problem.[1611] Testicular atrophy involving both the Leydig cells and the seminiferous tubules

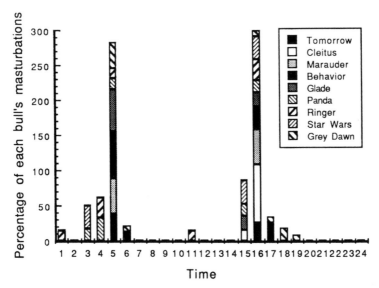

Fig. 4.8   The occurrence of masturbation by time of day. The masturbations observed are plotted by the hour of the day in which they occurred as the percentage of each bull's masturbations. Some bulls were observed longer than others, so it was necessary to use percentages rather than absolute numbers of masturbations.[884] (Copyright 1989, Elsevier Science Publishers.)

may occur and be recognized by the reduced size and soft consistency of the testis. This is one case in which androgen administration might be expected to lead to a return of normal sexual behavior. A sperm count is recommended, however, because a hypospermatic animal will still be an unsuitable breeder.

Management practices may influence male libido. A large bull may be unwilling to mount a teaser steer or a cow in an icy corral or on wet concrete floors. One or two slips may be sufficient to condition him to ignore the stimulus of the teaser. Distractions of other animals or human observers should be kept to a minimum; such distractions may present more of a problem for some bulls than others. By 2.5 years of age, most bulls are dominant over cows; before this age, a dominant cow may prevent a young bull from mounting. Restraint of the cow may be of value. Young bulls also lack experience, and their tentative approach while courting may stimulate aggression in a cow. If AI is not possible, and a proposed breeding is between animals far enough apart that one must be transported to the other, bringing the cow to the bull is advisable. Males seem more sensitive to environmental factors; a new or different surrounding may trigger a reluctance to mount. Fortunately, trucking a cow is usually easier than trucking a large, aggressive bull.

For reasons that must be classified as psychological, a bull trained to mount another male and ejaculate into an artificial vagina eventually may lose interest and refuse to mount, especially if he has been used too frequently. This inhibition may be overcome by changing the sexual stimulus to a new steer or bull. A new teaser, preferably a cow and even better an estrous cow, or a moderate change in the environment or location of the mating arena, may be sufficient to stimulate sexual behavior, but because of the risk of disease, cows are not allowed at AI centers. Other bulls are found to be more attractive teasers than steers. Although psychological in its origin, the Coolidge effect has a physiological limit. The maximum number of ejaculations will be the same as that obtained by electroejaculation.

Restraining the bull from the teaser or allowing him to watch another bull being collected also may arouse a previously disinterested male.[238,1006,1203] A caution regarding the latter technique must be made: A submissive or young bull allowed to observe an animal dominant to him may be further conditioned against servicing through intimidation. In most ungulate species, copulations are restricted to the dominant males. The lack of sexual activity in the remainder of the male population has been termed psychological castration, although the effect is usually and quickly reversed if the dominant individual is eliminated.

The buller steer. Although most problems of sexual behavior in food-producing animals are those of insufficiency, manifestation of sexual behavior in steers is also a problem. Approximately 3% of feedlot steers are buller steers that are mounted by other steers. Steers are implanted with various types of anabolic steroids, usually in combination; these include estrogen, progesterone, testosterone, trenbolone, or zeranol. Stilbestrol appears to stimulate bulling least.[62,229] Bulling occurs more often in steers that are implanted with stilbestrol or estrogen, but the level of hormone actually may be lower in the buller's plasma than it is in that of normal steers. The greater the number of steers, the larger the percentage of bullers. There is a large component of dominance-related aggression in the buller syndrome. Penile erection and anal intromission rarely occur. More aggressive animals mount and the rate of mounting increases dramatically when new steers are added.[1032] The syndrome is seen most frequently when groups of animals are mixed, especially in crowded conditions and in warm weather. The economic losses resulting from the syndrome are due to the increased activity of the mounting steers and the harassment of the buller steer. None of the animals will gain weight as they should.[932] The usual means of treating bulling behavior is to remove the steers involved; other solutions including metal buller rails under which the steer can hide, electrified wire placed above the pens so that a steer that reared to mount would be shocked, avoiding conflicts over food and water, and painting odiferous substances on the buller can be used to reduce the incidence of the behavior.[1004]

SHEEP

The ewe

Estrous cycle

Sheep are short-light breeders, that is, they usually cycle in the fall of the year as the light phase of the photoperiod decreases. The ewe is polyestrous and will cycle several times during one breeding season if not bred; the average cycle for the ewe is 16 days (range14–20). The actual period of estrous receptivity is 30–36 hours in the ewe. The duration of estrus in lambs and in the first estrus of the season is shorter than that of the normal estrus. Puberty is dependent on the time of birth. Females born early enough in the year will cycle their first fall season, indicating that puberty may occur as early as 4 months of age. Progesterone is necessary for estrous behavior, so the first ovulation of a ewe lamb is a "silent heat".[560] Other environmental influences affect the estrous cycle of sheep. Domestic sheep raised in the tropics and subtropics are non-seasonal breeders;[903] as with many other life forms in these areas, reproductive activity occurs all year.

Feral sheep display an even shorter breeding season than most of the domestic breeds, and it is likely that both predation pressures and the necessity of foraging over large areas for limited resources established estrous synchrony as an evolutionary stable strategy in the ancestral forms.

In feral sheep, the adult rams form a flock separate from that of the ewes and lambs and join the females only during the breeding season. Flocking tendencies are strong in sheep, and a ewe lambing after the remainder of the flock would be unable to keep up with the movements of the flock.

The ram effect. Most sheep breeding is still done naturally, with the rams pastured with the ewes all year or introduced in the late summer. The introduction of a ram, when the ewes have not been with one tends to synchronize estrus in a high proportion of the ewes 15–17 days later. The mechanism is through LH, a pulse of which is released within minutes of exposure to a ram. If contact with the male is maintained, a preovulatory surge of LH at around 36 hours occurs, accompanied by a rise in FSH. Ovulation occurs, but no estrous behavior (silent heat). Sexual behavior with subsequent ovulation appears 18 or 25 days after introduction of the ram. The ram effect occurs only in sexually experienced ewes. Continuous exposure to a ram tends to increase the incidence of estrus in the normally anestrous period.[1603] The presence of a ram also shortens the duration of estrus, but this depends on direct physical contact with the ram and probably on mounting of the ewe by the ram, rather than on pheromones.[1480] Rams that court more vigorously cause more ewes to ovulate than do less sexually active rams.[1496]

Estradiol-treated wethers can stimulate estrus in anestrous ewes, indicating that testosterone must be aromatized to produce the ram effect. The pheromone is present in the wool, wax, and anti-orbital gland secretion of the ram.[1040] The pheromone probably consists of more than one component.[365] Notice that in sheep, the odor of wool rather than of urine, which is so important in rodents, appears to be involved in both sexual and maternal recognition. There is some effect across species. Although ram wool does not stimulate resumption of cyclic behavior in does, buck hair increases LH levels and thus induces ovulation in ewes.[1458] Farm animals do not appear to be completely dependent on odor, however; for example, the ram effect can occur even in ewes without the sense of smell.[366]

Anosmic ewes exhibit the ram effect in response to a ram, but not to its fleece. Olfactory cues—the main olfactory not the vomeronasal organ—are not necessary, but they may be sufficient to stimulate estrus, because the synchronization of the first estrus of the breeding season in sheep can occur in the absence of direct contact or visual cues.[32] Synchronization of estrus is a desirable property of the ewe cycle for management purposes, because breeding may be accomplished in a short time and the lamb crop will be born synchronously and tend to reach market size simultaneously.

Synchronization may also be accomplished by using progesterone compounds, and this procedure is used more as the practice of AI in sheep increases. Estrus occurs 48 hours after withdrawal of vaginal progesterone sponges.[1885] Synchronization is more successful using these compounds if a male is added to the flock before the ewes come into estrus (120 hours) than if it is present only for the 48 hours after withdrawal of progesterone.[1616]

Courtship behavior

The estrous ewe can be identified because she follows or seeks out a ram, turns her head as the ram approaches, may circle, sniff the male's body and genitals and then thrust her head against his flanks, fans or wags her tail, and stands to be mounted. Estrous ewes will choose a ram on a two-choice test and will do so even on the basis of a photograph.[998,1875] She may call frequently with nonspecific bleats and be more active.[297] Standing occurs when the female is receptive, and she will look over her shoulder at the ram as he investigates and nudges her. Like cows, most ewes are in standing estrus at night.

The active role of the ewe in seeking the ram was demonstrated in an experiment in which two-thirds of a flock of ewes were inseminated even though the rams were tethered.[1157,1163] The ewes apparently use olfactory cues to locate the ram because anosmic ewes were unable to find tethered rams.[595] Even when a ram and ewe are both free, ewes initiate half of the contacts between the sexes.[1451] Ewes can be attracted to a male in the next field or to an infertile male, so ram seeking does not guarantee pregnancy. Ram-seeking behavior seems correlated with estrogen levels[1160] but does not occur without the visual and olfactory stimuli of the male.

Competition involving agonistic behavior has been observed between estrous ewes over access to a ram. Older ewes are generally more successful in gaining access to the ram; otherwise, experience does not seem to be an important factor in ewe sexual behavior, but maiden ewes should be kept in separate flocks from experienced ewes or the latter will out-compete the former for the ram's attention.[1191]

The ram

Sexual behavior of free-ranging sheep

The sexual behavior of the primitive and free-ranging Soay sheep may give some clue as to the optimal manner of raising breeding rams. Ram lambs remain with their dams from late spring when they are born until the following fall when they begin to chase ewes. They will be rejected by most adult ewes until they are larger. Meanwhile, the adult rams have been living in separate, all-male flocks on separate feeding sites. Before the ewes are in estrus, the rams begin to move toward the ewe flocks. They will chase away strange rams but remain on friendly terms with their own flock mates. As the season progresses, however, they will begin to fight with one another. The fights consist of head clashings in these horned sheep and nudging behavior similar to that seen in courtship. All this takes place before the ewes are receptive, although young rams will have harassed the ewes already. When the ewes come into heat, the sexual contests between the males have been settled and the males can turn their attention to breeding. The winner of the most contests between males breeds the most ewes, but he does so sequentially by tending each ewe for a day, or at least half a day, grazing with her and performing the courtship activities described earlier in this chapter for domestic sheep.[721] The rams graze and rest less while courting and fighting, and they may lose weight. These observations indicate that the best way to rear breeding rams would be to leave them with females for as long as possible, certainly until puberty, and then put them in an all-male group.

Domestic sheep

The reproductive capacity of the ram is not seasonally limited as is that of the ewe. Estrous ewes may be satisfactorily fertilized at any season, although semen quality may decline somewhat during the spring.[1493,1494] Thus, the breeding season in domestic breeds is primarily determined by the environmental input to the female's hypothalamic–hypophyseal tract. Although the ewe may seek out the ram, courtship is more elaborate in the male than in the female.

Courtship behavior

Rams need not have exposure to females as young lambs to have normal sexual behavior, but they should have exposure during adolescence. As does the female, the male spends a great

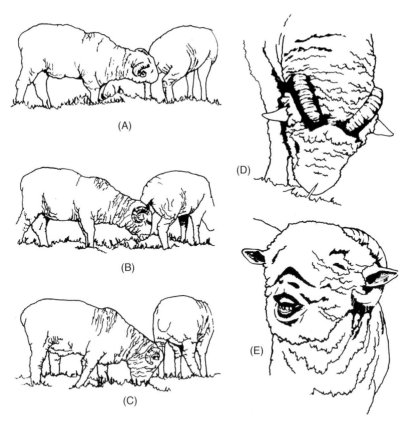

Fig. 4.9 Response of the ram to urine of an estrous ewe. (A) Urination by ewe, (B–D) ram nosing urine on the ground, and (E) the Flehmen response.[145] (Copyright 1964, with permission of E.J. Brill.)

deal of time sniffing the other's genitalia and urine; the flehmen response may be noted (see Fig. 4.9). As stated previously, the flehmen response has no visual communicative properties but may be a method of introducing material into the vomeronasal organ. Rams flehmen less frequently when ewes are in estros apparently because estrous ewes urinate less.[233] Urination appears to be a sign that the ewe is not in estros. The male may also lick the female's genitalia, a form of tactile stimulation that may also be part of the testing procedure. Normally, rams can discriminate estrous from nonestrous ewe urine using olfaction.[236] Bulbectomized (no olfactory bulb) rams in a range situation show some difficulty in identifying estrous females; they are nonselective in the ewes they approach and test but are able to identify estrous ewes, presumably via visual and auditory cues.[1159] In fact, confined rams may not use any sensory cue to detect estrus; they may rely entirely on the willingness of the ewe to stand. When given a choice of restrained ovariectomized ewes, rams sniffed, nudged, mounted, and copulated with ewes with equal frequency whether or not they had received estrogen; all had received progesterone.[1765]

Perception via the vomeronasal organ is important in that intact rams mount and ejaculate more than those with blocked vomeronasal organs.[1910] Ewes do differ in their sexual attractiveness to rams. This attractiveness is stable from estrus to estrus and depends, at least in part, on wool. Wooly ewes are preferred to shorn ones, indicating that wool and/or wax is an important

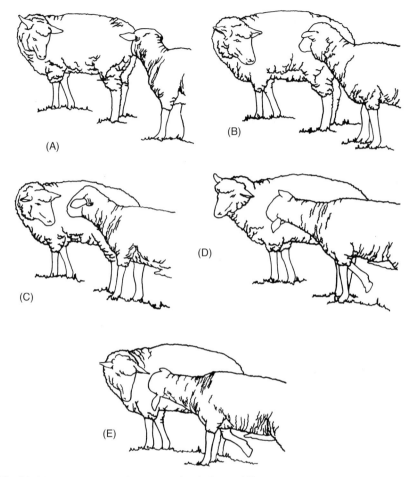

Fig. 4.10 Nudging sequence in sheep courtship behavior.[145] (Copyright 1964, with permission of E.J. Brill.)

source of attractivity.[1874] The attractiveness of estrous ewes for rams depends, in part on the bacterial flora present in their vagina. The bacteria may react with pheromones or themselves contribute to attractivity.[1911]

A ritualized kicking with a foreleg is performed as the ram orients himself behind the ewe; the leg is raised and lowered in a stiff-legged striking manner (see Fig. 4.10). Tongue flicking accompanies the nudging. Nudging is also stereotyped: The head is tilted and lowered while the shoulder is brought into contact with or oriented toward the flank of the ewe; simultaneously, the ram utters low-pitched vocalizations or gargling or courting grunts. Six nudgings of the ewe per minute are observed at the peak of the ram's sexual interest.[1864] Several abortive mounts may be made with pelvic thrusting but without intromission. When the tip of the glans penis contacts the vulvar mucosa, a strong pelvic thrust accomplishes intromission and ejaculation occurs immediately. After dismount, the ram may sniff the ewe's vulva, appear depressed, and stand near the female with head down; he may urinate.

The latency to ejaculation increases with the number of observed ejaculations during an observation period, but it is subject to large individual variation. The number of ejaculations that occur when a ram is presented with a large number of estrous ewes is similar to the number that occurs in response to an electroejaculator, indicating that physical capability rather than libido is limiting. Males show a reluctance to remate a recently mated female, whether or not the test ram was the male who inseminated her originally.

If rams are mated to sexual exhaustion with one ewe (usually three to six matings),[906] rapid recovery may be obtained by introducing a new ewe, whereas a much poorer recovery rate is obtained by removing and reintroducing the original ewe.[180] This effect of novelty already has been described here as the Coolidge effect. Another method of demonstrating this phenomenon is to present four receptive ewes to a ram; he mates three times as much as he does when only one ewe is in estrus.[32] There is some evidence that habituation to a sexual partner may last several weeks after a mating as measured by the degree of recovery in the sex drive following satiation. These effects make evolutionary sense to the species and are fortunate for the rancher. A ram is capable of something less than 20 ejaculations daily. If many of these copulations were repeat breedings to especially persistent ewes, the fertility rate for the herd probably would be low. This breeding efficiency allows a rancher to introduce only a few rams to service a flock. Ewes can produce lambs sired by different rams.[560] In wild or feral sheep, a dominant male can spread his genes over a much larger proportion of the population than if the mechanisms for reduced repeat breedings by either himself or subordinate males did not exist.

Serving-capacity tests. One serving-capacity test, which is predictive of the lambs sired, is to place a ram with three restrained estrous ewes and record mounts and ejaculations. The test is repeated nine times. To test for mate preference, the ram is observed with restrained rams and two restrained estrous females. When released with ewes, low sexual performance rams sired as many lambs as the female oriented rams, but the high sexual performance ram sired nearly twice as many.[1807] Rams do not discriminate between ewes in natural estrous and ovariectomized ewes treated with progesterone and estrogen,[1539] so either may be used for serving capacity tests. Rams show similar rates of ejaculation and mounting whether ewes are restrained or free to move in a pen; however, if copulation is prevented (by covering the perineum), there are many more mountings and foreleg kicks as well as buttings.[1541] Foreleg kicking and sniffing the anogenital area of the ewe are considered courtship behavior, whereas attempts to mount, mounting, and ejaculation are considered copulatory behavior. The courtship behaviors are a good measure of libido because when copulation or mounting is prohibited, males sniff and nudge more if they have higher serving capacity (that is, ejaculations).[1543]

Prenatal effect

The intrauterine environment influences subsequent ram sexual behavior. Rams born co-twin to a ram have a higher serving capacity than those born co-twin to a ewe. The larger the litter size, the higher the serving capacity of its male members.[591]

Rearing effects

It seems to be important for lambs to have heterosexual experience in the period between weaning and their first birthday in order for them to prefer ewes to rams as sexual partners. Ram lambs at 6 months will begin to exhibit adult sexual behavior sooner if they are exposed to estrous ewes for as little as 30 minutes per day for 4 days. By 8 months, exposure to estrous ewes does not result in an earlier onset of adult sexual behavior. This is important because the young ram lambs could be used for breeding before they are a year old. In addition to the immediate effects of exposure to females, delayed effects can occur. Exposure to estrous ewes for several hours at 10 months of age enhances sexual performance at 2 years in rams that were otherwise kept in all-male groups.[1544]

Dominance effect

When more than one ram is being used to service a flock, dominance effects may influence the percentage of the flock each ram inseminates. Mature rams may dominate younger rams and almost always will dominate yearling rams. Dominance orders, as determined by the number of butts each animal delivers when the animals are confined together, also exist and may be more marked between yearling rams. Rank in a food competition hierarchy corresponds to rank in the sexual hierarchy.[610] In a confined ewe flock, a dominant ram may copulate 12–15 times daily over the breeding season, whereas the subordinate ram(s) may average only two to five copulations daily.[902] The subordinate rams may service ewes, but this occurs mostly at times when pregnancy is not likely to result, that is, long after ovulation. In a feral population or a multi-ram pasture-breeding situation, a number of rams may copulate with a ewe. The ram who copulates between the ninth and fifteenth hour of estrus is most likely to sire the lambs because that is when the ewe is most fertile.[958] In less confined conditions, the monopolization of mating by the dominant ram may be restricted only to the harem of ewes he is able to hold.[1234]

Hulet[902] suggests using uniform age groups and allowing adequate space when groups of rams are to be used together in a mass-mating system. Three rams per 100 ewes or 20–50 ewes per ram has been suggested for a range-breeding situation. It is unwise to use a pair of rams to breed a group of ewes because agonistic activity may take precedence over mating behavior. Lindsay and Robinson[1162, 1163] showed that three rams served 50% more ewes than a single ram over a 4-day period. It is unfortunate that dominance or sexual aggressiveness does not necessarily correlate with fertility; the combination of dominance with infertility in a flock ram could be disastrous to a rancher.

In pen breeding, a teaser, or vasectomized, ram is used to mark ewes by means of a harness and crayon attached to his brisket. A ewe that is in estrus will be mounted and, therefore, marked.[1158] The marked ewes are then added to the breeding ram's pen. Problems can arise if the breeding ram is submissive to rams in nearby pens. He may be inhibited and not mount. Another problem is seen when young and mature ewes are added simultaneously. Rams prefer or are monopolized by the older ewes. For most effective pen breeding, ewes should be checked for heat at 12-hour intervals and the breeding rams should be free of disturbance from rams or ewes in adjacent pens.[1022]

The effects of the presence of the ram on the reproductive status of the ewe already have been discussed here. The ram is influenced in his turn by the presence of the ewe. Testosterone levels, testis size, and levels of aggressive behavior are all higher in rams in pens next to ewes than in isolated rams,[920] and rams thus stimulated show more sexual behavior when they have access to ewes.[1626] Rams, like ewes, prefer mates of their own or their dam's breed.[1008]

The effects of castration in prepubertal rams are extremely variable;[145] there may be some decline in, or the complete elimination of, sexual activity. Postpubertal castration causes decreased sexual activity in rams,[32] but erection and intromission may persist for years postoperatively, albeit with a marked decrease in frequency.

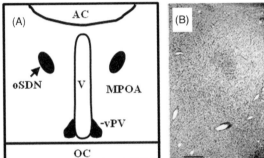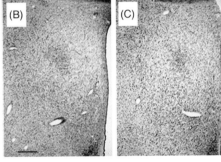

Fig. 4.11 (A) Schematic diagram of a coronal section through the sheep at the level of the optic chiasm (OC) and anterior commissure (AC). The position of the oSDN is shown bilateral to the third ventricle (V) in the central part of the medial preoptic nucleus (MPOA). The ventral paraventricular nucleus (vPV) is shown at the base of the ventricle. (B) Micrograph of oSDN from the left hypothalamus of a female-oriented ram. The third ventricle is at the right of the figure. (C) Section of a male-oriented ram comparable to that in (B). The photomicrographs are taken near the midpoint of the anterior–posterior extent of the oSDN. The scale bar is 1 mm. (Copyright 2009 with permission of Hormones and Behavior.)[1629]

Clinical problems of rams

Rams are often reared in large monosexual groups or individually, and Zenchak and Anderson[2082] have shown that the isolated males show some aberrations in behavior when first exposed to estrous females but most are eventually able to mate. The previously isolated rams were more proficient than rams raised in all-male groups.[295] Some of the rams raised in monosexual groups are sexually inhibited or show homosexual preferences and do so for long periods or permanently after maturity. In one study, after 9 days' exposure to estrous ewes, some rams (17%) still had not copulated.[905,1545] Continuous exposure to ewes eventually stimulates sexual behavior in most rams. About 6–8% of rams are male oriented. Even those rams who do eventually mate estrous ewes after several exposures continue to exhibit subnormal sexual performance, that is, they are not "cured."[1540] The frequency of mounting in an all-male group cannot be used to predict sexual behavior in a mixed-sex group. Homosexual rams have fewer estradiol receptors in the amygdala[24] and may have lower blood levels of estrone and estradiol.[1517] Aromatase activity, which converts testosterone to estradiol in the brain, is lower in male-oriented rams.[1628] There is a sexually dimorphic nucleus in the ovine brain and it is larger in female-oriented (heterosexual) than male-oriented (homosexual) rams (Fig. 4.11). These results indicate that male-oriented rams have not been masculinized completely.

Zenchak and Anderson[2082] argue that some individuals in the male groups learn to associate courtship and mounting activities with agonistic behavior, but the physiological data indicate an earlier neurological cause. It seems reasonable, nevertheless, to suggest not raising rams in monosexual groups in order to avoid sexual inhibition or the development of homosexual preferences. Mixed groups are probably ideal, with isolated rearing less preferable but acceptable.[988] Fence-line contact (separate sexes in adjacent pastures) only partially improves sexual performance of rams, and only those that are attracted to ewes on the other side of the fence exhibit normal male sexual behavior.[1540] The sexual performance is reflected endocrinologically. High-performing rams exhibit an increase in LH when allowed fence-line contact with ewes but do not respond hormonally to rams, whereas in low-performing or male-oriented rams, no change in LH occurred regardless of the sex of the animal on the other side of the fence.[25]

GOATS

Free-ranging goats

During the rut, feral bucks join female groups and fight for access to the estrous does. The most successful goats are 5–6 years old. Older males select groups in which they are more likely to be successful, that is, groups with few other males, whereas young males select the groups with the largest number of does.[498]

A detailed study of feral goats indicated that does permitted large, horned bucks to mount, but small, hornless goats were virtually excluded from breeding. When pursuing a doe, the buck would gobble, a sound produced by moaning and rapidly thrusting his tongue in and out. Courtship activity would cease when the buck exhibited the flehmen response to a nonestrous doe's urine. Although large males were usually able to chase off rivals, occasionally many males would mount a female in quick succession without regard to their position in the dominance hierarchy.[1738]

The doe

Goats, like sheep, are short-day breeders. Does in estrus show an increase in tail wagging, vocalization, urination, and mounting of other females. This is probably proceptive behavior in that it does not occur as frequently if males are in the same enclosure. Does are in estrus for 39 hours once every 20–21 days. There is a male effect in goats as well as sheep. Contact with bucks induces in anestrous goats an immediate increase of LH followed by ovulation. The bucks must be sexually active, that is, exposed to a light regime simulating fall, but they need be present only part of the day.[1608] In contrast to ewes, a large proportion of does exhibit sexual behavior with the first ovulation.[560]

The buck

Collias[372] noted the close relationship between agonistic and sexual behaviors in male goats. In general, billy goat or buck behavior is similar to ram behavior, kicking at the doe with the front legs and stretching his neck toward her and emitting the gobbling vocalization. The buck holds his tail straight up during courtship. A component of the mating sequence unique to the goat is the urination by bucks on their own forelegs and beards during courtship. This behavior is termed enurination. Occasionally, mouthing of the penis also occurs. Although various functions have been attributed to enurination, including increasing the intensity of the buck's odor and advertising his nutritional fitness, the behavior occurs most frequently in a situation of sexual frustration when the buck is restrained from mating. See Fig. 4.7 for normal caprine sexual behavior. Observation of does mounting one another or copulation by a male and female[1743] stimulates ejaculation sooner and with more frequency.

Goats reared in a group of males from the time of birth have fewer agonistic interactions with other bucks at puberty. The dominant goats initiate homosexual behavior toward the subordinate ones. Homosexual behavior does not interfere with their ability to ejaculate into an artificial vagina in response to the stimulation of an estrous female.[1452]

When semen is to be collected from bucks, their libido, as measured by the number of mounts before ejaculation and latency to ejaculate a second time, was better if they had a choice of two females, whether or not the second female was mounted. Postpubertal castration causes a decline in sexual behavior in goats, but wethers may still be sexually active, mounting half as many does as do intact bucks.[777,1883]

Clinical problems

The doe

Silent heat. The first ovulation of the season is often a silent heat.[224,344]

The buck

In contrast to sheep, bucks are unlikely to exhibit substandard sexual performance if denied heterosexual experience in their first year.[1542] Not all goats that mount homosexually in an all-male group will fail to mount heterosexually; those that do probably have a strong preference for one partner who happens to be male. The bucks that are mounted by other males are less apt to restrict their sexual activity to males. White bucks appear to be mounted more often than colored ones, which may be a function of the calm disposition of white Saanen goats rather than of coat color preference by the mounters.[1545]

HORSES

Free-ranging horses

Courting behavior

Free-ranging mares will often seek out a stallion during estrus and display the normal behavioral signs of estrus in front of him.[574,1909] It is unusual for free-ranging 2-year-old mares to breed (1%) and even uncommon for 3-year-olds to breed (13%).[1909] Stallions generally do not exhibit much interest in the sexual displays of young mares. Yearling mares may show very exaggerated signs of estrus and may attract males from bachelor herds. It has not been established whether the yearlings are in true or psychic estrus (see "Clinical Problems") because it has been most often observed in free-ranging horses. It is rare, but not unknown, for 2-year-old feral mares to deliver a foal, indicating that they can conceive as yearlings. It is hypothesized that the exaggerated signs of estrus in young mares may be a means of attracting stallions from a distance (that is, unrelated stallions). Incest is unusual in free-ranging bands; mares leave the band when sexually mature, are "stolen" by a stallion forming a new harem, or have their herd stallion replaced by a young stallion. Those that remain in their sire's herd have a much lower foaling rate than those who join an unrelated male's herd. Those who join a half-brother herd have an intermediate rate.[995] Stallions base their avoidance of incest on familiarity rather than on kin recognition.[214]

Free-ranging stallions rarely acquire a harem until they are five or 6 years old. The years between the time they leave their natal herd at age two and acquire their own mares are spent in bachelor herds. The stallion is the sire of foals born in his band in 85% of the cases. In the other cases, the mare has been bred by bachelor stallions or the stallion of another band.[986] In multimale bands, the dominant horse sires most of the foals as determined by electrophoresis of foal and stallion blood proteins. Dominant mares have dominant colts who sire more foals than do the offspring of subordinate mares.[570]

The mare

Estrous cycle

Mares show the opposite seasonality in estrous pattern to that of sheep and goats; that is, they are long-day breeders and cycle in the spring. Foaling season is late winter and early spring, and the 11- to 11.5-month gestation period has dictated a rapid recycling and rebreeding if foals are to be born to coincide with the spring grasses. Most free-ranging horses are probably bred on the first, or at latest the second, heat after foaling.[1909] If breeding does not take place, estrus recurs approximately every 21–24 days. The average length of receptivity is 5–7 days, longer than most ungulates. Breed differences in the length of estrus in different localities have been noted but are of uncertain significance, owing to the probable interplay of genetic and environmental factors, methods of testing for the presence of estrus, and statistical analysis.[1974]

Modern management usually isolates the stallion from the mares. Teaser animals are used to determine the receptivity of the mare. The teasers are usually stallions that are introduced to a mare across some form of barrier; the mare is restrained and sometimes hobbled. A nonreceptive mare will react to the teaser's advances by squealing, striking, kicking, and moving away. During full estrus, the mare indicates receptivity by her immobility and by permitting the teaser to nibble her rump and withers. The mare exhibits a characteristic breeding expression in which her ears are turned backward but not flattened and her lips are held loosely (refer to Fig. 1.6, in Chapter 1). She adopts a basewide squatting stance, urinates frequently, and rhythmically exposes the clitoris with a series of labial muscle contractions known as winking[97, 105] (Fig. 4.12A). Rectal palpation or ultrasonography may be helpful to ensure that follicular development coincides with the behavioral aspects of estrus. The optimal breeding time is usually the second or third day of estrus. In a pasture situation with 10–20 mares per stallion, a mare will mate six times in an estrous period.[401]

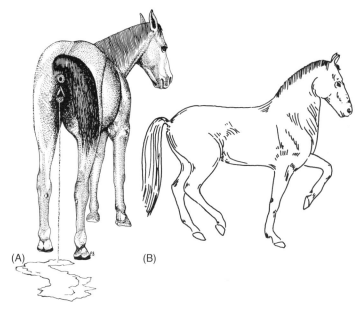

(A)   (B)

Fig. 4.12 (A) The posture of the estrous mare. The clitoris is everted and the tail deviated. (B) The prance, or piaffe, of the courting stallion.[867]

Mares show individual preferences for stallions, and the preferences are influenced by the stallion's vocal behavior. The more the stallion neighs, the more likely the mare is to approach him.[1514] The importance of vocal stimulation is demonstrated by playing a recording of a courting stallion's vocalizations and/or manipulating the mare's genitalia.[1242,1934] This makes it possible to detect behavioral estrus in the absence of a stallion. Exposure to male odor, a procedure that is effective in sows, elicits the signs of estrus in only half of the mares tested. Mounting of mares by other mares occurs, but rarely. The mounting mares are usually in the follicular phase and have a higher plasma testosterone.[672]

Foal heat

Foal heat following parturition is quite predictable, occurring usually 9 days (range 5–18 days) after foaling. Regular estrous cycles usually continue thereafter at approximately 21–22-day intervals, although a few mares appear to have a lactational diestrus due to maintenance of the corpus luteum following the foaling heat. Other mares are cycling but do not show estrous behavior in the presence of a stallion. Instead, the mares protect their foals. Habituation to the stallion might result in normal estrous behavior. Many mares are bred on the foal heat because it is predictable and easily detected and planned for, although the endometrial epithelium is rarely restored or complete at foaling heat and usually does not accomplish restoration until 13–25 days following the heat. The 30-day heat following foaling is a safer time to breed; a higher conception rate occurs.

Clinical problems of mares

Most of the sexual problems of mares occur at either end of the breeding season. Mares are seasonal breeders that come into estrus as daylight increases. Feral horses in the United States have a restricted breeding season. The foals are born in early summer and the mares are bred on foal heat. No doubt, if all domestic mares were pasture bred during the late spring and summer, they would be increasing in number at the same rate as the wild horses. Mares normally are anestrus from October to February; however, mares can and do show estrus and conceive all year around, especially if artificial light is used to simulate long days and the mares are well fed and well sheltered. Despite our ability to manipulate the equine reproductive cycle, seasonality is expressed in the large numbers of abnormal heats observed in mares.

Split and prolonged estrus. It is at the transitional periods, the beginning and end of the breeding season, that such sexual abnormalities as prolonged estrus and split estrus are usually seen. The length of estrus can be prolonged 5–7 days to up to 90 days. This may be accompanied by aggressive behavior. Other mares may show split estrus. Split estrus may consist of 1–2 days of "shallow" estrus in which the mare does not react to the stallion with vigorous squatting, tail deviation, and urination, but rather tolerates him and occasionally exhibits signs of estrus. A few days later, she may show strong signs of sexual receptivity. Both prolonged estrus and split estrus may be accompanied by active ovaries in which follicles are present but do not mature. In the fall, follicles may remain on the ovaries rather than regress, and this condition may be accompanied by complete anestrus or abnormal estrus. Mares that have either prolonged estrus or split estrus may begin to have normal cycles as the breeding season progresses and daylight length increases.

Anestrus. One of the most common reproductive problems of mares is anestrus. Mares may be either physiologically or behaviorally anestrous. The former includes mares with persistent corpora lutea and those with inactive ovaries. Older mares may have inactive ovaries due to degenerative changes in the endometrium and/or degenerative changes in the ovary itself. There may be senile changes in the ovaries, including the formation of germinal inclusion cysts. The age at onset of these senile changes varies from the mid-teens to well into the twenties.

A developmental cause of anestrus in mares is hypoplasia of the gonads and the reproductive tract. This condition, which is relatively rare, is similar to Turner's syndrome in humans because it is associated with an XO rather than the normal XX pair of sex chromosomes.

Although most pregnant mares do not show estrous behavior,[96] a few may. Hayes and Ginther[793] have shown that mares that show estrus while pregnant are carrying female foals. The sexual behavior is most likely to occur between 30 and 40 days of pregnancy, when accessory follicles are formed. The behavior of the pregnant mare can be distinguished from that of the nonpregnant estrous mare by the rapid tail lashing or wringing of the former as compared with the deviated tail of the latter. The pregnant mare will not usually stand for the stallion; she is not truly receptive. Her urine will be clear rather than cloudy, as is that of the estrous mare.

The common sexual behavior problems of mares are silent heat, psychic estrus, and excessive sexual behavior.

Silent heat. Behavioral anestrus is also known as silent heat. Palpation of the ovaries may reveal normal follicles. Ovulation will take place normally. There is physiological, but not behavioral, estrus because the mare will not accept the stallion. One reason for silent heat may be related to the fact that mares do show mate preferences. These preferences should be considered in teasing a mare in silent heat. More than one stallion should be used. Environmental factors can influence the behavior of the mare just as they influence the behavior of the stallion. A mare may not show estrus if she has just been trailered to a strange stud farm or handled by a strange person. If the mare does not show signs of estrus even in a familiar environment and with exposure to several stallions, she may still conceive if she is artificially inseminated or tranquilized, restrained, and forcibly mated by the stallion.

Psychic heat. Not all sexual abnormalities of mares are caused by a deficiency of sexual behavior; some result from an excess of sexual behavior. Some mares, for example, show estrous behavior without the normal physiological correlates of estrus. This abnormality is known as psychic heat. It may occur when any horse is brought into the environment of a solitary mare. In that case, it is usually a relatively short-lived phenomenon. Much more serious is psychic heat of performing mares. A mare that stops frequently to urinate and is attracted to stallions, geldings, or mares will not be a good competitive trail horse or show ring performer. Despite posture and behavior, the mare in psychic heat may not tolerate mounting by a stallion. Before psychic estrus is diagnosed, a painful condition of the pelvic area must be ruled out. Squealing and urinating accompanied by tail lashing is aggression, not estrus. A careful examination may reveal lower genital tract lesions.

Progestins such as altrenogest (0.02 mL/kg orally) or progesterone (0.4 mg/kg i.m. daily) have been used successfully to treat mares that show severe psychic heat. The progestins are believed to act on those neurons in the brain, probably in the hypothalamus, that control sexual behavior. Ovariectomy may be performed to treat psychic estrus or estrus related poor performance, but about 30% of spayed mares show constant estrus. If psychic estrus persists in an ovariectomized mare, dexamethasone may be used in an attempt to suppress endogenous adrenal steroids that might be inducing estrous behavior, but serious side effects can occur.

Excessive sexual behavior. Two pathological conditions of the ovaries can cause excessive sexual behavior in the mare. The abnormalities are granulosa cell tumors and persistent follicles. These conditions should be differentiated because one, granulosa cell tumor, should be treated surgically; the other, persistent follicles, usually resolves itself. The excessive estrous-like behavior of mares with persistent follicles is sometimes called nymphomania. The cysts will regress in time and do not need to be manipulated as follicular cysts of cows do. The persistent follicles may also be treated with gonadotropins, LH, or an increase in artificial day length to 16 hours or more.

Mares suffering from granulosa cell tumor can show a variety of signs. About 20% will show continuous estrus and 25% anestrus. About 40% of granulosa cell tumors also contain thecal cells that produce testosterone.[420] The affected mares will show stallion-like behavior, aggression, flehmen, urine marking (they straddle the urine of another horse as a stallion would, but their urine will be deposited behind rather than on the target), arched neck threats, mounting mares, and other symptoms. The affected ovary should be removed.

Effect of estrous cycle on performance. An owner who believes a mare's performance waxes or wanes with her estrous cycle should keep a daily record of her performance and have frequent veterinary examinations to determine when the mare is in estrus.

The stallion

Stallions exhibit libido throughout the year but show peak sexual behavior in the spring. Seasonal changes are also seen in sperm number and testosterone levels.[1515] Stallions with a harem have a higher level of testosterone than those in a bachelor herd, which in turn have a higher level than stalled stallions.[1257] This variation indicates the importance of the social situation. A stallion has three strategies: be a bachelor, be the dominant stallion in a band, or be a subordinate stallion in a band. The stallion has more chances of siring a foal as a subordinate than as a bachelor.[95,569] At times of turmoil, such as after a Bureau of Land Management roundup, the percentage of foals sired by stallions other than the dominant one is 30%.[268]

Sexual behavior was seen in 2- to 3-month-old colts, with full penile erection during resting, play fighting, or mutual grooming,[1909] but the age at the first successful copulation varied from 15 months to 3 years in the same study. Tyler[1909] also noted that stallions actively prevented young males from mounting females. When exposed to estrous mares, stallions raised from weaning in bachelor groups did not exhibit mounting until 2 years old.[1299,1302]

Courtship behavior

Courtship behavior will vary with the management practices involved. The following description assumes that the mare and stallion have free access to each other.

Driving, herding, or snaking with a distinctive head-down position is a behavior usually elicited by the presence of another stallion. Piaffelike prancing is also a display to other stallions (see Fig. 4.12B).

Intromission may be achieved only with a full erection, and this is correlated with the degree of sexual excitement. Thus, an adequate period of sexual foreplay is essential.[1974] Males may tend a female for several days before she is fully receptive. Nipping and nuzzling begins at the mare's head and proceeds gradually along the body of the mare to the perineal area. During this testing phase, he exhibits the flehmen response. As sexual excitement increases, the male calls with neighs and roars. The female allows the male to lick her around the rear legs and back. Full erection usually develops over several minutes in the mature stallion. Several mounts are usually made before intromission and ejaculation. During copulation, the stallion rests his sternum on the mare's croup and may reach forward to bite her neck. Ejaculation occurs around 15 seconds after intromission and after approximately seven thrusts,[1878] and intromission lasts less than 45 seconds.

Postcopulatory tending was not noted by either Feist and McCullough[574] or Tyler[1909] in their study herds in Wyoming and England, respectively. The male may sniff the mare's genital area and exhibit the flehmen response, but the pair soon separates. Under test conditions, sexual satiation occurs after 1–10 ejaculations (average, 2.9).[220] Although stallions usually are limited to a few hand breedings per week, a 6-year-old Belgian stallion bred 20 mares in 9 days, with an 85% conception rate. Prostaglandin had been used to synchronize estrus, so eight mares were in heat and were bred by the stallion on 1 day.[285]

Sensory stimuli

Visual and other sensory stimuli are probably vital to the display of sexual behavior; however, their importance may be modified through learning. Tyler[1909] believes that the visual stimulus of the mare's posture with raised tail is important for attraction and penile erection. This reaction may be generalized so that a dummy or phantom in the general shape of a mare will be mounted by a sexually experienced stallion. Inexperienced stallions will not mount the dummy.[2022] Experienced males will also mount a mare or dummy while blindfolded. The stallion is undoubtedly stimulated by olfactory information, but the stimulation may precede the copulation by several minutes to hours. Typically, a stallion will stop chasing an estrous mare to sniff and flehmen at the small volume of urine she has expelled. Odor stimulation of the vomeronasal organ may lead to an increase in LH and testosterone and consequently libido, so his behavior is synchronized with that of the receptive mare. Experienced males do not show any inhibition to mounting a mare or dummy when olfactory input is blocked, but inexperienced males will mount a dummy only when it has been sprinkled with urine from an estrous female.

Clinical problems of stallions

About 10–25% of stallions presented for breeding soundness examination have some behavioral problem. Those stallions most at risk are young and/or novice breeders, frequently bred stallions, those in a new environment, and those in transition from racing to breeding.[1256] Young stallions appear to be particularly affected by exercise; as little as 30 minutes per day of lunging can decrease libido.[466]

Some common problems of sexual behavior in the male are as follows:

- Stallions that show sexual interest in mares, but will not mount, or mount but do not ejaculate
- Stallions that have low or no libido, that is, do not show interest in a sexually receptive mare
- Stallions that will mount mares only when another specific horse is present
- Stallions that injure, or "savage," mares or handlers
- Stallions that self-mutilate
- Stallions that mount but do not intromit
- Geldings that behave like stallions.

Masturbation. Masturbation is normal behavior in a stallion. The stallion flips the erect penis against the ventral abdominal wall. Ejaculation rarely occurs. Stallions masturbate four times a day, spending 30 minutes with an erect penis sometimes, but not always, accompanied by masturbation.[1877] This behavior usually occurs in the resting stallion, even one at pasture with mares available. Masturbation may occur in association with recumbency.[2025]

Sexual experience and decreased sexual behavior. Too much serious sexual experience too early is very detrimental to normal libido. Many stallions overused as youngsters are presented with sexual behavior problems. The most common problems are impotence or low libido. Other stallions that are overworked as studs may bite the mares viciously or be uncontrollable by their attendants. It is not always clear whether the young stallions have had traumatic or unpleasant experiences. They may remember being kicked by a mare or they may simply remember that they were exhausted. The resultant loss of libido can persist indefinitely unless treated.[1516]

A typical case is that of a 4-year-old Arabian stallion that showed different behaviors to different mares. He mounted without erection and bit a Morgan mare with which he had been housed as a 2-year-old. His sexual behavior was normal toward another mare with which he had had no previous contact. He had been noted to display snapping (see Chapters 1 and 6) to the Morgan mare as a youngster and presumably was subordinate to her. As an adult he showed aggressive behavior toward her, perhaps because of an approach–avoidance conflict. He was sexually stimulated, but because she was dominant, he did not want to mount. His displacement behavior was aggression.

Stallions that are used as teasers, that is, to detect estrus in mares, but are not used for breeding, may eventually show a loss of libido. In addition, they may show stereotypic behavior, such as stall weaving. It has not been determined how often a teaser stallion should be allowed to copulate to prevent these abnormal behaviors, and there are, no doubt, individual differences in response to use as a teaser.

Stallions can learn to inhibit sexual behavior as easily as they learn to express it. Stallions may be fitted with stallion rings, devices placed on the penis that cause discomfort if erection occurs. They are used on stallions that are in training or in other circumstances in which sexual behavior would be inappropriate. Many stallions apparently can be fitted with these devices and learn not to respond sexually when wearing them and yet respond normally when the rings are removed. Other stallions have learned too well and are impotent even when the ring is removed. Stallion rings and belly brushes are also used to prevent masturbation, which, as already noted, should not be considered either abnormal behavior or a cause of infertility. Ejaculation rarely occurs, so the behavior is unlikely to lead to a drop in fertility; attempts to punish masturbation, however, do cause libido problems.

Physical impairment. The treatment of any behavior problem must begin with elimination, or at least identification, of any physical problem. The two most common physical problems associated with breeding are genital injury or limb injury. Any lameness or limb injury will inhibit the stallion's ability to mount, so he may exhibit normal libido and penile erection but will not mount. An older stallion with navicular disease or chronic arthritis is a typical example of the effect of organic limb disease on sexual behavior. When pain is the cause of libido problems, nonsteroidal anti-inflammatory agents such as phenylbutazone and flunixin meglumine may be of value. Another factor that may be responsible for failure to mount is improper flooring. If the flooring is slippery, for instance, the stallion will be reluctant to mount, especially if he has fallen when trying to mount a mare on other occasions. He is much more likely to mount if taken to an environment with a different substrate such as grass or tanbark. A stallion with a mild locomotor problem may mount but be reluctant to ejaculate in cold weather. In warm weather, when he is pain free, he will be normal.

Injury to the genitalia can be a cause of breeding difficulties. Naturally, a stallion will avoid intromission if his penis is painful. Stallions may be reluctant to copulate long after the injury is apparently healed because they may not have learned that copulation will no longer be painful. Any impairment of blood flow to the penis may produce behavior problems such as ejaculatory failure.

Stallions with physical impairment of the legs or back should be mounted on secure mounts, that is, sturdy mares. The flooring should be adequate and the mare should be the correct size so that the sternum of the stallion rests on her croup. Anatomical fit is important because even normal stallions may lose their balance and slide off a mare that is too small or too large. Physically impaired stallions can be trained to an artificial dummy mount that is secure when AI is permitted for the breed. At first, an estrous mare may have to be held next to the dummy, but stallions can, like bulls, be conditioned to ejaculate in the absence of the normal stimulus of the mare.

Breeding environment. The total breeding environment must be considered because another cause of injury to the stallion can be a low roof or an overhang. A stallion rearing on his hind legs to mount a mare is considerably taller than when he is standing on all fours. If a stallion strikes his head while mounting, he not only may sustain serious injury but also be inhibited from mounting on subsequent occasions.

Perhaps the most important aspects of the breeding environment are handlers. Handlers must be familiar with the routine of breeding and experienced in controlling horses. Some handlers are better able to calm stallions than others with equal experience, and the calmer the stallion, the less likely are accidents. Such simple arrangements as placing all attendants on the same side of the mare and stallion can facilitate communication between them and prevent difficulties. Most breeding injuries and accidents occur when an inexperienced, highly nervous, or nonreceptive mare is bred without adequate restraint or judgment. Because errors in detection of estrus can be made and because the situation is unnatural, mares should be hobbled beforehand breeding. Distractions in the form of extraneous people or animals should be avoided.

No single treatment exists for all abnormal sexual behavior in stallions. Patience and time are necessary with almost all cases. It is advisable to take advantage of the stallion's seasonal breeding pattern and institute behavioral therapy during the spring and summer. Advantage should also be taken of the stimulatory effect of the presence of other stallions. It already has been noted here that wild stallions are most likely to copulate when other stallions are present; the same appears to be true of domestic stallions. Some stallions have been known to breed mares only if another horse, even another mare, is present. The stallion may regard the second horse as a competitor—another stallion—or some other, unknown reason may be present.

The antianxiety drug diazepam (0.05 mg/kg slowly i.v.) has been used successfully to overcome impotence caused by pain associated with breeding and for the loss of libido shown in a novel environment.[1262, 1263] Imipramine (500 mg i.v.) has been used to treat stallions that will mount and intromit but not ejaculate.[1259] Gonadotropin-releasing hormone may act directly on the brain of horses to stimulate sexual behavior[1260] and could have clinical application.

Finally, some stallions have definite mate preferences, and they should be allowed to exercise these preferences while recovering from loss of libido or impotence. Tease the stallion with several mares and use the one to which he is most responsive for further treatment. A quiet mare is necessary for a stallion that has been injured by another mare. A stallion that will not mount a mare may ejaculate into an artificial vagina. He may gain confidence and overcome his fear by this process and can later be induced to mount a mare.

Vicious behavior toward the mare and the attendants is, like most other abnormal sexual behavior, most apt to occur when stallions are used for breeding outside the normal breeding season. Therefore, stallions may be unmanageable in January but well-mannered by May.

Overuse and rough handling. Overuse and rough handling are often the cause of misbehavior in stallions during breeding. They may bite the mare or be generally intractable. Attempts to improve the horse's breeding manners should be delayed until normal libido and copulation have been reestablished. Punishment of a horse with sexual abnormalities will retard its progress. If the stallion's viciousness is not attenuated as his libido improves, various physical devices, such as a muzzle and breeding bridle for him and a withers protector for the mare, may be used.

Self-mutilation. Self-mutilation is a very common behavior problem. Although it occurs in horses of both sexes, it is much more common in stallions.[470] The behavior consists of biting at or actually biting the flanks or, more rarely, the chest. The horse usually squeals and kicks out at the same time. The signs mimic those of acute colic, but can be differentiated because self-mutilation does not progress to rolling or depression and is chronic. It is extremely important to eliminate discomfort as a cause of self-mutilation because penile, testicular or urethral lesions, gastro intestinal pain, limb pain, bladder disease, etc. can cause self-mutilation.[1258] The cause of the behavior is unknown, but because it usually responds to a change in the social environment, it is probably caused by sociosexual deprivation. The behaviors observed in self-mutilating stallion mimic those of a stallion confrontation: sniffing and nipping at the genitalia, defecating and sniffing the feces, circling, and squealing. McDonnell[1258] has hypothesized that removing feces or skin secretion of the stallion, even his own, may reduce the arousal that precedes a bout of self-mutilation. Most breeding stallions lead deprived lives in that they are kept in stalls in isolation from other horses, particularly from other mares; however, most do not self-mutilate. The question arises as to whether stallions that self-mutilate should be used for breeding. Castration sometimes, but not always, stops self-mutilation. Preventing the behavior with the use of cradles and side poles does not remove the cause; the stallion will continue to vocalize and kick, so although he can no longer injure himself, he can still injure a bystander. A soft muzzle will prevent injury, slow down his prehension of hay and grain, but not frustrate his attempts to bite as much as other forms of restraint. Providing a stall companion such as a donkey will reduce the incidence of self-mutilation. Allowing the stallion to live on pasture with a mare will eliminate the problem in most cases. The chances that the stallion will be injured by the mare are less than the chances that he will injure himself or someone else by self-mutilating. Opiate antagonists will prevent self-mutilation.[473] Unfortunately, naloxone, the antagonist now available, is metabolized very quickly by horses and is quite expensive. (See Cribbing under Clinical Problems in Chapter 9 for a discussion of the involvement of endogenous opiates in equine "vices.") Simply reducing the grain in a stallion's diet and increasing his exercise and roughage can reduce self-mutilation.[1249]

Effects of castration. A horse that exhibits stallion-like behavior could be either a cryptorchid from whom the undescended testicle was not removed at castration or a gelding in which sexual behavior persists. A negligible plasma testosterone will distinguish the gelding from the cryptorchid stallion.[659] The testosterone response to gonadotropin administration is the best test for castration. Sexual behavior persists in more than one-third of geldings.[1164] The sexual behavior may be as innocuous as exhibition of flehmen or as extreme as mounting and intromission. The sexual behavior itself is usually not a problem, but aggression directed toward other geldings by the one who is acting like a harem stallion is. Another unwelcome stallion-like behavior is attacking foals, particularly newborn foals. Management can be used to prevent these problems. A gelding that acts like a stallion should be stalled alone or pastured only with other geldings and should not have access to foals.

Geldings may also self-mutilate. These are usually geldings that are displaying other stallion behaviors but, unlike intact males, they self-mutilate in the presence of mares. Stall confinement or pasturing without visual contact with mares usually reduces the incidence of self-mutilation. If not, progestins or cyproheptadine (8 mg increasing to 88 mg/day) may be used.

PIGS

The sow

As is the cow, the sow is a nonseasonal breeder. After regular cycling commences, the sow will cycle every 18–24 days (mean, 21 days) until bred. Puberty occurs at 5–8 months. The presence of a boar leads to the occurrence of estrus at an earlier age and in more gilts.[1867] Puberty is accelerated in gilts older than 160 days exposed to a strange male for 20 or more minutes per day.

Estrous cycle

As do females of other species, the sow shows an increase in activity as estrus approaches.[47] The increased motor activity eventually takes the form of searching behavior, which seems vital to the initial uniting of an estrous sow with a boar.[1768] Urination is frequent, as is calling to the male. The call is a soft, rhythmic grunt. An estrous female approaches the boar and sniffs him around the head and genitals. Estrous sows attempt to mount other estrous females, but subordinate sow rarely mount dominant ones.[1482] Olfactory stimuli alone will instigate this searching; anesthetized boars readily attract estrous sows. Olfactory bulbectomy drastically impairs the ability of the sow to discriminate between males and females.[32] Signoret and Mauleon[1769] have reported that bulbectomy also eliminates sexual behavior and prevents normal ovulation and estrus. This has not been confirmed by Meese and Baldwin,[1292] who found that bulbectomized females mated, conceived, and reared their litters, although there were deficits in maternal recognition (see Chapter 5, "Maternal Behavior").

This proceptive behavior can be used to detect estrus in sows using electronic monitoring to detect which sows visit a boar housed in a pen adjacent to the sow. Boars and sows show individual differences in mate selection; each animal has its favorite or favorites.[1852] Boars differ in the degree to which they attract sows, but this attractivity is not related to their libido.[821] Subordinate sows and gilts exhibit fewer signs of estrus and approach the boar less often, especially in crowded conditions.[1482] Even fear of humans can suppress estrous behavior.

Searching behavior appears to be under endogenous control and requires estrogen during behavioral ontogeny for full development. Gilts reared in isolation will show this behavior upon reaching puberty.[1768] The immobility response of the fully receptive sow, however, seems to require both tactile and olfactory or auditory stimuli. The specific auditory stimulus is the courting song of the boar (see later in this chapter).[1768] As with searching behavior, the immobility reaction does not seem susceptible to learned modifications. The olfactory stimuli to which the sow responds are pheromones present in both the saliva and preputial secretions of boars. The chemicals involved are metabolites of androgens and have been identified as 5α-androst(16-ene)3-one.[1303] These compounds have been used experimentally[1589] and are available commercially to elicit the immobility reactions.

Olfactory and auditory stimuli from adult boars, supplied by an aerosol spray and a tape recorder, will increase the proceptivity of gilts toward young boars.[900] Presence of mature boar can advance puberty and the onset of ovulation in weaned sows.[822] The presence of a boar has a slight effect on the rate of conception and number of piglets or the size of the litter.[820]

A robot boar—even with aldosterone and a recording of a boar's calls—is less effective than a real boar in stimulating immobility response and the duration of estrus is shorter.[682] Estrus is less apt to be detected in sows with less than 1 m² (11 ft²) of pen space and those living in pairs. It is also easier to detect estrus if the sows are housed across an aisle from a boar rather than in an adjoining pen. This may be because the sow has had close olfactory contact with the boar when the attendants were not present; she has shown the immobility response, but no person was there to notice.[816,819,820,823]

Clinical problems of sows

Aberrations are unusual, perhaps because of the somewhat rigid genetic control of sexual behaviors. Breed differences in the length of estrus are seen,[1766] but these are minor and unimportant clinically. Although not quantified, some sows seem to have decided mate preferences and display strong aversions to specific males.[1768]

Failure to reproduce in confinement. The most important problem is failure of reproduction in confined gilts. Confinement and the social environment appear to play a role in inhibiting estrus in young gilts.[603] Puberty is delayed in regrouped or crowded pigs or roughly handled pigs,[155,360,816] but accelerated by gentle handling. The stress of trailering can also stimulate the onset of estrus. It is interesting that chronic stress of overcrowding delays puberty, but the acute stress of transport accelerates it.

The boar

Pigs are unusual in that defeminization occurs well after birth and is under the control of estrogenic metabolites that act as late as 3 months postnatally.[14]

Courtship behavior

After contact with an estrous female has been made, the boar will pursue the female, attempting to nose her sides, flanks, and vulva (Fig. 4.13). Unique to the pig is the boar's "courting song," which is used during this phase of courtship. This is a series of soft, guttural grunts, about 6–8 per second.[1768] Tactile stimulation of the female continues and increases in intensity as the boar's sexual excitement increases. The boar usually emits urine rhythmically; pheromones in the urine may further increase the female's willingness to stand. Several mounting attempts may be made until the female becomes immobile, after which mounting and intromission follow rapidly. The boar's ejaculatory time approaches that of the dog, although no copulatory lock occurs in swine. Ejaculation occurs within 3–20 minutes, with an average of 4–5 minutes.[1768] Consort behavior continues for a short time following copulation. Burger[301] observed that boars mated an estrous female around 10 times over a 2- to 3-day estrous period. Although domestic pigs are not considered seasonal breeders, libido and testosterone levels increase earlier in prepubertal boars if the day is artificially lengthened to 15 hours.[847] Boars tend to have greater libido in a separate mating pen than in their home stalls.[817] Cortisol levels increase following mating.[1125]

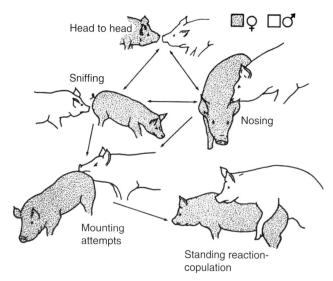

Fig. 4.13   The courtship sequence of pigs.[1768] (Copyright 1975, with permission of W.B. Saunders Co.)

Olfactory stimuli

Olfactory cues seem unimportant in stimulating a boar to mount a female or a dummy. Olfactory bulbectomy, for example, does not prevent normal sexual behavior.[251] Some but not all boars can distinguish between estrous and anestrous females from a distance, that is, on the basis of olfactory information.[1274] The initial contact with the sow, however, triggers a behavioral response from her: immobility, reflecting the degree of her sexual receptivity. It is this tendency toward immobility that seems to arouse the boar. As with the female response, this reaction is under fairly strict genetic control and not subject to much learned modification. Thus, what is noted by human observers as homosexual mounting or aberrant mounting of artificial stimuli is explained as being a normal response to immobile objects of approximately the correct size and shape. Although some breeds are easier to train for semen collection than others, training of a young boar to mount a dummy will usually be successful on the first few attempts.

Early socialization

In the boar, as in most species, the early social environment is important to later sexual behavior. Boars raised in isolation from 3 weeks of age copulated less often with estrous sows than did boars raised in groups. Boars with visual and olfactory contact with other boars were not nearly as inhibited as the isolates, indicating that contact with other pigs, even male pigs, is important.[820] Later, contact with females is also important because boars with visual and olfactory contact with sows copulated more often and ejaculated longer than boars kept in isolation or with visual and olfactory contact with other boars.[818, 824] This is probably a hormonal effect; testosterone and corticosteroid levels are higher in boars that are in contact with sows.[1169]

Clinical problems of boars

As with the other domestic animals, differences in the level of "sex drive" appear to be larger between individuals than between breeds. Low libido, however, has been associated with a high plane of nutrition, and, at least in the United Kingdom, is seen more frequently in Landrace than in boars of the large white breed.[61] Libido may be impaired through mismanagement of a young boar. A young male turned in with a group of gilts may be frustrated by excessive curiosity or bullied by the gilts. This incompetence or fear may become conditioned and a permanent problem. Supervision of early matings is recommended. A quiet sow or one recently serviced by a mature boar should be used for the first mating.[61] Another common problem is aggression by the boar toward humans. This is usually resolved by culling the boar, which removes the danger and prevents an aggressive animal from reproducing.

DOGS

The bitch

Estrous cycle

The domestic dog, unlike most of its canid relatives, is a nonseasonal breeder. The length of each estrous cycle is extremely variable from individual to individual and sometimes from one heat to the next in the same bitch. From one to four cycles yearly may be seen, with two being most usual. The basenji is an exception; one seasonal breeding per year is seen in the early fall.[653] Basenji–cocker spaniel crosses show both monocyclic and polycyclic activity, indicating genetic control of this aspect of the reproductive cycle. The proportion of urinations that are directed, that is, next to a conspicuous object, is higher during proestrus and estrus.[2049]

The onset of puberty also varies widely among individuals. No strict correlation of age at puberty may be made with either body size or conformation;[616] generally, however, the smaller breeds reach puberty earlier than the larger breeds. It would be very rare for a St. Bernard to reach puberty by 6 months, for example, but not unusual for a miniature poodle to do so. Thus, puberty onset for all dogs ranges from 6 to 15 months, with 7–10 months being the usual for the "average" dog.

Courtship behavior

The correlation of hormonal levels and sexual behavior in the dog are illustrated in Fig. 4.2. The first proestrus and estrus of a bitch's life are shorter than subsequent ones and the levels of LH and estradiol are lower.[338] She is less attractive to the male and less proceptive.[684] Courtship behavior is marked by play behavior in the proestrous part of the cycle, but this play behavior decreases during estrus. The female will run with the male, approach him using the typical play bow of puppies, and even whimper submissively. She will sniff and lick the male's body and genitalia. Urination becomes more frequent as estrus approaches and the posture used will frequently be the squat-raise (refer to Fig. 1.11, in Chapter 1). She may stand before the male momentarily during proestrus, but turns before the male can mount, often with a bark or growl.[356] Attraction of males and proceptivity appear in proestrus, but receptivity occurs later, during estrus.[173] During estrus, she stands more quietly to allow male investigation and eventually intromission toward the end of estrus. When the male touches her vulva, she will flex her body laterally;[770] while he is thrusting, she will move her perineum from side to side and ventrally, a motion that increases the probability of intromission. After the lock or the copulatory tie has been established, she may roll or twist and turn (the copulatory lock is discussed in the next section). Contractions of the constrictor vestibuli muscles and the anus occur as an after-reaction.

If the male does not mount, the female will "present" her hindquarters to him and even back into him and deviate her tail. An older and more experienced bitch may mount a young male and execute pelvic thrusts.[616]

Other social behaviors, in addition to sexual ones, are influenced by the reproductive condition of the bitch. Dominance relationships between females may shift, especially during metestrus. Males may defer to females in food competitions not because they are chivalrous males but because they are more motivated to mount than to eat.

Courtship in free-ranging dogs

Stray bitches avoid their male littermates but can be bred by a persistent brother. Estrous females attract two to seven males; they will show less proceptive behavior in the presence of many males and also less active rejection of nonpreferred males.

Clinical problems of bitches

Owners unfamiliar with canine courtship may be upset because the bitch appears to tease the male by soliciting and then threatening him if he mounts, but this is normal. Females may refuse males for any of several reasons. A bitch may display dominance over a male by not allowing the male to "stand over" her (a normal canine signal of dominance) or to approach from behind. Dominance relationships are learned, but can be established rapidly. Thus, dominance relationships probably help inhibit mother–son matings and may prevent certain sib–sib matings,[616] but may also develop quickly if an aggressive bitch is placed with a more submissive dog. Le Boeuf[1106] and Beach and Le Boeuf[178] demonstrated definite female preferences for certain males. Refusal can range from avoiding a particular male to actively chasing and biting him. Not all the females rejected a male to the same degree, and Beach[170] showed that dominant males were not necessarily chosen as preferred mates. Beach also found that sexual preference could not be correlated with social affinity outside the mating period.[170]

The dog

Sexual behaviors may appear in 5-week-old male pups, and mounting behavior becomes an important part of the male's social repertoire as it matures. As with many other mammals, mounting is used as a sign of dominance; a submissive animal will stand for a more dominant male, but standing over is not tolerated by the dominant animal. Fox and Bekoff[616] point out that most dogs are sexually mature physiologically long before they copulate for the first time. Perhaps the lack of dominance in young dogs inhibits early mating. Social contact is vital in the ontogeny of normal sexual behavior. Dogs raised in social isolation showed abnormal mounting orientation that persisted for longer than it did in dogs with similarly limited sexual experience but more social experience.[171]

Courtship behavior

Male dogs are attracted to estrous bitches.[174] Urine of the estrous bitch appears to be more attractive to the dog than vaginal secretions,[481,496] but a component of the vaginal secretions, methyl p-hydroxybenzoate, has been shown to induce male sexual behavior when applied to the vulva of an anestrous bitch.[702] The pheromone may be considered a "releaser" of sexual behavior in the male. Mammalian behavior is not as stereotyped as that of fish and birds, so although sexual arousal may occur in all male dogs exposed to the pheromone, the expression of that arousal may vary considerably; therefore, male courtship behavior is extremely variable. Males may show extreme interest or indifference to females, although mating may occur successfully in either case. Play behavior may be marked or absent. The male sniffs the female's head and vulva; he may lick her ears. While canids do not show the classic flehmen response of ungulates, it is possible that the "tonguing" response seen during this olfactory investigation accomplishes transport of pheromones to the vomeronasal organ in a manner similar to that postulated for ungulates. The length of the play activity and olfactory investigation probably varies with the past experience of the male and female, perceived degrees of dominance within the pair, stage of estrus, and sexual satiation of either partner. Bitches can be forced to accept copulation by a strong and aggressive male who chases her until she is exhausted and holds her with his teeth by the neck or with his paw on her back. Only half of the stray male dogs are able to copulate, and those under a year of age rarely do so.[684]

The male mounts in response to female immobility; he grasps her with his forelegs just cranial to her pelvis. He thrusts with his pelvis and when intromission has been achieved, the rate of thrusting increases. Engorgement of the bulbus glandis and contraction of the vaginal muscles following intromission result in the copulatory lock or tie, a phenomenon most closely associated with canids but not restricted to them. The male will usually dismount and turn around so that male and female are facing opposite directions while ejaculation occurs (Figs. 4.14 and 4.15). The lock may last 10–30 minutes (mean, 14 minutes[771]), after which the bulbus decreases in size and the pair separates. Following copulation, recovery from sexual refractoriness may be rapid. Fox and Bekoff[616] report records of up to five copulations by a male dog in 1 day.

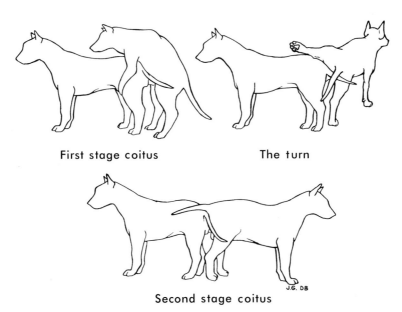

First stage coitus   The turn

Second stage coitus

Fig. 4.14   Coital positions of the dog.[708] (Copyright 1972, with permission of Vet. Rec.)

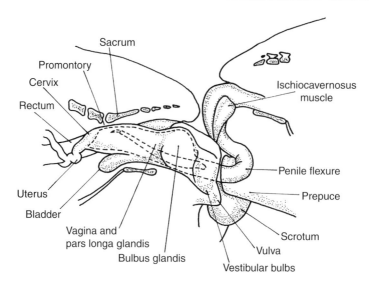

Fig. 4.15   Relationship of the male and female genitals during the copulatory lock of the dog.[708] (Copyright 1972, with permission of Vet. Rec.)

Clinical problems of dogs

Impotence. Male impotence or loss of libido can be the result of organic disease. Most commonly this would be musculoskeletal disease such as hip dysplasia, arthritis, or trauma-induced pain in the hindquarters. Balanoposthitis is generally a mild disease in dogs and unlikely to affect sexual performance, although a severe form could conceivably do so.

Lack of socialization. The lack of sufficient social contacts as a puppy may inhibit successful copulation. This becomes a very real problem, not only an experimental one, when a pup is ordered from a pet shop. Pups are weaned as early as possible (4–5 weeks) and shipped shortly thereafter to pet shops. The pup, if he survives transport, is kept isolated in the new owner's home, protecting him from infectious disease. When the owners finally do try to use their sheltered pet for breeding, they have great difficulty persuading the dog to perform or find it impossible to do so. Their dog has been essentially isolated from social contacts with conspecifics. Not only have the motor patterns of sexual behavior not been perfected, they have never been placed in a proper social context. Some dogs may overcome this void in socialization, but their sexual and other behaviors may never be normal in direction or quantity. An example of poor libido occurred in a pointer that was kept with his sister. Both the sister and his owners reprimanded the dog for sexual interest in his sister and when presented with an unrelated estrous bitch, he had no libido and seemed frightened. With increasing age and exposure to other bitches, his libido increased.

Timidity. Timidity, especially in poodles and German shepherds, may be both learned and genetic in nature. Affected dogs may be inhibited to the point of impotence. Leaving the male and female together for several days, rather than allowing only a short breeding period, has been suggested. This prolonged period of socialization could, however, exacerbate a potential problem if the female is dominant.

A conditioned fear of any phase of the breeding program may be inadvertently instilled in a stud dog. Analysis of breeding techniques and reversal of the conditioning may alleviate the problem successfully. Thus, a young dog forced to court a very aggressive female may associate the rough treatment he received with the breeding process in general, with a specific breeding location, or with a specific color or type of female. Young dogs may make some clumsy mounting attempts and may otherwise prolong courtship, but should successfully mount a bitch within the first few exposures to a female. If the dog is a persistently timid breeder, however, he should be dropped from the breeding program. AI is recommended if the timidity is suspected to be learned, or the result of the particular dominance relationship in the attempted mating. Most dogs will breed with most other dogs; therefore, mating problems with behavioral etiologies are unusual and require serious consideration.

Environmental disturbances. As are other male domestic animals, dogs are sensitive to environmental disturbances in the breeding process. If one member of a breeding pair must be transported to the other, the female should be brought to the male. Noise and other disruptions in the breeding area should be minimized. The rather curious insistence of some breeders on helping a male dog mount and copulate might actually cause more difficulties than it is thought to prevent. Besides the physical disruption of the observer–helper, the breeder will likely be dominant to the dog and thus be somewhat inhibitory to the male's sexual performance. A timid dog may require the owner's presence if his dominance over a female is doubtful; but, as already discussed here, the continued use of a dog this timid would be unwise because one doesn't wish to pass on genes for timidity. Slippery floors, such as waxed linoleum, may prevent mounting, but this problem should be easily avoided.

Masturbation. Masturbation is not an unusual problem in house dogs. Semen quality or value as a breeder are not affected, but the habit becomes an embarrassing or annoying one for the owner. Masturbation using inanimate objects is probably seen in most puppies, but will become an insignificant behavior in the normally socialized adult. Although mounting can be an aspect of sexual behavior, it is also a sign of dominance, so mounting of people should be discouraged. To resolve the problem, the owners should teach the dog submissive behavior by counter-conditioning the dog to stay down when it attempts to mount, as well as consistently punishing mounting. Castration may eliminate or decrease the problem (see the next section). Owners reporting homosexual behavior in their dog should also be informed that mounting of one male dog by another is probably a sign of dominance.

Sexual behavior after castration. Prepubertal castration greatly reduces sexual interests. Because mounting is an integral part of the dog's behavioral ontogeny and is used in agonistic interactions, all sexual behavior will probably not be eliminated. Hopkins et al.[854] studied the postoperative effects of castration on 42 postpubertal dogs in normal home situations (Fig. 4.16). They found that 90% of the dogs castrated to control roaming showed a rapid or gradual decline in this behavior. Inter-male aggression was reduced noticeably in only 60% of the dogs and urine marking in the home only 50%. About 67% of the dogs showed a decrease in mounting behavior following surgery; mounting of people was reduced in seven of eight dogs castrated specifically for that problem. Mounting of other dogs was reduced in only one of four dogs castrated for that reason. The authors do not report any changes in the owners' handling or attitude toward their dogs following surgery, however, which might have been responsible for some of the behavioral changes noted. Age at castration was not correlated with the noted effects. Although in no cases did the occurrence of an objectionable behavior return to its preoperative level, some behaviors appeared intermittently for long periods following castration. Hart[771] reported that castrated dogs may retain sexual mounting behavior, with intromission, lock, and ejaculation for several years postcastration or indefinitely, although the frequency of the behaviors decreased.

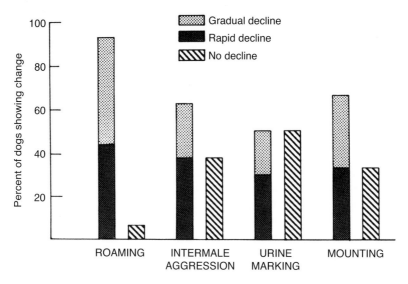

Fig. 4.16   Percentage of dogs experiencing rapid decline, gradual decline, or no change in four behaviors after castration.[854] (Copyright 1976, with permission of the School of Veterinary Medicine, University of California at Davis, and J. Am. Vet. Med. Assoc.)

Castration reduces aggression to people in only 30% of dogs, and the effect is independent of age at castration or duration of the aggression.[1404] Although aggression to males is decreased, aggression to bitches persists.[1194]

CATS

Free-ranging cats

In a feral situation, one estrous female will be surrounded by a group of males. Tomcats will knock one another off an estrous queen or mount the tom that is mounting the female, but little overt aggression takes place during courting. A male dominance hierarchy, based on size and age, gives the dominant tom priority of access to females. Dominant males tend to be closer to estrous females than are subordinate males, but they do not mount more frequently.[1400] Fifteen copulations will occur in 24 hours.[435] Groups of cats living on farms seem to have only one sexually active tom. Although pair-bonding does not occur in the domestic cat, short-term consort behavior occurs normally. A male and female may remain together for several hours or days, mating many times. Juvenile males tend to move away from their birth area before their third year.[1137]

The queen

Estrous cycle

The queen is seasonally polyestrous, and most cats will cycle at least twice yearly if not bred. Although population peaks occur in mid-January to March and May to June in the Northern Hemisphere, individual cats may be in estrus at any season. The nadir for reproductive output of a population is late fall, making the availability of kittens as Christmas presents very unreliable.

If unbred, the cat will cycle every 3 weeks for several months. Actual estrus lasts 9–10 days without copulation and around 4 days if the cat is bred.

Most felids, including the domestic cat, are induced ovulators, thus breeding may be accomplished whenever the female shows receptivity. Owners unwilling or unable to have a pet cat neutered may use this feature of the reproductive cycle to shorten estrus; artificial stimulation of the vagina using a cotton-tipped applicator stick will induce ovulation and shorten the receptive time. This is an especially useful procedure in terminating repeated heats.[611] Females will usually reach puberty at 6–10 months, but females born in April may not cycle until the following year.[611] Eckstein and Zucker man[523] report that free-ranging cats may not reach puberty until 15–18 months, although "barn" cats born in May to July in Ithaca, New York, routinely give birth to their first litter 12 months later.

There appears to be avoidance of incestuous mating in that estrous females will travel farther from home if the closest male is related.[1137]

Catnip. Nepetalactone, a volatile terpenoid found in the catnip plant (Nepeta cataria),[1967] and estrus elicit similar behaviors, and there has been continued debate as to whether this is a release of sexual behaviors or a nonspecific pleasure inducer.[768, 782, 843, 935, 1135, 1471, 1882] As Hatch[782] points out, however, estrous behavior is similar to, but not identical with, catnip-induced behavior. Catnip does not cause vulvar presentation, vocalization, or foot treading, and cats in estrus do not head-shake as do cats exposed to catnip. Also, male cats respond in an identical manner. Todd[1882] found that the body-rolling and head-rubbing behaviors characteristic of both the estrous and catnip-induced states could be induced in males and females by an extract of tomcat urine. As Hart[768] concludes, nepetalactone may be mimicking one of the compounds in male urine to which an estrous female may be especially primed, but to which most or all cats are sensitive. The response to catnip depends on the main olfactory system, not on the vomeronasal organ.[778]

Courtship behavior

An estrous female will call and purr. She is restless and shows increased general motor activity. If she is a house cat she may run from one room to the next, stopping to call at each door or window. She may be very affectionate toward the owners. Urination occurs frequently, and she may spray. She rubs her head and flanks on furniture; glands in these areas may produce pheromones that contain information announcing the presence of an estrous female. She crouches, elevates her perineal region, and treads with her back legs.[2006] This will usually be accompanied by a rhythmic opening and closing of the claws of the front feet. Rolling, squirming, and stretching are seen. This activity occurs whether or not a male is present but becomes synchronized with male behavior when the female is interacting with the male. During proestrus, she will roll and solicit the male's attention but act aggressively if he mounts.[1316] This may be termed postural acceptance and affective rejection. When fully receptive, she becomes immobile and stands crouched in lumbar lordosis and with her head held on the ground between her forelegs (Fig. 4.17). Her tail is deviated to one side, and she allows the male to mount. This latter sequence may be stimulated in an estrous female by scratching her over the dorsal tail base.

An estrous female may show a darting behavior in the presence of several tomcats. She will repeatedly run a short distance from the toms, and this may be her means of assessing the relative strength of the males as they chase her and try to displace one another.

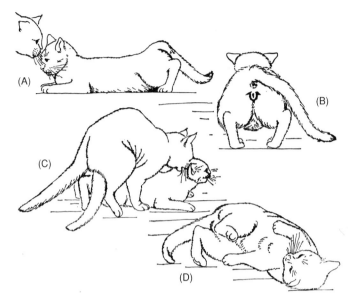

Fig. 4.17   Sexual behavior of the female cat. (A and B) The typical posture adopted by the queen in full estrus. Note leg flexion, lordosis, and deflection of the tail. (C) Tom holding queen with neck grip during intromission. (D) Postcoital rolling by the queen.[1718] (Copyright 1970 and 1987, with permission of Lea & Febiger.)

Clinical problems of queens

Female–Female. Female–female mounting behavior is seen only rarely and usually in colony situations. Two estrous cats may try to squirm underneath each other when presenting to an inaccessible male; one may mount the other and perform male-like pelvic thrusts. Leyhausen[1133] reports definite examples of female mate preferences in colony cats. He does not offer a clue as to the mechanisms of this selection but does observe that the dominant members of the colony were sometimes bypassed as mates.

Effects of ovariohysterectomy. Spaying (ovariohysterectomy, or less commonly, ovariectomy or tubal ligation) is performed quite commonly on the domestic house cat. Spaying eliminates sexual behavior but may affect other behaviors. Care must be taken not to ascribe changes in behavior to surgery, when the changes might be caused by maturational changes in the cat or changes in the cat's environment. A common behavior problem following spaying is an increase in aggression between cats in a multicat household, resulting either from the lowered progesterone levels of the spayed cat and/or the change in her odor that precipitated attacks by the other cat. Maternal behavior has also been observed in newly spayed cats, perhaps triggered by the fall in ovarian hormone levels—which is similar to the fall that occurs at parturition—and the presence of neonatal kittens.

The tom

Courtship behavior

The male probably locates an estrous female via olfactory cues deposited as pheromones in the urine and by some sebaceous gland secretions. A male placed with a female in a mating arena will spend some time investigating and marking the area with urine and anal gland secretions before mating. The cat shows a flehmen response, or gape, similar to that of ungulates (refer to Chapter 1, "Communication," Fig. 1.13). He calls to the female, circles her, and sniffs her genitalia. A nonreceptive female will actively, even violently, rebuff a male. When a female is receptive, the male approaches her from the side and behind and grips her neck in his mouth. He then mounts with the front legs, then the hind, and rubs her with his forepaws. Intromission follows a forward stepping with arched back and pelvic thrusts.[611] Ejaculation occurs seconds after intromission, and intromission usually lasts less than 10 seconds. The penis is covered with numerous small spines that apparently cause an intense stimulation as evidenced by the loud copulatory cry of the female with intromission. With retraction of the penis, the female rolls and claws at the male. The male will often lick his penis after copulation. Copulation may occur every 10–15 minutes for several hours. A seasonal variation in sexual readiness with a decline in the fall is seen in the male cat under experimental conditions.[94]

Clinical problems of toms

Reluctance of the male to breed a female is usually the result of the female's being nonreceptive and thus aggressive toward the male's advances. Inexperienced males may be especially intimidated by the aggressive responses of a proestrous female. In a laboratory, only one tom in three will consistently copulate with fully receptive queens. It is not surprising, therefore, that many visits to the tom are necessary before successful breeding takes place. Estrous females may indicate a mate preference by actively rebuffing one male or staying near another.

Effects of castration. Castration is a widely accepted procedure for the pet cat. Prepubertal (6–8 months) castration generally eliminates sexual behavior. Fox[611] points out that although testicular androgens are secreted by 4 months, mating behavior does not develop until 8–9 months. Some owners object to a feminine-appearing male and so delay castration until 12–14 months, or the first serious fight abscess. Rosenblatt and Aronson[1633, 1634] and Rosenblatt[1632] point out that the effectiveness of castration in eliminating mating behavior depends on the previous level of sexual experience. Thus, owners should be advised to restrict the access of their cat to females until after surgery unless they do not mind the cat's continued sexual interests. Early castration when the kitten is less than 4 months old virtually guarantees that he will not spray as an adult. No negative side effects occur from early neutering in male cats, so it should be recommended highly.[1791]

Hart and Barrett[772] studied the effects of postpubertal castration on fighting, roaming, and spraying. Castration seems much more effective in reducing or eliminating these behaviors in the cat than it is in the dog. About 88% of cat owners interviewed 23 months after having their cats castrated reported a rapid or gradual decline in fighting, 92% reported the same for roaming; and 87% responded favorably for spraying. The failure of surgery to eliminate these behaviors completely probably is due to the learned components of the behaviors. Mounting behavior, either mounting inanimate objects, other cats, or the owner, occurs in 25% of castrated male cats. See Chapter 1 for treatment of spraying by neutered cats. It is interesting that the copulatory or consummatory aspects of sexual behavior, but not the appetitive activities such as roaming, persist.

5 Maternal Behavior

Maternal behavior is influenced by hereditary, experiential, and hormonal factors. Primiparous females are most likely to neglect or attack their offspring. During a sensitive period soon after birth, the mother of a single or small number of young forms a bond with her offspring. Three important time intervals occur: (1) the length of time after parturition when a neonate will still be accepted, (2) the length of time during which the dam must be exposed to the neonate before she recognizes it as her own, and (3) the length of time the mother and offspring can be separated after the initial bond is formed before the mother will not recognize or accept the offspring. The offspring may take somewhat longer to recognize its mother than the mother to recognize it. Litter-bearing animals such as pigs, cats, and dogs are not as exclusive in their bonds. Nest building occurs in pigs and to a lesser degree in dogs and cats. Nursing is less frequent in hider species such as cattle and goats than in followers such as horses and sheep. Weaning time depends on the number of offspring and the availability of food. Artificial weaning is almost always earlier than that seen in free-ranging animals.

INTRODUCTION: GENERAL PRINCIPLES OF MATERNAL BEHAVIOR

Internal factors that elicit maternal behavior

Hormonal and neural controls

Maternal behavior is characterized by sudden onset. One day we own a single cat who spends her day eating, sleeping, grooming herself, and hunting or playing. The next day, we own five cats, four of which are kittens, and the original cat now spends almost all her time feeding and grooming the kittens. This behavior will gradually subside but is remarkably persistent in contrast to some other behaviors. Aggression, for example, may be sudden in onset but does not persist very long. Other adult behaviors seem to have been rehearsed by the developing animal in play. Play includes elements of aggressive and sexual behavior, chasing, and fleeing, but not of maternal behavior.

What then is the basis of maternal behavior? It is certainly an innate behavior pattern, although experience does play a role, as is discussed later in this chapter. Even if a behavior is innate, that is, a genetically programmed response to a certain set of stimuli, the behaving animal must be physiologically prepared to respond to the appropriate stimuli. In trying to determine the biological basis of maternal behavior, we investigate the hormonal basis of maternal behavior and the learned aspects, as well as those features of the neonate that may serve to release maternal behavior.

The combination of the proper hormonal milieu and the stimulus for maternal behavior, the neonate, plus prior experience of being a mother can elicit maternal behavior. The stimulation of maternal behavior appears to be under both hormonal and neural control. Estrogen rises and progesterone falls at parturition in sheep. Estrogen appears to facilitate, and progesterone to inhibit, maternal behavior in this species.[1758] In regard to neural control, one of the sequelae of parturition is cervical stimulation. Vaginocervical stimulation for 5 minutes will result in the reflex that stimulates oxytocin release. Oxytocin is released not only from the posterior pituitary into the bloodstream, but also from the terminals of cells whose cell bodies lie in the periventricular area of the hypothalamus, the axons of which can stimulate the neural mechanism underlying maternal activities in other parts of the brain. Brain oxytocin levels increase at parturition, at suckling, and when the vagina is stimulated,[1002] and increasing oxytocin in the cerebrospinal fluid can stimulate maternal behavior.[1001] Six weeks of treatment with intravaginal progesterone and estradiol, plus cervical stimulation at the time of introduction of the lamb, stimulated normal maternal behavior in anestrous ewes, indicating the importance of both hormonal and neural factors. Cervical stimulation will also cause a ewe that is already selectively maternal toward one lamb to be maternal toward another, alien lamb.[1007]

Hormonal priming by estrogen and progesterone, plus vaginocervical stimulation, is necessary in order to reduce aggression toward, or withdrawal from, alien lambs by ewes. Experience is also necessary for full expression of maternal behavior because only multiparous ewes would show positive maternal behavior licking, sniffing, and low-pitched bleating after the combination of hormonal and vaginocervical stimulation.[1000]

The fact that primiparous ewes routinely reject their lambs if they have been delivered by Caesarian section also indicates the importance of neural stimulation by the passage of the lamb through the vaginal canal. The fact that multiparous ewes will readily accept their lambs even if they have been delivered by Caesarian section indicates the importance of prior experience in ovine maternal behavior.[35]

Learning

The evidence for the role of learning in maternal behavior is found mostly in higher primates and rodents. Monkeys that had been artificially reared made very poor mothers and very reluctant sex partners.[761] Apparently, a monkey must have been mothered in order to be a good mother spontaneously. It is interesting that monkeys that neglected or even killed their first offspring exhibited normal maternal behavior after the second pregnancy. This aspect of maternal behavior has not been well investigated in domestic animals; it is worth noting, however, that most problems in maternal behavior are seen in primiparous animals. Ovine maternal behavior, in particular, seems to be more independent of physiological changes after the ewe has mothered one lamb. The quality of maternal behavior in artificially reared cats, dogs, or sheep has not been documented. When maternal behavior in beef and dairy cattle is compared, the beef cattle exhibit more maternal behavior. These animals, at least on the range, raise their calves, and adequate maternal behavior is necessary for their calves' survival. Artificial rearing of dairy calves has been practiced on many generations of cows; consequently, few dairy cows have had much experience at mothering or at being mothered.

Concaveation

The presence of neonates can induce maternal behavior in virgin females and even in males. This phenomenon is called concaveation. When exposed to rat pups daily for 7 days, virgin female rats, and even male rats, will begin to retrieve the young, lick them, and even huddle over them in the typical nursing position. Mice will show similar behavior with no latency whatsoever as long as the pups presented are only 1 or 2 days old. Maternal behavior can, therefore, be induced in these rodents in the absence of hormonal stimulation, although hormonal stimulation accelerates the appearance of maternal behavior. The phenomenon of concaveation is used to force acceptance of alien (not the female's own) or rejected young. It is used to treat lamb and foal rejection.

Recognition of the young (individual signature vs. maternal labeling)

It is not clear whether licking the neonate imparts the mother's odor to the offspring or consumption of her milk imparts a recognizable odor to the offspring's feces. If that is the basis of recognition, it is maternal labeling. Another possibility is that the mother learns the individual olfactory signature of the offspring.

External factors that elicit maternal behavior

What stimuli emanating from the neonate are important in maternal behavior? Some of these stimuli are presumably olfactory, such as the smell of a small conspecific wet with amniotic fluid. The appearance of the newborn may also serve as a visual stimulus, for Lorenz[1179] has hypothesized that the short forehead, cheeks swollen by sucking fat pads, and the erratic gait of the neonate elicit maternal behavior in a number of species, including humans.

Summary

To summarize our somewhat sketchy knowledge of the biological basis of maternal behavior, we conclude that hormonal priming can lower the threshold for the initiation of maternal behavior that can be brought on and maintained as a response to the stimuli characteristic of the neonate even in the absence of the appropriate rise and fall of gonadal and pituitary hormones and cervical stimulation. Animals, especially those believed to be higher on the phylogenetic scale, can learn to be good mothers both by having been mothered themselves as infants and by having been mothers previously. Vaginal stimulation and oxytocin release appear to be important in sheep and horses; otherwise, the hormonal and central nervous system control of maternal behavior in domestic animals is virtually unknown and is a field that demands more attention from biological scientists. Fig. 5.1 summarizes the factors involved in maternal behavior.

PIGS

The free-ranging sow

Maternal behavior in sows can be divided into two prepartum behaviors: nest site seeking and nest building, as well as the postpartum behavior of nursing. One day before farrowing, free-ranging sows will leave their herd and their normal home range, traveling as little as 50 m (153 ft) or as far as 7 km (4 miles). They will build several rudimentary nests before selecting a final site at which they dig a hole, which typically is 10 cm (4 in) deep and 1.5 m (4.5 ft) wide. They will bring grass and sometimes sticks to the nest.[953] The nest is usually located under protective overhead cover, usually in a forested area.[1390] The sow will spend more and more of

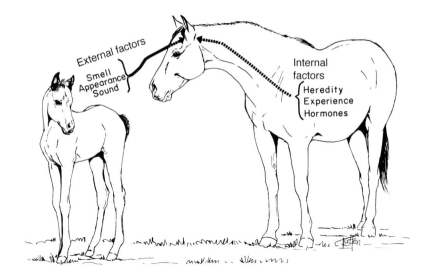

Fig. 5.1   Factors that influence the expression of maternal behavior. The horse is used as an example, but there are similar influences on maternal behavior in all domestic animals.[886] (Copyright 1979, with permission of Veterinary Practice Publishing.)

her time building her nest during the day of parturition. Usually, 3–7 hours elapse between the onset of nest building and farrowing. Oxytocin increase may inhibit nest building.

The sow stays with the piglets for the first 2 days and then leaves to forage for short periods. The nest will be defended against the sow's juvenile offspring and against other adults. Failure to defend the nest results in crushing of the piglets and a consequent threefold to fourfold increase in mortality.[1411] Nursing takes place every 45 minutes. Piglets do not all suckle simultaneously at first, but later their behavior becomes more synchronous. For the first 2 days, the sow initiates all nursing, but after that the piglets initiate at least half of the nursing bouts. On day 7, the piglets leave the nest and the sow rejoins the herd. By day 9, the piglets sleep in the herd's communal nest. The pigs are weaned at 14–15 weeks.[950]

The group-housed sow

Sows housed in group pens become more aggressive as parturition approaches.[76] Gilts, but not sows, prefer an enclosed area in which to farrow. That is probably an innate behavior related to the behavior of the free-ranging sow that leaves her herd to farrow.[1509,1802] Group-housed sows nurse as frequently as single-housed females, but terminated the bouts more.

The confined sow

Farrowing crates

Modern husbandry practices have all but eliminated most porcine maternal behavior except nursing. Sows are placed in farrowing crates that prevent them from turning around or touching the sides of the pen; consequently, the piglets are protected from crushing. Most crushing takes place when the sow lies down, especially when she lies down on her side rapidly. Sows lie down in five steps: (1) One foot is lifted and placed before the other until she in kneeling on one limb and then the other limb is advanced until she is kneeling on both limbs, (2) there is a pause, (3) the sow slides one knee forward along the floor and rotates her head and upper body until her shoulder and head rest on the floor, (4) another pause may occur, and (5) the sow lowers her hindquarters, rotating slightly, causing the rear legs to slide sideways and the hindquarters drop so that the upper thigh lands on the floor. This takes between 7 and 20 sec. The slower the sow is to lie down, the less risk to her piglets. If she leans against the wall or a rail of a farrowing crate, she is less likely to crush the piglets.[426] Sows that lie on their sides during the immediate prepartum hours rather than nest building are more likely to crush their piglets.[1484]

Because crushing of piglets by the sow is such a common cause of piglet mortality, it is interesting that sows do not respond to the feel or sight of a piglet under them; they do respond to the sound of a piglet squeal, although it must be loud.[916,917] Sows respond by standing up or rolling to only half of the calls.[922] Sows that crush their piglets have less maternal behavior in general; they spend less time building a nest prefarrowing and respond less to play backs of piglets distress calls.[50] Maternal response to piglet vocalizations both an unrelated piglet and their own declines with parity.[811] Sows are most responsive to piglet squeals on the first 2 days postpartum, the time when piglets are in the most danger of being crushed if the sow lies on them.[914]

Crushing of piglets is reduced but not eliminated by farrowing crates. Sows can be kept in an ellipsoid crate that allows them to turn around but does not result in any more crushing of piglets than does a traditional crate.[1181] Losses can be reduced further using a device that shocks the sow's belly when a piglet screams; however, the sow may also be shocked when extraneous noises trigger the device.[647] Another approach to preventing crushing is to attract the piglets away from the sow with a simulated udder, a warm, resilient, sow-scented area under the heat lamp.[1103] Because most piglets are crushed as the sow lies down, it is important that she lies down against a wall, which not only protects the piglets, but also supports the sow. Sows prefer the back wall of the pen, so a solid wall with no protuberances should be available there.[427]

Nest building

The use of farrowing crates for nursing sows has resulted in much lower death rates for piglets because the sow rarely can crush or cannibalize her young, but farrowing crates prevent sows from building the elaborate nests used by wild and feral swine; all that remains of the nest-building behavior is a futile pawing at the floor of the crate. The restlessness, which increases linearly during the last 48 hours prepartum, probably represents attempts at nest seeking and nest building. If sows are introduced to farrowing crates the day before farrowing, they had more still-born piglets, indicating that environmental changes can be detrimental.[1483]

Nest-building behavior consists of two distinct factors, gathering nest material and arranging it by rooting and nosing. Environmental factors, temperature, and udder comfort influence nest building.[43] Sows gather more material when no artificial shelter is available.[949] When given access to an earth floor, sows will excavate a nest 8 hours before farrowing and farrow in it.[915] Sows in a pen provided with material (straw is preferred) build nests the day before (16 hours before parturition) and for several days after parturition.[756,1085,2016] Nest building is triggered initially by endogenous factors including prostaglandin F2 alpha[302,303] and prolactin, which stimulate nosing and rooting, but external stimuli, that is, nest material, is necessary for pawing, carrying, and arranging; that is, pigs do not engage in carrying nothing to their nest.[335] If the pig has a preformed nest, nest building is increased, not decreased.[949] For example, if a hollow in the sand filled with 23 kg (50.7 lb) of straw is available, sows begin to nest build earlier and root more but do not carry as much straw to the nests.[75] Provision of sawdust to preparturient sows increases nesting behavior, shortens their labor, and may result in fewer piglet deaths.[397] In the natural situation, sows use branches to build their nests, and provision of branches in addition to straw apparently causes sows to be satisfied with their nests in that they do not continue to nest build after their first piglet is born, as many sows that have access only to straw will do.

Parturition

Most farrowings take place in the afternoon or night.[1768] After labor begins, most sows lie in lateral recumbency. The sow will swish her tail violently as abdominal straining takes place. Parturition usually takes 3–4 hours, but varies considerably with litter size and the condition of the gilt. If parturition is interrupted by moving the pig to a new pen after one piglet is born, a delay of hours occurs until the next piglet is born. Opiates released in response to the stress of moving inhibit oxytocin release; however, exogenous oxytocin will reinitiate labor.

Behavior of the sow toward the neonate

Maternal behavior in sows is composed of three main factors: (1) calmness (low cortisol response to minor stressors), care when lying down to avoid piglets, few changes in behavior, and remaining in the nursing posture following milk ejection; (2) protectiveness (response to piglet squeals and human approach to piglets); and (3) nursing activity.[1796]

When not confined, the sow will eat the placenta. The function of placentophagia remains unknown. It may be a recycling of nutrients or a form of defense against predators by removing odors. Placentophagia enhances analgesia in rats.[1062] The question of whether this occurs in domestic animals as well deserves investigation.[1101] Parturition is painful, so the use of analgesics is warranted. In fact, piglet crushing can be reduced by treatment of the sow with butorphanol probably because the sows were less active.[1103]

Sows do little licking of their newborns even when not confined in a farrowing pen. Therefore, human attendance at parturition is recommended. Although most piglets begin to breathe and quickly struggle free from the fetal membranes, a few will not. The removal of membranes, clearing of the airway, and stimulation of respiration can save a piglet that would otherwise die.

Behavior of the neonatal piglet toward the sow

Piglets make a most startling transition from fetal to independent existence. They may be apneic for 5–10 seconds after birth. Then, they give a few gasps before beginning to breathe regularly. Their eyes and ears are open, and they are able to walk immediately, although their gait is staggering for the first few hours. The firstborn may be slow to find the udder, but later-born pigs apparently respond to the voices of their littermates and quickly begin to seek the udder. Most piglets are nursing within 30 minutes of birth.[825] During farrowing and for some time afterward, piglets can suckle continuously, presumably because oxytocin levels are high; thus, they are rewarded for each suckle in the correct place, that is, on a teat.

Piglets are attracted to soft, warm surfaces,[1991] pig vocalizations, and the sow's odors, and they move in the direction of the sow's hair growth.[1615] Washing the udder with an organic solvent delays nipple location, as does blocking the piglet's sense of smell, indicating the importance of odors.[1370] Texture may be even more important because piglets are more attracted to a cloth covered artificial udder than to one to which sow odor has been applied [1895] The firstborn pigs appear to use thermal, tactile, and olfactory cues to find the udder, whereas the later-born probably respond to the suckling sounds of their older littermates and walk straight to it because social facilitation is strong in pigs at birth. Suckling attempts are probably stimulated by tactile contact with a protuberance (the teat). Piglets rarely attempt to suckle on a haired portion of the sow; they will suck on the snout or the tip of the sow's vulva. Piglets nose the udder and intersperse nosing with gapes, the behavior in which the piglet opens its mouth as if to grasp a teat. Larger pigs do more gaping, which may account for their success in reaching teats. The nosing behavior of lighter pigs declines more rapidly than that of heavier pigs.[1615] The piglet may find the udder, give a few inept sucks at a teat, and then make another circuit or two of the sow before it settles down to nursing.

Experiments using artificial sows have revealed that the piglets are attracted to the voice of the sow and to either end of the udder, but they avoid the middle and quickly abandon teats that give no milk.[956] Competition during formation of the teat order is intense, and only one-third of pigs end up on the teat initially chosen. After a teat has been chosen and won by competition with other piglets, it is recognized by odor rather than visual cues.[957]

Nursing

Nursing causes release of opiates so that sows are less reactive to painful stimuli at that time. The opiates stimulate prolactin and somatotropin release.[1664] Approximately 10 hours after the birth of the first pig, nursing becomes cyclic.[1132] Nursing bouts occur approximately every 45 minutes. The interval between nursing is longer at night than during the day. Small litters suckle less frequently than large.[2040] The sow ordinarily calls the piglets to suckle with a low-pitched rhythmic grunting. Piglets can initiate nursing by giving high/deep grunts. As the piglets begin to massage the udder with their snouts, the frequency of the sow's grunts increases from one per second to a peak of 10 per second. The more pigs massaging the udder, the faster the sow grunts and the less time until the release of oxytocin, which occurs at the peak of grunting followed in 25 seconds by milk letdown.[42] Piglets grunt faster and faster as they await milk letdown, but there is no increase in grunting rate preceding an unsuccessful suckling bout (no milk letdown).[924] Sows may stretch a foreleg and rotate it toward the udder while the piglets are massaging the udder (foreleg rowing). Rubbing of the udder of a lactating sow can induce her to lie down and begin to give the nursing call. Stimulation of the anterior half of the udder and, especially, rubbing of the nipples in that area can increase the grunting rate.[633,634,638] Rubbing of the belly has a calming effect on even immature or male pigs and can be used to great advantage in handling swine.

A suckling bout is divided into four phases: (1) an initial massaging of the udder for 1 minute; (2) a quiet phase during which the piglets' ears go back and they stop massaging, which may correspond to the peak of the sow's grunts; (3) true suckling for approximately 14 seconds while the milk is ejected, during which the piglets' ears are back, their tails are tightly curled, and their front legs are in rigid extension; and (4) a final massage phase that is quite variable in length, 2–15 minutes.[689] The massage stimulates prolactin release, which will increase milk production. The less weight a piglet gains, the more it will massage the udder after suckling, indicating that hunger drives this behavior.[1794] These slow-growing piglets also suckle more between nursing bouts.[1891] Young piglets often fall asleep on the nipple or curled beside the udder, whereas older pigs will nose the udder and pull the teats for some time.

Not all nursing bouts are successful. In 22% of the nursing bouts, the sow may call the piglets, which approach and massage the udder, but no milk is ejected. Unsuccessful nursing usually occurs less than 40 minutes after a successful bout. The piglets leave the udder as they do after a successful nursing but return much sooner.[632] The proportion of unsuccessful bouts increases if sows are moved to an unfamiliar pen.[1665] Apparently, unsuccessful nursing bouts occur in free-ranging sows.[954] Unsuccessful nursings can also occur when the sow terminates the bout by changing position. She may be responding to the vocalization of piglets fighting for a teat.[921]

The strong social facilitation and dependence on vocal communication exhibited by pigs can be used to practical advantage. If one sow in the farrowing house calls her litter to nurse, soon all the litters will be nursing. Nursing rates and weight gain can be increased by playing tape recordings of nursing noises to the sows at more frequent intervals than they normally nurse.[1817] A talented manager can imitate the noises and accomplish the same thing.[779] Piglets can also initiate suckling by their calls and persistent nudging at the sow. If half a litter has been fasted, the hungry piglets will induce the sow to lie down, and then all the piglets will nurse, although the nonfasted piglets will consume less.[876]

Despite the apparent low level of maternal activity in sows, piglets separated from their mother for even a short time (a few hours) exhibit considerable distress. They vocalize with either squeals or closed-mouth grunts[637] up to 21 times per minute. The vocalizations increase with the length of isolation. The vocalization changes to a higher-frequency, quacking vocalization when the piglets can hear their mother's voice, which they can discriminate from that of another sow.[1753] If the piglets are in a strange pen, they will make persistent efforts to escape, and they often urinate. The vocalizations are reduced if the piglets are isolated as a litter rather than individually. The effect of the presence of littermates is additive with that of the sow, so a litter placed in a strange pen with their mother gives only closed-mouth grunts and a few squeals. The olfactory cues are not sufficient to prevent vocalizations because the presence of the sow's bedding has no attenuating effect on vocalizations.[637] If the separated litter is closely confined and provided with a heat lamp, they are much quieter, and weight losses, especially due to urination, are reduced. Similarly, cuddling of a piglet will reduce the number and volume of its squeals.

Mutual recognition

Sows and piglets apparently use olfaction to identify one another but need more than 1 day and possibly as long as a week to learn. The piglets can identify their dam's feces, milk, and urine odors,[858, 860, 1371] as well as her vocalizations.[858] Sows respond to playbacks of piglet separation calls by vocalizing,[1983] but cannot discriminate their own from other piglets on the basis of their voices. They can identify their own piglets by the time they are a week old on the basis of olfaction.[859] Piglets can easily be fostered onto another sow when they and the sow's litter are less than a day old. After that, the fostered piglets walk around, vocalize, and are reluctant to suckle, perhaps because they have already formed a bond to their dam.[1544]

Sows will reject strange piglets older than 2 days. The rejection is based on olfaction, for Meese and Baldwin[1292] found that anosmic sows would accept strange piglets.

Defensive reaction

Sows normally exhibit strong defensive reactions when their piglets are threatened. They give a crescendo of barks, open their mouths, and attack. Only when pigs are defending their young are they really dangerous. The use of the farrowing crate has had a definite effect on the maternal behavior of sows. The sows can do nothing if their piglets are handled or hurt despite the piglets' loud distress calls. In herds in which the piglets are handled often and by many people, as in university or research institutions, the sows become accustomed to the distress calls of their pigs. A sow may even continue to sit on a piglet that is screaming loudly and eventually smother it.

Weaning

Weaning begins at five weeks when the sow begins to aggress against the piglets; however, the piglets continue to suckle for 80 days. Although the number of nursing bouts (approximately 20/day) does not change much from day 3 to day 30 of lactation, the duration of individual nursing bouts decreases from 7 to 5 minutes. The number of nursing bouts terminated by the sow increases.[1918] When able to leave piglets behind by stepping over a barrier, sows spend increasing time away from their piglets; the amount of time varies with litter size.[1466,1982,1983] Surprisingly, those sows who spend most time away from their piglets respond most to calls of isolated piglets.[241–243,1520] Some sows that have the opportunity to leave their piglets may do so, but confining sows with their piglets reinstates normal maternal behavior.[242] This fact indicates that contact, particularly visual contact, with the piglet is necessary to sustain the maternal behavior.

Under modern management techniques, piglets are weaned at four weeks or even younger. Early weaning (at 3–4 weeks old) of piglets is often practiced in order to decrease the interlitter time.[1529] Early-weaned pigs massage and nibble on one another, yet spend less time rooting or nibbling on other objects. If placed in cages, early-weaned pigs dog-sit (on their haunches) seven times more frequently than do piglets in straw-bedded pens[1927] which indicates that flooring type, as well as age at weaning, influences behavior. Aggression is higher when pigs are weaned at four weeks than if they are weaned at three weeks, but it decreases with time.[376] The piglets spend approximately 70% of the daylight hours lying down, 13% exploring, and 9% feeding.[17]

Because piglets eat little solid food at two weeks of age, weaning at this time is more stressful and is associated with greater inhibition of growth than is weaning at four weeks.[1314] The younger the piglets are when they are weaned, the more they squeal and "quack" and the higher pitched the squeals, declining from eight to one squeal per hour after 4 days of separation.[1979] Piglets weaned at three weeks are still vocalizing 6 days after weaning in contrast to pigs weaned at four weeks [376] Improvements in diet for young piglets[1979] has led to the practice of segregated early weaning (SEW). One of the behaviors observed in piglets weaned at one or two weeks of age is belly nosing. About 81% of the piglets engage in this behavior, which occupies 2.4% of their time. The behavior gradually increases, peaking by day 26 and decreasing by day 33. It is associated with social interactions with other pigs and so may not be a nursing attempt.[1136] Piglets that spend more time suckling before weaning are less likely to belly nose.[1892] Enrichment in the form of a foam rubber mat on the pen wall decreases belly nosing, but neither a rubber teat nor soil in which to root deceases the behavior.[210] These pigs eat less, especially when first weaned, and gain less.[2063]

To prevent piglets from sucking on one another and to prevent spread of gastroenteric diseases that plague artificially raised piglets, they can be housed separately. Pigs reared without the sow would defecate in the nesting area, whereas normally raised pigs do not.[127] Piglets raised in germ-free isolators give distress calls almost continuously during handling and feeding; conventionally raised pigs give distress calls only when hurt.[1432] Piglets weaned at 6 days show an initial increase in cortisol. A week after weaning, their urinary norepinephrine is lower than those of pigs weaned at 28 days, possibly indicating adrenal exhaustion.[792] Food intake can be increased and aggression decreased by application of the synthetic porcine pheromone to the pigs' snouts or to the feeder.[1272]

Weaning at four weeks is also stressful, particularly if the piglets of one litter are mixed with those of another. Aggression occurs, but can be reduced by pairing enrichment, in this case, a novel palatable food with an acoustic signal. This classical conditioning leads to more play and less aggression,[490] presumably as a response to the anticipation of the enrichment. Enrichment alone was less effective. Another method of reducing aggression and increasing weight gain at weaning is to allow litters in adjacent pens to interact so that they are "socialized" to one another before weaning.[836] Little cross suckling occurs.

In the United States, the majority of sows have been kept in gestation crates during pregnancy in order to prevent aggression among sows and to allow intake to be monitored. Because these sows cannot walk or turn around, group housing is now being considered. Effects of the sow's housing environment on their offspring's behavior have revealed that piglets of group housed sows gain more weight, do not have to be hand fed at weaning, and are less stressed by isolation.[1789]

Clinical problems

Cannibalism

Cannibalism occasionally occurs in sows; nervous primiparous gilts are the most likely offenders. Cannibalism is responsible for 4% of piglet deaths and occurs in 18% of litters.[398] The most common occurrence is immediately after parturition. In fact, many sows will bark at the first piglet that walks by their heads after parturition.[1574] Farrowing crates successfully prevent cannibalism unless an unwary piglet walks right in front of the sow. The tranquilizer, azaperone 2.2 mg/kg, has been used to treat cannibalistic sows.

Refusal to nurse

A more common problem is seen in sows suffering from mastitis; a sow that is normally a good mother will attack her litter whenever they attempt to nurse. This early behavioral sign warns of disease before many physical signs can be detected. This type of behavior is seen in sows that become afflicted with mastitis late in lactation, after the farrowing crates have been removed. Sows that have the mastitis metritis syndrome shortly after farrowing are usually too ill to protest when the piglets suckle. The failure of the sow to eat and of the piglets to gain weight is the best clinical evidence of the latter syndrome.

SHEEP

Maternal behavior in sheep has an important clinical aspect, as most lamb mortality occurs within the first week of life in range-reared sheep. Mortality rates are from 5 to 15%, rising to as high as 50% in huge flocks in bad weather, even in the absence of predators.[1363] Ewes do use shelters more after lambing, probably as predator avoidance behavior.[1527] Abnormal or weak maternal behavior accounts for parts of these high losses and perhaps for some of the losses attributed to coyote predation. Most maternal rejection or simply poor mothering without absolute rejection occurs in young ewes and in those that had difficulty at parturition.[1966]

Parturition

Lambs may be born at any time of the day or night, with peak frequencies being noted at 9–12 a.m. and at 3–6 p.m.[1154] A few days before parturition, the ewe withdraws from the flock, if on the range, and seeks some sort of shelter. Shelter seeking by the ewe improves the environment into which the lamb is born so that its chances of survival are greater; however, the ewe is responding primarily to her own thermoregulatory needs whereby shorn, but not unshorn, sheep seek shelter.[1190] Allelomimetic behavior is so strong in sheep that some of the flock may follow her. In a pen, the ewe will withdraw from social contact and seek a corner.[279] She will show restlessness, circle, vocalize, rub her head on her flanks, lick herself, and paw at her bedding 60–90 minutes before parturition.[522] Grazing and ruminating ceases. The older the ewe, the shorter the lapse of time between the onset of restlessness and the onset of labor. The interval between onset of labor and the appearance of the lamb can vary, but is usually 30–60 minutes.

Even before parturition, 20% of ewes show maternal behavior toward other lambs.[84] This prepartum maternal behavior results in lamb stealing (discussed later in this section). The amniotic fluid dripping from the vagina to the ground attracts the ewe. She will sniff and lick at bedding contaminated with amniotic fluid. This attraction to amniotic fluid can be used to predict parturition because only ewes close to parturition will eat food mixed with amniotic fluid. Ovine or caprine,[1129] but not bovine, amniotic fluid is accepted,[91] indicating that some species specificity exists. The attraction of the ewe to this fluid may serve to keep the ewe in the area where the birth will take place, ensuring that the lamb will not be abandoned before it can get to its feet.[1780]

Behavior of the ewe toward the newborn lamb

Licking and bleating

When the lamb is born, the ewe begins to lick it for 80% of the first hour after parturition.[511] Simultaneously, she emits a special parturition call that is a very low-pitched gurgle or rumble, a call that also may be given before parturition. Primiparous ewes bleat more, and hill breeds bleat more than Suffolks, perhaps reflecting the greater risks of losing lambs in the harsher hill environment.[514,515] The call is heard only at parturition in domestic sheep, but it persists in the feral Soay sheep as a close-contact call.[1756] The lamb's behavior influences that of the ewe. If the lamb is inactive, the ewe will cease licking. Licking of the lamb can be very important in cold or windy weather because it serves to dry the neonate; it additionally serves to stimulate the lamb. While the lamb is recumbent, the ewe licks its head, even restraining the lamb with a front leg to prevent it from standing. Licking of the perineal area stimulates the lamb to rise. After the lamb is standing, usually within 30 minutes,[1966] the ewe continues to lick it, but mostly on the hindquarters. If the ewe stops licking, the lamb gives distress calls.[149] Finally, licking of the lamb by the ewe establishes the maternal–offspring bond, for the ewe will be able to identify her lamb by smell and taste. Usually, the fetal membranes are licked off the lamb and ingested, but the placenta is not eaten (Fig. 5.2).

Lamb licking rate is correlated with estrogen levels at parturition. Circulating estrogen and the ratio of estrogen to progesterone ratio in late pregnancy are higher in sheep with good maternal behavior.[516] Ewes are less attentive to embryo-transferred lambs of a breed different from themselves.[512] Although mothers of twin lambs spend more time licking their offspring than do mothers of singletons, the increase is not double; so, twin lambs, especially the second

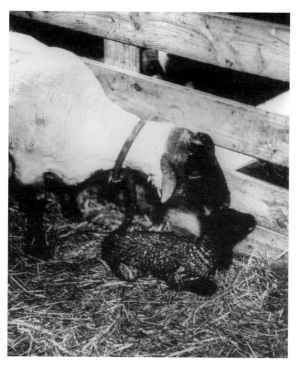

Fig. 5.2 Ewe licking the head of her newborn lamb. (Courtesy of Dr. Martin Siegel, Annandale, NJ.)

born, are licked less than singletons.[1440] The lack of licking is reflected in the longer interval to successful suckling in twins.

The lamb raises and shakes its head, rolls onto its sternum, and bleats. It rises to its knees and stands first on the hind limbs and then both fore and hind. Although lambs are able to stand within 30 minutes or an hour of birth, it may take 2–3 hours before they find the udder.[40, 1966] The ewe plays a part in the search. She may either facilitate or inhibit teat seeking.

Suckling

The ewe is most attracted by the head of the lamb. As she circles to maintain head-to-head contact, she moves her hindquarters and udder away from the lamb, which hinders the lamb's attempt to find the udder. The innate pattern to which lambs appear to respond is the curved underline of the ewe. The newborn lamb moves toward the ewe's head and toward her udder—both areas appear to be attractive (Fig. 5.3). After the lamb has established contact with an underline, odor, texture, and temperature probably serve to guide him.[1948] The warmest surface of the ewe is her woolless inguinal area; furthermore, the lamb is attracted by the odor and resilience of the inguinal wax.[222, 223, 1950, 1951] Having its face contacted stimulates the lamb to push its head up and forward. Contact with the lips causes it to open its mouth and protrude the tongue.[1191, 1949] Contact with its tongue causes the lamb to curl the tongue into the suckling position.[1951] This series of innate responses serves to bring the lamb to the ewe, then to the udder, then to the teat, and finally to suckle the teat.

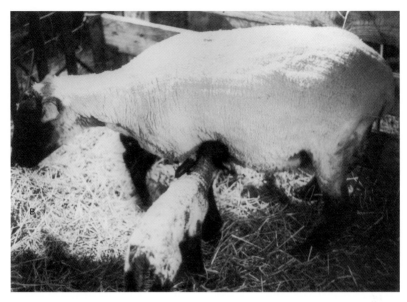

Fig. 5.3 Initial orientation of the lamb to the ewe's underline, but in the axilla rather than the udder. (Courtesy of Dr. Martin Siegel, Annandale, NJ.)

Lambs whose dams are stanchioned take longer to locate the udder,[40] indicating the active role the ewe usually plays. The drive to suckle is inhibited, but not eliminated, by intragastric loads of milk; consequently, hunger is not the lamb's only motivation.[39] After the udder has been located, the lamb uses visual cues to relocate it for subsequent sucklings.[150] "The ewe signals that she is prepared to nurse by standing with her head up and/or vocalizing. Ewes refuse far fewer suckling attempts if those ewe behaviors precede the suckling attempts.[513]

Advantage can be taken of the features to which a lamb responds to build a colostrum feeder from which the lamb will suckle without human aid. The colostrum feeder consists of a fleece-covered horizontal ledge through which soft rubber teats protrude at a 45° angle, 50 cm (20 in) off the ground.[639]

After suckling has begun, it occurs with great frequency; twin lambs suckle 22 times during 16 hours of daylight, and single lambs, 6–14 times.[477,1385] Newborn lambs may nurse for as long as 3 minutes in one bout; later, the duration falls to 20–40 seconds. Frequency of suckling and suckling duration both decrease with age. By the end of the first week, lambs suckle hourly, and by nine weeks, every 3 hours.

Triplets nurse less often and for shorter duration than singletons or twins.[552,555] Probably because they are not receiving adequate nourishment from their dams, they are most likely to try to suckle an alien ewe. During the first 2 weeks, the ewe will allow one twin to suckle without the other. Later, the ewe will walk away when the lamb nudges her in the inguinal area and will refuse to let one twin nurse until the other is also present. If the ewe is lying down, the lambs will not only nudge her but also jump on her back and paw at her in an attempt to make her stand. The ewes will call their 5-week-old lambs to them and then refuse to let them nurse. Such behavior encourages the lambs to stay in close contact.[551] As suckling decreases, grazing by the lambs increases. Although the ewe stays within 10 meters of the lamb the first few days, she will increase her distance from it as the lamb ages. During the first month of her lamb's life, the ewe will leave the flock to seek out her lamb if it has strayed. Thereafter, she will bleat but remain in the flock.

Acceptance of the lamb

The "critical period" during which a ewe will accept a lamb is the first several hours after parturition.[372,1781] Normally, a ewe will stay within two meters of her lamb for most of the first day.[1190] If a ewe's lamb is removed immediately after birth and before she has licked it, the ewe will accept any lamb presented to her. After the ewe has spent 30 minutes to 2 hours with a lamb, her own or a substitute, she will not accept another. If the lamb is removed 4 hours after birth, the ewe will continue to exhibit maternal behavior if it is returned within 24 hours.[1126] If the lamb is removed 7 days after parturition, the ewe will accept it when it is returned after 36 hours, but not after 72 hours by which time her maternal behavior has ceased.

The importance of olfactory cues in the establishment of the bond is demonstrated by the fact that ewes will temporarily accept strange lambs that have been rubbed with the ewe's placenta. Ewes can also be induced to follow their placentas.[372] Primiparous ewes will not accept a lamb whose wool has been washed free of amniotic fluid, whereas multiparous ewes will,[1128] indicating both the importance of amniotic fluid and the importance of prior experience at mothering. Olfaction is necessary for normal maternal behavior in primiparous, but not multiparous, ewes.[1127] If the ewes could not smell the lambs, they bleated less and licked the lamb less; the lambs took longer to suckle.

In hilly country, newborn lambs may roll down the hill away from the site of their birth. The ewe may neglect the lamb because the odor at the birth site is more attractive than the lamb itself. In this situation, a weak lamb, or the weaker of a pair of twins, is most likely to roll away and not be licked. A more vigorous lamb will survive and seek out the ewe. If too long a time elapses between parturition and the presentation of the lamb, the lamb may be rejected.

Mutual recognition by the ewe and lamb

Recognition of the lamb by the ewe. Recognition of lambs depends on at least three senses: olfaction, audition, and vision. The wool of the lamb contains the odor used by the ewe to identify her own lamb.[28,34] Apparently, ewes base their recognition of their lambs at a distance on vision and hearing and at a close range, 0.25 m (10 in) or less, on smell,[28,1161] recognition cues being reinforced each time the lamb suckles. By 6 hours postpartum, the ewe can recognize her lamb at a distance[1431] During nursing, the ewe sniffs at the tail and perianal area of the lamb. Olfactory bulbectomy eliminates the preparturient lip licking observed in Soay sheep, as well as the licking of the newborn and normal lamb recognition. The bulbectomized ewe will accept other lambs indiscriminately.[140] After a month of exposure to their lamb, anosmic ewes do not accept alien lambs as readily, although they still allow more contact and show less aggression than normal ewes.[580] Other senses can compensate in part for olfaction.

At least two senses must be impaired before ewes are unable to find their lambs.[1364] Visual cues may be most important, as indicated by ewes having had more trouble finding a hidden lamb than a silent one.[31] By changing the appearance of various portions of the lamb's body, it was found that maternal recognition was most impaired by altering the appearance of the head.[30] Although it represents only 12% of the body surface, the head is apparently the area that the ewe uses to identify the lamb visually. Evidence also shows that ewes use the color of their lambs to identify them. They reject their own lambs when they are dyed, and, if they do reaccept them, they will choose lambs of the same color when their own is not available.[28] Laboratory experiments (Chapter 1, "Communication") indicate that sheep can perceive color; the studies on lamb recognition indicate that sheep use color vision.

The strong individual recognition of her lamb by a ewe, however, can break down. Multiple-birth lambings of three, four, or more lambs are not uncommon, especially in Finnish Landrace sheep. As sheep are bred to produce litters, there may be changes in maternal behavior. The ewes rearing three lambs bleated less and approached a solitary lamb less often than ewes with singletons or twins.[1526] If several ewes and their litters are penned together, the ewes may not distinguish their own lambs from the others; communal suckling of all lambs by all ewes results.

Recognition of the ewe by the lamb. A signal originating from the lamb's gastrointestinal tract can be the mechanism for recognition of and preference for the dam. Lambs given their dam's colostrum by stomach tube and with no experience suckling from her chose her instead of an alien ewe at 24 hours of age.[706] The bond of the lamb to its mother is stimulated by colostrums ingestion, which leads to release of cholecystokinin and stimulation of vagal afferents.[1431] (Fig. 5.4) Without that stimulation, the lambs do not prefer their mother. They can learn which ewe will allow them to suckle while giving low-pitched bleats and which will butt them away while giving high-pitched bleats. They detect their own mothers faster and more accurately with age. During their first several days of life, lambs are not able to discriminate their mother from other ewes very well except at very close range. A lamb separated from its mother will rush up to the nearest ewe and attempt to suckle, only to be butted aside. Lambs can distinguish their dam from an alien ewe at 24 hours of age by approaching her pen, but, if tested again, will approach the same pen whether or not their dam is there. That indicates that after they have learned where

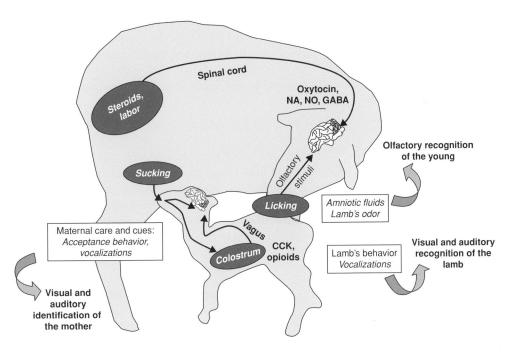

Fig. 5.4 The bond of the lamb to its mother is stimulated by colostrum ingestion, which leads to release of cholecystokinin and stimulation of vagal afferents.[1431] (Copyright 2007, with permission of Elsevier.)

to find the dam, they have difficulty finding her in a different location. By 3 days, they are able to recognize their dam from a distance, but they do not appear to use olfaction to recognize their dams even at close range. Vision and hearing are more important.[1430] Given a choice between their own mothers, similar (same breed), or dissimilar ewes (different breed), they will continue to be more attracted to similar rather than dissimilar ewes.[29,1754]

The importance of hearing was demonstrated by Arnold et al.,[80] who found that lambs were more apt to approach a ewe that was not their mother when the voices of the ewes were muffled. Technical advances in reproduction have allowed advances in understanding of auditory recognition. Most Dalesbred and Jacob lambs born after embryo transfer to Dalesbred ewes could identify the ewe on the basis of her voice, whereas most of those born to Jacob ewes could not.[1752] Sonographic analysis indicated more intersheep differences among bleats of Dalesbred ewes than among Jacob bleats.[1750,1751]

As lambs mature, visual cues become more important. A lamb less than a week old is not affected by a change in his dam's coat, such as shearing or blackening, but a 2-week-old lamb may hesitate to join a visually altered dam.[26] Covering the pens in which the ewes were restrained slows the approach of their lambs.[1755]

A critical period within the first few hours after parturition may exist for acceptance of lambs by ewes; however, the lamb is not restricted in time as far as his social attachments are concerned. The tendency to follow any large moving object is most marked during the first 3 days of life; for the next 3 days, fear responses predominate, but from 6 days to 2 months, lambs will continue to follow even an artificial sheep model.[2041] Lambs tend to follow large moving objects, but imprinting in the avian sense does not occur, for a lamb's attachment can be quite impermanent. Lambs easily can become attached to a nanny goat or to a human who feeds them. Lambs that had been normally reared with ewes quickly formed attachments to dogs when one of each species was penned together. Within eight weeks, the lamb would follow the dog, vocalize if the dog was removed, and even run a maze to be reunited.[310] After living in a normal situation for 4 months, the lambs no longer preferred dogs to sheep. Therefore, social attachments in lambs seem to be relatively easily formed and equally easily dissolved. This phenomenon of attachment can be used to bond sheep to cattle. The cattle deter coyotes from attacking the sheep. See Chapter 2, Aggression and Social Structure, referring to the section "Guard Dogs for Predator Control."

Weaning

Weaning does not exactly parallel decline in milk production. Milk production falls gradually, but suckling stops abruptly when milk production reaches a threshold.[86] A study of free-ranging Soay sheep found that the ewe–lamb bond ceased just before the estrous period. The ewe lambs continued to follow their dams but the ram lambs did not. None of the lambs slept touching their dams as they had done previously. The young sheep associated with their peer groups, the ewes remained in the dam's home range groups, and the rams wandered off to join a ram group.[722]

Artificial weaning

Weaning lambs at 2 days causes a rise in cortisol and immune suppression. Lambs weaned at 2 or 15 days do not gain weight as quickly as unweaned lambs.[1397] When weaned at three weeks, lambs will bleat, but the bleating rate is lower if they are paired with another lamb, especially if that lamb is its twin.[1533] Lambs remember one another and are less stressed, that is, emit fewer distress vocalizations if they are with a lamb they lived with a week before separation from ewe. They show a preference for familiar lambs, but treat lambs they have lived with recently similarly to those they had lived with previously; that is, they remembered them.[1150] Two-stage weaning in which the lambs are prevented from suckling for a week by a udder net before separation from the ewe results in less stress as evidenced by less agitation and fewer vocalizations than one-stage weaning in which the lamb is simply removed from the ewe.[1697] Inducing estrus in the ewes and tethering rams in the enclosure with the ewes reduces weaning stress and vocalizations by the ewes.[1495]

Clinical problems

Poor maternal behavior is often seen in ewes that have been in labor more than 30 minutes. The corticosteroid levels of such ewes are elevated, indicating that they are stressed.[279] Poor maternal behavior may vary; the ewe may reject the lamb outright, but more frequently she will lick it in a desultory fashion only and nervously avoid the lamb's attempt to nurse.

Great breed differences appear in the frequency of abandonment of one of a pair of twin lambs. Merino sheep are much more likely to abandon one of their twin lambs than are Dorsets or Romney.[37]

Cross-fostering

The problem of cross-fostering of lambs is a common one. In general, older ewes will more readily accept lambs than will younger ones.[1781] Fortunately, if a ewe is exposed to young of its own species long enough, maternal behavior will occur. The process (concaveation) may take weeks, and the ewe should be stanchioned or somehow restrained so that the lamb will not be badly butted in the interval before maternal behavior appears. Tranquilization of the ewes with pherphenazine will facilitate acceptance[1402] but does not facilitate fostering of alien lambs onto ewes with their own lamb present.[1886] Diazepam administered after parturition will facilitate acceptance of an alien lamb by a ewe and could be used to facilitate cross-fostering as well.[579] A variety of methods have been used to facilitate cross-fostering. The time-honored method is to tie the skin of the ewe's own lamb over the lamb to be fostered. There are, however, quicker and easier methods of providing olfactory cues from the ewe's own lamb that do not depend on skinning a dead lamb. These include pouring amniotic fluid on the alien lamb, washing the lamb,[36] and putting a garment worn by the ewe's own lamb inside out on the alien.[33,38,1546] This method of transferring the familiar scent to the alien lamb also is successful in fostering a second lamb onto a ewe.

Visual cues should also be altered. Either the lamb can be tied so that it cannot stand, thus mimicking the attempts of a neonate to stand, or visual cues can be eliminated. Stanchioning the ewe is effective because the ewe cannot move away from the lamb or butt it, and if her view of the lamb is also blocked (eliminating visual cues), fostering is facilitated.[27,1545] Advantage should also be taken of cervical stimulation, as already discussed here, to facilitate fostering.[998] The technique of slime grafting, in which the vaginal fluid of the ewe is rubbed on the lamb to be fostered, probably owes its success to the consequent vaginal stimulation in addition to, or instead of, the transfer of her odor to the lamb.

Mismothering

Mismothering, that is, maternal behavior directed toward a lamb that is not the ewe's own, is a common problem, especially in large flocks in which ewes are not penned separately for parturition. Up to 15% of lambs may be raised by ewes that are not their mothers. Many combinations exist. A ewe's lamb may be born dead and the ewe will steal another ewe's lamb. She may steal a lamb before parturition, have one of her own, and be credited with twins. Although stolen lambs may survive, it is impossible to make accurate statements about productivity of a given ewe under these circumstances. A shepherd might cull a productive ewe and keep one that never produces twins but often acquires them.[1992] The opportunities to mismother are increased when sheep are confined at parturition; however, if cubicles are provided, the incidence of mismothering is considerably lower in those ewes that choose to lamb in them,[697] but if isolated from their flock mates for 24 hours, lambs fail to differentiate their mother from other ewes.[1930]

Oral vices of artificially reared lambs

Artificially reared lambs suck one another's navel or scrotum and eat feces. Such behavior may cause injury or interfere with weight gain.[1812]

GOATS

As parturition approaches, does, especially multiparous ones, leave the herd and seek a sheltered place, almost always near a vertical object, to kid. The does will defend this area and the kid both before and for the first day after the kid is born. A doe is usually very agitated vocalizing, urinating, and moving, but this response disappears just before parturition.[1525] Vaginal cervical stimulation can induce maternal behavior in goats as well as sheep. Parturition is most likely to occur during the day at a time when goats are generally inactive. As parturition approaches, they grunt, paw the ground, kick, and lick their backs.[1569] Does usually lie down to kid. After parturition, the kid will be sniffed and immediately licked; the head is the primary target. The licking continues for 2–4 hours. Although the total time licking twins by the mother is longer, it is not twice as long; therefore, twin kids are licked less than singletons.[1570] The doe will vocalize frequently, using a low-pitched bleat similar to the rumble of periparturient sheep. Vaginocervical stimulation can be used to induce a recently parturient doe to accept an alien kid.[1618] There seems to be a critical period of an hour for acceptance of the kid; kids removed at birth and presented to the doe an hour later may be rejected.[748,1617] The doe must have contact with the kid for more than 5 minutes to become not only maternally responsive but also selective in that response, that is, accepting only her own kids.[260,725,1619] Olfaction seems to be important for selective maternal behavior; anosmic goats accept all kids, rather than only their own.[1038,1617] Within 4 hours after the kid's birth, the doe can recognize it by sight and sound. The small ruminants seem unable to distinguish between species: lambs can easily be cross-fostered onto goats and vice versa.

Intensive maternal behavior is short lived in goats because within a day (or after 3 days in some goat populations), the kid will have left the doe to hide. Hiding can last as long at 6 weeks. Some does are stayers, remaining close to the area where the kid is hidden, but others are leavers, travel a considerable distance from the kid. The doe will approach the hidden kid several times a day and call to it. The kid will answer and emerge to suckle as infrequently as twice a day. In the absence of a proper hide, a dim area with vertical sides and a roof, hiding behavior may not be recognized, but it has persisted in domestic as well as feral goats.[1140,1657]

Goat kids should stand within 20 minutes and suckle within an hour.[44,834,1139] The kid seeks the udder and usually searches the axilla first because the doe is turned toward the kid licking it. The kids of does with udders transplanted to the neck region located the udder as quickly as the kids of normal does.[1814]

Two-day-old kids can identify their mothers visually; apparently they use their dam's pelage for recognition.[1141,1660] Twin kids are slower to learn to recognize their dam than singletons.[104] Nursing of twin kids in a domestic situation or after the hiding period occurs every 30 minutes the first week, but falls to once every hour or two by 1 month.[451] Kids are more apt to be farther from their mothers than is the non-hiding lamb that develops visual recognition only slowly.

Weaning in the wild occurs between 3 and 6 months. It is interesting that prolactin release occurs in response to suckling by any kid—own or alien—but oxytocin release occurs only in response to suckling by the doe's own kid. Maternal behavior is maintained by the visual, auditory, and acoustic cues from the kid; suckling is not necessary.[1525]

Clinical problems

Kid rejection

The importance of olfactory identification of the young is emphasized by the following case: a week-old kid was castrated; an open castration technique was used in which incisions were made and the testes removed. When the kid was returned to the doe, she took one sniff and rejected it. The kid had to be hand raised (Dr. Mary Smith, personal observation). The smell of the fresh wound was probably responsible for the rejection response. Closed castration techniques should probably be used in suckling kids.

CATTLE

Some of the signs of imminent parturition are relaxation of the sacrosciatic ligament, slackening of the tissue of the perineum and vulva, distention of the udder and teats, and mucous discharge from the vulva. Unless the afternoon body temperature is below 39°C (102°F), parturition is unlikely even in the presence of all the other signs.[553] The normally lower body temperature of cattle in the morning interferes with the predictive value of temperature at that time.[491,493] Cow will alternate standing and lying much more frequently in the hours before parturition.[1961]

Parturition

The majority of cattle do not leave the herd to calve. This is probably an example of flexibility of behavior that takes advantage of geography. When trees or rocks are available, the cow leaves the herd and hides, but in an open pasture, the risk of predation is less if she stays with the herd.[1148]

Cows choose dry, elevated areas with shelter available, so those are the areas where one should search for lost neonatal calves. A periparturient cow will sniff and lick other calves, especially if she is within 24 hours of parturition and the other calf has just been delivered, whereas after parturition, all her activities are directed toward her own calf. Licking of alien calves does not cause rejection of the cow's own calf nor does suckling of an alien mother cause a calf to fail to suckle its own dam.[923] Other cows will sometimes push or butt a newborn calf. In a study of Hereford cattle, George and Barger[680] found that 82% of all parturitions take place between noon and midnight. Parturition times are distributed throughout the 24 hours, but dystocias occur mostly at mid-day.[1462,2070] During the first stage of labor, heifers were more restless and pawing than older cows. When introduced into a calving box during first stage labor, all cows explored the pen and most sniffed. They tended to build a nest by pushing the straw into a pile and lying on it; most got up again before calving. Cows that had a dystocia were more likely to rub against the walls and urinate during the first stage of labor.[1987]

A greater proportion of births will take place during the day if cows are fed late at night.[1183] Arching of the back and an elevated tail occur for 1–3 hours before the chorioallantoic membrane ruptures. When the membrane ruptures, the cow often licks the fluid and tends to stay near the spot, now attractive to the cow, where the fluid fell. Attraction to amniotic fluid begins up to 12 hours prepartum.[1518] About 95% of all cows are recumbent at the actual time of delivery.[1727] Approximately 100 minutes elapse from the rupture of the membranes to the birth of the calf. Placentophogia occurs in 82% of cattle. Parturition is longer in cows that give birth to large calves and in nervous heifers. In fact, labor may cease if nervous heifers are disturbed.[492] Handling of the cows at the time of calving appears to result in improved behavior at milking.[817]

Bonding

Contact between the cow and her calf for as brief a period as 5 minutes postpartum results in the formation of a strong, specific maternal bond. Cows groom their calves during the early postpartum period, concentrating on the back and abdomen. Licking the calf occupies up to half the cow's time during the first hour postpartum; heifers lick less.[526] Licking not only dries and stimulates the calf but also results in analgesia in the cow. Opiates are released at parturition and their analgesic effect is enhanced by ingestion of amniotic fluid.[1519] If contact between cows and their calves is delayed for 5 hours postpartum, 50% of the calves will be rejected; therefore, the critical period for formation of the cow–calf bond must be the first few hours postpartum. When the calf is removed after a brief initial contact, the cow vocalizes and is restless; however, after 24 hours, she can no longer distinguish her own calf.[898] There appears to be a sensitive period for calves to bond with cows. If calves are fed colostrum by bottle for 3 days, they suckle less and rub or lick the foster cows less than do calves who had suckled their dam before being placed with a foster cow.[1915]

Cows do not show kinship recognition of their calves. When twins were created by transferring an embryo into the uterus of already pregnant cows, the unrelated calf was treated just like their own calves.[1968] Maternal experience is also important in that maternal protectiveness increased with parity.[855] Calves can recognize their dams but make many errors when trying to identify their dam from 20 other cows. They tend to choose a cow of the same coat color as their mother.[1387] Advantage can be taken of the cow's nonselective maternal behavior to foster several calves—up to four onto one cow.

Suckling

The newborn calf shakes its head, snuffles, and sneezes. This behavior may begin during parturition as soon as the calf's shoulders are free of the mother's vulva. Some calves will remain motionless for up to 30 minutes after birth, but within an hour most calves can stand. A calf may take 30 minutes to an hour to locate the teats, and the cow's conformation may not provide the higher recess that the calf appears to seek. Passive transfer of immunity to calves is poor in cows that have had dystocias, presumably because the calves did not suckle as much or as often.[476] Most calves suckle within 3 hours, but up to a third of calves may not suckle within

6 hours of birth. This is particularly apt to be the case when the cow has a pendulous udder.[525] After the teat has been located for the first time, the calf will be able to locate it much more quickly at subsequent nursings. As the calf suckles, the cow will lick the perineum, stimulating urination and defecation by her calf. Calves that have not suckled for the first 6 days of life cannot learn to suckle.[583] Younger calves or those that have had suckling experience can learn to suckle from another cow.

When suckling, calves assume a particular stance with spread legs so that their shoulders are lowered, allowing them to butt upward at the udder. The butting appears to function in the stimulation of milk flow.[736] Similarly, artificially reared calves butt as they would butt the udder when milk flow is slow from an artificial teat.[742] As do other young ruminants, they nuzzle and lick along the cow, especially in high recesses such as the axilla and groin, and will mouth any hairless protuberance as they seek the udder.[1728] They appear to be confused when they encounter a hairless, teat-like object that does not supply milk. They wag their tails while suckling, although not at as high a rate as that of lambs. Newborn calves normally suckle 5–10 times a day.[754] Usually, the number of suckling bouts decreases with age, but beef calves may actually suckle more frequently with age, possibly because the milk supply of the beef cow is small.[736,1443] The most regular suckling time is at daybreak, with other bouts occurring between 9 a.m. and noon, 3 and 6 p.m., and 10:30 p.m. and 1 a.m.[1964] Most suckling takes place during the day.[1693] Suckling bouts are long, approximately 6–12 minutes, and do not seem to vary with frequency of suckling.[671,734,1502,1788] When housed in groups, calves will allosuck (suckling on a cow that is not their dam), usually from behind rather than in reverse parallel position. The calves that do so may not be obtaining adequate nutrition from their dam because they tend to be lighter weight.[1942]

It is now possible to produce twins in beef cattle by embryo transfer. These twins, like triplet lambs, suckle more often and are more apt to suckle from an alien cow. They usually approach the udder from the rear rather than in the normal antiparallel position. The smaller of the twins is the most likely to suckle from an alien cow, and the cow suckled usually has a single calf.[1548] The twins are groomed less than single calves.[1546]

When calves are raised artificially on a nippled feeder, they show similar rates of nursing when the milk is similar in concentration to cows' milk, but nursing increases in frequency when the milk is diluted. The calves often stand touching the wall while sucking from the feeder, just as they would touch the side of the cow if they were nursing. Calves weaned from a milk diet to solid food call less if the transition is made by supplying water rather than milk from the nipple feeders [300] or by reducing the amount of milk they receive in proportion to the amount of grain they consume.[1643]

Most dairy cows do not suckle their calves, but they are still physiologically responsive to calf stimuli. Playing tape recordings of hungry calves during one milking increases milk production in the following milking.[1252] One result of the increased popularity or organic products is that dairy calves may be raised more naturally, that is with their mothers. Calves allowed to suckle for 20 minutes twice a day grew as well as calves feed milk and crosssuckled less.[648] Cows that are allowed to suckle their own calves for 10 weeks produce more milk than do cows whose calves are removed. Although the suckled cows produce a large supply of milk, some of the total goes to the calf, and they do not compensate with marketable milk for all that the calf consumes. Calves allowed to nurse only twice a day gain more weight than those fed from buckets and those with continuous access to their dams.[548] Calves allowed to remain with their mothers in an automatic milking system lay down more and ruminated more but ate solid food, moved, socialized, and explored less than calves fed from an automatic milk dispenser. They did not exhibit stereotypic tongue rolling as the artificially fed calves did.[649]

Weaning

Cows do not break the bond with their yearling calf when their next calf is born; they may even allow the yearling to suckle, although they are more aggressive toward the yearling than they were before the birth of the younger calf.[1938]

In Bos indicus, bull calves are weaned at 11 months, but heifer calves are weaned much earlier, at 8 months.[1591] The cow apparently invests more of her resources in a son that can produce many offspring per year than in a daughter that can produce only one.

The shorter the time that a dairy cow and calf have been together, the less the effect of weaning; weaning at 6 hours results in fewer vocalizations by both the cow and the calf than if they were separated later.[1980] Beef calves are weaned at 200 days, much closer to the natural weaning age, but still show a reduction in growth. Allowing the calves fence-line contact with their dams reduces the negative effects of separation. The calves spend nearly half their time within 3 m (10 ft) of the fence separating them from their mothers.

When calves are weaned from a foster cow, the process can be done in two steps. In the first step, the calves are fitted with a nose flap to prevent suckling and in the second step they are separated. They are less stressed as measured by behavior and cortisol levels than abruptly weaned calves.[1175, 1176]

Clinical problems

Sucking problems

Nonnutritional intersuckling is a very frequent problem when calves are raised in groups, especially if they are pail, rather than nipple, fed. Some calves raised by cows intersuck even before weaning and will continue to do so afterwards. An inadequate diet increases the frequency of intersuckling.[991] Nonnutritional intersuckling can occur 78–300 times a day.[734] Skin irritation or even hernias can result from prolonged sucking by one calf on the umbilicus or sheath of another. Calves that engage in nonnutritive sucking often fail to thrive.[1811] The incidence of intersuckling on British dairy farms is 13%. If the problem exists on a farm, as many as 30% of the calves and 11% of the adult cows may be affected; there is apparently social facilitation of the behavior.[2057] Most dairy farmers solve the problem by penning calves separately, but they may still suckle on buckets or themselves. Non-nutritive suckling on inanimate objects or self-suckling may be decreased by providing a dry teat for the calf to suckle. The component of milk that stimulates nonnutritive suckling is not fluid, fat, protein, or calories per se, but lactose.[443] Calves that can suckle dry teats are calmer.[1937] When this is not feasible, however, other procedures are available that may prevent the behavior, such as muzzles, or application of unpalatable substances to the part sucked, and changing to dry food rather than milk. To reduce intersuckling, serrated rings are placed on the suckler's nose so that the suckled animals will be prodded and rebuff the suckler. None of these methods reduce the calf's motivation to suckle. Most nonnutritive suckling occurs immediately after feeding, so provisions of nipples in the feeding area will decrease self-, or auto-suckling, and allo-suckling.

Calves weaned after 6 days are more apt to suckle one another than are calves weaned earlier. A related problem is that of self-suckling. Various harnesses and even surgical procedures, such as splitting of the tongue, have been devised to deal with the problem.

Cross-fostering

As noted previously, cross-fostering can be accomplished by draping the calf with the skin of the cow's dead calf, if that is available. A more difficult problem is convincing a cow to accept a foster calf in addition to her own offspring. Fostering calves onto dairy cows is fairly easy because they have not been selected for maternal behavior that includes rejection of alien calves. Beef cows have been selected for these traits; hence, it is much more difficult to foster additional calves onto them. There are practical reasons for wishing to do so; a well-fed beef cow has a milk supply large enough for two calves. Dairy calves can be fostered onto these beef cows and will, when raised in this manner, suffer far less from maternal deprivation and from the respiratory and enteric diseases to which artificially reared calves are susceptible.[897,1012]

Persuading the cow to accept the dairy calf presents difficulties. Although the cow–calf bond is presumably formed when the cow first encounters the fetal fluids and the newborn calf, a beef cow may reject a dairy calf even when its own calf has been removed immediately after birth and when the foster calf is rubbed with fresh amniotic fluid. The cow apparently still can discriminate between a newborn and the older, larger, more active foster calf, probably on the basis of visual cues; blindfolding the cow may help.[1012] Substituting one calf for another is possible by removing the cow's own calf 48 hours postpartum, leaving the cow with no calf for 3 days, and then returning her own calf plus the alien calf. The bond to the original calf has been broken, but maternal responsiveness persists.[1005] Placing a jacket worn by her own calf inside out on the calf to be fostered is helpful; the same technique is used in sheep.[831]

Much obviously remains to be learned about the basis of maternal bonding in cattle. Some cows will grudgingly foster the dairy calf and mother their own calf. Others will become promiscuous mothers that allow four or more calves to suckle.[1018] The maternal bond has been broken in these cases and replaced by nondiscriminative tolerance. The promiscuous mother may suffer teat or udder damage when too many calves suckle. There is also the danger that mastitis may be passed from nurse cow to nurse cow by the calves. It is not necessary to find a foster mother who has recently calved; cows will accept foster calves as long as 178 days after separation from their own calves, but their milk production will be lower.[1174] Cows that live in a group with their foster calves continuously present are more likely to be maternally selective than those cows that are exposed to the calves only for nursing periods twice a day.[1516]

HORSES

Parturition

The onset of parturition in mares is heralded by waxing of the udder, but the length of time between the appearance of udder waxing and the appearance of the foal may be quite variable, up to 21 days. The calcium level of the milk increases as foaling approaches and can be used as a predictor. Body temperature is lower the day prior to parturition.[1741] The mare will walk more and stand less the evening of parturition. In the free-ranging situation, only primiparous mares leave the herd to foal; multiparous mares remain with the herd.[214]

In the first stage of labor, which lasts for about 4 hours, the mare is restless and will crouch, straddle, and urinate. The smell of fetal fluids is attractive to parturient mares. The mare will exhibit the flehmen response in response to amniotic fluid that is expelled. Sweat will appear on her elbows and flanks.[627]

During the second stage of labor, the mare will lie in lateral recumbency. This second stage is very violent and very short in horses, lasting less than a half hour. For that reason, it is important to have a veterinarian in attendance when complications are expected. There will not be time for professional help to reach the mare if problems develop in the course of labor.

Mares are notorious for their ability to thwart observation of their parturition. Although most mares foal at night, some will wait until they are released from their stalls in the morning in order to foal in the solitude of the pasture. Thus, parturition appears to be under some type of voluntary control in such mares, but the evidence is all anecdotal.

The most exciting findings in equine maternal behavior is that lactation can be induced using the dopamine antagonist sulpiride and that maternal behavior to an alien foal can be stimulated by vaginal stimulation of those mares induced to lactate. The process of stimulating lactation takes a few weeks, but could be used to produce nurse mares without producing unwanted foals.[1396]

Postparturient behavior

Ordinarily, the foal is delivered in such a way that the mare need only turn her head to meet her foal muzzle to muzzle. The establishment of the selectivity of maternal behavior is still uninvestigated in horses. It may be based on olfaction, because the mare licks the fetal membranes and then the newborn; licking behavior usually is confined to a few hours after parturition.

Licking, as well as sniffing, is concentrated first on the head of the foal and later on the hindquarters, particularly the perianal area. The rate of licking decreases markedly during the first hour postpartum. Although the period for bond formation has not been identified in horses, the first hour is probably critical for the mare to learn to recognize her foal selectively. The foal appears to take much longer, perhaps as long as a week, to recognize the mare. The foal will follow any large, moving object. The mare is usually very aggressive toward other horses and sometimes toward people for the first day or two after foaling. This behavior serves to keep away other horses that the foal otherwise might follow.

Suckling

Standing and suckling occur within the first hour after birth for pony foals and within the first 2 hours for Thoroughbred and Saddlebred foals.[320,1640,1973] Many managers of brood mares guide the foal to the udder and place a teat in its mouth in order to ensure the foal obtains colostrums. This appears to have a detrimental effect on the foal because it will remain closer to the dam and play less months later [785]

Foals suckle four times per hour at one week of age and gradually decrease the frequency to once per hour by 5 months[328,329,404,1909] (Fig. 5.5). Mares spend approximately 2 minutes nursing, during which the foal spends less than half the time actually suckling. The rest of the time is spent in nuzzling the teat and butting the udder.[148] The mare usually flexes her hind leg on the side opposite the foal, possibly conserving energy by shifting her weight to the stay apparatus.[2039] (Fig. 5.6) Subordinate mares have shorter nursing bouts because dominant mares aggressively disrupt nursing and nursing attempts.[1668] High-ranking mares are closer to their foals and in late lactation allow their foals to suckle more.[808] Nursing also occurs after any separation, even a very brief one, or after the foal has been frightened. When a foal approaches its dam to nurse, it often shakes its head and nickers or crosses in front of the mare. Foals turn their heads sideways to nurse, especially as they grow larger.

Fillies suckle longer but obtain no more milk than colts.[313] Colts may suckle more frequently than fillies when food is a limiting factor.[214,503] There appears to be more investment in a colt by mares in good body condition and more in fillies by mares in poor condition, which is explained by Trivers'[1900] hypothesis that a surviving son will father many or few offspring depending on his success, whereas a daughter always produces for a small number of offspring.[311] Nursing is often terminated by the mare, not by aggression but by simply walking away from the foal. This behavior occurs most frequently during the first month of the foal's life.[404] The foal may

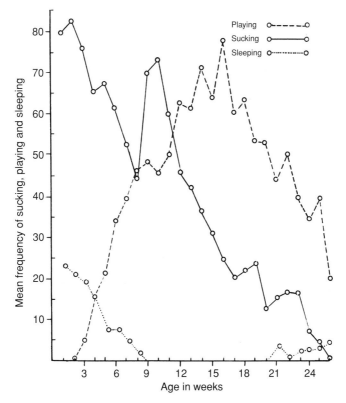

Fig. 5.5 Changes with age in frequency of sucking (solid line), playing (dashed line), and sleeping (dotted line) of free-ranging pony foals.[1909] (Copyright 1972, with permission of Academic Press.)

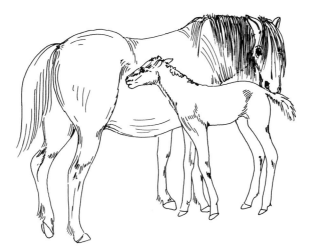

Fig. 5.6 Identification of the foal. The mare sniffs the anal area of the foal. The hind leg on the side opposite the foal is flexed to facilitate nursing.[867]

be forced to practice following the mare as a result of her behavior. The more skilled the foal is at identifying and following his dam, the more likely he is to survive. Mares do aggress toward their foals during nursing, but the aggression appears to be a response to bunting of the udder and does not prevent or shorten suckling bouts.

Weaning occurs at 40 weeks when the mare is about to foal, but is prolonged beyond a year if the mother is not pregnant.[503] Under domestic conditions of abundant food, foals continue to suckle for 3 or 4 years, even when they are larger than their mothers. Orphaned or newly weaned foals will often attempt to nurse from nonlactating mares, suckle the sheaths of geldings, and investigate the inguinal area of any horse.

Mares seldom venture far from their foals throughout the first few months. Foals spend several hours per day lying down. During these periods, the mare remains with the foal, either grazing in circles around it or standing next to it. This behavior, the recumbency response, which probably functions to protect the foal both from predators and from becoming lost, wanes as the foal matures. When the foal is awake, it is responsible for maintaining contact with its dam.[403] The mare is within five yards of the foal 94% of the time during the first week and 52% of the time the fifth month of the foal's life. The typical equine family group will travel in the following order: mare, most recent foal, yearling foal, and then the other offspring in the order of increasing age.[1691]

Mares are very protective of their foals, especially during the first few hours of a foal's life. Mares may be dangerous to humans at this time, even familiar ones. Good maternal behavior including protecting a foal from aggression by other horses as well as predators is important for foal survival, especially in the first month. Older mares spend more time defending their foals during this period, which may account for their greater reproductive success.[311]

Weaning

At least five different methods of artificial weaning are available: (1) removal of the foal from the mare and confinement of the foal by himself; (2) removal of the foal from the mare and confinement of the foal with another foal or foals; (3) interval weaning, in which the mare alone is removed from the pasture while the foal remains with the other younger foals and their dams. The other mares are removed gradually in order of their foals' ages; (4) separation of mares and foals into adjacent corrals for one week and subsequent removal of the mares; and (5) feeding mares and foals separately and gradually increasing the duration of separation. This latter method is particularly valuable for the owner of a single mare–foal pair. Although pony foals seem less stressed when weaned as pairs rather than singly,[870] Thoroughbred foals are more stressed, apparently because more aggression takes place between members of the pairs. In addition, separation of the two foals may also be stressful. Weaning by the fourth method, in which the foals can see and hear their mother but cannot make direct contact (or suckle), appears to be less stressful than methods in which the mother cannot be seen, probably because weaning is more gradual.[1247] Weaning from the mother as a food source occurs before weaning from the mother as a social companion. Feeding concentrates before weaning appeared to reduce stress.[849] Interval weaning is associated with fewer gastric ulcers and cribbing than weaning into a stall and feeding of concentrates.[1977] Creep feeding foals a high fat and fiber diet decreased activity in newly weaned foals.[1416]

Mutual recognition

The roles of the three senses, vision, audition, and olfaction, in the mare–foal bond is complex. The neighs (or whinnies) of the separated mare and foal are impressive, and horses make use

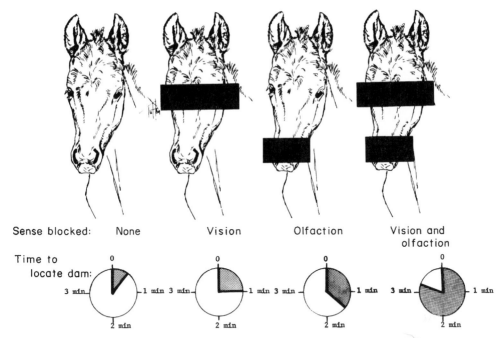

| Sense blocked: | None | Vision | Olfaction | Vision and olfaction |

Time to locate dam:

Fig. 5.7 The effect of masking vision or olfaction or both on the time that a foal takes to locate its dam.[886] (Copyright 1979, Veterinary Practice Publishing.)

of these calls to locate one another. The more frequently a mare neighs, the more quickly her foal will find her. The mare's neighs are not specifically recognized by the foal, but the mare neighs more often to her own foal.[2055] Changing a mare's or a foal's appearance by hooding, blanketing, and bandaging does not interfere with recognition; yet, visual cues must be involved because both foals and mares have difficulty finding each other when one is in a closed stall. They orient toward whinnies but need visual confirmation of the dam's or foal's presence.

Olfaction is also important. Mare and foal sniff each other's heads, and the mare sniffs the anal region of the foal (see Fig. 5.6). Masking olfactory cues with a strong odor greatly retards location of mares by foals, especially in the absence of visual cues.[2055] Thus, olfactory and possibly vocal cues (nickers) are used for close-range identification, whereas other vocal cues (whinnies) and visual cues are important for more distant communication of identity or presence (Fig. 5.7). Visual cues are probably not of vital significance; many blind mares have raised foals successfully even in seminaturalistic conditions.

Clinical problems

Mismothering

Mismothering can occur in equids, although it is much rarer than in sheep. A female mule adopted and successfully raised a foal; only examination of the foal's karyotype revealed that the foal was a Shetland pony, one of a pair of twins born to a pony mare in the same pasture as the mule.[530] Mules may be particularly prone to this behavior; in another case, a mule stole a calf from its mother and raised it.[1740] Mules have successfully raised Thoroughbred foals born to them after embryo transplant, but a donkey foal was rejected.[1740]

Foal rejection

Some mares resent manipulation of the inguinal fold—not the udder itself; these mares can be treated quickly by negative reinforcement. The mare is made to trot on a lead line until she will allow rigorous manipulation of the inguinal fold. (Jeannine Berger, personal communication) There are three types of foal rejection that occur immediately after foaling: (1) rejection of suckling, (2) fear of the foal, and (3) attacking the foal. All three forms are more common in the primiparous mare, but the third form may occur again and again.

In the first type, many mares lick the foal and appear attracted to it but will not tolerate suckling. They will kick the foal if it persists. These mares can usually be treated successfully either by tranquilization and/or by milking the mare while holding the foal next to the mare and feeding the milk to the foal from a bottle held in the inguinal area. The newborn foal normally nurses every 15 minutes, so this exercise should be repeated many times in order to nourish the foal, transfer colostral antibodies, and teach the mare that milking relieves tension on the udder. Gradually, the foal should be encouraged to suckle the teats, and less and less restraint should be applied to the mare until the pair can be left alone safely.

In the second type of foal rejection, the fearful mare tries to escape from her foal and may injure him by running over him. She will kick when the foal approaches her. Several behavioral methods can be used to stimulate maternal behavior. Turning the mare and foal out in a paddock so that both the mare and the foal can avoid each other may lessen the mare's fear. Adding another horse may stimulate the aggression that periparturient mares normally show, and this may be followed by acceptance of the foal. A large dog has been used for the same purpose, that is, stimulating maternal defensiveness.

In the third, and most dangerous, type of foal rejection, the mare actively attacks her foal, usually biting him in the withers and throwing him across the stall. These mares act toward a foal as foal-killing stallions do. She will not have licked the fetal membranes or the foal. She will also kick if the foal approaches her. Tranquilization with acepromazine and passive restraint for as long as three weeks, immediate punishment of aggression, and administration of oxytocin and progestins can result in acceptance. This problem can be seen in any breed of mares but is most common in Arabians that reject 5% of their foals in comparison to less than 2% of Paints, indicating a genetic component.[973] Passive restraint is best obtained by placing a pole across a box stall so that the mare cannot move sideways, forward, or backward. She can still bite, but the foal can escape and soon learns to avoid her head. She can kick forward, that is, cowkick, but a persistent foal can suckle. Usually, the mare will accept the foal after a week or two of restraint. These mares tend to be merely tolerant of their foals, and some may relapse after a few weeks. Mares that reject their foals have lower levels of progesterone before parturition than normal mares.

Pain, such as that associated with passing the placenta or with uterine contractions caused by suckling-induced oxytocin release, may result in aggression toward the foal. Removing the source of pain eliminates the aggression. Maternal rejection may occur after foaling. Too much disturbance of the mare and foal has been implicated, as has changing the odor or appearance of the foal. A common clinical problem is rejection of the foal that has had to be separated from its mother for treatment of a medical problem. The foal is changed in odor and may have had its appearance altered by clipping and bandaging. Allowing the mare to have visual contact with the ill foal may help to prevent rejection even if the foal is too weak to suckle for many days.

Redirected aggression also occurs. A mare may be aggressing against another horse and then bite or kick her foal. More frequently, the foal simply is kicked accidentally during a fight.

Occasionally, a mare may aggress against her own foal when an alien approaches – a failure of recognition.

Some mares do not reject their foals but do not respond vocally to them when they are separated. This can lead to injury to the foal because it will approach other mares and be attacked or will try to jump a fence or gate to return to the stall where it last saw the mare. Although this would be presented clinically as accidental trauma to the foal, it is the result of poor maternal behavior.

Mares can be vicious when protecting their foals, but they can also be vicious when weaning them. When the foal attempts to nurse, a mare may bite not only the foal but also a nearby person. This behavior also may be caused by mastitis or injury to the udder, or may have an unknown cause.

CATS

Parturition

Gestation is 63–66 days in cats. Births have a seasonal distribution, with the greatest number of litters being born in the summer and the least in autumn and early winter.[1537] Cats rarely deign to use the boxes carefully provided for parturition by their owners. Most cats will choose a cave-like place, such as a closet or a linen cabinet. A cat is attracted to the smell of the amniotic fluid at the birth site, so moving the kittens to a more suitable location will not entice her from her chosen spot. Parturition in the cat is characterized by a great deal of licking by the queen: self-licking mostly directed at the belly and genital area, licking of the fetal fluids from her body or the floor, and licking the kittens. The queen is responding to the fluids, rather than to the kittens, at this time.

The queen is typically very restless, and a normal protocol will list lying down, sitting up, licking of the vulva, squatting, bracing lordosis, circling, walking around the cage, lying down again, rolling, licking of a kitten, and so on. No consistent pattern emerges, and the behavior of the queen varies with the endogenous stimuli (from the uterus) and exogenous stimuli (from the birth fluids and kittens). The uterine contractions of labor can be distinguished from fetal movements because the raised hind legs of the queen usually flex when she is in labor.[1700]

Most cats prefer solitude, though some highly socialized ones seem to be content only when the owner is present. Cats, with the exception of Siamese, are usually quiet during parturition. The restless behavior of the queen serves to stretch the umbilical cord of the newly delivered kitten. When the placenta is delivered, the queen will eat it and part of the cord with the same tilt of the head and pronounced chewing motions that she shows when consuming prey. In the process of eating the placenta, the queen stretches the umbilical cord so that little bleeding occurs when the cord is severed. It is rare for the eating to extend to cannibalism of the kitten. The interval between kitten births can be as long as one hour even in normal births but is usually much shorter. As already mentioned here, the queen seems unaware of the kittens despite her bouts of licking them, as demonstrated by her inadvertent stepping on them in the course of her pacing, as well as her ignoring of their cries. The bursts of activity are interspersed with periods of fatigue.

When the last kitten has been delivered, the queen directs her attention to her litter. She lies down with an encircling motion, positioning her legs in such a way as to form a U around the kittens. For the next 12 to 24 hours, she rarely leaves the newborns and then only for brief intervals to eat, drink, and eliminate. Each time she returns, she arouses the kittens by licking them, after which she encircles and then nurses them.

Suckling

Finding the teat

Most kittens are suckling within an hour or two of birth. The cues used by the neonate to find the mammary glands are unknown in this species as well as in the other domestic species. The kittens probably use temperature cues but also the mobility and responsiveness of the adult cat to locate her. Kittens who are blind and deaf at birth apparently use smell and, probably to a greater extent, tactile sensations to locate the nipple. Kittens with anesthetized tongues can find the nipple but cannot suckle; kittens with anesthetized lips cannot locate the nipple but can suckle.[1760] Olfactory bulbectomy also eliminates the ability of kittens to find the nipple,[1054] but damage to the olfactory bulb eliminates more than the sense of smell alone.

Kittens locomote by pulling themselves along with their front legs while paddling with the weaker hind legs. As they crawl forward, they turn their heads from side to side. When they encounter the nipple, they pull their heads back and lunge forward with open mouths. Eventually, the nipple is secured in the mouth. The position of the mother facilitates locating the mammary region. The responses of the kittens to the areola and nipple appear to be innate, almost reflex in nature.[1880]

Experiments conducted on artificially reared kittens revealed that before their eyes were open, they followed a path produced by their own body odors to find the nipple of the brooder. The kittens could also make tactile discriminations under these experimental conditions, learning to choose a nipple with bumps on it over one with concentric ridges when the former was associated with milk reinforcement.[1700]

Prolonged experience with suckling from an artificial teat (one to three weeks) delays, but does not abolish, the kitten's ability to initiate natural suckling.[1631] Milk reinforcement is not necessary for suckling, because intragastrically fed kittens will initiate suckling on the teats of a nonlactating cat as rapidly as on a lactating cat, even on repeated trials.[1044] The ability to initiate suckling disappears after 22 days of age if the kittens have been fed intragastrically.

Teat order

By the second day, kittens have a teat order determined, which is usually but not always followed. The largest kittens, however, do not appear to be those that acquire the best producing glands, in contrast to the teat order in piglets.[557] In some litters, no regular teat order is formed. After the teat order is established, a kitten can use the presence of its sibling on either side to help guide it to the proper nipple, though sometimes the kittens obstruct more than facilitate one another's progress. Kittens massage the udder with treading motions of the paws. Treading on soft surfaces persists in the adult cat, presumably as a pleasurable activity or in pleasurable situations.

The feline nursing period has been divided into three stages: stage 1, 1–14 days: mother initiates nursing; stage 2, 14–21 days: both mother and kittens initiate nursing; stage 3, 22–35 days: kittens initiate nursing. In the hormonally primed queen, the suckling of kittens is probably tactilely pleasant. However, as kittens grow older and their feeding demands become more persistent, the female develops an approach–avoidance type of behavior toward her kittens; she discourages their attempts to nurse from the third week onward by moving away. In a home situation, she could easily escape from the kittens, whereas in a cage, she can only jump to a shelf to which the kittens can soon gain access as their locomotor skills improve. Another ploy by the mother is to lick the kittens vigorously, thus preventing them from nursing. Figure 5.8 illustrates the change with time in the queen's relationship with her kittens. In a two-kitten litter, the time of

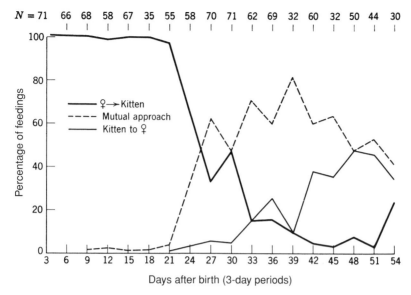

Fig. 5.8 Approach of the queen to her kittens and kittens to the queen during the first eight weeks of life.[1700] (Copyright 1963, with permission of John Wiley & Sons.)

weaning occurs later.[1226] In the single kitten, these stages are not as discrete. The queen spends less time with a single kitten initially (30% versus 70% of her time), but she continues to allow it to nurse long after a larger litter would have been weaned. Apparently, a single kitten is less attractive than several kittens but also less aggravating. From the fourth week on, "barn" cats will begin to bring live or dead prey to their kittens (see Chapter 6, "Development of Behavior"); however, these females sometimes allow intermittent nursing until the next litter is born.

Homing and retrieval

Even before the opening of their eyes, kittens can return to their nest from several feet away. Apparently, they use olfactory cues; a washed floor between the kittens and the nest prevents them from finding their way back.[1700]

Feline retrieval behavior is quite different from the canine form. Queens retrieve their kittens in response to auditory, not visual, signals. The more the kitten vocalizes, the more apt the queen is to retrieve it.[781] The queen usually picks the kitten up by the scruff of the neck, though occasionally she grasps the skin of the back of the head or even the kitten's whole head. Queens are able to lift and even jump several feet carrying large kittens. In fact, the peak of kitten carrying occurs when they are three weeks old. Picking up by the scruff is an effective means of establishing dominance even over an adult cat, probably because the cat is being treated like a kitten.

Communal nests

Cats frequently move their kittens to new nests, moving four to nine times before the kittens are weaned, a phenomenon many cat owners have observed. Various hypotheses have been put forth, such as avoidance of predators or infanticidal males (if indeed there are any such males).

In a semi-natural situation, the nests are moved closer to the food source.[576] A queen may share a nest with another lactating female where the kittens are suckled communally and where one cat can remain with the litters while the other hunts. The cats that share litters are members of the same group but might not be related. Communal nesting has advantages to the kittens; they leave the nest earlier (20 days) than do kittens in single-litter nests (30 days). Kittens in communal nests are moved to different nest sites more often than those in a one-litter nest.

Grooming

Grooming plays as important a part in feline maternal behavior as in most other species. Queens lick their kittens frequently and in particular lick the perineum to stimulate urination and defecation for the first 2–3 weeks of life. In common with most carnivores, female cats ingest the kittens' urine and feces for several weeks postpartum, thereby keeping the nest clean.

Acceptance of kittens

Cats will accept alien kittens that are not too much older than their own at the time of parturition. Maternal behavior persists much longer in cats than in ungulates, so a queen whose kittens were removed at birth will accept one kitten weeks later and encircle it. Three kittens will be avoided or actually attacked under the same circumstances.[1700] In general, species that produce litters are more willing to accept foster young than are those that produce singleton or twins, probably because the mothers of litters do not discriminate between individual offspring.

Clinical problems

Few clinical problems of maternal behavior arise in cats. In fact, the efficiency of feline reproduction is much more of a problem. Occasionally, a queen may reject her litter, but this happens less frequently than in other species.

Infanticide

Tomcats may kill kittens, an abnormality of paternal, not maternal, behavior. Infanticide by males is rare in cats; there is only one authenticated case. There is no particular reproductive advantage to the male from infanticide in feline society, where many males can mate with each female[1398] (see Chapter 4, "Sexual Behavior"). Infanticide and cannibalism by the queen, although infrequent, does occur, usually at parturition or shortly thereafter.

Mismothering

Cats sometimes care for one another's kittens or nurse communally.[1196] An interesting variation of this behavior occurred in a newly spayed cat that stole the kittens of another cat in the household. The problem was easily solved by shutting the natural mother in a room with the kittens. This case indicates that maternal behavior is independent of ovarian hormones and/or is stimulated by a dramatic decline in estrogen and progesterone levels as occurs at spaying and at parturition.

Overgrooming

Some primiparous cats trim their kittens' whiskers; others chew their claws.[527] Overgrooming to the point of removing the kitten's fur in spots can occur.

Nonnutritive suckling

The nutritional, but not the social, development of orphan kittens will be adequate if they are artificially fed. Because cats socialize with one another almost exclusively as kittens, orphan kittens should probably be placed with the litter of another lactating queen if possible. Sometimes, older kittens will show suckling abnormalities. They may suckle on one another, on a human skin or hair, on cloth, and on wool. The latter is a particular favorite of Siamese (see Chapter 8, "Ingestive Behavior: Food and Water Intake"). Occasionally, this behavior can be related to early weaning, but more commonly, no explanation is immediately obvious. The suckling is usually not injurious to the kittens' health and will gradually diminish in frequency.

DOGS

Parturition

The pregnant bitch gives little indication of her condition for the first 30 days. Late in pregnancy, her activity decreases and her appetite increases. In the last weeks, she may wish to eat small but frequent meals as abdominal pressure increases. She may grunt each time she sits, especially if she is carrying a large litter. The slow development of the fetuses during the first half of pregnancy allows the bitch in the natural state to hunt and forage as well as ever. She is encumbered for only the last two weeks of the 60–63-day gestation period. During that time, she may even urinate or defecate in the house unless she is taken out frequently.

In contrast to the more independent feline behavior, when a nest box is provided, bitches usually will use it. If nesting materials, such as strips of rags or paper, are provided, the bitch will make a nest. Like the sow, she will make digging attempts in the absence of nesting material. Restlessness, inappetence, and a drop in body temperature are the cardinal signs of impending parturition. After labor begins, the bitch usually lies in lateral recumbency. As labor progresses, her hind legs twitch and she shivers; several strong abdominal contractions are visible just before the puppy is expelled. The fetal fluids appear to be attractive to the bitch. She licks herself, any soiled bedding, and, almost incidentally, the puppy. The pup's head, umbilicus, and perineum are the areas most frequently licked. The bitch cuts the umbilical cord with her molars and then licks the stump. She may recut the cord if it is too long. If the placenta has not been delivered, she may extract it by pulling on the cord. The placenta is then nearly always eaten. She is usually silent as labor progresses, unless dystocia occurs. Adult male dogs, if present, often whine.[235]

Pups are usually born at 30-minute intervals, but delays of a few hours are not pathological. Labor can be interrupted if the bitch is disturbed; the disturbance can be as mild as the entrance of another human observer. If she is resting between deliveries, the birth interval will be lengthened; if she is in the middle of labor, it may stop. Depending upon the temperament of the dog, 15 minutes to an hour are required for normal parturition to proceed.[235]

Amniotic fluid is very important because if pups have been cleaned the bitch will not accept them.[1] Although the bitch licks the neonatal puppy dry, she pays little more attention to it until all the puppies are born. In fact, she may step on the puppies and ignore their cries at this time.

After all the puppies are born, she lies quietly and allows them to nurse. She helps to orient the puppies to her by licking.

Suckling

The puppies move forward by paddling and turn their heads from side to side, as they cannot lift their bodies from the floor yet. If they encounter a wall or any cold object, they will change their direction. After they encounter the mother's body, they nuzzle through the fur, usually attempting to burrow beneath her. High-chested breeds such as Shetland sheep dogs present much more of a challenge to the pup seeking a nipple than do flat-chested breeds such as cocker spaniels. When the pup locates a nipple, it does not immediately grasp it but rather noses it from beneath. Unless the pup opens its mouth at the same time as the nipple moves past, it will not succeed in grasping it. Puppies improve markedly in the first 2 or 3 days of life in their ability to locate nipples. After it locates the nipple, the pup jerks up with its head, pushes at the mammary gland with its front feet, and arranges its hind feet to support itself against the mother.[1600] All this is not proceeding in a social vacuum; the other pups are also struggling for positions. The efforts of one will dislodge the other, and whining and scrambling will ensue. The supposedly serene maternal scene is, in fact, noisy and tumultuous. Puppies do not appear to have as definitive a teat order as cats or pigs. The inguinal mammary gland is the preferred one and is the one approached by a single pup.[612]

Puppies have two vocal signals, the whine and the grunt. The whine is emitted whenever the puppy is cold, hungry, or separated from its litter or mother. Whining stops immediately if the puppy's head and neck are covered with a warm towel or if it is again placed with its litter. Puppies show a distinct preference for soft surfaces; they spend more time on a cloth-covered versus a wire-covered artificial mother.[919]

Textural, as well as olfactory, cues may help puppies locate their mother and her mammary glands. The grunt is apparently a pleasure communication that occurs when sought-after warmth or reunion is obtained. Despite the puppy's loud vocal response to separation, the bitch appears to notice that a puppy is missing when she sees it rather than when she hears it.[235]

Licking

Bitches lick their puppies a great deal. Licking serves three functions in puppies: two are common to other species and one is unique to dogs. The licking arouses the pups to eat, and, when it is directed at the anogenital area, it stimulates urination and defecation that would otherwise not occur spontaneously. The bitch keeps the nest area clean by consuming the urine and feces of her puppies for at least the first 3 weeks of their lives. The third function of licking is retrieval. Bitches seldom carry their puppies. Instead, they lead them back to the nest by licking the pup's head. The pup will orient toward the bitch and move toward her. The bitch will back toward the nest, continuing to lick the pup that follows until the nest is reached. Licking can be reinstated by substituting young (2- to 3-day-old) puppies for older ones.[1052]

Differences in maternal behavior, especially licking, can lead to differences in stress response and fearfulness. The more an offspring is groomed, the less fearful and reactive to stress it will be. Increased grooming causes an increase in hippocampal glucoreceptor number, and, therefore, greater negative feedback sensitivity of glucocorticoid secretion.[1684] Furthermore, rats groomed often by a foster dam as pups will groom their own pups more, indicating the behavior need not be transmitted genetically.[621]

Weaning

During the first few days, the bitch spends most of her time with the pups (22 nursing bouts per day). Nursing reaches a peak at the end of the first week. The amount of time that she spends with them decreases with time (Fig. 5.9). The undisturbed litter is weaned gradually by the bitch; weaning usually is complete by 60 days by the well-fed laboratory bitch but is delayed by 3 weeks in stray bitches in India, who remain with the puppies for 13 weeks. Males, presumably the sires, remain with and actively guard the puppies for six weeks.[1468]

During early lactation, the bitch always approaches the puppies to initiate a nursing bout. By 3 weeks, the puppies have opened their eyes and can locomote well. They then approach the bitch and initiate most of the nursing bouts. Bitches rarely punish their puppies until the third week. Even during the weaning process, the punishment is mild enough that it may momentarily deter the pups' attempts to nurse but will not inhibit them from trying again. The punishment may consist of a growl, a snarl, or an inhibited bite. The level of aggression of the bitch toward her puppies increases and the number of nursing bouts per hour decreases after the puppies' third week.[2035]

Some bitches, and all stray Indian dogs, may regurgitate food for their pups during the weaning process at four to six weeks.[1211,1212,1231,1468] This behavior, commonly seen in wild canids, helps to maintain adequate nutrition in the young during the transition from a milk diet to a raw meat diet, when their powers of mastication and digestion may not have matured enough

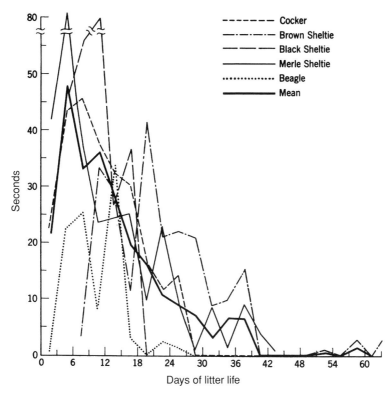

Fig. 5.9 The decrease in licking of the puppies by the bitch as the puppies mature.[1600] (Copyright 1963, with permission of John Wiley & Sons.)

to enable them to survive on the raw meat.[612] Wolf pups beg for regurgitated food by licking at the mouth of the adult. This behavior is occasionally seen in domestic dogs and may be the basis of face licking and licking intention movements directed toward people by adult dogs.

Clinical problems

Pseudopregnancy

Pseudopregnancy in the intact, nonpregnant bitch during the luteal phase of the canine reproductive cycle is so common that it may be normal behavior. Bitches do vary, however, in the severity of the behavioral signs. Some dogs show only slight enlargement of the mammary glands, whereas others go through pseudoparturition at 49 days postestrus and actually lactate. The pseudopregnant bitch becomes less active, mimicking the slowing down of the truly pregnant animal. She may make a nest, usually either in her own bed or in some cave-like environment, under a table, or in a dark corner. She may adopt a toy, a leash, a shoe, or some other object to mother. She not only will place it in her nest and assume a nursing posture next to it but also often defend it. Serious problems with aggression can arise in the pseudopregnant bitch. She may be generally aggressive but, more commonly, she attacks only when her nest is invaded or her "offspring" are threatened. Mibolerone, an androgenic anabolic steroid, will relieve the signs of pseudopregnancy, but ovariohysterectomy should be recommended. The bitch who shows recurrent cycles of pseudopregnancy is prone to uterine infections, pyometra in particular. It is advisable to wait until after the behavioral signs of pseudopregnancy have passed before performing the ovariohysterectomy, as protective behavior persists if the animal is operated upon while pseudopregnant (B.L. Hart, personal communication). Pseudopregnant bitches can adopt and successfully raise foster puppies.[615] A bitch spayed during late metestrus may also exhibit lactation and maternal behavior, including maternal aggression, for a few weeks.

Maternal rejection

Maternal rejection also occurs in bitches. It is most common in dogs that have undergone cesarean section and have been anesthetized during the time they would normally be licking and smelling the neonatal puppies. It rarely happens if the bitch has delivered a puppy normally before surgical intervention was necessary. She may lick the puppies if amniotic fluid or even water is applied to them; this will improve chances of acceptance. The bitch may tolerate the first nursing better if some milk is expressed from the engorged glands before the pups suckle. She can be restrained while they nurse for the first time and sedated lightly if necessary. Attacking of puppies at some time after parturition is less common but does occur.

Moving pups

A nervous bitch, especially one housed with other dogs or in an area with too much commotion, may repeatedly move her puppies. They will not be nursed often enough. Providing a nest box in a quiet room with no other animals and minimal visitors can solve the problem.

A related problem is continued carrying of pups in circles and without much other maternal behavior. Isolation and tranquilization may be helpful.

6 Development of Behavior

Ontogeny in all the domestic species involves a decrease in time spent close to the dam and in sleeping. Especially in ungulates, time spent foraging for food or grazing increases. Time spent with peers increases, and much of the time is spent in play. Sex differences appear in play; males spend more time play fighting and mounting than females. In cats and dogs, a sensitive period for socialization has been identified. These periods probably exist in the more precocial species as well, but occur within the first days rather than within the first months of life.

INTRODUCTION

One of the most pleasant aspects of owning animals is watching the young develop. Even in a world overpopulated with cats, kittens have not lost their attraction. The gangly foal and the playful kid are also very appealing. The veterinarian or animal scientist will find that more questions are asked about normal developmental behavior, when to take a puppy home, and when to start various types of training than are asked about adult behavior. To answer these questions correctly, the clinician should be familiar with the neurological development and behavioral maturation of various species because owners spend more time observing infant than adult animals.

DOGS

Critical or sensitive periods

During the past 40 years, the behavioral concept of critical periods has emerged, a concept that has had a strong impact on practical dog handling. Recently, the term sensitive period has replaced critical period. Nevertheless, socialization can occur in older animals, albeit with difficulty. For that reason, Bateson[163] has suggested that the adjective sensitive, rather than critical, be used with these periods. A sensitive period is a time in the life of an animal when a small amount of experience (or a total lack of experience) will have a large effect on later behavior. The sensitive periods for dogs are defined as the neonatal period (1–2 weeks), the transitional period (3 weeks), the period of socialization (4–14 weeks), and the juvenile period (14 weeks to sexual maturity).[642,1708,1715] The sensitive periods are not sharply defined and may vary among breeds that are fast or slow to mature. Cocker spaniel puppies appear to mature more

Domestic Animal Behavior for Veterinarians and Animal Scientists, Fifth Edition by Katherine Albro Houpt
© 2011 John Wiley & Sons, Inc.

slowly than do basenjis, for example. Marked neurological changes appear during development and have been well described by Fox.[613] See Fig. 6.1 for a canine development chart.

Neonatal period

The neonatal period, during which the puppy is deaf and blind and able to find the nipple only through tactile and olfactory cues, is described in Chapter 5, "Maternal Behavior." Most of the puppy's time is spent eating and sleeping. The sleep is characterized by a high proportion of rapid eye movement (REM) or stage IV sleep. Urination and defecation do not occur spontaneously but can be elicited by stimulation of the anogenital area; usually such stimulation is supplied by the mother's licking. Puppies locomote with their front legs, pulling their hind legs along.

During this period, several reflexes are present that will gradually disappear as the central nervous system matures. One can use the presence or absence of these reflexes to determine the age of a normal puppy and to assess development if pathology is suspected in a puppy of known age. For the first 3 days, puppies show flexor dominance; that is, when picked up by the scruff of the neck, they will flex their legs. From 3 days until the fourth week of life, extensor dominance occurs; that is, the puppy will extend its legs when it is picked up. Gradually, normotonia appears.

The Magnus reflex is present for the first 2 weeks. The reflex is demonstrated by turning the pup's head to one side. The front legs and hind legs on the side toward which the head is turned are extended; the legs on the opposite side are flexed. The crossed extensor reflex is also demonstrable for the first 2 weeks. The reflex is elicited by pinching on a hind foot; that foot is withdrawn while the opposite leg is extended. The rooting reflex is best demonstrated after the puppy is a few days old. The puppy will push its face into a cupped hand and crawl forward. This is the reflex utilized by the mother to retrieve a puppy (see Chapter 5). Like the Magnus and crossed extensor reflex, the rooting reflex will wane by the fourth week.

Transitional period

During the transitional period, the puppy begins to be bombarded by many more stimuli as his sensory organs develop. The eyes open between 10 and 16 days, although visual acuity is poor and puppies will not follow visual stimuli when the eyes first open. As vision improves, the puppy no longer swings its head from side to side as it locomotes. The ears open and a startle response to auditory stimuli can be elicited at 14–18 days. By day 16, sound can be localized.[99] The crossed extensor reflex disappears from the front legs first, as does the Magnus reflex. Urination and defecation occur spontaneously; the bitch continues to ingest the excreta for several weeks. When kept in a kennel, the puppies will begin to leave the nest to eliminate and will use the same area as that of the bitch. If the bitch is paper trained, this is the ideal way to train a puppy, long before it can follow its mother outdoors. The puppy can support its weight on all four legs by 12–14 days, although normal adult sitting and standing will not be seen until 28 days. Tooth eruption begins to take place during the transition period, and the pups will chew on one another, begin to play clumsily, and growl.

Socialization

The third period, socialization, is the most important from a behavioral viewpoint. During this time from the fourth to the 14 week, pups learn about their environment, about their

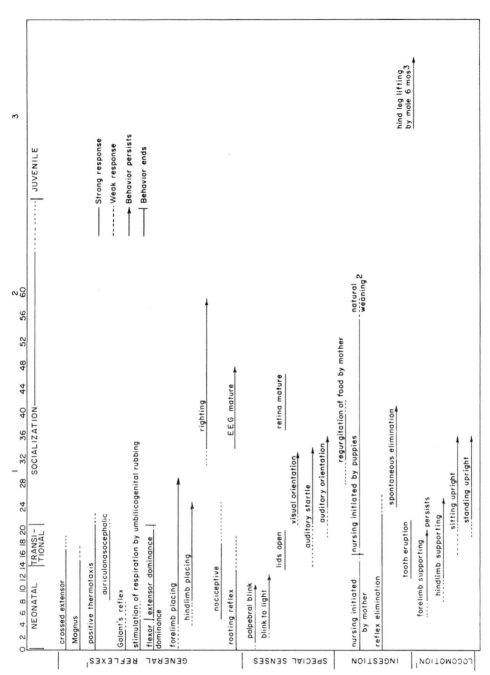

Fig. 6.1 Behavioral development of the dog. The superscript numbers refer to the references (1),[613,616] (2),[1599] (3),[212] (4),[235] (5),[1714] and (6).[619,620].

173

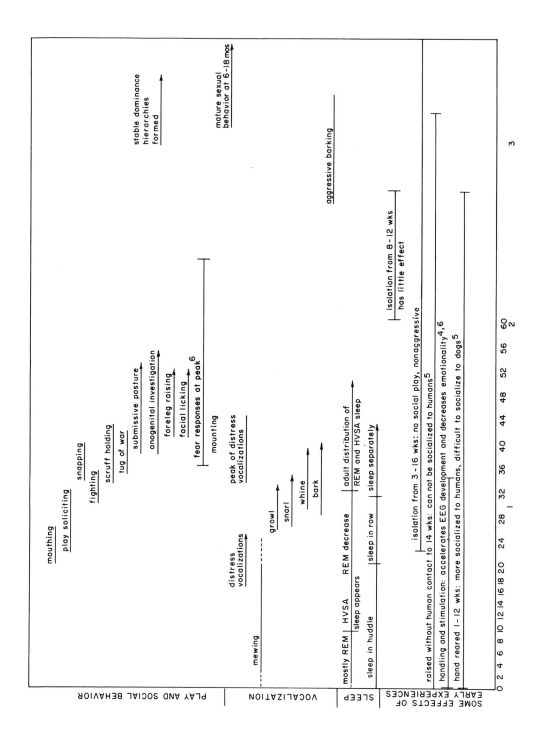

littermates and mother, and about humans. Play begins and has its highest frequency in the socialization period. Canine play is discussed in more detail later in this chapter. Dominance hierarchies are formed. Strong avoidance behavior develops, and by 8 weeks, fear reactions are seen.

This period is also most important from a clinical standpoint. Puppies weaned and removed from the company of other dogs before the period of socialization will, as adults, often be difficult to handle in the presence of other dogs. They will either be frightened of other dogs or, less commonly, too aggressive. They will not be able to play with other dogs and will be difficult to breed. A dog that has not had the opportunity to interact with other dogs will be too human oriented. Male dogs may direct their sexual attentions toward humans. Unfortunately, playing with other puppies and being handled by other people ("socialization") in the puppy socialization classes will not change the dog's innate response to social stimuli such as strange dogs or people.[1726] Puppies from pet shops and those ill as puppies are more apt to have problems.[1733]

Normally, pups are not weaned before 4 weeks of age, but they may be weaned even earlier if the bitch has died and the puppies must be hand fed. The nutritional requirements of the orphan puppy can be met, but many of the tactile and social requirements may not be. Hand-fed puppies usually will suck more on fingers and other objects than will normal puppies, indicating that the need to suckle has not been met, despite scheduled bottle feedings.[1636] It would be best to foster a litter of orphan pups onto another lactating bitch. If this is not possible, the litter should be kept together and separated only for an hour after feeding, when suckling on one another is most apt to occur. A similar situation may arise if the bitch has lactation tetany, in which case the litter may have to be weaned quite early. Again, the litter should be kept together at least until the puppies are 6 weeks old.

The importance of social contact to the puppy during this period is demonstrated by the emotional reaction to separation from the litter. Six-week-old beagle puppies yelp 1,400 times per 10 minutes when placed in a strange pen. Older and younger dogs are less disturbed[534] and, therefore, less vocal (Fig. 6.2). Surprisingly, human contact is more effective than canine contact in alleviating separation distress in 4–8-week-old puppies.[1503,1639] By 7–8 weeks, a fear posture, tail tucking, is first seen in beagle puppies.

Socialization to humans is equally important. A dog that has had little contact with humans until 14 weeks rarely becomes a good pet.[1714] This is, of course, typical of kennel-raised, rather than family-raised, dogs and is sometimes called kennelitis. Such a dog is well socialized to other dogs but has had limited experience with humans. The dog, depending on his genetic background, may be over-timid or most difficult to control. Although normal dogs find contact with a human rewarding,[1805] the dog that has not been socialized with humans will not; it will, therefore, be a much more difficult animal to train.

A substantial amount of experimental evidence supports the sensitive period hypothesis. Most impressive is the effect of early isolation.[16] If puppies are completely isolated from the third to the twentieth week of life, they are markedly disturbed. Their learning ability is impaired.[1304,1868,1869] They are socialized to neither humans nor dogs, and their response to either species is fear. Even a week in isolation will produce changes in the canine electroencephalogram (EEG),[613] although the changes are transient.

Complete isolation is rarely, if ever, imposed on puppies except for experimental purposes, but exclusive human, dog, or cat contacts do occur. Dogs raised with cats prefer the company of cats to that of dogs and fail to recognize a mirror image.[613] Hand-raised or early-weaned (by 3.5 weeks) puppies will approach a human much more quickly than will dogs that were weaned at 8 weeks with little human contact before that time.

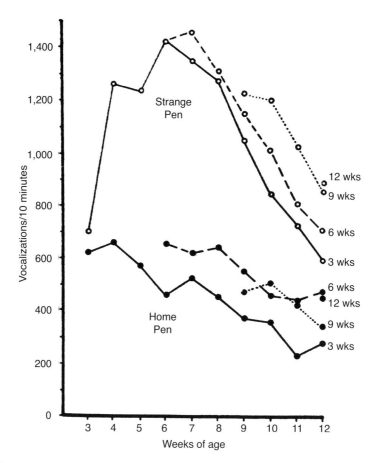

Fig. 6.2 The average number of vocalizations by puppies at different ages and in two environments. Note that vocalization of a puppy alone in the home pen is consistently lower than that of one in a strange pen. Puppies whose tests were begun when they were older than 3 weeks showed a slightly higher rate of vocalization, but the curves are parallel.[534] (Copyright 1961, with permission of the Helen Dwight Reid Educational Foundation, published by Heldref Publications, 4000 Albemarle St., N.W., Washington, DC, 20016.)

Not only the presence or absence of human contact but also the quality of that contact will affect the puppy's later behavior. It has been shown in many species that early handling can influence emotionality in later life; the dog is no exception. Dogs were subjected to varied stimulation (exposure to cold, vestibular stimulation on a tilting board, exposure to flashing lights, and auditory stimulation) from birth until 5 weeks of age. The stimulated pups differed from controls in several physiological and behavioral parameters. They showed earlier maturation of the EEG, larger adrenal glands, and lowered emotionality, which enhanced problem-solving ability in novel situations, than the nonstimulated pups. Most interesting was the finding that they were dominant over nonstimulated controls in a competitive situation.[613] Some effects of early stimulation are not permanent. Development is accelerated, but the nonstimulated animal eventually catches up. Not only social deprivation but also food deprivation during early life can affect later canine behavior. Food-restricted puppies were more attached to their handlers during the period of deprivation and later showed increased eating rates and increased intake of highly palatable food.[533] The effect of early illness on aggression and other problems in adulthood is discussed in Chapter 2, "Aggression and Social Structure."

Puppy socialization classes, usually held as soon as the dogs have had at least one vaccination, are useful in that dogs learn obedience easily at that stage, but it has no effect on their later behavior toward strange dogs or people.[1726] It does indicate owner motivation, and, therefore, puppies taken to socialization classes are more likely to remain in that home. Other factors important for retention are being female, wearing a head collar as a puppy, sleeping on or near the owner's bed, and living in homes without children.[508] German shepherds who attended a puppy class were more likely to be confident and less likely to be nervous.[650]

Juvenile period

During the juvenile period, a dog increases in size and in competency at adult activities. Puppies begin to show adult sexual behavior at 4–6 months when they begin to show greater attraction to estrous bitches than to spayed ones. This attraction increases with age until they reach 2 years old, at which point dogs are fully mature.[172] Although considered to be adult at puberty, most dogs do not mature socially until 18 months or later.

Conclusions

The conclusion to be drawn from the experimental studies and clinical observations of the sensitive periods of the development of dogs is that dogs should be exposed to both dogs and humans during the period of socialization. The exposure to both species should be pleasant because fear responses are also strong during this period. The effects of isolation are most pronounced in dogs that have been isolated during the period of socialization; however, isolation, or even partial isolation, in a boarding kennel for several weeks during any portion of its first year can reduce the sociability of a dog and increase its fearfulness. The importance of human socialization to canine training is exemplified by the study of Pfaffenberger and Scott,[1504] in which 90% of the dogs (mostly German shepherds) that were home raised from the twelfth to the fifty-second week of life were trainable as guide dogs for the blind. Dogs that remained in the kennel for the same period failed the training program. Properly socialized dogs will be much more willing to work for a reward as simple as verbal praise or even reunion with the human handler.

Neurological development

There is an old adage that "One can't teach an old dog new tricks," but it is equally difficult to teach a very young one. As discussed in Chapter 7, "Learning," 6-week-old puppies could not solve a barrier problem, nor could 4-week-old puppies (even after 13 days of training) remember the location of hidden food for more than 10 seconds, although 12-week-old puppies could remember for 50 seconds. Puppies less than 21 days old cannot learn to pull food into their cage with a ribbon, 13 and 5-week-old puppies took twice as long to learn a visual discrimination as 12-week-old ones.[613] Neonatal puppies, however, can learn to avoid an aversive stimulus.[1804]

The poor performance of the young puppy is not surprising in light of the stage of development of its nervous system. The brain consists of only 10% dry matter at birth. The adult percentage (19) is not reached until the fourth week of life.[613] Myelin is almost completely absent from the newborn puppy's brain and appears gradually over the next 4 weeks. Conduction speed along nerves is related to the presence of myelin, and the more rapid reactions of the month-old puppy attest to the myelinization of its central nervous system. At birth, the length and width of the canine brain are nearly equal. The increase in length of the brain with age is due to an increase of the frontal and occipital areas. A great increase in the complexity of the gyri and sulci also occurs.[613]

Placing measures the ability of a dog to put its paws onto a table when held up to it, usually without visual contact. Placing reactions mature in the following order: chin placing (if the dog's chin makes contact with a surface, he will reach for it with his paws), visual placing (if the dog sees a surface, he will put his paw out), contact forelimb placing (if the dorsal surface of the paw is touched to the lower surface of the table, the dog will place the paw on the upper surface), and contact hind limb placing and tail placing (if a dog's tail makes contact with a surface, the dog will reach toward that surface with its hind legs). By 6–9 weeks, all these reflexes are functional.[418]

Sleep

Sleep shows many changes in duration, type, and posture with development. The newborn puppy spends most of its time (96%) sleeping except for brief nursing bouts. Most of the sleep in the neonate is REM or stage IV sleep. Only 1% is slow wave sleep (SWS). REM sleep is associated with dreaming in the adult human, but one wonders what the newborn puppy dreams of, given that its experience is limited to intrauterine life. Owners are often concerned about the twitching exhibited by puppies during the neonatal period, but this is normal.

Newborn pups sleep in a heap, which may serve to prevent heat loss. A puppy removed from its littermates will wake and whine until it is either returned to the litter or placed on a soft, warm surface. Holding a puppy will often calm it, probably because of the warm body contact. As puppies mature, the percentage of time spent in REM sleep drops from 85% at 7 days to 7% at 35 days. Meanwhile, the percentage of time that the dog is awake has increased to 62% by day 35, and SWS occupies the other 31% of the 24 hours.[618] By 3.5 weeks, puppies sleep in a row with side contact only. Later, they will sleep apart but may sleep against a wall for contact.[1600] Even adult dogs often try to maintain contact while sleeping by curling against their owner or simply lying on the owner's foot. Much of the nocturnal distress of the newly weaned or separated puppy can be alleviated by providing it with a warm "companion" such as a hot water bottle or even an old, and preferably dirty, sweater with lots of olfactory stimuli.

Play

Puppies, kittens, lambs, and even foals are attractive both because their foreshortened faces and awkward gaits inspire maternal, or at least protective, attitudes in humans[1179] and also because they play. Play remains an enigma not because we do not know how animals play, but because we do not know why they play. Play appears to be important in the development of the social organization of animals, but that does not explain solitary play. Play may be important simply as a form of exercise or perhaps as a means of practicing and perfecting the skills necessary for the hunt, in the case of carnivores, or the escape, in the case of herbivores. None of the preceding reasons explains adult play and why it persists more in some species and in some individuals than in others. Finally, play is presumably pleasurable and may, therefore, be its own reward whatever the ultimate value to the organism may be.

Play in puppies begins when they are about 3 weeks old, with mouthing of one another. The mouthing is concentrated on the head region of the opponent. This should not be surprising because it is the cranial nerves that are most myelinated in the suckling animal. The biter and bitten will get maximal sensory input from play that involves the puppies' heads. As the puppies' strength improves and as their teeth erupt, the mouthings become genuine nips. Four-week-old pups may nip painfully, but the violent reaction of their littermates and, in particular, their mother to painful bites soon teaches them to inhibit the force of the bites. The early-weaned or orphaned pup will not learn to inhibit its bites; it is up to the owner to punish, albeit mildly, the painful nip. The worst disfavor one can do a puppy is to wear heavy gloves when playing with it; the dog will not learn to play gently or to be submissive to humans. Safe chew toys should be substituted for human hands.

Play fighting

By 4–5 weeks, play fighting becomes more skilled as the puppies' motor and perceptual skills improve. Male puppies play more than females.[1467] Scruff holding and shaking or worrying appear. Pouncing, snapping, and growling occur in the course of play. The facial expressions of the adult dog replace the mask-like expression of the younger pup. Tug of war is a favorite game with littermates. Wrestling bouts occur with the puppies alternating the standing-over and lying-on-the-back positions.

Sexual play

Elements of sexual behavior appear at 6 weeks but the frequency of sexual play never equal that of social play and—like social play—decreases in frequency from week 10.[1467] The puppies will mount, clasp, and perform pelvic thrusts without regard to the sex of the partner. Male puppies, in particular, exhibit this behavior. Dogs deprived of all play experience and social contact as puppies can mate but are often misoriented when they mount and, consequently, achieve fewer intromissions.[171] The poor sexual performance of socially isolated dogs indicates the importance of play in puppyhood to normal adult behavior.

Characteristics of play behavior

It is important to the participants, as well as the observer, that play be distinguished from serious behavior. This is particularly true of fighting behavior. By 3.5 weeks, puppies can effectively signal that "what follows is play." The signal most often used is the play bow, in which the dog lowers its forequarters and often paws at its own face while wagging its tail (refer to Fig. 1.10, C, in Chapter 1). The play bow is an innate, not a learned display, for it occurs in hand-raised puppies.[200] The play face is distinguished by an open mouth and erect ears. Other signals are the exaggerated approach, repeated barking, approach and withdrawal, slapping the forelegs on the ground, and pouncing and leaping. A submissive dog is more successful in soliciting play than is a dominant one. Perhaps this is because the dominant dog usually is taken seriously by its subordinates.[201] In another demonstration of theory of mind, dogs rarely give play signals to an inattentive dog, for example one that is facing away. Instead, they make exaggerated approaches or retreats, pawing, presenting the rear quarters, bumping, leaping on, or even biting the inattentive dog. When that dog turns to face its tormentor, play signals ensue.[857]

Play in the dog, as in all species, is characterized by actions from various contexts (aggressive, sexual, and so forth) incorporated into unpredictable sequences in which the actions are repeated and performed in an exaggerated manner. A typical sequence would begin with a play bow, followed by an exaggerated approach, veering off, a chase, general biting, head shaking while biting, rolling and wrestling, reciprocal chasing, more wrestling, inhibited biting, rearing, and pushing with forepaws. Typical bouts last for 5–15 minutes in puppies between the ages of 3 and 7 weeks. The more play exhibited by young canids, the less true aggression is manifested, as shown in a comparison of the pups of three canid species: dogs were the most playful, coyotes the least, and wolves were intermediate. An analysis of play and fighting can be used to identify canids of unknown genotype.[202]

Play is valuable not only for the development of normal behavior but also for its diagnostic use. Play occurs most often in the warm, well-fed, healthy puppy. The absence of play behavior in 3–9-week-old puppies is an indication of pathology. Social play is the most common form in dogs, but solitary play does occur. The dog's pouncing upon and carrying a stick is an example. Tail chasing occurs in the absence of another puppy to chase. Games of fetch between owner and dog are the outgrowth of chasing play. If the game is not initiated during the period of socialization, it is very difficult to teach,[1714] especially to a dog that is not genetically a retriever.

Exploratory behavior may be classified as a thrill-seeking type of solitary play. Exploratory behavior increases with age, in contrast to social play, which decreases after 10 weeks of age. By 6 weeks of age, the puppy has mastered many of its social skills. It can signal play and aggression. It approaches another dog and investigates the inguinal area. It is beginning to form a dominance hierarchy. It eliminates in the same area as its mother and littermates do. It can eat food and sleep alone. In the next week or two, it should be ready to become socialized with humans.

Toys are important to adult dogs, who spend 24% of their active time using toys, but this can actually result in a decrease in time spent playing with other dogs.[895] Nylon bones are used longer than rawhides, although the latter are preferred initially. There are dogs that prefer to play tug of war and those that prefer to retrieve a ball. They don't differentiate between their owners and an unfamiliar person as a play partner. Dogs that prefer tug of war are more reactive, but no matter which game they prefer, dogs highly motivated to play are not fearful.[166,1896]

Puppies left alone vocalize, lip lick, yawn, and scratch. Puppies younger than 3 months were most apt to exhibit these behaviors. Over time, they will be inactive more often, and explore and play less.[623]

CATS

See Fig. 6.3 for a feline development chart.

Sensitive periods

Feline sensitive period for socialization, occurring at 2–7 weeks, is earlier than that of dogs.[1907] A litter of kittens isolated for the first month will be reluctant to approach people even if they are genetically friendly (see later in this chapter). Handling for 15 minutes per day from 2 to 6 weeks will result in friendly kittens.

The most detailed study on the role of early experience in adult feline behavior was that of Seitz,[1725] who separated kittens from their mothers at 2 days, 6 weeks, or 12 weeks. Kittens

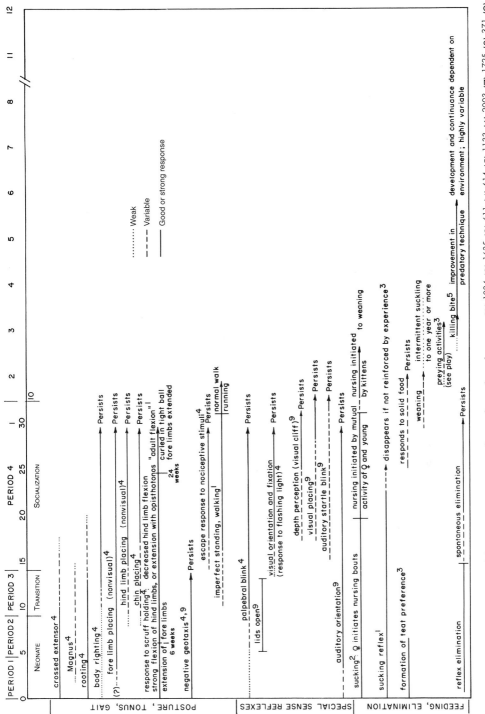

Fig. 6.3 Behavioral development of the cat. Superscript numbers refer to the references: (1),[1034] (2),[1635] (3),[611] (4),[614] (5),[1133] (6),[2003] (7),[1725] (8),[371] (9),[1944] and (10).[1907]

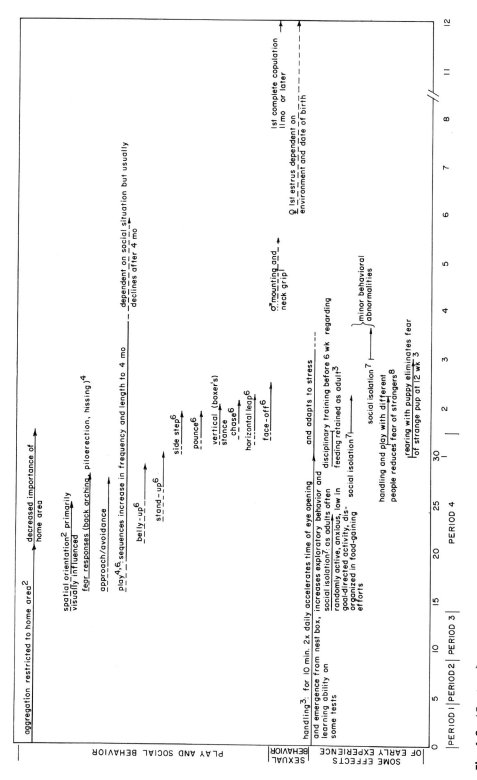

Fig. 6.3 (Continued)

weaned at 12 weeks did not cry upon separation, even though they had been living on their mother's milk alone. Kittens weaned at 6 weeks cried for a day or two. Those weaned at 2 days and fed by dropper cried for 1 week. As adults, the early-weaned kittens showed the most random activity, such as trying to escape from a carrying cage, and were most disturbed by novel stimuli. When tested with food, they were most persistent in trying to obtain food secured under a wire cover but least successful in competing with other cats for food. The early-weaned cats were also the slowest group to learn to associate the sight of a light with food.

Konrad and Bagshaw[1049] also weaned kittens at 2 days of age. The kittens were fed by nipple and handled as little as possible. When tested in an unfamiliar room, the cats raised in the restricted environment explored, played, and approached less than conventionally reared cats. Kittens raised in isolation from 40 days of age spent more time close to another cat than did kittens raised communally, but all the cats spent more time with another cat as they grew older.[322]

Handling kittens each day for the first month accelerates eye opening and EEG synchronization. Such cats are more active and aggressive when confined and are quieter in a novel environment.[1296] In another study, Meier and Stuart[1297] found that cats that had been handled and raised in a stimulating environment made fewer errors in a visual discrimination task. Kittens raised with their mothers and without handling were very slow to approach humans. Handling of the kittens appeared to impair their ability to learn some tasks several weeks later.[2033] Handling of kittens also affects their personalities: More handling before 8 weeks increases boldness for the first year, but thereafter the genetic component is more important, a trend seen across species.[1182]

It appears to be difficult to slow a kitten's development. Neither limitation of food nor severe hypoxic episodes affected kittens' development, although treatment with a goitrogen did delay development of solid food ingestion and locomotory skills, and resulted in slow physical development.[217]

The physiological basis of the behavioral abnormalities seen in early-weaned kittens may be inferred from the changes in the function of the visual pathways observed in cats reared either in the dark or in an environment in which they had no, or very limited, visual stimuli, such as horizontal or vertical lines. Both behavioral and neurophysiological evidence demonstrated that the visual system, especially the cortical components, does not develop normally; cats exposed only to horizontal lines show little response to vertical lines.[232] Kittens raised without opportunity to see their front paws because they were either in darkness or wearing Elizabethan collars have difficulty in visual placing. They extend their paws appropriately, but may miss a small target that normally reared kittens reach 95% of the time.[805] Kittens must learn to match paw position to target position. Similar changes occur in more complex behaviors: A cat that never had the opportunity to play as a kitten does not respond to the appropriate play signals as an adult. Kittens have adequate genetic capabilities to form the neuronal connections necessary for normal vision or social behavior, but the complex connections between cortical neurons form with visual or play experience during a critical period.

Neurological development

The neurological development of the cat has not been studied as systematically as that of the dog. The kitten shows a dominance of flexor tone for the first 2 weeks of life and then a dominance of extensor tone for the second 2 weeks. The motor cortex involved in forelimb movement develops during those first 2 weeks and cortical control of the hind limbs in the second 2 weeks.

This is reflected in the locomotion of the kitten. It drags itself by its forelegs at first, but later the pushing movement of the hind legs grows stronger.[611,1601] The eyes open at 7 days (range, 6–10 days), and orienting responses to auditory stimuli develop a day or two before.[607] Between the third and sixth week, cats develop the ability to land on their feet (air righting).

Visual acuity improves 16-fold between 2 and 10 weeks of age. The development of the cytoarchitecture of the sensory cortex is interesting in that the cortical layers of the kitten brain are arranged in an orderly fashion with few dendrites linking the cells. The adult cat brain possesses disordered layers with many dendritic processes on the cells, which apparently pull the cells out of the original orderly alignment. It is hypothesized that the interconnecting dendrites form with increasing sensory experience.

Adult cats and dogs will respond to a silhouette of their own species as they would to a real animal. Five-week-old kittens do not even orient themselves to a cat silhouette, but 6-week-old kittens do, and the frequency approaches the adult level by 8 weeks. Adult cats are apparently threatened by silhouettes and will show piloerection toward a silhouette on its first presentation. Five-week-old kittens show no piloerection and 6-week-old kittens show very little, but 8-week-old kittens show the adult response to silhouettes.[1045] Hypothalamic stimulation does not elicit adult-like affective response with piloerection and enlarged pupils until 3 weeks, although sensory motor responses, such as arching and jaw movements, can be elicited at 4 hours.[1033]

Adult cats show a unique expression, the gape, to conspecific urine (refer to Fig. 1.13B, in Chapter 1). This response is not seen in kittens less than 5 weeks old and is essentially similar in frequency and performance to adult gaping at 7 weeks.[1045] Kittens can make ultrasonic vocalizations. In general, the frequency limit and range fall with age. Deafened kittens produce vocalizations similar to those of normal kittens, indicating that learning is not important; however, their calls are louder than those of normal kittens, indicating that feedback through the auditory system normally occurs.

As kittens mature, they become more proficient at finding their way back to their home area. They also vocalize less when placed on a cold surface (30 cries per minute at 1 day of age as compared with 17 cries per minute at 15 days). After the eyes have opened, the kittens use visual cues to find their nest; prior to that time they use olfaction. Very young kittens will become less active and less vocal when placed on a warm rather than cool surface, but the calming effect of thermal stimuli is lost after the first week.[643,644,1630] Isolation produces most vocalizations (4 cries per minute) at 3 weeks of age; younger and older kittens vocalize less. Response to restraint remains high and unchanged (5 cries per minute) throughout development.[781]

Sleep

Sleep in kittens also shows a developmental pattern. For the first 3 weeks, the EEG cannot be correlated with the other behavior defining the different sleep stages, such as eye movements and muscle quiescence. Although the percentage of time that kittens are awake remains constant, the percentage of active REM sleep decreases and that of quiet sleep increases. Muscle twitching, which is characteristic of REM sleep, also decreases with age. The sleep cycles are also much shorter than those of the adult cat. Kittens also pass directly from the awake state to REM sleep; adult cats almost always pass through SWS sleep before entering REM sleep.[1268] Not until 3 months of age do forebrain maturation and environmental influences mediate a mature sleep–wake cycle.[856]

Play

Play in kittens is first seen at the beginning of the third week at the same time that the queen begins the process of weaning by repulsing the kittens' attempts to nurse (see Chapter 5). Play in cats has been most thoroughly studied by West,[2003, 2004] Caro,[324–326] and Martin and Bateson.[1228] Although severe malnutrition leads to a suppression of play, less severe restriction of the food of a lactating queen leads to more play, especially more contact play, by her kittens. This is presumably in response to milk deprivation of the kittens and may be a form of early weaning or preparing the kitten to hunt for its own food.[165] Perhaps some of the kittens whose play is too exuberant for their new owners were deprived while suckling. Certainly, this appears to be true of hand-reared kittens.

Play in kittens begins with gentle pawing at one another. As kittens improve in coordination, biting, chasing, and rolling replace simple pawing. One kitten is usually in the belly-up position (kitten lies on its back with all four legs held in a semivertical position). Social play increases from 4 to 11 weeks and then declines relatively rapidly (Fig. 6.4). At first, three or more kittens may play together, but by 8 weeks, almost all play is between pairs of kittens. A reliable sign of play is the arched back and tail, but a definite play signal has not been defined in cats, although tail position and movement have been suggested.[2003]

Play periods

Usually, four play periods occur per day. Almost an hour a day is spent in play at 9 weeks of age. Most kitten play bouts begin with a pounce and end with a chase. In between, the kittens frequently face-off, hunching forward with tails arched out and down. They may bat at one another. Kittens also assume a vertical stance in play, rearing back on their hind legs, sometimes standing up by extending the legs. Various leaps are seen also. Kittens are much more apt than puppies to paw rather than bite at one another. The prevalence of pouncing, stalking, and chasing in feline play may be evidence that it is practice for hunting. Play bouts may have one chase per minute. Play may occupy 9% of the kitten's total time and only 4–9% of its energy expenditure, indicating that play may be important, but it is not calorically costly.[1227]

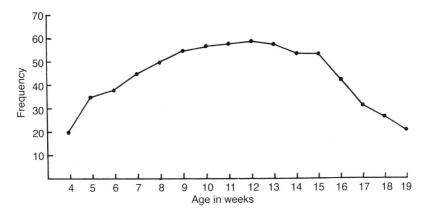

Fig. 6.4   The change in playing behavior of kittens with age. Social play reaches a peak at 12 weeks and then declines. Frequency refers to the percent of the daily 90-minute observation period in which play was observed.[2003] (Copyright 1974, with permission of Am. Zool.)

Predatory play

The mother plays an active role in the development of her kittens' predatory behavior. Mothers not only attack and eat prey in front of their kittens but also vocalize to attract the kittens' attention to these activities. These behaviors occur when the kittens are 4–8 weeks old. After that, the mother defers to the kittens in that she rarely kills and almost never eats the prey. The kittens are more apt to interact with the prey if the mother has just been interacting with it than if a littermate has, indicating that the mother has a greater influence.[324,326] Kittens also learn other tasks better from watching their mother than from watching another cat.[347]

A very definite increase in predatory activity occurs around 8 weeks. At that time, most kittens will kill and eat mice, and most of their behavior is directed toward prey than toward playing with one another. After the prey is dead and eaten, the kittens return to playing with one another, indicating that the motivation to play is still present but is overridden by the motivation to hunt. Social play and predatory play are not correlated and probably are controlled by different systems.[325] By 2 months of age, those kittens that will be frightened rather than aggressive toward prey and toward other cats can be identified; these same kittens are reluctant to explore and to relax with people in a new environment.[7] This is unfortunate because some people prefer that their cat does not hunt, and many wish their cats to be less aggressive toward other cats; but almost all owners want their cat to be friendly, even in a novel environment. Play can be encouraged in adult cats by a pause of 5 minutes after a 2-minute play bout and by changing toys.[747]

Sexual play

Elements of sexual behavior are not seen in kitten play, but one sex difference appears in feline play. Males show more object contact than females; females with male littermates play with objects more than do females with no male littermates.[157] Play may be more important for intraspecies socialization in cats than it is in other species because the ancestral species are solitary for much of their adult lives.

Solitary play in kittens also begins to decline at 4 months, but the decline is much more gradual.[2003] Kittens will chase small rolling objects or even a moving string. They particularly like to bat at suspended objects, such as window shade pulls or tassels. Many of the pounces and face-offs of social play may be performed by solitary kittens with "imaginary" playmates, a mirror, or their own shadow. Solitary play persists in many adult cats. Playfulness is a factor for which breeders should select because it enhances the pleasure a cat gives to its owner as well as to itself. Social play may also occur between species. Cats will often play with dogs with which they are familiar. Interspecies play consists mostly of chases by the dog and pounces by the cat.

Several factors may contribute to the decline of play in kittens. Subadult cats begin to sleep more during the day. Older cats tend to spend more time sitting quietly but alertly. Male kittens show sexual activity by 4.5 months and attempt to mount and bite the scruff of females, who will reject these attempts until they reach sexual maturity a few months later. Young feral cats may also devote more time to finding their own prey. When canine and feline play are compared, dogs are found to chase (especially in a group), mouth, wrestle, shake, and indulge in solitary play more than cats. Cats stalk and ambush more frequently.[22]

Relationships with humans

Handling of kittens during their sensitive period of socialization from 2 to 7 weeks is important.[985] Handling kittens for less than 30 minutes twice a week from the time the kittens are

5 weeks until they are 8 weeks does not increase their friendliness.[1594] More handling beginning at an earlier age does, especially if the kittens are genetically inclined to be friendly.[1253]

Clinical problems

Two common clinical behavior problems in cats are aggression between two or more cats in a household and rejection of the tom by the estrous queen. Both may be related to failure to socialize adequately to other cats as kittens. Kittens usually are removed from the mother at 6 weeks, long before the peak of playful interactions at 11 weeks. Cats that have remained with other kittens longer than 6 weeks may be more tolerant of other cats, including courting toms, as adults.

Playful behavior itself can be a behavior problem, particularly if it occurs in the middle of the night.[187] This is most apt to occur when the kitten has been alone, and probably asleep, most of the day and has not had much opportunity to play. Punishment may inhibit the kitten's play, but it is more likely simply to move out of range and to continue racing about and knocking over objects. A scheduled play period in late evening is the best treatment. Cat toys also help. Adding a second kitten might help because two kittens usually play with each other, they will not interact with humans as much as kittens and the cats may become incompatible as adults. Hand-reared kittens frequently bite hands, possibly in response to the frustration of lack of suckling as a kitten, to ambivalence toward stranger's hands as providers of food, but also as frightening objects, or to a lack of bite inhibition due to lack of play experience with other cats.

HORSES

The foal's first day

First hour

The perinatal behavior of foals has been described by Waring,[1972] who studied American saddlebreds, and by Rossdale,[1640] who studied thoroughbreds and ponies. The foal can move its head and legs immediately after birth. The suckling reflex appears within the first few minutes. The suckling reflex is elicited by anything put into the foal's mouth. Righting itself to sternal recumbency and the first attempts to stand occur within the first 15 minutes, but the foal will fail in a dozen attempts, so an hour may elapse before the foal stands. Pony foals can stand at a younger age than those of the long-legged breeds.

The foal begins to use all its senses within the first hour. It experiences tactile stimulation from its mother's licking and will begin to respond and orient to visual and auditory stimuli within the first hour. Within the first hour, it will begin to communicate by nickers to its mother and by snapping (see Fig. 6.10, later in chapter) at any fearful object. The foal can walk soon after it can stand, although it will not be well coordinated for another few hours. As soon as the foal can walk, it begins to search for the udder. It may attempt to suckle from the walls of the stall or from inappropriate parts of its mother, as well as suck when no oral contact has been made (vacuum suckling). The feature that the foal innately seeks is an underline, so it will attempt to nurse from the axilla as readily as the inguinal region. Defecation also occurs within the first hour.

The rest of the first day

Successful suckling is the major event of the foal's second hour of life. Although pony foals suckle within the second half hour of life, a further 30 minutes is necessary before saddlebred and thoroughbred foals are able to suckle. By the second hour, the foal has also begun to follow its dam or any other large moving object. Lying down is another difficult task for the foal to master but is usually accomplished within the second or third hour. The foal will then sleep; a few foals will sleep standing up if they have not been able to lie down but will fall down if they go into REM sleep. By the third hour, the foal can also groom itself and gallop. Within the first day, the foal can play, urinate, flehmen, and graze as well as communicate, suckle, and locomote; in other words, it is already a well-coordinated, functional horse. See Fig. 6.5 for the behavioral development of the foal.

The first year

The behavior of foals is well illustrated in McDonnell and Poulin.[1264] The ontogeny of the foal has been extensively studied in Welsh ponies,[403,410,412] New Forest ponies,[1909] Camargue ponies,[269] thoroughbreds,[1076,1079,1081] and Belgians.[148] Little difference appeared in the time budgets and rate of development among these five types of horses even though the environments varied considerably in the degree of confinement and amount of forage available. Thoroughbreds and other horse breeds are more apt to be managed intensively than ponies; therefore, differences in time budgets are more apt to reflect artificial feeding and stall restraint rather than breed differences in ontogeny. For example, Kusunose and Sawazaki[1076] found that thoroughbred foals lay down more often while stalled at night than during the day on pasture, whereas foals on pasture 24 hours per day distribute their lying time more evenly.

The mare–foal bond

The distance between a mare and her foal is proportional to the age of the foal, that is, young foals are closer to their dams than are older foals. The foal is responsible for this proximity in most circumstances. It follows the mother; this changes when the foal lies down. Then the mare remains close to the foal either stand resting or grazing in circles around the foal.[403] This behavior—the recumbency response—wanes as the foal matures, but one can almost guess the age of the foal by how close the mare remains while the foal sleeps. The other circumstance in which the mare follows the foal is when the young foal ventures more than 10 m (33 ft) away.[403]

Grazing

Foals at first must spread and flex their legs in order to graze, especially if the grass is short; later, their necks lengthen in relation to their legs and they can graze more comfortably. Foals gradually increase the length of time that they spend grazing, from 4 to 16 minutes per hour during the period from birth to 4 months. Thereafter, the increase is more rapid, reaching adult levels (60–70% of the time) at natural weaning (40 weeks).

   The development of feeding behavior is interesting because social facilitation plays such an important part. Foals graze only when their mothers are grazing[412] (Fig. 6.6). This fact illustrates the importance of providing creep feed for a foal in a location from which the foal can watch his mother eat. Drinking may not occur in foals on lush pasture. They obtain all their water needs

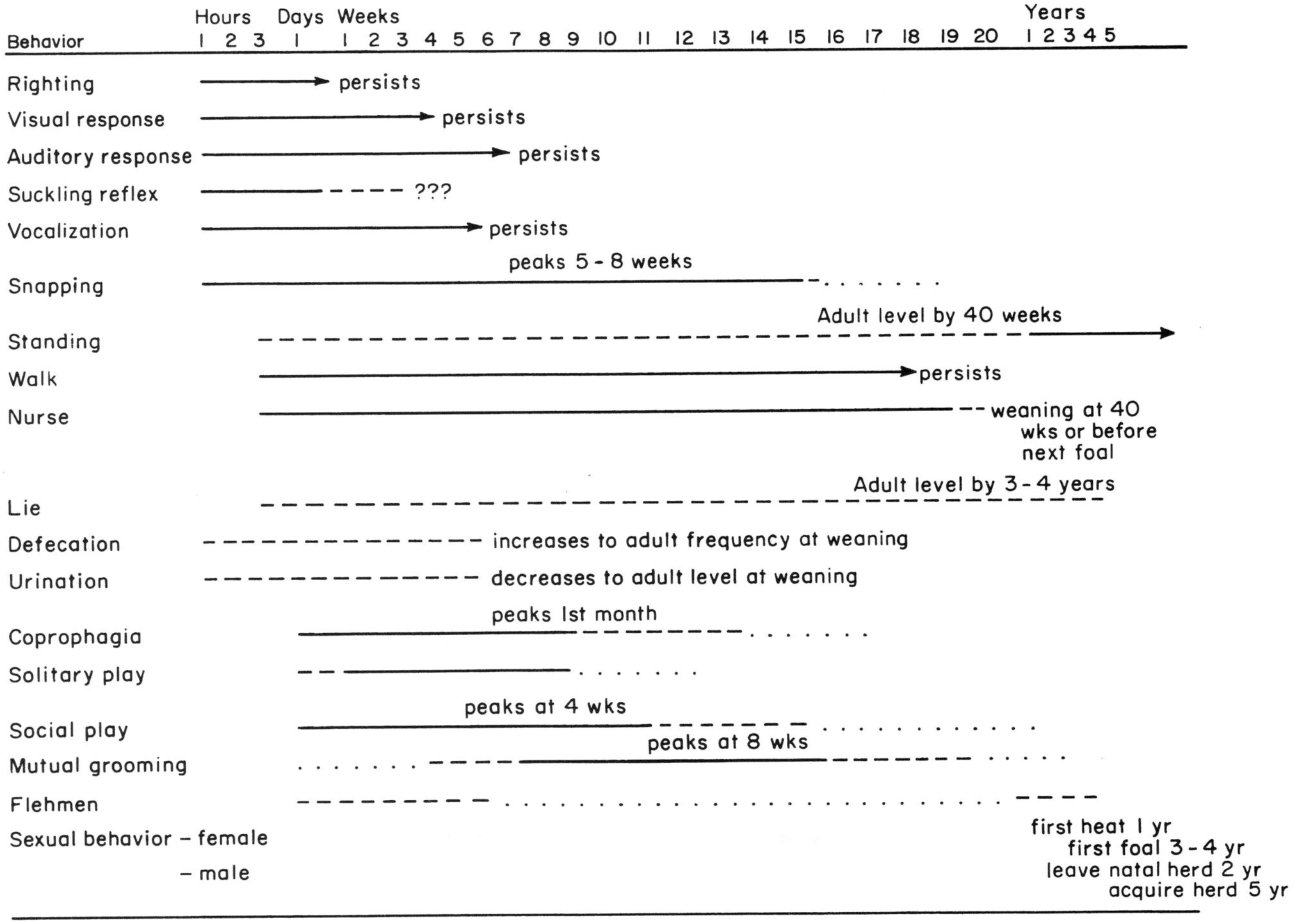

Hours Days Weeks   Years

Behavior 1 2 3 | 1 | 1 2 3 4 5 6 7 8 9 10 11 12 13 14 15 16 17 18 19 20 | 1 2 3 4 5

Righting → persists

Visual response → persists

Auditory response → persists

Suckling reflex – – – ???

Vocalization → persists

Snapping peaks 5 - 8 weeks .... Adult level by 40 weeks

Standing → persists

Walk – – weaning at 40 wks or before next foal

Nurse

Lie Adult level by 3 - 4 years

Defecation – – – – – – – – increases to adult frequency at weaning

Urination – – – – – – – – decreases to adult level at weaning

Coprophagia peaks 1st month ....

Solitary play peaks at 4 wks ....

Social play peaks at 8 wks ....

Mutual grooming ....

Flehmen – – – – –

Sexual behavior – female first heat 1 yr
first foal 3 - 4 yr
       – male leave natal herd 2 yr
acquire herd 5 yr

Fig. 6.5 Behavioral development of the horse. 214, 408, 410, 412, 413, 501, 1973

189

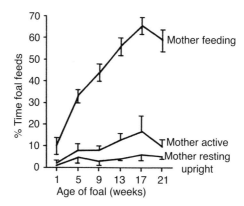

Fig. 6.6 The mean percentage of time the foals spent feeding when their mother was feeding, active, or resting upright.[412] (Copyright 1985, with permission of J. Anim. Sci.)

from their dams' milk and moist grass, and although they follow their dams to water, they do not drink. In arid areas, foals do drink.[272]

Adult horses normally will avoid feces,[1442] but coprophagy is a normal ingestive behavior of foals, although its function is unknown. Both negative and positive consequences may occur: The foal may ingest ova of parasites, but it may also ingest bacteria and protozoa that inoculate its gastrointestinal tract with the proper flora. The dam's feces are consumed in preference to those of another horse.[407,408,622]

Sleep

Foals rest either standing or lying. As foals develop, they spend less time lying down and more time resting upright.[402] They spend a great deal more time lying than adult horses. The percentage of time spent in lateral recumbency decreases with the age of the foal from 15% (first month) to 2% after weaning.[269] Resting in sternal recumbency does not change very much throughout the foal's first 6 months (averaging about 15% of its day) and is still higher than adult levels in 2- and 3-year-olds. Resting while standing also occurs in foals. The foal usually stands beside the mother, often facing in the opposite direction in order to take advantage of her tail to ward off flies.

Play

As the foal matures, it spends less time resting; it suckles less and grazes more. In between these activities, it plays. For the first 2 weeks, play is solitary. Foals gallop away from and toward their mothers, which may be a form of exploration or even thrill-seeking behavior.[22] Play in foals is one of the best examples of play as exercise. About 70% of locomotion in foals is in a play context.[562] Foals at first play with their mothers by nibbling at their legs and mane. Later, this will become true allogrooming. Social play with other foals gradually increases with age, and solitary play declines; by 8 weeks, solitary play rarely is seen (this, of course, would not be true of foals that do not have companions available; see Fig. 6.7). In lone foals, solitary play persists and social play may include dogs and humans.[1691] Foals may also play with inanimate objects, such as twigs, by tossing them into the air.

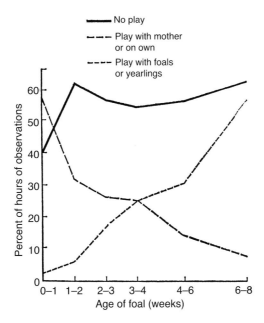

Fig. 6.7   Changes with age in foal's choice of play partners. As play with the mother decreases, play with other foals increases.[1909] (Copyright 1972, with permission of Academic Press.)

At 20 weeks of age, foals still spend more than half of their time within 5 m (16.4 ft) of their mothers, although they are most apt to leave her to play.[403] Definite sex differences appear in play: Colts mount and fight; fillies chase and mutually groom one another. Play in foals often centers about the head. Nipping of the head and mane, including gripping of the crest, accounts for the greatest number of play sequences. Rearing up and mounting is frequently seen, especially in colts. Properly oriented mounting is seen even in very young colts. Chases are a common play sequence.[1701] Side-by-side nipping can progress to circle fighting in which each foal attempts to bite the tail and legs of another. When colts do mutually groom, they tend to groom fillies rather than other colts.[411] Grooming the mare is part of the courtship behavior of the stallion. These sex differences in play may prepare the animals for their adult roles.

Figure 6.8 illustrates the types of play seen in pony foals on pasture. Play in horses reflects their dam's investment; colts of feral mares in good body condition play more and are larger at 1 year than colts of mothers in poor condition. In contrast, fillies of mares in poor condition play more. In either case, the mother of the foal that plays more loses more body condition, reflecting her investment in the foal.[312] This may reflect the sociobiological position that the mother should invest more in a son when she has plenty of resources because he can sire many offspring, but should invest more in a daughter when resources are scarce because a daughter is likely to foal at least once if she survives for a year, whereas a stunted colt may never sire a foal because he can't win mares from stronger stallions.

Foals have a dominance hierarchy that is related to their age and their dams' rank. The effect of birth order disappears postweaning when foals are all about the same size. Colts receive more aggression than do fillies. Fillies are more likely to kick; colts, to bite.[67,1986] Foals are most likely to have as a preferred associate the foal of their dam's preferred associate.

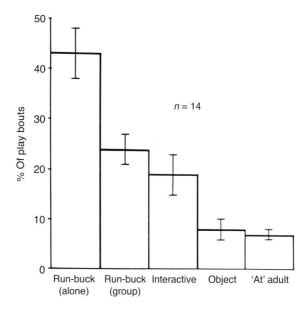

Fig. 6.8 Relative frequency of various types of play. The mean percent of total play bouts by 14 foals in which the type of play was running and bucking alone, running and bucking as a group, interactive, manipulation of an object, or play with an adult. Standard error of the mean is shown as a vertical bar.[413] (Copyright 1987, with permission of Elsevier.)

Flehmen and snapping

Flehmen behavior is also much more frequent in colts than in fillies. It is probably investigatory behavior. Flehmen peaks during the colt's first month, possibly because his dam will be in estrus then and/or because he is still somewhat precocially masculinized owing to his prenatal hormonal environment[412] (Fig. 6.9).

The facial expression of snapping (also known as tooth clapping or champing) occurs almost exclusively in foals and subadult horses (Fig. 6.10). This expression persists in zebra and donkeys as yawing, the mouth movements associated with estrus. In fact, the facial expression of snapping and that of yawing occur in the same circumstances, that is, an approach–avoidance situation. A colt is most apt to snap when approaching a stallion to whom he is apparently attracted, but who is also frightening. The estrous donkey and zebra mares, and, rarely, a submissive, estrous mare[2062] may be attracted to the stallion but may also be frightened. Snapping in foals is likely to occur when a stallion is courting the mare. The rate of snapping falls rapidly with age from one every 3 hours during the first month to one every 20 hours during the sixth month. The peak of snapping is during the foal's second month of life.[410]

The juvenile period

Play and activity in general decrease with age; 2- and 3-year-olds are more active than adults. About 97% of colts and 81% of fillies leave their natal band.[1669] Fillies leave their herd and tend to join bands with familiar females, but unfamiliar (that is, unrelated) males.[1351] The age at which colts leave depends on whether there are colts of the same age in the band; if so, the colts stay longer. The first male offspring of a mare may leave and return several times, indicating

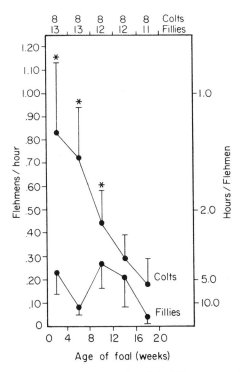

Fig. 6.9   Rate of flehmen by foals of various ages. Colts exhibit flehmen more than fillies only during the first few weeks. Asterisks indicate significant difference.[409] (Copyright 1985, with permission of Academic Press.)

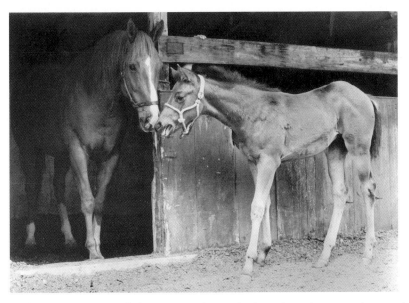

Fig. 6.10   Submissive snapping of the immature horse. Foal on the right approaches its dam while snapping.[2055] (Copyright 1980, with permission of Elsevier Science Publishers.)

a particularly strong bond.[1009] Colts also are influenced to leave by scarcity of food as well as by the birth of siblings. The colts may join wandering female, juvenile, and adult mares, mixed-sex groups (juvenile and adult mares plus juvenile males), or all-juvenile male bachelor groups.[992,1010] Bachelor males spend much time playing, half of which is play fighting.[351] Those colts that remain in their natal herd do not have this experience and appear to be slower to mature. The peak of colt play occurs at 3 years. At 5 years, he will begin to show adult male behaviors such as marking of urine and feces, true aggression toward other stallions, and driving of mares.[848] At five, he is able to take over his own herd either by defeating an infirm harem stallion, replacing a dead one, or competing successfully against other bachelors for a filly that has left her natal herd.

PIGS

Pigs are intermediate in their development at birth. They can walk, albeit unsteadily, within a few minutes of birth; they can see and hear. Their brain development is not complete at birth, however, and some homeostatic mechanisms, such as temperature regulation, are not yet mature.

The neurological development of the pig has not been extensively studied despite the considerable clinical application such a study would have. Piglet mortality is very high, approaching 20%. Some of this mortality is due to infectious disease, but a considerable number of deaths are "accidental." The piglets may wander out of their pen and drown in a gutter or simply become chilled and die from exposure, or they may wander in with older pigs that maul them to death. Other piglets are crushed by the sow even though she is in a farrowing crate. Normal piglets do not wander; they stay close to their littermates, the heat source, and the sow's udder. Piglets, especially those among the last delivered, may suffer various degrees of brain damage as a result of hypoxia during birth. If these brain-damaged pigs could be identified and hand reared or otherwise given extra protection, piglet mortality would fall.

When piglets are castrated, they stand and suckle less and lie down more.[1275] This response occurs in piglets castrated at any age from day one of life, indicating that they are able to perceive the pain. They vocalize more at the time of castration, and the vocalizations are more high pitched, another indication of the painfulness of this procedure.[1855]

Piglets have some unique physiological problems that affect their behavior. Piglets are born almost hairless and with little subcutaneous fat for insulation. Their small size, lack of insulation, and low energy reserves leave piglets very vulnerable to hypothermia.[1376] Piglets solve the problem of heat conservation behaviorally rather than metabolically. They huddle with their littermates, thus decreasing their surface area and, in effect, making one large animal from 12 small ones. If a heat source is provided, they lie next to it. Unless the environmental temperature is over 26°C (79°F), a heat lamp should be provided.[1879] Piglets that do not huddle or that persist in wandering away from the sow and the heat source have very likely been brain damaged at birth. A quick inspection of the farrowing house can enable one to determine whether the temperature conditions are correct: If piglets are sprawled on the floor in extension, they are warm enough; if they are crouched on their sterna with their legs drawn under them, they are too cold.

Sleep

As with most newborns, piglets tend only to eat and sleep. Piglets sleep for 16 minutes of every hour. The number of REM bouts decreases with age, but each bout remains of similar length.[1071]

Teat order

Nursing behavior has been described in Chapter 5. The teat order is formed on the first day. The peak of aggression occurs 1 hour after birth. By day 6, only 10% of the piglets change teats.[825] To reduce injuries to the sow's udder or to the piglets that may occur during the formation of the teat order, it is common to clip the incisors and canines of day-old pigs.[635]

Feeding

Piglets rest for most of the day during the first week but are active most of the time by their eighth week. Piglets begin to eat creep feed around day 12; their intake is less than five grams per day, but within a week they are eating 10 times as much.[1465] Intake can be increased by providing more feeders so that advantage can be taken of social facilitation.[65] The time spent eating the creep feed was greater when the feed was available on flat trays rather than troughs.[1978] Piglets who start consuming solid food earlier will consume more.[64, 245] Piglets that had access to the most productive teats gained less weight when first weaned. They had not learned to eat solid food as soon as their hungrier littermates.[41] Piglets are more apt to eat solid food if the food is sweet, because suckling piglets possess a well-developed sweet taste preference.[873]

Piglets will begin drinking from a bowl at 15 days of age and drink mostly right after suckling.[452] Pigs weaned at 27 days did not eat for almost 20 hours, although they spent more time drinking than they did on the second day.[517] When pigs are weaned and housed with other pigs, there is considerable fighting. One method of alleviating that problem is to mix the litters before weaning. This also results in fighting, but may not be as serious when not combined with the stress of separation from the sow.[1476] In a seminaturalistic environment, piglets begin to graze by 4 weeks, and the percentage of time spent in this activity rises from 7 to 42% by 8 weeks.[1499]

Play

In a seminatural environment

When sows leave the maternal nest and rejoin the herd, the piglets are gradually integrated into the social life of the older animals.[1500]

In a confined environment

Piglets begin to explore their environment by rooting, biting, and chewing within the first days postpartum. They also play alone, jumping and running. Play with the sow, nudging, climbing, and biting as well as naso–naso contact begins in the first 2 days of life. Social play with littermates begins at 3–5 days[230] (Fig. 6.11). Male piglets play more frequently than females, and play occurs more frequently between same-sex pairs than mixed-sex pairs. Play in piglets is characterized by play fights. These fights are usually head-to-head confrontations in which each piglet chews and roots at the other's shoulders and neck. In older pigs (3–4 weeks old), chases and gamboling can be observed. At about the same age, the typical porcine startle reaction (a woof and freezing behavior) can first be elicited. Failure to play is of diagnostic value in determining the seriousness of neonatal pig disease.

Exploratory behavior is very pronounced in piglets and consists of rooting and mouthing anything that is new in the environment. Pigs in an environment enriched with straw, logs, and

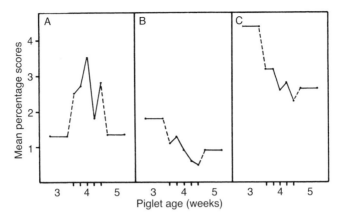

Fig. 6.11   The change with age in play fighting and solitary play in piglets. The graphs give the mean percentage of minutes in which early-weaned piglets were scored as (A) biting littermates, (B) scratching their bodies, and (C) scampering during the first 5 weeks of life, expressed as a percentage of the number of minutes in which the animals were scored as active. Piglets were weaned at the end of the third week.[230]

branches spend less time manipulating the sow's udder and later spend less time nudging or tail biting.[1501] In the absence of manipulatable objects, piglets chew the floor and walls of their pens and one another; therefore, toys should be provided. Pigs prefer hourglass rubber dog toys to chains, ropes, or rubber hoses.[63] Pigs prefer shredded paper to rope as toys.[1130] Hanging toys are preferred to the same toys on the floor of the pen.

Straw bedding seems to be the most effective enrichment in that penmates are not manipulated. The piglets will spend 18% of their time in straw-directed behavior. Piglets will choose to investigate a novel object, and other forms of play, such as scampering, increase in the presence of novel objects.[2061] The novelty of an object wanes with exposure after 2 days.[687]

Elimination

Pigs begin to eliminate only at the edges of their pens as they mature.[2007] In pet minipigs, this behavior can be used to facilitate housebreaking. Defecation is more frequently performed in brightly lit areas,[1854] so a darker rest area might encourage elimination away from the bedded area.

Relationships with humans

An investigation into the effect of early handling revealed that piglets handled daily were not larger than nonhandled littermates but were more aggressive when penned with strange pigs.[1702] The effects of human handling depend on the quality of the handling and can have economic importance. For example, Hemsworth et al.[815] found that pigs treated pleasantly (stroked) grew more rapidly and had better feed conversion than those treated unpleasantly (pigs were shocked if they approached the handler). Handling of pigs from 0 to 3 weeks or from 9 to 12 weeks reduces their fear of humans.[814,816] Gently handled pigs not only were less afraid of humans than harshly handled ones, they also came into estrus sooner. More intensive handling by an individual resulted in pigs spending more time with humans, avoiding them less, and being easier to catch.[1851] Unfortunately, few farmers would be able to spend 10 minutes a day with each pig. Boars handled 10 minutes per day for the first 14 days gained less weight in the following 7 months and had a greater ACTH response at slaughter. In contrast to handled rats, handled pigs did not have an increase in hippocampal glucocorticoid receptor.[1984]

RUMINANTS

Very few behavioral studies of development in ruminants have been done. Despite the detailed knowledge we possess about growth rates in these food-producing animals, next to nothing is known about the daily activity of young ruminants or how their relationship to their environment and their peers changes with maturity. The change in suckling patterns with age is discussed in Chapter 5. Some general statements can be made. Young ruminants are born in an advanced state of development; they are true precocial animals. They can stand and walk within a few hours of birth and can apparently see and hear.

Lambs

By 30 days of age, young lambs will spend 60% of their time with other lambs, but for the first few weeks they stay quite close to their dams. This behavior is to be contrasted with the behavior of the kid, who is much more apt to stray. The lamb may depend on its proximity to its mother for protection, whereas the kid uses its own behavioral pattern, that of freezing, to protect itself. Handling by humans seems to affect artificially raised lambs more than ewe raised lambs in that the artificially raised lamb investigate more.

Play

By a month of age, play is well developed in lambs.[1363] Play begins with investigation of one another when the lambs are only a few days old. Play consists of intentional butting, vertical leaps, rearing up on the hindquarters, which may be a play signal, and twisting the forequarters and kicking. Play may be centered around rocks or mounds so that one lamb can butt others from above. The lambs push one another, lay their heads on one another, and mount each other. Male lambs mount much more than females and are the only ones to "nudge," raising a foreleg under the belly of another lamb while standing close behind it. The sex differences in lamb play are mediated by prenatal testosterone.[1451] Male lambs behavior is less synchronized with that of their dams than female lambs and, therefore the males are at greater risk of predation.[1235]

Lambs form groups by a few weeks of age and rest, graze, and play together. Disportive or solitary play also occurs in which lambs gallop and leap. Adults may join the lambs in play. Lambs are especially playful in the evening. By 4 months of age, play begins to wane.[722]

Feeding

Lambs tend to prefer foods their dams eat, rather than avoiding what she rejected.[1341] Lambs will eat less of a shrub avoided by their dams,[1342] but this may not apply to more palatable foods.[1870] They will eat low-quality roughage diets if their dams have done so.[468]

When suckling lambs were offered creep feed at 3 weeks of age, their intake was variable and they did not consume the solid food on a daily basis until 2 weeks later.[562] Grazing times of lambs who had had a week of experience with pasture prior to weaning were twice as long as those of naive lambs. Exposure to a novel flavor (onion and garlic) from a month of age for 3 months resulted in only a temporary preference for those flavors.[1426]

Social relationships

The social relationships of sheep are formed in the first few weeks and appear to persist for life in the undisturbed flock, but this may vary with breed and environment. Twin lambs are less upset if their twin is visible, indicating that they use vision and olfaction to identify each other.[1534] Whether a yearling ewe associates with her mother may depend on environmental factors such as high population density. The yearling who remains with its dam may gain more weight, and the ewe will incur no costs. The ewe is followed by her lamb, and the lamb is submissive to her. Even as adults, daughters will follow the mother, and their lambs will be close at the heels of their respective dams.[1710,1713]

Sexual behavior

Sexual behavior develops gradually in ram lambs. Despite the sexual elements of play, six-month-old lambs rarely even investigate a ewe in estrus. At 10 months, they investigate ewes in estrus, and at 13 months will mount; but only at 17 months is the complete mating sequence, including copulation, seen in all rams.[2042]

Sleep and activity patterns

Sleep can occupy up to 40% of the lamb's day, but only 15% of the adult's.[1656] Grooming behavior, scratching with the hooves or teeth, occupies as much as 9% of the lamb's time, but far less of the adult's.[722]

Relationship with humans

Restraining lambs in a head gate (stanchion) and handling them did not increase their tendency to approach people, allowing the lambs to approach on their own did.[1233,1533] Lambs who had been bottle-fed for their first 3 weeks, after 3 weeks with no visual contact with humans, could recognize the shepherd who fed them at 6 weeks of age but not at 14 weeks.[249] Apparently, it is the tactile contact with humans that is important because lambs held separately from feeding were as likely to approach the handler as bottle-fed lambs, although bottle-fed lambs interacted more than lambs who were only held.[1847]

Kids

Lickiter[1138] has described changes in activity patterns of goat kids. Lying decreases markedly around 4 weeks from 60 to 70% of the time to 30% for the next few months. Ruminating begins at about 4 weeks as they begin to graze. It is apparent that the change to a herbivorous ruminant accounts for the biggest change in behavior during development. Presumably, this is true of all ruminants and contrasts with the more gradual changes that can be seen in the foal. Standing increases somewhat at the time that lying decreases. By 15 weeks, grazing is the predominant activity, and behavior of the kid is synchronous with that of its mother.

Play

Kids appear to be much livelier than lambs. Even in the confined environment of a pen, they will play a game that can only be described as "king of the mountain," as each kid leaps onto the highest available horizontal surface, which may be an overturned bucket or even another animal. Other types of play consist of short bursts of running (less than 15 seconds), leaping into the air, kicking, butting and mounting (more in males than females), mouthing objects, and standing on the hind legs with the forelegs against a vertical object. Play occurs most at dawn and dusk in 1-hour periods separated by a period of rest. Restraint in a pen or other forms of play deprivation are followed by a rebound of play in which play may last for 3 hours.[346]

Vocalizations

The call of the kid changes during development. The fundamental frequency falls from 600 kHz on the first day to 250–350 kHz on the fifth day. By 4 weeks, sex differences appear, with the male voice being three octaves below the female voice. Call lengths vary. The orienting call is 1 second in duration, the distress call, 1.5 seconds.[1119]

Social relationships

Two-week-old kids separated from their dams for 10 minutes exhibit increased cortisol, epinephrine, and norepinephrine, but decreased dopamine levels in their blood.

The pattern of older animal dominant over younger is true of a stable herd of goats, but not if strange adult animals are mixed.[1816] The dominance that an adult nanny shows over an alien kid is apparently never challenged by the kid even when it is itself adult.

Calves

The development of calves has not been studied in great detail. In particular, beef calves have not been studied, so most of the descriptions of play and ontogeny are based on Brahma or Masai cattle (Bos indicus) or on the primitive Maremma cattle (Bos primigenius taurus).

Calves, as with other ruminants, must change in a few weeks from simple-stomached milk-drinking animals to grazing ruminants. Rumination increases to occupy 7 hours per day by 7 weeks of age in calves kept on pasture. Sleep time declines to 4 hours per day. Calves tend to sleep in groups or "kindergartens." This attraction of calves for one another results in the calves' spending more than half of their time 15 m (49 ft) or more away from the mother. The mothers leave their usual sleeping areas to rest near their calves.[1591] When calves that had been suckling were separated from their mothers, they spent more time with other calves. This effect is due to social rather than nutritional needs; if the dams remained, but nursing was prevented by cloth placed around the udder, the calves did not shift their social contact to their peers but instead maintained close contact with their mothers.[1939]

Feeding

Most female dairy calves are weaned at birth, given colostrum, and raised in single calf hutches with milk replacer as their diet. Calves are normally fed 10% of their body weight per day, but would consume twice as much and gain four times more weight. The restricted calves stand more, engage in more nonnutritive suckling, and make more unrewarded visits to the feeder.[444]

Group housing of calves allows more normal social interactions, but problems can arise when calves less than 2 weeks old cannot compete for access to automated milk dispenser.

Play

Calves play most in the morning and at feeding times and are active about 20–30% of the time, but only a fraction of that time is spent in play.[947] Play in calves has been studied by Brownlee.[294] Calves, as well as older cows, have a special play vocalization, the baa-ock. Calves play in a variety of ways, often trotting or galloping with the tail elevated. They often buck, kicking up and to the side with both hind legs, but these kicks are not aimed at anything in particular. Directed kicking, which is playful rather than aggressive, may be aimed at a stationary or moving target. Calves also play by making noise with inanimate objects, such as buckets or latches. They may be increasing their auditory stimulation level just as children increase their vestibular stimulation level on slides, swings, and merry-go-rounds.[22] At 7 weeks, about 3 minutes per day is spent in play.[1646] This type of play, solitary play, is more commonly seen in young calves. Social play, especially frontal butting and mounting, predominate in the older calf. Play tends to occur during grazing bouts.[1957] Calves head butt with each other or with inanimate objects. This is the same action used by adult cows in dominance interactions. They may prance, paw the ground, or gore as adult bulls do, and even threaten human attendants. Soft snorting noises may accompany play. Mounting behavior is also seen in calves. Mounting and pushing play decrease with age, whereas butting increases.

There are sex differences in bovine play. Male calves play more than females, the same pattern that is seen in most animal play. Exploration peaks later than play; yearlings are more apt to investigate a novel object than older or younger cattle.[1386] Males mount, push, and exhibit the flehmen response more than females, but butting and social licking are seen equally in both sexes. Mounting and pushing by bull calves is usually directed toward other males, but the flehmen response is directed toward females.[1592]

As in other species, play can be used as a diagnostic criterion, for calves play more when well fed and healthy than when malnourished or ill. They also play more often in fine weather than in foul. Play is stimulated in calves by any change in the environment. They play most when let loose from confinement, after gaining access to new terrain, or even when new bedding is placed in their stalls. A new pen mate, the arrival of a human attendant, or even the stimulation of scratching their backs may set off a play bout in calves.

Activity patterns

Weaned calves raised in individual pens spend their time in the following manner: standing, 40%; ruminating, 28%; feeding, 22%; grooming, 5%; and drinking, 2%. When calves feed from a teat were compared to those fed from a bucket and those suckling from their dam, the artificially fed calves had more sleep bouts and more fragmented sleep than dam fed ones. The calves spent 70% of the day and 80% of the night resting and lay in lateral recumbency more often at night.[754] Such calves quickly learn to anticipate feeding times and become restless at those times.

Many calves are able to make contact despite being penned separately, by making tongue contact through the opening where they are fed.[1023] Calves raised in single pens are most likely to associate with the calves that had been in adjacent pens when they are released in pasture. The singly raised calves rarely associate with group-raised calves. There is no difference in weight gain between the groups.[289] Dominance hierarchies are not stable even though artificially fed calves may compete fiercely for access to their feed.[321] Calves raised in isolation for the first 10 weeks of their lives had higher cortisol values when stressed as yearlings than did calves raised with the opportunity to interact with other calves,[393] indicating the long-term effects of stress during development.

Social and sexual behavior

Bulls mount females by 9 months of age but do not usually achieve ejaculation until they are a year or older. Aggressive behavior increases markedly among bulls from 9 to 18 months, but stable hierarchies have not formed by 2 years.[1549]

Cattle remain in the same general vicinity (less than one kilometer) that they experienced as sucklings, although drought can cause them to travel elsewhere.[894]

Relationships with humans

Handling influences cattle more if the breed has not already been selected for docility.[248] Handling in the first 10 days, or for 10 days when the calves are 6 weeks old, or just before or after weaning at 8 months, all seem to eliminate aggressive behavior. Handling 6 weeks after birth and after weaning appears to be most effective.[247] Calves raised artificially are friendlier to humans if they were handled (feed, milk, and stroked) on the first 4 days of life than if they were handled later (days 5–14) or not handled.[1064] About 90 seconds a day of stroking was enough to cause calves to be easier to load and to have a smaller increase in heart rate, but not all studies have found an effect of handling.[939,942,1120,1659] Calves are easier to handle when they are out of visual and auditory contact with other calves.[718] Calves raised in isolation are more friendly to humans and learn more quickly; they are not handicapped in achieving dominance but may initially be fearful of other calves.[948,1561] Calves change with age in their latency to interact with a startling object. They become less willing to approach a novel object.[1096] The older calves are slower to learn which teat to suckle from an array of two blind and one open nipples.

Behavior problems

One problem of raising calves in groups is that they will suckle on one another, particularly on one another's mouth and ears and the scrotum, and, rarely, on the prepuce. The suckling occurs most frequently in the 15 minutes after a milk meal;[457] weaning from milk to grain reduces the frequency of cross suckling.[1147]

Nonnutritive suckling is observed in calves following a milk meal drunk from a bucket. The motivation to suckle after drinking milk lasts for less than an hour. Calves who are hungrier before they drink the milk will suckle more afterward.[1662]

The drastic changes that are taking place in management of young ruminants have resulted in a much higher incidence of infectious disease. The role of behavioral stress in the etiology of neonatal pneumonias and diarrheas remains unknown. The economic value of these animals would dictate that more information is needed on their behavior in both naturalistic and highly artificial environments in order to best advise.

7 Learning

Learning occurs in all animals, but it is particularly important for the usefulness of dogs and horses. Testing relative intelligence among species and breeds is controversial, but all species tested can be operantly and classically conditioned and can form taste aversions. Housebreaking is the one essential task a pet dog must learn, and several methods are presented. The distinction between negative reinforcement and punishment is important because most horse training depends on the former, not the latter. The ability to reason—nonassociative learning—was once thought to be reserved for humans, but recently has been extended to dogs and horses. Theory of mind, that is, consideration of another's thoughts, is also present to some extent in domestic animals.

INTRODUCTION

Types of learning

Learning in animals can be classified into various types. Horses are used for most examples.

Habituation

Habituation, considered the simplest type of learning, is the long-term, stimulus-specific waning of a response, or learning not to respond to stimuli that tend to be without significance in the life of the animal.[1872] Horses habituate to the feel of a halter on their heads just as we habituate to the feel of glasses on ours. We make use of habituation when we try to desensitize horses to the sound of crowds at a horse show. Another example of habituation is a horse's response to traffic on a road beside its pasture. When first put in the field, the horse will react to traffic on the nearby road; later, it will not. Other examples of habituation are found in pigs that soon ignore a sparkler over their feed trough[439], sheep that become more willing to approach humans within and across tests,[540] or dogs that are not repelled after a few exposures to a dog olfactory repellent.

Classical conditioning

Classical conditioning or signal learning was first demonstrated in dogs by Pavlov. An unconditioned stimulus (UCS), such as the sight of meat, which produces a response (R) by the animal, such as salivation, is paired with a conditioned stimulus (CS), for example, the sound of a bell. The stimuli are paired repeatedly until the CS alone elicits the response; the dog salivates when the bell is rung. Because horses do not salivate at the sight of food (the food must be in

Domestic Animal Behavior for Veterinarians and Animal Scientists, Fifth Edition by Katherine Albro Houpt
© 2011 John Wiley & Sons, Inc.

their mouths before salivation is stimulated), it is interesting to speculate on what might have happened to the field of psychology if Pavlov had used horses rather than dogs.

Perhaps the best illustration of classical conditioning is the release of oxytocin in response to the jangling of milk equipment; oxytocin causes contraction of the myoepithelial cells of the mammary gland, or milk "letdown." Cows normally release oxytocin in response to suckling on the teats by the calf or squeezing of the teats by the negative pressure of the milking machine or the hands of the milker. When a cow has been milked in the same environment a number of times, the sounds of the approaching machinery and milk cans will have been paired with the milking process, and those noises alone will elicit oxytocin release.[537] This type of classical, or Pavlovian, conditioning reduces the time required to milk a herd of cows.

A pet animal's fear reaction to the smell of a veterinary hospital or the sight of a person in a white coat is often a classically conditioned response. The dog or cat responds to a painful stimulus (UCS) with the fear or escape response (R). The hospital and the professional staff are the CS. It does not take many pairings of these stimuli to produce a fear response (R) whenever the animal encounters the conditioned stimuli. It is somewhat disheartening for veterinarians to discover that many of their patients turn tail and hide whenever they approach, sometimes even outside the veterinary clinic. The behaviorally oriented clinician will make every effort to reduce the painful and frightening incidents, especially during a young animal's first visit, so that a conditioned fear response will not develop and hinder future patient–veterinarian (not to mention client–veterinarian) relationships. Figure 7.1 shows classical conditioning of the goat.

Operant conditioning

The third type of learning is called operant, or instrumental, learning. Operant conditioning was first demonstrated by Thorndike,[1871] using cats as experimental animals. Hungry cats were

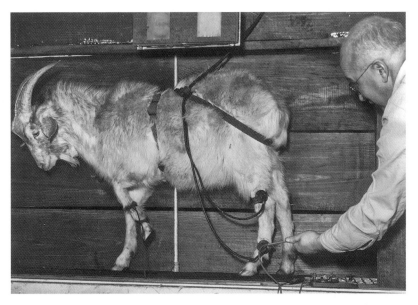

Fig. 7.1 Classical conditioning. Pairing the sound of the metronome with shock to the foreleg conditions a goat to lift its leg when a metronome ticks. Also shown is the late Professor Liddell, who compared the rate at which various species of farm animals learned a classical conditioning.

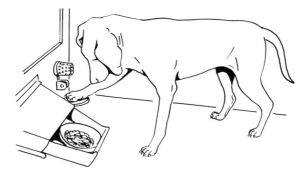

Fig. 7.2   Operant conditioning. The dog pushes a pedal (operates on the environment) to obtain a dish of food.[866] (Copyright 1978, with permission of Veterinary Practice Publishing.)

placed in slatted boxes. Food was available outside the box within sight and smell of the cats. At first, the cats struggled vigorously to reach the food. Eventually, some of them, by chance, pulled a latch string that opened the box door. The cats were then free to consume their reward. Each time a cat was replaced in the box, it took a shorter time to escape, making fewer and fewer extraneous motions, until eventually it pulled the latch string immediately upon being placed in the box.

Operant conditioning is also called instrumental learning because the behavior is the instrument by which the reinforcement is obtained. A laboratory example of instrumental learning is a rat in a "Skinner box," named for the psychologist who popularized the technique,[1775] in which an animal presses a bar to obtain food, water, or electrical stimulation of its brain. Figure 7.2 demonstrates a dog using a Skinner box to feed itself.

Operant conditioning is also used on the farm. Swine use electronic feeders. Horses use automatic waterers, and cows can be taught to enter an area to be milked by a robot, that is, the cows milk themselves.[2048] Operant conditioning devices that dispense food when a cat or dog presses a switch are sold as novelty items.

Chaining

A fourth type of learning is chaining. Chaining is the performance of a series of operant responses in sequence. A good example is goats who were trained to jump three hurdles, walk on a raised walkway, pass through two barrels, and press a lever 10 times.[1746] Many dog owners inadvertently chain obedience commands, with the result that the dog sits, shakes, lies down, and rolls over when the owner says "sit." The owner always gives the commands in the same order, and the dog has chained the responses.

Discrimination learning

A fifth type of learning is discrimination learning. Animals can learn to discriminate between various visual, auditory, or tactile cues. One of the simplest tests of visual discrimination in horses, cattle, and sheep was done by Gardner.[665–669] Her studies revealed that all three species could learn to choose a feedbox covered with black cloth instead of two uncovered feedboxes. With increasing trials, the number of errors decreased. The animals retained the discrimination when tested over a year later.

Conceptual learning

The highest type of learning, that is, the one that demands the most intelligence, is conceptual learning. The simplest form of conceptual learning is the ability to respond to a common quality or characteristic shared by a number of different specific stimuli. We are most familiar with this from the children's shows on TV in which toddlers are exhorted to tell, "Which of these is not like the others?" In that case, difference is the concept.[1685] Horses can form that concept. They were taught to touch two cards with the same symbol rather than a card with a different symbol even when the symbols were novel.[593]

Apparently, horses can form the concept of triangularity. The experiment was an operant conditioning task. The horse simply had to push one of two hinged panels. The correct panel was unlocked, allowing the horse access to a bowl of grain. The incorrect panel was locked, but a bowl of grain was locked behind it to ensure the horse did not choose the panel because it could smell the grain. The correct choice was not always on the same side. The first problem was a simple discrimination between a black panel and a white panel. Next, it had to discriminate between a cross and a circle. The third problem was to distinguish a triangle from a rectangle, and the next was to discriminate triangles from half circles and various other patterns. In the true test of conceptual learning, the horse had to choose between two shapes it had never seen before: one triangular and the other nontriangular. It learned the task quickly but was not correct on the first trial. Horses can also categorize by learning the concept of filled versus empty symbols, such as circles, squares, triangles, trapezoid, etc.[752]

There appear to be other types of learning that are difficult to classify, such as taste aversion, imprinting, and imitation.

Imprinting

As defined by Lorenz,[1180] imprinting is a special process that (1) can occur only during a definite and short period of the animal's life; (2) is irreversible; (3) involves an attachment to an object that will later evoke adult behavior patterns, including sexual behavior; and (4) involves reactions to a particular object that can be generalized to all objects in that class, for instance, all humans or all duck decoys. Subsequent laboratory studies have revealed that in ducks, imprinting does not appear to be irreversible or to influence any adult patterns of social behavior.[1348]

Imprinting is often misused and confused with socialization. Imprinting occurs most commonly in birds and involves a following response. Ducklings will follow their mother because she is the first moving object they see. If a red ball is the first moving object they see, they will follow that. Imprinting probably occurs in horses, too. Neonatal foals will follow any large moving object. That is the reason they may follow a human if the mare has not yet risen after foaling. Imprinting occurs more rapidly in frightened animals, which explains why a newborn foal may follow a horse that has been biting him. Mares may have developed the tendency to guard their foal against any animal or person who approaches, not only to defend the foal from predators, but also to prevent the foal from following the wrong animal.

The few studies done to date indicate that the following tendency is not irreversible. Cairns and Johnson[310] showed that normally reared lambs that presumably followed their mothers began to follow dogs when the two species were housed together, but they lost the response after returning to the company of other sheep. Scott[1710] hand raised a lamb that subsequently showed abnormal social and maternal behavior. The lamb's situation was quite comparable to that of the geese that were hand raised by Lorenz.[1179] Sambraus and Sambraus[1676] have shown that in order for goats, pigs, and other domestic animals to direct sexual behavior toward humans, the animals must have been isolated from conspecifics and been in close association with humans.

Dr. Robert Miller[1329] has popularized "imprint training" in foals. His technique involves habituation and probably learned helplessness when practiced on a foal too young to stand or otherwise resist. The foal is not really imprinted on humans. Mal et al.[1208] found that foals handled for 10 minutes twice a day during their first week and then weekly until weaning at 4 months of life were no more likely to approach people than were foals that received only routine and emergency veterinary care. Simpson[1771] and Williams and Friend[2029] found that imprint-trained foals were calmer and friendlier to humans (would approach sooner) but did not accept hoof handling and other management techniques any better than untrained foals. Both these studies employed mare–foal pairs that were pastured soon after birth of the foal. Whether imprint training would be more or less important to foals that were raised in box stalls has not been determined. Foals handled for 10 minutes per day (alternating rubbing, touching, and picking up feet) 5 days a week beginning at two weeks of age were easier to catch and handle than those reared in a stall, but without intensive handling, which in turn were easier to handle than those who had been running free for 10 months.[959] Even more extensive training beginning within 7 hours of birth and continuing for two weeks resulted in easier handling of the foals. They were tested at 16 days, 3, 6, and 12 months and their behavior compared to unhandled foals. The handled foals were easier to handle (halter, pick-up hooves, lead) at 16 days, but by 1 year, there was no difference between handled and unhandled foals. As yearlings there were no differences in discrimination and spatial learning between the handled and unhandled foals.[1092] See Table 7.1 for the results of imprint training on foal behavior.

One of the most interesting findings is that interacting with the mare, not the foal, is as powerful, and much less difficult, than imprint training. Grooming the mare for 15 minutes per day for 5 days after the foal's birth had long-lasting consequences. At 1 month, the foals whose mothers had been brushed accepted a saddle pad on their back more quickly and tolerated it longer as well as being more likely to approach a person. The reaction to humans persisted in those foals as yearlings.[828]

Later handling, of course, can be used to increase tractability and reduce fear. If weanling horses are stroked for 5 minutes twice a day for two weeks they are more likely to approach a strange person than unhandled or those stroked only when they approached a person voluntarily.

Table 7.1 Results of imprint training.

Imprint age	Repetitions	Test	Age	Author
14 days	Until 24 weeks	Hoof[a] lead[a] approach[a]	6, 12, 18, 24 months	Jezierski et al. 1999
24 hours	Daily for 42 days	Halter, lead[a]	85 days	Mal et al. 1996
10 minutes	24 hours	Restrain halter Worm Vaccinate hoof	90 days	Spier et al. 2004
Birth	Daily for 7 days	Approach responses to stimuli	120 days	Mal et al. 1994
2–8 hours	Daily for 5 days	Approach[a] stimuli	4 months	Simpson 2002
45 minutes	12, 24, 28 hours	Approach stimuli	1, 2, 3 months	Williams et al. 2002

[a]Significantly better performance by imprint trained foals.

Most important, they were much less apt to kick when approached and haltered 4 months later.[1149] Thoroughbred yearlings were tested before and after a 6-week training period of 45 minutes duration in which they were haltered, groomed, and received veterinary examinations. It is not surprising they were less nervous and more likely to approach an unfamiliar human if they had been handled daily.[1339]

The pretraining environment is important because pastured horses were more easily trained using a round pen technique than were stalled 2-year-olds.[1609]

Imitation

Animals can learn by imitation, that is, by observing others. This form of learning has been most thoroughly studied in cats, cattle, and horses and is discussed in those species' respective sections on learning in this chapter. The most interesting finding, albeit in only one dog, is imitation of human action—carrying bottles across a room and putting them in a cabinet.[1320]

Conditioned taste aversion

Taste aversion, or bait shyness, is the process by which an animal learns to avoid a food not because it tastes bad, but because it associates it with illness, particularly gastrointestinal malaise. This form of learning has long been recognized by those attempting to rid farms of rats. When first used, a poison usually kills many rats; but after the first application, very few rats are killed. The animals that survive will no longer eat the bait. The same phenomenon occurs when rats are exposed to radiation and at the same time offered a novel food. They soon avoid the food that they associate with radiation sickness.[663]

Three unique characteristics of taste aversion differentiate it from classical and operant conditioning. One is that it appears to be specific for taste and olfaction; other stimuli such as visual or auditory cues will not be avoided. Rats will learn to avoid the taste of saccharin, which they normally like, but not a blue solution. On the other hand, birds readily learn to avoid novel-colored foods; avian species, which possess few taste buds, apparently depend more on sight than on taste for food identification. Second, the illness must be of internal origin, a general or gastrointestinal malaise. External injury, as from electric shock to the feet, is not a sufficient stimulus. Third, the novel taste and the illness can be widely separated in time, and learning will still take place. This is in contrast to both operant and classical conditioning, in which the stimulus and the response must be close together in time for learning to take place. Sheep and cattle can form taste aversions to a particular food even when the illness follows the ingestion by as much as 8 hours, but the aversion is weakened if the food is present in an unfamiliar location or in the presence of conspecifics that are consuming the food.[305,307,1066] Taste aversions can be formed even if the animal is anesthetized during the time illness was present. Anesthesia blocks other forms of learning, so taste aversion may be noncognitive learning.[1556] It is always difficult to know how an animal feels, particularly when the sensation is something subtle, such as nausea in an animal that cannot vomit. Anesthesia does not prevent taste aversion, whereas an antiemetic does, indicating the critical importance of nausea.[1556] The higher the doses of toxin and, presumably, the sicker the animal, the stronger the conditioned taste aversion. The concentration of the flavor is not important, but sheep will generalize from one food to another if the flavor is the same.[1097]

Taste aversion has four uses, one experimental and three practical. Experimentally, taste aversion can be used to determine what substances an animal can taste or perceive. An animal will show an aversion to a substance at concentrations far below those at which it would show preference or aversion if the taste had not been paired with illness. Practically, taste aversion has been used to teach coyotes to avoid lamb. Repeated pairing of lamb infused with lithium chloride, which produces nausea and vomiting, resulted in a definite aversion to live or dead lambs by the coyote.[730] Taste-aversion techniques have not been successful on a large scale to reduce livestock predation by wild coyotes. The second practical use is to teach livestock to avoid a poisonous plant. Many poisonous plants, such as larkspur, do not make the animal nauseated, but instead are chronic poisons. The cattle or sheep can be taught using another emetic to avoid that plant before they encounter it on the range. Finally, taste aversion can be used to prevent wildlife from eating agriculturally or ornamentally important plants. Four important factors arise in teaching a flavor cue: novelty of the cue; the dose and pharmacology of the toxin used as the UCS; availability of alternative foods; and social facilitation, that is, other animals avoiding the plant.[1026]

Formation and strengthening of a learned task

Shaping

In teaching an animal an operant task, one can wait until the animal performs the desired activity or one can speed up the process by shaping the behavior. If, when teaching a dog to heel, the trainer first rewards the dog for staying within a yard of his side, then a foot, and finally only when the animal walks quietly exactly beside the trainer, he is "shaping" the dog's behavior.

Circus horses are usually shaped by being rewarded for a simple task such as trotting around the ring and then for trotting close to another horse. Later, the horse is rewarded for rearing on command, perhaps with special urging with a whip to get the first rearing motions. At last, the horse can be induced to rear up and put its legs on the horse in front. Then, the various movements are chained.

Animals that are trained to perform complicated and relatively unnatural tricks are usually reinforced with food rewards and reinforced for each correct response at first. The same techniques are used to teach chickens to play baseball or to teach pigs to put giant coins in a bank.[280]

Autoshaping

Autoshaping is a phenomenon whereby an animal makes a response directed toward a stimulus that precedes a reinforcement. If a light signals that food will be delivered in a few seconds, pigeons will peck at the light and dogs will lick the response keys. An attempt to autoshape horses failed.[483]

Reinforcement schedules

When operant conditioning is employed, a variety of schedules of reinforcement can be used. The animal can be rewarded, for example, after every response, after every 10, or after every 20 responses. These schedules are called fixed ratios or FR1, FR10, and FR20, respectively. This technical detail is important because the higher the fixed ratio, the faster the animal will respond; even more important, the longer it will take for the response to be extinguished or forgotten. The animal will go on responding for some time after it is no longer rewarded. Many situations arise in which owners inadvertently put their animal on high FR schedules. Take, for instance, the dog that barks while its owners are eating. They may have given it food once or twice when it barked, until they became annoyed at the behavior. The dog continues to bark while the owners try to ignore him. Finally, they relent and give it some food; they have just increased the ratio. Dog and owner may adjust to this new level, but often the adjustment is temporary and the level of response (barking) needed for reward increases again. Dogs have been trained in the laboratory to bark 33 times for each small food reward and cats to meow 15 times.[1347,1675] The problem dog at the dinner table may continue to bark hundreds of times even though its owners do not give it any more food.

Another type of reinforcement is called fixed interval (FI). In this case, the animal is rewarded for a response that occurs after a certain period of time has elapsed since the last reward. Animals do have a good time sense, and their rate of responding will slow down after a reward and then increase sharply just before the end of the time interval. If animals can learn to respond in this manner, it is not surprising that they learn to expect their owners home at a given hour. Another variant of reinforcement ratios is the progressive ratio (PR) in which, for example, the animal must respond once for the first reward, twice for the second, four times for the third, and so on, until the break point, which is the number of responses (the price) that are too high for the animal to make (pay). The number of responses per reward increases progressively. This technique is used to measure the strength of preferences for food or other commodities.

A more long-lasting response, that is, more difficult to extinguish, follows a variable interval (VI)-reward schedule. Here, the reward follows the first response after 1 minute has elapsed, then after 3 minutes, then after 5 minutes, and so on. The highest response rate follows variable ratio (VR) reward. The owners of the barking dog may find themselves rewarding their dog on this type of schedule if they inconsistently reward the barking, depending, perhaps, on their own mood on any particular evening or on which family member gives in to the pet. A high rate of barking may contribute to the owners' giving in sooner, but the owners are probably not counting barks; they are merely "holding out" for as long as possible, a war of nerves that the dog invariably wins.

Obviously, however, a VR-reward schedule is to be recommended in routine animal training; after a task has been learned using continuous reward, owners should supply verbal or food rewards sporadically during a training session rather than after every trick.

One of the most difficult tasks for the animal trainer is to get the animal to understand the experimenter's instructions.[691] Dogs, for example, have remarkable olfactory acuity and can be taught to detect gas leaks, hidden narcotics, and fatty acids at very low concentrations, but Becker et al.[194] found it extremely difficult to get dogs to learn to turn right in response to an olfactory cue. It is also important to know what is rewarding for an animal. Dogs learn faster when the reward is simple contact with a passive person than when the reward is stroking or picking up.[1805]

Effect of drugs

Dantzer and his colleagues have studied the effects of various drugs on learning in pigs.[430–434,1365,1366] Dantzer[431] has found that pigs treated with diazepam will press a panel more times for food than untreated pigs; diazepam stimulates feeding (see Chapter 8, "Ingestive Behavior: Food and Water Intake"). The muscarinic receptor antagonist scopolamine slowed maze transit by sheep;[1108] cholingeric mechanisms have been identified as part of the learning process. Administration of a tranquilizer facilitated operant conditioning of a genetically nervous pointer. Petting has a physiologically demonstrable calming effect and can be used to facilitate learning. For example, dogs classically conditioned to expect a shock following a tone have a higher heart rate during the tone,[657] but heart rate declines if the dogs are petted during tone presentation.[1192]

Rewards

Positive and negative reinforcement

An animal will learn for both positive and negative reinforcement. Positive reinforcement is a reward, usually food but sometimes social interaction, for performing a response. Negative reinforcement is something aversive applied until the animal makes the response. One pulls on the horse's mouth until it stops, or the rat is shocked until it moves to the other side of the cage. Many field dogs are trained using negative reinforcement varying from a pinch to a shock collar. The use of electric shock to train animals is controversial. There are definitely correct and incorrect ways to use shock. The best way is negative reinforcement in which the aversive stimulus (pain) is applied until the animal does the desired action. For example, cattle can learn to avoid a trough of hay if the shock ceases as soon as they turn away. When the shock continues whatever the animal's does, they don't learn as well.[1111] When beagles were able to clearly associate the electric stimulus with their action, that is, touching a rabbit, and consequently were able to predict and control the stressor, they were not stressed, but beagles shocked randomly or for failure to come on recall were stressed.[1694]

A practical application of negative reinforcement (shock avoidance) learning is now commercially available as "invisible fences." Dogs, goats, and cattle can learn to avoid shock from a collar by heeding a auditory warning signal.[1109,1110] Some dogs become fearful of the boundary or even of the yard when improperly trained; others tolerate the shock to reach the target of their aggression.

One of the most difficult concepts for owners to understand is the difference between negative reinforcement and punishment.[258] Punishment is something that occurs after an action as a consequence. The dog chews the slipper and the owner hits him. Timing is very important. Punishment will not decrease the frequency of the behavior unless it occurs when the animal is misbehaving or within a second or two of the termination of the behavior. Most owners feel that they can punish a dog hours after it has chewed a slipper or eliminated in the house, and they are surprised when the dog does not learn.

Learned helplessness

A phenomenon that has considerable application to practical animal training has been discovered in dogs and cats. This phenomenon is learned helplessness.[1090] Normal, naive dogs, when first placed in an active avoidance situation in which impending shock is signaled, at first escape the shock after it has begun, and later avoid the shock by performing the necessary task, such as jumping over a barrier during the signal before the shock begins. Dogs that previously have been exposed to unavoidable shock act in a quite different manner. They not only fail to learn to avoid as naive dogs do, but also fail to escape; they simply sit and take the shock. These experimental findings indicate that the same form of aversive stimulus should not be used first as inescapable punishment and then later as negative reinforcement that the dog should learn to avoid. Improper use of the popular shock collars or invisible fences may produce learned helplessness in dogs, and any form of inescapable punishment may inhibit later learning. Pigs apparently do not suffer from learned helplessness as dogs do.[1366]

COMPARATIVE INTELLIGENCE

Which animal species are the smartest?[226] This is a question commonly asked by lay people. Although knowledge concerning the IQ of the pig may not contribute much to one's medical or husbandry skills, a well-informed discussion of the facts and the pitfalls involved in assaying relative intelligence will be appreciated by the questioner. Furthermore, in species that are commonly trained, such as dogs and horses, many of the behavior problems revolve around learned tasks or, more frequently, tasks not learned. A dog that refuses to be housebroken and a horse that runs out of a jump are good examples. Volumes have been written on training horses and dogs, so only the underlying principles are discussed here.

Methods of measurement

Brain weight to body weight ratio

An anatomical approach to intelligence can be used. There may be a correlation between brain size and intelligence.[1598] The brain-weight to body-weight ratios in decreasing order are human, 2%; cat, 1%; mongrel dog, 0.5%; rat, 0.3%; goat, 0.3%; horse, 0.1%; and pig, 0.05%.[437] Figure 7.3 illustrates the brains of domestic animals.

The brain- to body-weight ratios of various breeds indicate that increases in brain weight are not linearly related to increases in body size. The smaller the dog, the higher the brain- to

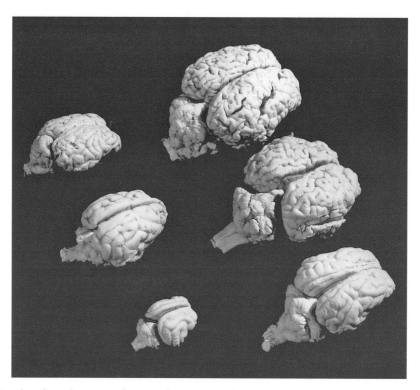

Fig. 7.3 The relative brain size of various domestic animals. Right row, from top to bottom: horse, cow, and pig; left row: dog, sheep, and cat.

body-weight ratio. The toy poodle and Pekinese have ratios of more than 1%, whereas the Saint Bernard and Great Dane have ratios of 0.2%; the medium-sized breeds such as the cocker spaniel have a ratio of 0.6%.[288]

Pigs and most other animals have suffered by domestication in this regard. Pigs have been bred for larger bodies, so wild pigs tend to have larger brain-weight to body-weight ratios. The fallacy of using so labile a parameter as body weight to judge intelligence is manifest when one realizes that the malnourished pig, which shows definite intellectual impairment,[151] has a greater brain-weight to body-weight ratio than the well-nourished pig. This occurs because the brain appears to be spared when the rest of the body is stunted by malnutrition.

Problems of cross-species comparison

Learning rates

Another way in which intelligence might be measured is to compare learning rates of various species on the same task. Many confounding factors exist that may invalidate this approach, also. The task must be physically possible for all species tested. A task requiring manipulation with the forelimbs, which a rat could perform with ease, would be nearly impossible for any ungulate. Scaling also presents a problem. Is a 60-ft maze appropriate for a cow if a 6-ft one is for a cat? Similarly, one must be careful that one is not measuring athletic ability rather than intelligence. A dog that can run fast may complete a task before a slower animal that actually made fewer errors. The task to be learned should also be within the normal behavioral repertoire of all species to be tested. A cat can easily be taught to pounce on an object; a cow rarely performs such actions.

Classical conditioning

Liddell and Anderson[1145] and Liddell et al.[1146] used classical conditioning to measure comparative intelligence. They compared the number of trials necessary to produce leg flexion in response to the CS, the sound of a metronome. The UCS was a shock to the foreleg. Dogs were most easily conditioned. Pigs were the most easily conditioned of the farm animals, followed by goats, sheep, and rabbits.

Delayed response method

Several experiments comparing intelligence in a variety of species were done early in the twentieth century.[1265] For example, Hunter[908] used the length of time an animal could remember which of three boxes identified by a brief illumination held the food reward. This technique, called the delayed response method, revealed that a rat could delay its response for 10 seconds; a raccoon, 20 seconds. Children 2 years old could delay their responses for 25 minutes; dogs, 5 minutes. In other experiments, it was found that cats can remember for 6 minutes, adult dogs for 18 minutes, and goats for 30 minutes, although the goats had a more intensive signal to remember than did the other species.[1787] Of two horses tested by Grzimek,[724] one could remember for only 15 seconds, the other for 60 seconds. The delayed response time is quite variable, however; the delayed response time for cats varied from 18 seconds to 16 hours, depending on the test and the investigator.[1207]

Multiple-choice method

Hamilton[748] used a multiple-choice method to test comparative intelligence. The animals could escape from the apparatus through one of four doors; the correct or unlocked door was never the door that had been unlocked on the previous trial, the win-and-shift strategy. Humans were superior in this test, followed by monkeys, dogs, cats, and the one horse tested. The horse engaged in stereotypic behavior, making repeated attempts to escape through the door that had been unlocked on the previous trial, the win-and-stay strategy. Monkeys did as well as pigs in choosing doors when the correct response was the second door from the end, but an orangutan did poorly.[2072]

Avoidance–response method

Willham et al.[2027] have suggested another method to measure learning ability both among and within species. An avoidance response is taught using a shock for the UCS and a buzzer for the CS. The animals must cross a barrier either to avoid or to escape shock.

   Cats had to undergo 12 trials to learn to avoid a shock by jumping on a shelf.[438] Dogs needed only four trials to learn to avoid a shock by jumping a barrier; pigs, ten; and horses, eight. This does not necessarily mean that dogs are more intelligent than horses and that horses are more intelligent than pigs. A much higher level of shock was used on the dogs and pigs than on the horses, and this factor may have increased or decreased the learning rates.[733,1058,1786]

   Even very young animals have been tested. Newborn kittens cannot learn to escape an aversive stimulus (an air blast),[106] whereas puppies can.[1804]

Maze learning

Gardner[665] compared the learning ability of cattle, sheep, and horses and found that the horses and cows learned visual discrimination better than sheep. Maze learning has been used to assess species differences in learning ability. Karn and Malamud[983] found that dogs learned a double alteration maze better than cats. In a series of maze tests using the Hebb-Williams maze, in which different configurations are made and in some of which the animal can see the solution whereas in others it is hidden from view (see Fig. 7.4A), children made the fewest errors; dogs, cows, goats, and sheep made approximately the same number of errors; pigs and cats made more. Horses made more errors than pigs or cats (see Fig. 7.4B).[1138]

Object permanence

Cats, dogs, and goats have been shown to comprehend object permanence. They will watch the place where an object disappeared from view and go to that place to find the object.[658,1865] This means that these animals have the ability to represent objects in their brains when they are not visible. Out of sight is not out of mind. This is the level of insight usually obtained by 12–18-month-old children.

Social cognition

There is considerable interest in whether animals are aware of the intentions or thought processes of others (theory of mind). For example, will pigs follow another pig that knows the location of

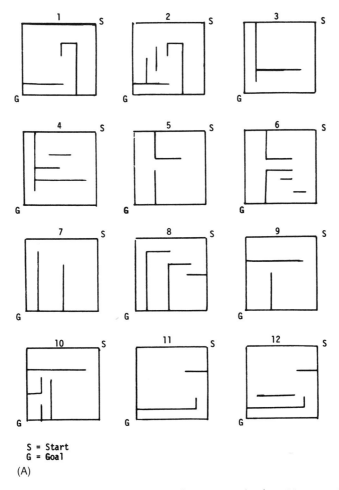

Fig. 7.4 (A) The Hebb-Williams maze. Partitions can be rearranged to form 12 or more barrier problems. Each day, the animal has a new problem to solve, with 10 trials on each problem. The number of errors is used to compare with that of other species[1246] (Copyright 1981, with permission of J. Anim. Sci.).

hidden food? The answer is yes.[812] Dogs are better than horses and even better than primates in finding hidden food cued by pointing or even by gaze.[757] See "Dogs" later in this chapter.

Decision making or cognitive flexibility

Hunting animals must frequently reassess situation when their prey changes direction or is momentarily hidden. On one hand, cats will reassess a situation and may choose a different target if it is closer or more visible than their original target. On the other hand, dogs choose the more distant target. Cooperative hunters such as dogs need to consider not only the target, but also their conspecifics, whereas the solitary hunters, such as cats, need to consider only the target.[494]

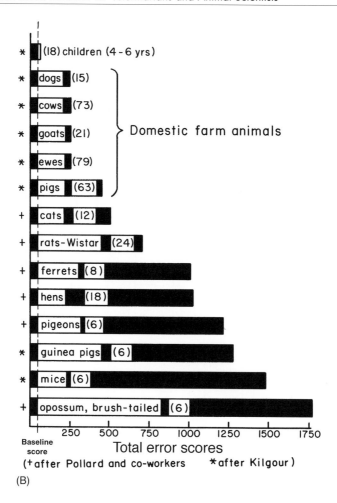

Fig. 7.4 *(Continued)* (B.) Comparative maze learning in various species of animals. Children made fewest errors and opossums the largest number of errors in a Hebb-Williams maze. (Courtesy of Dr. Ron Kilgour, Ruakura Animal Research Station, Hamilton, New Zealand.)[1017,1528]

Episodic memory

Episodic-like memory requires the hippocampus and involves simultaneous recall of three aspects of a past event—what, where, and when. Pigs exposed to various objects in a different position or a different context (room) would explore them more, indicating that they remembered the object, its position, and where it had been last seen.[1053] Dogs, or at least one dog, could remember which room one of 6 toys was.[976]

Summary

One might also answer the questioner on comparative intelligence with the observation that each of the domestic species has apparently had enough intelligence to survive for several million years on its own and several thousand years with people. Nevertheless, studies of comparative intelligence can, if performed properly, answer some questions as to the role of particular learning abilities in the survival of a species.

PIGS

Pigs can be conditioned to salivate in response to a bell[1831] and increase heart rate in response to a metronome tick that signals shock.[1217,1218,1355] Early work also indicated that they could run a maze for a food reward[1391] or choose one of a series of doors to gain access to food.[2073] Difficulty was encountered in teaching a concept such as "center" to the pigs; they could choose the middle of three, but not of five, doors.[2073]

Influences on porcine learning

In the years since the pioneering studies already described here, pigs have been used in many types of learning situations to validate or cast doubt upon concepts developed using laboratory species. Pigs learn to make more correct responses when trials are spaced in time rather than grouped. As had been shown in other species, four trials a day for 10 days produces learning superior to that shown by pigs given 40 trials in 1 day.[980] Classical conditioning occurs more quickly if the interval between the UCS and the CS is not longer than 2 seconds.[1424] Although pigs usually require a food reward, they will swim a maze when the reward is reunion with their littermates. The speed and accuracy of solving a water maze is not correlated with the pig's ability to learn to avoid shock by jumping over a small barrier.[750]

Although season of testing, body weight, and age of dam do not account for variation in avoidance learning,[2026,2027] pigs from large litters ran a maze more quickly than pigs from small litters.[2018] Apparently, when the reward for completion of the maze was a return to the company of littermates, social isolation was more severe and the reward of reunion greater when the litter size was greater.

Operant conditioning

Pigs will not perform an operant response for some types of sensory reinforcement, such as pig noises,[128] but will for others, such as light[137] and brain stimulation.[139] Older pigs (40–150 days) learn to avoid shock less well than do younger pigs (three weeks)[1058] (Fig. 7.5A and B).

Operant conditioning of pigs is used for a variety of purposes: on the farm, in animal acts, and in the laboratory. Feeders with hinged covers that the pig must open with its snout are a good example of a very simple operant response that pigs learn rapidly, and they can learn to use electronic feeding stations. In a more complicated system, pigs can be taught to approach whichever feeder emits a certain sound that indicates that food is available for that pig alone. Such a system reduces competition at a feeder and also reduces fearfulness.[1559]

Pigs prefer the place where they received a reinforcement after a delay in comparison to a place where they received an immediate reward. This conditioned place preference indicates that pigs find anticipation of the reinforcement rewarding.[449]

Consideration of the anatomy and normal behavior patterns of pigs indicates that it would be much easier to teach them to manipulate their environment with their snout than with their feet. Consequently, pigs have been taught to push a panel with their snouts for either a food reward[142] or for heat in a cold environment.[133] To measure a pig's motivation for various sweet solutions, a PR technique has been used.[1003]

A conditioned anxiety reaction can be produced in pigs by training them to press a panel for a food reward and by then adding a tone that signals a shock if the animal presses the panel.[142] The pigs learn to inhibit panel pressing; although experimental neurosis is sometimes produced,[416]

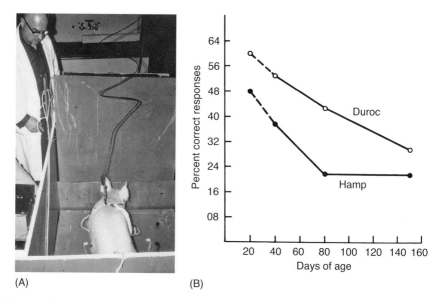

Fig. 7.5   Avoidance learning in pigs. (A) To avoid a shock, the pig must jump the barrier when a buzzer sounds. The late Ulric Moore, who performed some of the early experiments on learning in pigs, is shown. (B) The ability to learn to avoid shock decreases with age in Duroc and Hampshire pigs.[1058]

tranquilizers do not reduce the inhibition of responding.[433] Conditioned anxiety does lower heart rate[432] and increases endogenous levels of corticosteroids, but the rise in corticosteroids is not as great as when the pigs are exposed to cold or chased with a goad.[141]

Visual discrimination

Pigs are better at spatial (right versus left) than at visual discrimination tasks and must be taught to make visual discriminations before 20 weeks of age.[1037] A discrimination task can be used to show that pigs do have color vision.[2002] Pigs have difficulty in reversal learning of either a visual or spatial discrimination; they abandon the original correct response, but their performance remains at chance levels for many trials. Overtraining, training carried beyond criterion on the first task, does improve reversal learning.[2002,2002] Most visual discrimination tests involve pressing one of two panels for the reward. If the animal has learned the discrimination, it will get a reward after six responses on FR6, but if it has not learned, it will take many more responses, an average of 18, to get a reward by chance. Pigs may fail to learn a visual discrimination not because they are unable to either learn or to see, but because they are willing to work very hard (respond many times) for one food reward. They will tolerate being rewarded at a chance level, whereas another species will expend the minimum amount of energy.

Effect of malnutrition on learning

Avoidance learning has been used to study the effects of malnutrition on brain function. Barnes et al.[151] demonstrated that pigs previously malnourished but subsequently rehabilitated for several months show poorer avoidance learning than do well-nourished pigs.

Theory of mind

Pigs can learn that one of them knows where food is hidden and will follow that pig to the food source. If the follower is dominant, it will "scrounge"—take the food from the subordinate pig. That pig will learn to avoid approaching the food source if the dominant pig is close enough to take the food from him. Both pigs seem able to interpret the intentions of the other.[812]

Effect of a barren environment on learning and memory

Pigs raised in a barren environment—the typical pig pen—could learn a maze as easily as those raised in an enriched environment (larger pen with straw), but 10 weeks later they did not remember the maze as well.[442]

DOGS

Housebreaking

The first task that all house pets must learn is voluntary control of the anal and urinary bladder sphincters. There are probably as many methods for housebreaking dogs as there are books on dog training. Both classical and operant conditioning methods have been recommended.

Immediately after a meal, the gastrocolic reflex operates to increase motility of the large colon and rectum. As a result, filling of the rectum will stimulate relaxation of the smooth muscle of the internal anal sphincter and the striated muscle of the external anal sphincter. If a dog is taken outside after every meal, the CS of being outside will soon replace the UCS of the gastrocolic reflex. Some clinicians recommend the use of glycerin suppositories after a meal when the dog is taken outside. The principle is the same; the suppository is the UCS and is more reliable in action than is postprandial defecation.

Operant conditioning is more useful in teaching voluntary control of urination for which no reliable UCS exists. Newspapers are spread all over the room where the puppy is confined. Gradually, the area of newspaper is decreased; the puppy is placed on the newspaper when it squats to urinate and praised when it urinates in the proper place. The newspaper can then be laid outside the door to encourage the dog to go outside to urinate and even to whine to go outside. In other words, the puppy behavior is shaped by first being rewarded for a general action; later, the reward is contingent on more and more specific actions of the animals. It is often valuable to continue to reward the use of newspaper in case the dog must be left indoors for longer periods than one can expect it to retain a bladder full of urine. (Be consistent: Do not punish the animal if it uses the daily paper that has been left on the living room carpet inadvertently.)

Still another method takes advantage of the innate reluctance of animals to soil their sleeping quarters. The puppy is put in a small cage or crate and kept there except for trips outside to eliminate every hour or two as well as play sessions. The premise is that the dog will not urinate or defecate in the cage, and after the animal can control its bowels and bladder for long periods, it will generalize the control to the whole house and will no longer have to be closely confined. It would be asking too much of a young puppy to wait an entire night without eliminating; its control is not good enough yet. Besides being cruel, this expectation may only condition the pup to accept urine and feces on its bed and itself. This technique has merit for those who can stay home with their puppies or for an older dog that is still poorly trained.

Whichever method is used, the trainer must use appropriate and consistent rewards and punishment. Verbal praise and a perfunctory pat are ample reward; in fact, as already mentioned, Bacon and Stanley[107] and Stanley and Elliot[1805] found that dogs will learn to perform better when simple contact with a passive person is the reward than when stroking and picking up is the reward.

Punishment of the animal for misbehavior must come as soon as possible (a second) after the offense. The UCS is the punishment, and the response is avoiding the pain. Unless the CS, inappropriate urination or defecation, is closely paired in time with the UCS, the animal will not learn. If it is punished 10 minutes after it has performed its misdeed, the likely result is for the punisher, not the act of elimination, to become the CS. Dogs who act "guilty" are those in whom this kind of conditioning has taken place. They have learned to associate the presence of a pile of feces in the house with a painful experience; they have not learned to associate their act of eliminating with the painful experience.

Although taking the puppy outside to eliminate is a good method of training, a common mistake that owners make is to put the dog outside for longer and longer periods. The dog does not know what it is to do outside and, if it should eliminate, the owner is not there to praise it. Praising the dog when it returns to the door is a good way to teach the dog to return home but not to housebreak it. Still another complication is that of the dog who is walked on a leash, but whose walks always end as soon as it eliminates. It learns to avoid eliminating in order to prolong the walks. Walk lengths should not be contingent on elimination. A dog may also be afraid to eliminate when the owner is present because it has been punished when "caught in the act." The dog has learned to avoid eliminating when the owner is present, rather than to avoid eliminating in the house.

The problems of housebreaking have been covered in great detail because they represent 20% of the behavioral complaints from dog owners.[1959] Owners will tolerate many defects in their animals, but few will tolerate house soiling, as a case of a Lhasa apso donated to a veterinary college illustrates. The dog suffered from lissencephaly (absence of normal gyri and sulci) (Fig. 7.6) and had many learning disabilities and visual deficits, but the owner's reason for donating the dog was its inability to learn bowel or bladder control.

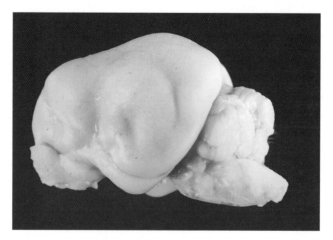

Fig. 7.6   An example of a learning deficit associated with organic disease of the central nervous system, showing the brain of a Lhasa apso terrier that suffered from lissencephaly and could learn neither bowel nor bladder control.

From the clinician's point of view, house soiling in a previously well-trained animal indicates a medical problem. A dog with diarrhea will not be able to retain voluntary control of its irritated intestines. Ulcerative colitis must be treated as both a behavioral and a medical problem; stress should be reduced and the appropriate drugs prescribed. Dogs with chronic nephritis do not concentrate their urine, so they must excrete large quantities of dilute urine and will not be able to retain or limit their maturations as well as they could when healthy. Many diseases can cause polyuria. In addition to medical problems, old dogs may suffer from cognitive dysfunction syndrome (see below), which is similar to human senility. A common sign of cognitive dysfunction is house soiling.

Navigation

Dogs usually relate environmental information to their own body in space (egocentric) rather than by the relation of two environmental objects to one another allocentric.[587] They seem to be able to determine the direction in which they saw an object disappear rather than the distance.[587] They can be taught to use landmarks—for example a wooden rod demarks which cup holds the food, but as soon as the landmark is moved away from the cup, performance falls.[1326] They can find their way back to a target when deprived of visual and auditory cues, presumably by direction and speed of travel on the outward journey.

Dogs have difficulty in generalizing from one situation to the next. For example, if a target is inside a V-shaped barrier, they have more trouble reaching it than if the target is outside.[1320] Because they communicate well with humans, dogs when given a choice of a cup full of food or an empty one can be enticed by a human who calls his name, looks at the dog, and at the empty cup. Under those conditions, the dog may choose the empty cup rather than the full cup.

Dogs can learn by the model rival technique in which the trainer and a colleague call the object by name and ask one another for it. This method was used to train the African Grey parrot Alex a large number of words and colors. The dogs may actually be responding to stimulus enhancement because they will retrieve an object if they watched a person handle it just before they are asked to retrieve it.[391] Because social facilitation is strong in dogs, slow dogs tend to run faster with another dog than they do alone.[1958] This is in contrast to cats, who run slower for a food reward in the presence of another cat.

Dogs can form the concept of dog and no dog. They were trained using pictures projected on a touch screen and they could discriminate a novel dog in a landscape from a landscape.[1579] Unfortunately, dogs can also learn that there will be no drugs in a given area and will fail to detect drugs there.[676] This phenomenon is called context specificity and is analogous to the superior response to commands that many of our dogs show in the kitchen.

Young dogs can learn faster when given the drug selegiline, which increases brain dopamine, but only if a food lure is visible; otherwise, they actually learn more slowly than placebo-treated dogs. This indicates that dopamine enhancement helps only rewarded behavior.[1332]

Canine intelligence has been a subject of much interest recently as more and more human-like abilities are discovered in dogs. There are two hypotheses: Dogs have lost intelligence during domestication; or possibly have gained the ability to understand the minds of humans (social cognition), but certainly have gained the ability to read very subtle signals. The evidence for the first hypothesis is that dogs that live with their owners don't solve problems—such as gaining access to food by manipulating a bowl—as well as dogs who live outdoors. In addition, dogs selected for independent behaviors, such as pointers, do better than other breeds.[1888] The evidence for the second hypothesis is that dogs do better than chimpanzees on finding a human-cued reward—based on pointing, tapping, or direction of gaze of humans.[758,759] They also do better than wolves on human-cued tasks, whereas in simple delayed response, wolves and dogs perform similarly, and in tests of problem-solving, wolves do better.[625],[757] The ability to interpret human gestures and a human gaze is innate, not learned, in domestic dogs; kennel-raised puppies perform as well as family-raised puppies. Puppies do not improve with age in these tasks between 9 and 26 weeks.[757]

Dogs can learn by observations, and the demonstrator can be a human[1530] or another dog, especially a familiar dog such as the mother.[1777] The dog will learn from a dog that is dominant to him, but not from a subordinate.[1532] Dogs can learn by observation and can even learn complex tasks such as narcotics detection by observing their mother from 6 to 12 weeks despite the fact that they were not trained until 3 months had elapsed.[1777] Dogs can learn by observation of a human demonstrator, but it is the subordinate dog in a household who learns, not the dominant one.[1531]

Dogs can not only interpret human gazes but also "show" humans where to get an object that is inaccessible to the dog. They gaze at the owner and then quickly at the food or toy and back again.[1321] This is called functional referential communication. Dogs have numerical competency. If they are shown two bones that are then hidden by a screen, they are surprised if one or three bones are there when the screen is removed. Surprise was measured by how long the dog looked at the bones—the same method used for assessing surprise in preverbal infants.[381],[2005] Dogs can make discriminations between our verbal commands so that they can retrieve objects by name: spoon, brush, and pin.[2074] The record is a border collie that could remember over 200 objects by name[975] and when an unfamiliar word was used, he would fetch the novel object, possibly because dogs prefer to interact with novel toys[989] or because of reasoning by exclusion.

Inferential reasoning by exclusion

Dogs and children can learn to choose a symbol as positive and another as negative (no reward). If a novel stimulus is presented with a negative stimulus, half of the dogs and all the children will choose the novel stimuli, having learned the significance of the negative one. When given a choice between the formerly novel stimulus and another stimulus they haven't seen before, they chose the formerly novel stimulus. This ability is called inferential reasoning by exclusion, demonstrating that they understood that the formerly novel stimulus belonged to the class of rewarded stimuli excluding the new stimulus.[103]

The importance of social cues is the response of dogs to the command (Down for lie down). When the owner faced the dog, most lay down on the first or second request, but if the owner was hidden behind a screen or if the owner faced another human rather than the dog, the dog rarely obeyed.[1952] This means that dogs understood the focus of the human's attention. Dogs are able to assess quantities and will choose the greater number of pieces of food, but if the owner seemed to favor the smaller quantity by exclaiming over it, most dogs will choose that the smaller over the larger. When the two choices are of equal size, more dogs choose what the owner favored, but older dogs and highly trained dogs were more likely not to choose the owner-favored bowl.[1536],[1971]

Mean-end connection is another measurement of comparative intelligence. A treat is placed behind a barrier. The treat is attached to the end of a string. Dogs can retrieve the treat by pulling on the string, but only if the string is in on a straight path (perpendicular to the barrier) to the treat. If the string is displaced or if two strings cross, the dog makes errors, indicating that he does not understand means–end connections involving strings.[1456]

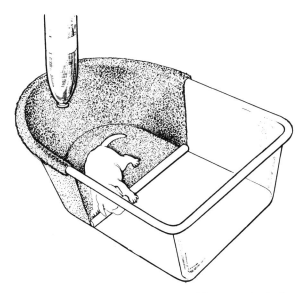

Fig. 7.7 Learning in neonatal dogs. The puppy learns to avoid the textured side, for which puppies have an innate preference, if that side is associated with a blast of air.

Fox and Spencer[617] have shown that dogs improve in their ability to make a delayed response. If puppies were trained for 13 days beginning at 4, 8, 12, or 16 weeks, all increased the interval over which they could remember during testing, but the 4-week-old puppies could never remember longer than 10 seconds, whereas the 12-week-old dogs could remember for 50 seconds. Sixteen-week-old dogs did not perform as well; they made many errors. Fox and Spencer[617] explain the poor performance at 16 weeks by postulating a lack of inhibition at that age. Stanley et al.[1803] also studied the ontogeny of learning in dogs. They found that puppies less than a week old could be conditioned to suck more from a nipple when milk was the reward and to inhibit sucking when a quinine solution was the aversive stimulus, although earlier studies had found that puppies less than 18 days old could not be conditioned.[654] Stanley et al.[1804] also found that puppies less than a week old can learn to escape from a cold stream of air and will even move from a comfortable, carpeted surface to a hard, cold one to do so (Fig. 7.7). Puppies less than 2 weeks old could also learn to choose a wire or cloth model that contained a nipple for a milk reward if given five tests a day, 2 hours apart.

Training is easier if the innate responses of dogs to auditory signals are used. Dogs will increase their activity to high tones and inhibit it to low tones,[1250] and this is reflected in the signals shepherds use to signal their dogs.[1251] Dogs can learn landmark discrimination, that is, they can learn that a third object placed on or near one of two identical objects indicates the reward. It is difficult for dogs to learn this unless the landmark is close to the object.[1324] This type of learning is called allocentric (two things relative to each other, as opposed to egocentric—things relative to the dog) learning and involves the parietal not the frontal cortex as egocentric learning does.[586]

Military dogs are trained fairly forcefully with leash corrections. Pats were the only rewards, but those rewarded dogs perform better than those only corrected. Perhaps they were rewarded more because they performed better, but it does indicate the value of rewards.[788] Puppy tests can be used to identify dogs that will be successful police dogs. Puppies that are heavier, have high prey drive chasing a ball and playing tug and respond less to sound and are low activity when negotiating obstacles.[1835]

Geriatric cognitive dysfunction

Old dogs may have physical problems such as deafness, cataracts, heart disease, or arthritis, but many old dogs are euthanized for behavioral reasons. They forget to be housetrained, or they pace and whine at night. Old dogs are also slower to learn new things. Older dogs have learning deficits that can be measured in objective laboratory tests such as delayed nonmatching to sample. The dog is shown an object, such as a circle, and then after a delay of 5 seconds is given a choice between a circle and a rectangle. It must choose the rectangle (nonmatch) to be rewarded. Beagles over 10 years old could not learn this.[1325] The behavior of old dogs differs from that of younger ones; when unstimulated, that is, in their home cages, old dogs (over 9 years) are less active than younger ones.[1774] At least some of these changes may be due to oxidative damage to the central nervous system. Many otherwise healthy dogs may be euthanized because of the age-associated behavior changes, especially if the owner's sleep is interrupted. Owners complain that old dogs are less affectionate, less active, lose housetraining, pace and vocalize at night, and may seem disoriented (getting lost in their own yard). About 28% of 11–12-year-old dogs and 68% of 15–16-year-old dogs have these signs.[119,1405] Intact male dogs may be less at risk.[767] There is Alzheimer's-like pathology—amyloid deposits in the brains of old dogs—that may account for the signs.[414] Three treatments are available: selegiline (Deprenyl®), a monoamine oxidase inhibitor that increases the availability of dopamine in the synapse; a diet (b/d® Hills) supplemented with antioxidants, vitamin E, lipoic acid, carnitine, and so on, which reverses the learning disability in old laboratory dogs and many of the signs in pet dogs; a supplement Senilife® with vitamin E, phosphatidylserine, a component of neural structures, ginkgo, resveratrol from grapes that also appears to reverse the signs of cognitive dysfunction.[800]

CATTLE

There have been few studies of learning ability in cattle, and most of those published described attempts to increase production or reduce labor on the farm.

Operant conditioning

Kiley-Worthington and Savage[1016] have trained cows to come in to be milked when an automobile horn connected to a timer and the electric fence was sounded. Albright et al.[20] trained cows to come into the barn in a given order, but the cattle reverted to their original order, probably based on dominance, as soon as the trainer was absent. Wieckert et al.[2019] also trained cattle to come to a feeding trough when an auditory stimulus was delivered to the cattle from a small, timer-activated tape recorder attached to the cow's halter.

Offord et al.[1446] conditioned cattle to eat in response to an auditory stimulus and then attempted, unsuccessfully, to increase food intake in the cattle when they were free-feeding by playing the auditory stimulus. Dairy cows have also been taught to press a handle with their muzzles to obtain food and to make right- and left-handle discriminations. The most difficult task was to accustom the cows to lifting, rather than lowering, their heads for food because they were accustomed to eating from the floor.[2012] Cattle have also been taught to use individual feeders that open only when the animal inserts the electronic collar around its neck into the feeder.[984] These systems are now widely used because cattle can be group-housed, yet feed themselves individually. Other cattle have been taught to enter a feeding stall when one signal, a bell, is presented and to leave the stall when another signal, a buzzer, is presented.[1742] Cattle could not learn an operant task by observation.[1935]

Moore et al.[1356] taught seven Jersey cows to press a panel for a food reward. The cattle learned to respond to various schedules of reinforcement: a fixed ratio, in which a certain number of presses resulted in the food reward; a FI, in which food was delivered at intervals and only one panel press at the appropriate time was necessary for the food reward; a VR; and a VI. The VR schedule produces the highest response rate in cattle, as it does in other species.

Cattle can learn both radial-arm mazes and parallel-arm mazes, that is, they learn that food will not be in a location they have previously visited even if visits were separated by as much as 4 hours, but not by longer intervals. Kilgour[1017] found that Jersey cows learned 12 detour problems in the Hebb-Williams maze (refer to Figs. 7.4A and B) and made few errors after four runs of a given detour test.

Cattle can be clicker trained to touch a target, but teaching the same animals to eliminate on concrete rather than their bedding using a clicker was not successful.[2010]

Conditioned avoidance

Many farmers teach their cattle to defecate in the gutter behind their stanchions rather than on the stall floor by running an electrified wire (cattle trainer) that shocks the cow whenever it arches its back to eliminate in the wrong place. Because cattle defecate seven times a day, the cows learn quickly, and the average fecal output of 60–80 pounds is deposited in the gutter.

Cattle sometimes receive shocks through milking machines. Cows were taught to press a bar for food in order to determine how large a shock had to be before it disrupted a cow's feeding and other behaviors. They stopped bar pressing when a shock greater than 7 mA was applied to one teat or 6 mA to all four teats.[2014] This type of conditioning can be used to determine what is painful to cattle.

A practical application of bovine avoidance learning is to train cattle to respect electric fences by confining them in a pen with a sturdy fence beyond the electrified wire. The cattle will then respect an electric fence even in a new environment and will not be in danger of breaking through it.[1254]

Taste aversion

Cattle can form a taste aversion to alfalfa pellets and corn (Fig. 7.8). Cattle can be taught to avoid licorice-flavored alfalfa pellets, but the aversion is much weaker than that to beet pulp even when the same illness—that produced by lithium chloride—is associated with the taste.[1565] This demonstrates the general rule of taste aversion learning: that it is harder to learn to avoid a very palatable food. Older cows are easier to teach a taste aversion than younger ones. Social facilitation can outweigh aversion learning in cattle as well as in sheep.

Visual and auditory discrimination

One of the earliest studies of learning in cattle is one of the most extensive in that large numbers of cattle were tested. Gardner[666,668] studied the ability of cows to discriminate a box covered

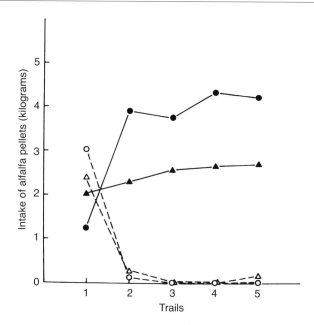

Fig. 7.8 Taste aversion learning in cattle. On day 1 (trial 1), the experimental cows (open symbols) were offered alfalfa pellets. After they had eaten the food, LiCl (lithium chloride), which produces mild gastrointestinal malaise, was infused into the rumen through a fistula. The control cows (closed symbols) were infused with 0.9% NaCl. Four days later (trial 2), when all cows were offered alfalfa pellets, the cows that had been treated with LiCl ate almost nothing, whereas the controls ate more than they had initially. The experimental cows learned to avoid a feed associated with illness.[2079] (Copyright 1977, with permission of Baylor University Press.)

with black cloth, which contained feed, from two empty and uncovered boxes. The errors per trial fell as the trials proceeded. The cows had retained the learning when tested a year later. More errors were made when the cloth was moved below or, in particular, above the feed box. Calves have been taught to make shape and orientation discrimination.[124] See the next major section, "Sheep and Goats," for further discussion of visual discrimination in ruminants.

Effects of age

When the ability to remember the location of a feeder was tested over a period of 5 days, heifers learned more quickly than older cattle, but cows after the second calving remembered the location best when tested six weeks later. In both tests, primiparous cows were intermediate in performance.[1055] Stress appears to enhance learning because newly weaned calves learned a T maze more quickly than those weaned a month before training.[1121] Cattle can learn to shift from one arm of a maze to another (win-and-shift strategy) if they ate all the food in the initial arm on the previous trial.[864] It is interesting to compare the behavior of cattle in the very artificial maze situation to that on pasture. When tested in a pasture with high-quality forage, they display the win-and-shift strategy, but on a poorer pasture, they display the win-and-stay strategy.

From a practical point of view, cows can be "trained" to use cubicles to rest as adults by providing experience with cubicles as heifers.[1439] Cows can learn to activate a robotic milking machine for "on demand" relief of mammary pressure. They are variable in their requests to be milked but averaged three times a day.[2048] No milking was done from midnight to 6 a.m., and the system was timed so that a cow could not be milked more frequently than every 4 hours.

SHEEP AND GOATS

Sheep and goats can be classically conditioned to flex a front leg in response to a ticking metronome that had been paired with an electric shock, although the small ruminants did not learn as quickly as pigs or dogs.[1146] (Fig. 7.1) Sheep can learn simple mazes[1142] and will run a maze to be reunited with a cohabitant, whether the animal was another sheep or a dog.[310]

Operant conditioning techniques have been used to study thermoregulatory behavior. The sheep learned to activate a heat lamp by sticking their muzzles through a slit to break a photoelectric beam. Unshorn sheep did not learn to turn on the heat at 5°C (41°F), but shorn sheep, deprived of the thermal insulation of their fleece, did.[144] Sheep have also learned to press a bar for reward in response to a tone signal and to refrain from pressing the bar for 30 seconds after each reinforcement.[1681–1683]

Sheep will learn to move faster through yards (chutes and alleys) with experience and will do better than inexperienced sheep months later, but training in moving a different way through the same yard is worse than no training.[913] Apparently, the sheep have to forget their previous experience. Giving the sheep a food reward at the end of a yard is an efficient way of speeding their movement though it but will not help if an unpleasant experience, such as restraint, is also associated with the same movement.[912]

The ability of sheep to perform operantly conditioned tasks has been used in experiments with sodium-deficient sheep. These sheep learn to press a bar for sodium bicarbonate in proportion to their sodium deficiency. Sheep can also learn to discriminate which of five feeders contain food.[2083] Sheep have also been studied by Gardner[665] and Liddell,[1143,1144] as was discussed in the section "Comparative Intelligence" previously in this chapter. Sheep have the ability to form spatial memory so that they can locate food faster after several days experience. The sheep appeared to learn better when the resource density is low. When it is high, the sheep need not try to relocate the food, but rather find another location.[1623]

Sheep can form taste aversions.[2080] In a range environment, sheep are exposed to various toxic plants including locoweed. They can be trained to avoid locoweed, but may form only weak aversion to another food, presumably due to the negative central nervous system effects of swainsonine (the alkaloid in locoweed).[1505]

Goats can learn to press a bar for the reward of electrical stimulation of their brain[1497] and press more than a 1,000 times in 45 minutes for a food reward.[1746] Sheep and goats can learn to make fairly fine visual discriminations between different shapes and different orientations of the same shape. For example, they can learn to discriminate not only between a circle and a square but also between a triangle pointing right and one pointing left.[124,125] Their learning rate improves with additional discrimination tasks, indicating that these ruminants form a learning set, or can learn to learn.[1089]

Goats can learn which food is associated with illness—which food makes them sick; but if both foods and illness occur on the same meal, the goat will respond by eating a little of each food.[499] Learning a conditioned taste aversion has been used to prevent goats from eating Leucaena, a palatable, but poisonous plant that is a goitrogen and a depilatory.[704] Unfortunately, conditioned safety, taught by feeding increasing percentages of sagebrush in the diet before goats were released on the range, did not cause the goats to eat any more sagebrush than inexperienced goats when they were free to select a diet on the range.[1604]

HORSES

The horse is, like the dog, a species that is useful to humans only if trained. In fact, despite their aesthetic value, few horses are kept as pets unless they can be ridden or driven. Myriad volumes have been written on the training of horses, and it is appropriate to mention only a few of the basic principles. Nicol[1415] has reviewed the subject.

It is easiest to teach a horse a natural response; consequently, horses can be trained to race at a very early age. Two-year-old horses on the racetrack are very common; a horse under age five in a dressage class is a rarity. Most horse training is based on negative reinforcement: applying an aversive stimulus until the horse performs the response. The best approach to horse training is to try to substitute conditioned stimuli (a voice command or subtle pressure from the rider's legs) for unconditioned stimuli (the painful flick of a whip). In this manner, neck reining can replace direct reining. When punishment must be given, it should be applied as soon as possible after the misdeed. A slap on the pony's muzzle 30 seconds after it has nipped will only serve to make it head shy; a blow 1 second after the nip may inhibit further aggression.

Round pen training or natural horsemanship has become very popular. It is another form of negative reinforcement in that the horse is chased and learns that if he doesn't move in response to subtle movements of the trainer's body a more aversive stimulus such as a the lash of a whip may occur. The response of running away seems to be avoidance of a predator. The reward for the horse is not having to move quickly. The trainer must keep behind the horse's withers in order to stimulate it to run and can move ahead of the shoulder to slow the horse. Horses can be taught quickly to reverse to the outside or to the inside. An untrained animal can learn to tolerate a saddle and then a rider in 1 day. There has been no study of the relative value of this type of training over conventional training. Pastured horses learn in a round pen more quickly than stabled ones perhaps because they are more respectful of humans when they don't see them daily. When the trainer stops driving it forward, many horses will approach the trainer, especially if he or she avoids eye contact and backs slowly away from the horse. This is the phenomenon of "Join up."[1067]

Perhaps the best example of intelligence in horses is Clever Hans. This nineteenth-century Arabian stallion could perform mathematical problems by tapping out the answer with its hooves. The horse was able to give the correct answer whether or not his trainer was present. It was finally discovered that someone had to be present who knew the answer to the problem. The horse was able to perceive some subtle change in the person when it reached the correct number. Clever Hans was more clever at interspecies communication than he was at mathematics.

See the section "Types of Learning" in the introduction to this chapter for examples using horses.

Operant conditioning

A single horse was taught by Myers and Mesker[1392] to make a typical operant response, pushing a lever with its muzzle for a half cup of grain. After the horse had been shaped using continuous reinforcement, the schedule was changed to three and then to eleven responses for every reinforcement. The horse increased its rate of responding as the FR ratio (fixed ratio of responses per reward) increased. When a fixed-interval schedule was imposed, the horse at first "sulked" by refusing to turn toward the lever, but later responded with the scalloped pattern typical of laboratory rodents on fixed-interval schedules. The practical application of the study is that a horse will perform better when it is not rewarded for each performance.

Operant conditioning is used to evaluate drugs in equine pharmacology.[2059] The horses are usually conditioned to break a beam with their head for a food reward. The rate of responding will be lower if a depressant, such as acepromazine, is given and will be higher if a stimulant, such as methylphenidate (Ritalin), is administered. The action of an unknown drug can be tested by comparing its effect on responses to that of other, known, drugs. Using this technique, one can determine whether the horse is being stimulated or depressed, that is, whether the horse's performance is being improved or worsened. Operant conditioning has also been used to measure environment preferences of horses for such things as food and exercise.[531,872,1113]

The basis of most horse training is negative reinforcement, but in most instances a secondary reinforcement of the sound of a clicker and positive reinforcement also can be used to train horse to lead and to load. The methods are equally successful in training, but the positively rewarded horse appear more eager.[930] A secondary reinforcer did not improve learning or retention of a visual discrimination task, but was very effective in improving learning rate of a second visual discrimination task.[2028]

Horse that exhibit stereotypies (see Chapter 9) such as weaving and cribbing are slower to learn the task of lifting the cover of a feedbox and a greater proportion never learn.[784]

Visual discrimination

Visual discriminations have been used extensively to study learning in other species and therefore were applied to horses. Gardner's studies[667,669] revealed that a horse could learn to choose a feedbox covered with black cloth and containing food instead of two empty feedboxes. With increasing trials, the number of errors decreased. The horses retained the discrimination when tested over a year later, but, as did cattle, they found it difficult to choose the correct box when the cloth was moved to a position above or below the box. In general, the horses made slightly more errors than did cows in a similar situation.[666,668] Using figures on the covers of feedboxes, Giebel[686] was able to teach ponies to discriminate between many pairs of figures to obtain feed. If the symbols used were too similar to be perceived as different by the ponies, they would exhibit weaving behavior, swaying from side to side over the boxes without making a choice. As in Gardner's study, the discriminations were well retained for long periods. Fat horses make more errors on a simple visual discrimination test than do thin ones, which is probably a result of poorer motivation for the food reward rather than intellectual deficit.[1243] Mules are superior to both ponies and donkeys in visual discrimination learning. They learn more pairs and are more accurate.[1554] Horses seem to be able to learn spatial (left–right) discriminations better than visual discriminations (light on or off).[1230] Horses can remember which of a pair of visual stimuli was rewarded 10 years later and one horse could remember the concept of larger (the larger of two novel symbols was correct) 7 years later.[753]

Maze learning

Yearling quarter horses can easily learn a simple right- or left-turn maze and can learn to turn in the opposite direction (reversal learning). Punishment did not improve performance.[1059] Ponies

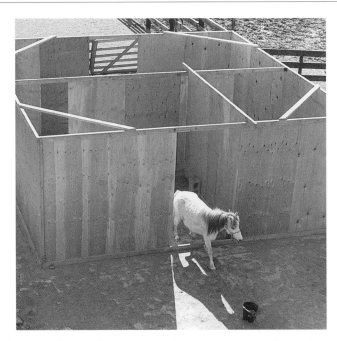

Fig. 7.9 Maze learning in horses. The horse enters the maze and must make a right turn in order to leave the maze and receive a food reward.

who learned a maze reversal (to turn right rather than left) most quickly also learned to avoid a shock in the least number of trials. There was, however, no correlation between learning ability in either task and position in the dominance hierarchy.[733] The maze is shown in Fig. 7.9. In a study of warmbloods, Visser et al.[1956] found no correlation between avoidance learning (negative reinforcement) and learning for positive reinforcement. Horses that had been operantly conditioned to push one of two levers for a food reward when a particular stimulus (a striped piece of wood) indicated which lever was associated with the reward were no quicker than naïve horses in learning that the same stimulus indicated the correct side of a maze.[1244]

Horse can learn that choosing one side of a maze will lead to being ridden in the Rollkur (extreme neck flexion) posture, whereas the other side leads to being ridden in an ordinary bridle. They avoid the Rollkur.[1960] Horses can solve barrier problems and learn to open a chest with their noses when a human demonstrates the task (but not if a horse demonstrates) and the offspring of some stallions are more successful than the offspring of others.[2053] Horses can also learn to form taste aversions,[2078] and practical use of this has been made to teach horses not to eat locoweed (Oxytropis sericea).[1506]

Observational learning

Three unsuccessful attempts have been made to demonstrate observational learning in horses. In two cases, the horses, young quarter horses, watched another choose one of two feed buckets. In neither case did the horses that observed perform any better than those that had not had the opportunity to observe.[111,120] In the third case, horses watched a demonstrator horse step on a pedal to open a feed bin. Observers did no better than naïve horses.[1155] This is particularly interesting because horse vices, in particular cribbing, are believed to be learned by observation.

There has been as successful demonstration of observational learning in horses. Horses learn join up more quickly if they observe a horse dominant to them perform; watching a subordinate confers no advantage.[1067] This is similar to the interaction of social rank and learning by observation in dogs.

Influences on learning

Handling

Mal et al.[1209] and colleagues[1208] have shown that early handling (imprint training) does not influence trainability but that extensive handling for the first six weeks is more beneficial than the same amount of handling later in the foal's life.

A moderate, but not an extensive, amount of handling improves a young horse's performance in a maze-learning test.[806] Perhaps the most useful information is that handlers can predict trainability after working with a horse for 10 days, and although another interpretation might be that handlers determine performance, these scores are correlated with trainability under saddle as judged by different people. The more emotional a horse, the poorer its learning ability.[590,807,1204]

Age

Weanling foals learn to make the correct choice in the maze shown in Fig. 7.9 with fewer errors than adult mares, but the latter move faster, so despite entering the wrong side, they reach the food just as quickly as the foals. Orphan foals do not appear handicapped in their learning ability but move even more cautiously than normally reared foals.[881]

Frequency of training

In general, pauses between training bouts result in faster learning, apparently because the biochemical processes involved in learning do not happen instantaneously. Learning must consolidate a process that involves formation of new protein in the relevant part of the brain. The problem is that, although the horse spends less time in training to learn optimally, more days have elapsed. Nevertheless, as Rubin et al.[1650] demonstrated with avoidance learning, spacing training bouts is more efficient than crowding them into a few days. When given 17 days of training to lead, to lunge, to be driven, and to be ridden, yearling thoroughbred horses that were trained every day learned better—with fewer errors—than those trained for 4 days and then given a 3-day break and then trained for 4 days, and so on.[1078] How many repetitions of a task should each training session contain? Sixteen seems to be the optimum when negative reinforcement is used.[1248]

CATS

Dogs were the animals used in the earliest experiments on classical conditioning,[1481] whereas cats were studied in the first experiment in operant conditioning.[1871] Cats learned to operate on their environment in order to escape from puzzle boxes. They also learned to pull strings to which a piece of food was attached, selecting from the one attached to the meat from among several others.[8] Manipulating strings is a task that dogs perform poorly (see earlier discussion in "Dogs"); cats may be more anatomically than intellectually suited to the task. Cats can be classically conditioned,[762] and experimental neurosis can also be conditioned in cats, as in most species,[56] by requiring them to discriminate between two very similar stimuli (auditory, in this case).

Discrimination

The cat's ability to learn discrimination has been used to great advantage by psychophysicists in studying vision. For example, color vision can be studied by teaching cats to discriminate between two symbols and then to discriminate between the symbols when they differ only in hue. Cats can, in fact, make this discrimination but only after 1,400 trials; they do have color vision, as both behavioral tests[1721] and electrophysiological studies[367,1605] attest. The color stimulus must be large (that is, a big object) before the cat is able to make use of the hue. Nonneman and Warren[1427] used a two-cue discrimination to measure the salience or importance of various sensory modalities to cats. The animals were taught to feed from one of two feeders, which emitted a buzzing noise and a flashing light associated with it. Later, one feeder flashed and the other buzzed; the cats went to the flashing feeder, indicating that auditory stimuli are less important to cats than visual ones when both are carefully equated for intensity.

Rewards

Unlike dogs, cats will not usually perform in order to be reunited with the experimenter. They will perform for food rewards. Feline finickiness can even interfere with the reward value of food, but in general, cats will work harder for food rewards if the experimenter is the one who feeds the cats in the home cages. It is even more difficult to teach a cat to press a bar for water; water must be withheld for a week.[117] Kittens will learn more quickly when the reward is freedom to explore a room than when the reward is food.[1323] Kittens learn to make a light–dark discrimination more slowly than do 35-days-old cats.[373]

Conceptual learning

Cats are able to form learning sets, that is, to form concepts. Warren and Baron[1975] showed that cats could learn to solve a problem, such as choosing the object on the left when identical black squares were the stimulus, and would learn much more quickly on the next problem to choose the object on the left when white triangles were presented. After four problems, the cats' errors fell to 36% of the original errors, and only 58% of the number of trials originally necessary were needed to reach criterion. Cats seldom show insightful behavior; they do not learn to move a light box under a suspended piece of fish in order to reach the fish.[8] Captured feral cats learn a discrimination more quickly than cage-reared ones.[2024] These findings indicate that a varied environment or experience may lead to an increased learning ability in cats. When trained in a progressive elimination task in which there are many sites with food, but once the food has been consumed the cat must look elsewhere (win shift). In these tests, cats chose the site closest to the start point.[478]

Imitation and observation

Learning by observation and imitation takes place in cats. Cats watching a cat press a bar or jump a barrier to obtain food learned to press the bar or jump the barrier much faster than did cats that did not observe a trained animal. Cats can also be misled. If the cats watched a cat that obtained food by simply approaching but not pressing the bar, they learned to bar press for food more slowly than nonobserving cats.[961] Kittens can also learn by observation, and they learn more readily by watching their mothers than by watching another adult cat.[347]

Both cats and dogs can be taught to make auditory discriminations and to lift the lid on a food pan when one pitch but not another is sounded. When the two sounds are too close to be discriminated (less than one-third or one-quarter tone apart), the animals exhibit experimental neurosis. The cats respond to all tones as positive, and most dogs refuse to respond to any.[509] Early visual experience can influence a cat's performance on visual discrimination tasks.[2076,2077]

Cats cannot remember the location of a disappearing object very well with a rapid decline between 0 and 10 seconds, despite visual cues, whereas dogs show a gradual decline between 0 and 30 seconds, Nevertheless, the cats' accuracy remained above chance at 60 seconds.[585]

Illness or age affects feline learning abilities. Immunodeficiency virus (FIV)-infected cats make more errors on a learning test.[1806] FIV-infected cats showed a higher activity level and more distractibility than healthy cats. They explored more, but were more likely to return to previously baited cups, and they had more difficulty traversing a narrow plank.

Old cats (10–23 years) do not learn as well as younger cats. They are most apt to fail to learn, even after 1,000 trials, if the CS begins too far in advance of the UCS but did well in a spatial learning task.[766]

Cats do show changes in behavior when older than their late teens. The signs are a decrease in activity, an increase in vocalization, especially at night, and house soiling, in particular defecation, outside the box. Cats develop amyloid plagues.[798]

A final note on performance of cats: Dogs tend to run faster when competing with other dogs, whereas cats do not; in fact, they may refuse to compete for food in a runway situation.[2047]

8 Ingestive Behavior: Food and Water Intake

A variety of factors influence feeding in animals. Some of these factors act in the short term, others in the long term; still others are operational only in emergency situations. Taste can either stimulate or inhibit intake. Gastric factors, particularly gastric fill, can suppress feeding and the hormone ghrelin can stimulate it. Changes within the intestinal tract, such as an increase in osmotic pressure and release of the hormones cholecystokinin or PYY, can bring a meal to an end, thus inhibiting intake. These are all short-term factors. Eating in response to a lack of metabolizable glucose is an emergency mechanism that is probably not involved in meal-to-meal initiation of eating. Increasing blood levels of glucose does not suppress feeding. When food is freely available, animals, including carnivores, eat many meals a day. Under these circumstances, initiation of a meal is probably a response to waning of the satiety signals. The long-term controls of feeding in which intake is controlled as part of the regulation of body weight or body fats are obviously operational in pigs and other domestic animals. The feedback from fat cells to the brain is a protein, leptin, which inhibits intake. All these signals are integrated in the brain, in which a variety of neurotransmitters and anatomical sites are involved in feeding. The finding that depressants introduced into the brain stimulate feeding reinforces the concept that hunger occurs when satiety signals weaken.

Drinking is associated with eating or stimulated by an increase in osmolality or a decrease in blood volume. Salt intake is controlled by the angiotensin aldosterone system.

INTRODUCTION

General

Animals typically show a growth curve that includes a short, dynamic phase in which weight gain per day is large and a much longer static phase in which there are no major gains or losses in weight but rather oscillation around a mean or set point of body weight. Most domestic animals grow rapidly for several months or the first year following birth and then plateau at a mature body weight.

Animals treated by veterinarians fall into two general categories: either food- and/or fiber-producing animals or companion animals. The problems of ingestive behavior of animals differ from category to category. Animals used for human food rarely survive much beyond the dynamic phase of weight gain. The objective of the producers and the veterinarians who advise them is to maximize weight gain per unit of time. The dairy cow presents a special case. She

Domestic Animal Behavior for Veterinarians and Animal Scientists, Fifth Edition by Katherine Albro Houpt
© 2011 John Wiley & Sons, Inc.

must be a good producer of milk and therefore must increase her food intake, yet she should route that increased energy intake not to body fat but to milk production.

A quite different problem is presented in some companion species, especially household pets and horses. In a seminaturalistic setting, such as a pasture, a horse can be fed ad libitum, but when presented with an energy-rich concentrate diet that it would not have encountered in the wild, the horse may overeat. Acute problems such as colic or laminitis (founder) may result. Chronically, a simple shift upward in body weight, obesity or metabolic syndrome, may result. Dogs and cats face a similar problem. They can maintain their body weights on relatively unpalatable, dry chow diets but may succumb to obesity or digestive upsets when offered a highly palatable diet ad libitum.

The physiology of the controls of food and fluid intake has been studied extensively by such diverse scientific groups as nutritionists, physiologists, animal scientists, and psychologists. Knowledge of the physiological mechanisms involved in hunger and satiety will enable us to stimulate intake for maximum yield or to control body weight without inducing hunger in an animal that tends toward obesity. The physiology of hunger is reviewed here, using the pig as an example; next to the laboratory rat, the domestic pig has been more thoroughly studied in this regard than any other animal. What is known about ingestive behavior in other species is then discussed, and the unique control of food intake in ruminants is described.

The central nervous system controls of feeding are complex. Neuropeptide Y (NPY) and agouti-related protein (ARP) stimulate feeding, whereas cocaine and amphetamine-related transcript (CART) and melanocyte-stimulating hormone (MSH) suppress feeding by their actions in the hypothalamus. Consideration must also be given to the mechanism by which these influences are integrated in order that animals not only survive but maintain an optimal and nearly constant body weight. Until recently, there was a missing link between body fat stores and the brain. The question was how the animal "knows" that it is becoming fatter. An obese strain of mice (obob) differing from lean controls (Ob-) in one gene was discovered. The product of the gene found in normal mice is formally termed ob protein, but popularly called leptin. Leptin is carried to the brain, and as a result, feeding signals are inhibited (NPY and ARP) and food intake decreases. In addition, the sympathetic nervous system is stimulated, with resultant lipolysis, via ß-adrenergic receptors. In this way, less food is taken in and more fat is broken down, thus decreasing fat stores. Advantage has already been taken of ß-adrenergic effects on fat stores. Pigs are fed ß-adrenergic drugs such as clenbuterol to decrease fat deposition, thus

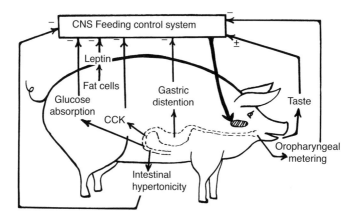

Fig. 8.1 Integration of physiological factors that stimulate and depress food intake in the brain. (Drawing by Dr. T. Richard Houpt.)

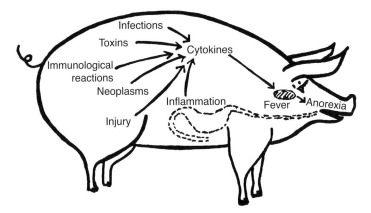

Fig. 8.2 Integration of pathological factors that depress food intake. (Drawing by Dr. T. Richard Houpt.)

sparing calories for lean meat, that is, muscle growth (see Fig. 8.1), but they tend to be more aggressive and nervous than untreated pigs. Another feedback system is peptide YY (PYY), a peptide released from intestinal cells when ingested fat enters the cells, suppresses feeding.

One of the first signs of illness is lack of appetite (see Fig. 8.2). For example, pigs infected with porcine reproductive and respiratory syndrome virus (PRRSV) reduced the time spent eating and food intake while lying more often in ventral recumbency.[543] This lack of appetite or anorexia is caused by cytokiness. Cytokines are polypeptides produced by one cell that influence other cell factors. There are numerous cytokines with numerous functions, but one of those functions is relevant to feeding behavior. Cytokines such as interleukin-1 can reduce food intake and rumination in goats without producing fever.[1924]

CONTROL OF FOOD INTAKE IN PIGS

Meal patterns

Pigs are essentially diurnal animals; therefore, most feeding takes place during the day.[102] Feeding behavior is a circadian rhythm modified by environmental temperature. Pigs avoid eating when daily temperatures are highest and therefore eat early in the morning and late in the evening.[568] They tend to eat every 45 minutes during the day and every two-and-one-half hours at night.[1361] Pigs eat meals in which eating bouts are interrupted for short periods when the pig may drink. The meals are separated by long intervals (90 minutes) from the next meal.[967] When meals of individual pigs were recorded, the pigs were found to eat 8–12 meals per day, with the number of meals decreasing as the pig grew larger. Many "snacks" of less than 50 g are also eaten.[221]

About 75% of feeding takes place during the day in lactating sows. They consume eight meals a day.[484] Younger pigs eat about 14 meals a day.[1360] If food is available from a ball that dispenses it only when the pig moves it, foraging in the bedding decreases. This means of obtaining food results in a more natural feeding behavior in which the appetitive behavior is combined with the consummatory behavior, ingestion of food.[2075] When deprived of rooting for 24 hours, sows will compensate by rooting more. If pigs have access to a substrate for rooting, such as spent mushroom compost, they spend 3–4% of their time rooting, but if food had been hidden in the substrate previously, they root less when the food is consumed.[181]

Electronically controlled feeders have enabled animals, especially cattle and swine, to be kept in groups; yet all have access to feed, and their individual intake and meal patterns can be evaluated. No consistent rank order of entrance into electronic feeders exists, but groups of sows that have been in a pen longer eat before more recently added sows.[282] Few pigs forage for their food under domestic conditions, but they have preserved the ability to forage optimally. If they have to work harder to move from one patch of food to another, they spend longer at each patch.[729] They also can remember and prioritize food sites of different value, choosing the site with the larger quantity of food.[810]

Social facilitation

Two animals housed together usually eat more than the sum of their intake when each is housed separately. This is true of most social animals. Social animals tend to do things as a group; therefore, when one pig goes to the feeder, all the pigs go to the feeder. Cole et al.[370] have demonstrated that group-penned pigs eat more than separately housed pigs. The same phenomenon, social facilitation, leads all pigs to attempt to eat from one set of feeders while ignoring other feeders. Social facilitation of eating begins early; all members of a litter nurse together.

Social facilitation may increase food intake, but this tendency can be offset by the opposing tendency of subordinate pigs to eat less in the presence of dominant pigs. Pigs may refrain from eating even in the absence of overt aggression by the dominant pig.[135] When housed in groups, the pigs tend to eat at separate times, probably to avoid competition at feeders, whereas individually housed pigs tend to eat at the same time as their neighbor.[696] Piglets housed in groups eat more if more feeders are available because they are socially facilitated to eat but need not compete as much for a feeder.

Palatability

The adult set point of body weight (see the section "Defense of Body Weight" later in this chapter) applies to an animal on a given diet. An increase in palatability can result in a shift upward in body weight set point. More simply put, animals eat more and gain weight when their food tastes good. Sows prefer high concentrate to high-fiber diets in short-term, two choice feeding tests[726] despite the findings that higher fiber diets are associated with lower levels of stereotypic behavior.

Pigs show a marked preference for sweet substances,[981,1003] consuming up to 17 L of sucrose solution per day. Advantage has been taken of this preference to increase intake.[21] The intake and weight gain of pigs are not affected by the addition of a substance that tastes very bitter to humans, indicating a species difference in taste perception.[231] Pigs appear to separate sweet-tasting (to humans) flavors into two groups, with the first consisting of almond, raspberry, and peach, which are highly preferred, and the second consisting of vanilla and strawberry, which were not as attractive. Carrots are a preferred food and, pigs will work as hard to obtain carrots buried in sand as for easily accessible ones.[851] Some bitter compounds, such as caffeine and sucrose octaacetate, are consumed, whereas eugenol, benzaldehyde, and anise are not.[967] Texture, color, and odor are important factors in palatability. For example, sows avoid blue food.[916] In contrast to anosmic rodents, anosmic pigs ate with the same meal pattern as that of intact pigs, indicating that odor is not too important.[129]

Newly weaned pigs often show a drop in weight gain, and sweet pig starters are used in an attempt to stimulate intake. Although suckling neonatal pigs show nearly as strong a preference for the various sugars as do adults,[873] these attempts are not always successful. A more rewarding approach may be to add to the sow's feed a flavor that will appear in her milk and then to add the same flavor to the pig starter. Pigs will learn to associate a given flavor with a familiar food (in this case, sow's milk), and they will ingest that flavor more rapidly in solid food than they would a strange flavor.[315] As a result of testing 129 flavors, McLaughlin et al.[1286] found that one, a cheesy flavor, would increase intake of newly weaned pigs.

Environmental temperature

Food intake is inversely related to environmental temperature; therefore, in hot weather, animals eat less. The classic explanation is that "animals eat to keep warm and stop eating to prevent hyperthermia."[286] Certainly, inhibition of food intake in hot weather reduces specific dynamic action and other metabolic heat as further heat loads to the animal. Under normal conditions, food intake increases or decreases in response to environment rather than body temperature; but when body temperature rises to pathological levels, as in fever, food intake also decreases.

Food intake is also stimulated by cold environmental temperature. This thermostatic control of food intake is part of body temperature regulation. When more energy must be applied to maintain body temperature, more energy is taken in.[928] Changes in temperatures of the brain are not correlated with the initiation and termination of meals; and thermostatic eating is a response to changes in ambient or environmental temperature, not to changes in body temperature within the physiological range (Fig. 8.3). If cold temperatures are too extreme, the animal will not be able to compensate for the energy lost by increasing its intake and will lose weight.

Gastrointestinal factors

An important hormone is grelin, which, when the stomach is empty, stimulates intake and growth hormone release.

Gastrointestinal fill alone is not important. High-fiber diets do not suppress intake or motivation for food.[1571] The most likely candidates for the meal-to-meal controllers of intake are those factors that are closely associated with the act of eating. Following a meal, changes occur in the gastrointestinal and plasma level of various constituents, any one or several of which might influence food intake. Food intake ceases before intestinal absorption is complete.

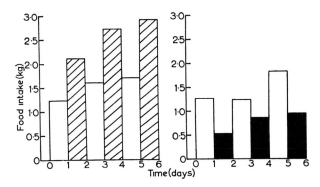

Fig. 8.3   Daily food intake of pigs fed ad libitum. Pig on left was subjected on alternating days to temperatures of 25°C (white) and 10°C (hatched). Pig on right was subjected on alternating days to temperatures of 25°C (white) and 35°C (black).[928] (Copyright 1974, with permission of Pergamon Press.)

If it did not, animals would consistently overeat because food would continue to be ingested during the lag between ingestion of food and its absorption. Gastrointestinal hormones are released as soon as food is present in the upper gastrointestinal tract; they may be satiety signals. Of the many gastrointestinal hormones, such as gastrin, secretin, and enterogastrone, cholecystokinin–pancreozymin (CCK) is the one that holds most promise as a satiety agent.[685] The hormone is released from the mucosa of the upper gastrointestinal tract. CCK has several physiological actions: it stimulates contraction of the gallbladder; it stimulates release of pancreatic enzymes; and it has been shown to inhibit food intake in hungry animals, including pigs.[875,889] Further, CCK acts on the stomach, presumably by slowing gastric emptying, to produce feelings of satiety. CCK is bound by two types of receptors: CCK-A and CCK-B; CCK-B receptors are found in the brain and mediate panic behavior, whereas CCK-A receptors are found peripherally in the gastrointestinal tract as well as in the brain stem. Agonists of CCK-A, but not CCK-B, suppressed feeding in pigs.[1477] Fat in the intestine suppresses intake out of proportion to the caloric value of the fat,[715] and a CCK antagonist prevents that suppression.[1586] Immunizing pigs, but not lambs, against CCK results in a significant increase in intake and weight gain.[1487]

Removing the gastric contents before a meal has little effect on pigs' meal size. There are gastric influences on feeding, but they do not act instantly. Satiety after meals high in protein or fat is probably mediated through the release of CCK, but another satiety mechanism may exist for high-carbohydrate foods. Suckling pigs show a depression of food intake following gastric loads of isotonic glucose solution, but not following gastric loads of isotonic sodium chloride solutions, indicating that there may be glucoreceptors in the gastrointestinal tract[876,1810] that produce satiety. Hypertonic solutions of either glucose or sodium chloride depress intake of both suckling and more mature pigs.[876,890,892] As food is being digested, the osmotic pressure in the intestine rises and stimulation of osmoreceptors in the intestine may be part of the basis of pre-absorptive satiety (Figs. 8.4 and 8.5).

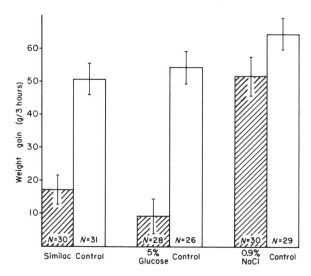

Fig. 8.4 Effect of various gastric loads on 3-hour intake of suckling pigs. Note that milk (Similac) and isotonic glucose, but not isotonic saline, depressed intake.[873] (Copyright 1976, with permission of Oxford University Press.)

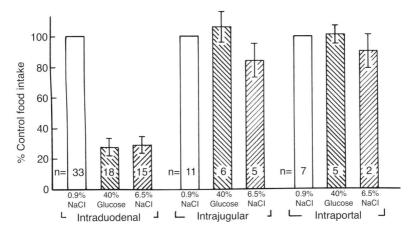

Fig. 8.5   Effect of hypertonic injections administered into the duodenum (left), the jugular vein (center), or the portal vein (right) on subsequent food intake of pigs. Only intraduodenal injections depressed intake relative to saline-injected controls.

Hormonal effect

When female pigs are in estrus, food intake is depressed and activity levels rise. Gilts eat 4 kg (9 lb) less during a week in which they are in estrus than in weeks when they are in another stage of the reproductive cycle.[646] The increase in activity has been quantified: Sows in heat walk 1,400 steps per day, whereas sows that are not in heat walk 5,000 steps per day.[47] Observation of the food intake and general activity of a sow can assist the producer in identifying a female in estrus.

Feeding at parturition

Sows fed ad libitum during gestation have almost complete anorexia on the day of parturition, and although their food intake increases during lactation, it does not reach gestation levels for several weeks. In contrast, sows fed half of their ad libitum intake eat on the day of parturition and ate more than previously ad libitum-fed pigs during lactation when feed was available ad libitum.[1993] This could be a result of depleted fat stores and decreased leptin production in the restricted sows, or increased insulin resistance and reduced mobilization of non-esterified fatty acids in the ad libitum-fed pig.

Imbalance of dietary amino acids

Animals generally show nutritional wisdom in that they select an adequate amount of protein. For example, growing pigs given a choice of a protein-free or an adequate-protein diet ingested sufficient protein for maximal weight gain.[461] In certain circumstances, however, nutritional wisdom is not shown and pigs will choose a nonprotein diet over a protein diet.[1612] This occurs when the protein contains an imbalance of essential amino acids. The explanation for the marked depression of food intake seen when the imbalanced diet is the only one offered, or for the selection of no protein rather than an imbalanced protein, is unknown. It is speculated

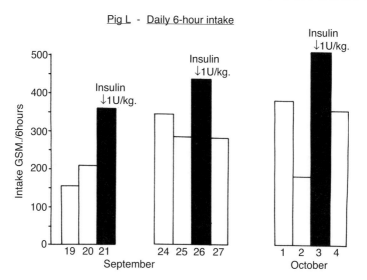

Fig. 8.6 Intake of a pig following injection of saline (white) or insulin (black).

that an imbalance in essential amino acids leads to an imbalance in central nervous system neurotransmitters. Accumulation of a neurotransmitter might depress intake.

When tryptophan is deficient in the diet, the concentration of serotonin for which tryptophan is a precursor is low and food intake is suppressed.[1425]

Glucose utilization

Animals increase their food intake when the rate of glucose utilization in the brain falls. Experimentally, this phenomenon can be demonstrated by administering a competitive inhibitor of glucose, 2-deoxy-glucose (2 DG), which decreases glucose uptake in the brain.[1809] Similarly, food intake can be increased by administering an agent that markedly lowers plasma glucose (Fig. 8.6), such as insulin. Although eating in response to a lack of utilizable glucose (glucoprivation) can be readily demonstrated in a variety of species, it is probably not a practical method for stimulating intake because the dosage necessary to stimulate food intake is perilously close to the dosage that produces hypoglycemic convulsions. Eating in response to glucoprivation is an emergency mechanism the animal uses when its endogenous energy supply is approaching exhaustion. It probably is not involved in initiation and termination of meals in the free-feeding animals.

Defense of body weight

The constancy of body weight in the adult animal is believed to be the result of an innate set point for body weight or, perhaps and more likely, a set point for total body fat stores. The set point is most easily detected when body weight is artificially manipulated. For example, if an animal is starved for a few days it will, when food is again freely available, eat more than it did before the fast and rapidly regain the weight lost during the fast. In some cases, pigs show compensatory increases in intake after food restriction; in other cases, they do not increase their intake over that of nonrestricted controls, but their weight gain is greater, presumably owing to increased efficiency or decreased energy output.[1311] When diets are diluted with noncaloric bulk, intake rises so that caloric intake remains constant.[1327,1460] Conversely, if the animal is force-fed, it will gain weight but will decrease its voluntary intake while being force-fed.[1325] Similarly, animals that have gained weight while being injected chronically with insulin will, when treatment ceases, decrease their intake, losing weight until their weight is at the preinjection set point. The leptin system described earlier is probably the mechanism in pigs but has not been studied in that species. Set point is also maintained by adjustments in energy output that can be varied both by changes in motor activity and by metabolic changes in heat production.

The set point of body weight is more difficult to determine in the young, rapidly growing animal because it is being adjusted upward. The set point can be changed by manipulation of the neonate's nutrition. The starved piglet may remain stunted for the rest of its life.[2015] Similarly, overfeeding of piglets, as may occur in a small litter, may result in a permanently higher set point of body weight. If a young growing pig is fed 120% of its normal intake intragastrically, it will grow faster, indicating that appetite, rather than genetic growth potential or gastrointestinal fill, limits the rate of growth.[1486]

In response to changes in consumer preferences, pigs are now selected for leanness, so the set point for body fat is low and an obese pig is rarely seen on the farm. There are, however, genetically obese strains of pigs maintained for experimental purposes.[841,1229] Obesity can also be produced by dietary manipulation in young, meat-type pigs.[728] The number of fat cells did not increase in these pigs exposed to a palatable, high-carbohydrate diet, but the fat cells were larger, that is, they contained more fat. Pet minipigs must be maintained on an amount of food far below their ad libitum intake to prevent obesity. As a result, they may become destructive in their efforts to find food.

In general, intake can be stimulated in the adult animal by any manipulation that lowers body weight or body fat stores beneath the set point. The neonatal piglet can respond to fasts of short duration with an increase in food intake, but longer fasts may produce irreversible hypoglycemia, coma, and death.

Integration of factors that stimulate and inhibit intake in the central nervous system

Central nervous system stimulants, in particular amphetamines, have been used extensively in human medicine to treat obesity. Less stimulating and less abused but less effective drugs, such as phenylpropanolamine, are also used as over-the-counter aids to dieting. Amphetamines apparently have their effect on neurons or neurotransmitters that mediate satiety or determine set point. Stimulants increase satiety and lower body weight set point.

A drug that inhibits microsomal triglyceride protein, which assembles lipids with protein to form chylomicrons—the structures that carry fat in the blood stream—has been marketed to increase satiety and, therefore, decrease hunger in dogs. Domestic animals' weight is controlled by the owner, and in rapidly growing meat-producing or lactating animals, depression of food intake is generally avoided. Unlike insulin, central nervous system depressants, in particular the benzodiazepine tranquilizers that affect the gamma amino butyric acid, or GABA, receptor, such as diazepam and elfazepam, can probably be used to stimulate food intake when given as food additives to pigs, cattle, and horses.[293,1287] Elfazepam, for example, has been shown to increase pigs' mean intake from a control level of 220 g/h–570 g/h.[1287] A GABA-A receptor agonist increases feeding, and GABA receptor blockers decrease feeding.[131]

Whether use can be made of the effects of barbiturates and tranquilizers to increase food intake of food-producing animals economically and safely remains to be seen. All those interested in manipulating serotonin (5HT) function as a means of decreasing aggression should also be aware that agonists of the 5HT receptors increased spontaneous feeding in pigs, although intake may be suppressed by the same drug when food-deprived pigs are again offered food.[130,520] Kappa opiates increase feeding in pigs, and opiate blockers inhibit feeding.[132,138] It is somewhat confusing that there is a post-feeding opiate-mediated hypoanalgesia.[1663]

The controls of feeding in pigs have been reviewed by Houpt.[887] All the factors that have been discussed here—environmental temperature, rate of glucose utilization, palatability, social factors, estrus, gastrointestinal hormones, and the presence of glucose or hypertonic substances in the gastrointestinal tract—are operating at the same time. The information is integrated, presumably in the brain, and the animal eats more or stops eating accordingly. The role of the various neurotransmitters remains unclear.[936] Such factors as social facilitation and avoidance of protein-imbalanced diets are mediated through the cerebral cortex. Changes in food intake in response to temperature are mediated through the anterior hypothalamus.

Clinical problems

Polydipsia

Scheduled induced polydipsia has been produced experimentally in pigs; that is, when food is available only intermittently and in small quantities, the pig will over-drink.[1813] Sows in a farrowing crate may show polydipsia, perhaps because the waterer may be the only thing available for them to manipulate.[1661] Pigs that are fasted or on a severely limited ration may also increase their water intake (that is, show polydipsia).[2067,2068] Note that in the free-feeding pig or one that is food deprived only for a few hours, drinking accompanies eating, but in a very hungry one, drinking occurs as a compensation for lack of food.

Effects of diet on stereotypies

Adding fiber does not decrease motivation for food 4–23 hours after the meal[1571] but does appear to reduce psychogenic polydipsia and stereotypic behavior in sows.[1610] High-fiber diets reduce rooting behavior, whereas low-protein diets increase rooting.[291] There is considerable evidence that feeding sows free choice will reduce or eliminate stereotypic behavior.[1861,1862] Feeding the limited ration all at once (drop feeding) results in more oral–nasal stereotypic behavior in crated sow than providing the same amount of food over 30 minutes.[901] This bar biting behavior often alternates with drinking, a behavior the sow may substitute for eating when fed only one-third of voluntary intake, which is the standard diet for gestating sows.

CONTROL OF FOOD INTAKE IN DOGS

Meal patterns

Dogs that have free access to foods 24 hours a day eat many small meals a day, mainly during daylight hours.[1379] This meal frequency indicates that dogs are diurnal, rather than nocturnal, and that once-a-day feeding is not "natural," or at least not preferred, by dogs. Beagles living in individual kennels with dry food freely available tend to eat three times a day, at dawn, at dusk, and whenever fresh food is given.[1581]

Social facilitation

Many animal owners have noted anecdotally that the addition of another animal to the household increased the original pet's interest in food. At times, the increase can be a pathological hyperphagia or excessive food intake.[615] Social facilitation of food intake has been quantitatively measured in puppies.[941]

Palatability

Taste preferences must be determined for each species; one cannot assume that because something tastes good to humans, it tastes good to animals. Dogs prefer meat to a high-protein, nonmeat diet, and they show preferences for one meat over another. These preferences, in order, are beef, pork, lamb, chicken, and horse meat.[871,1178] Not only flavor but also the form in which the food is offered is important in palatability. Dogs prefer canned or semimoist food to dry food.[1031] They prefer canned meat to the same meat freshly cooked, and prefer cooked to raw meat, despite the claims made for the Bones and Raw Food diet.[1178] Dogs do not prefer familiar food; in fact, they prefer a novel flavor of canned food. Puppies also tend to prefer novel food, but palatability and maternal effects may outweigh these[581,1379] (Fig. 8.7). Dogs familiar with semimoist food eat only a little canned food at first, when both are available, but soon show a preference for the canned. Dogs also have an innate preference for sucrose in liquids or solid food.[707] They are unusual in preferring fructose to sucrose (humans and pigs prefer sucrose). Lactose, but not maltose, is also preferred.

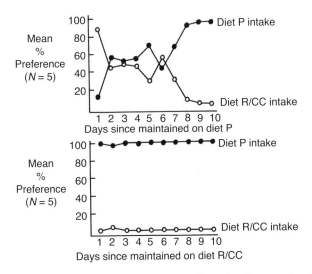

Fig. 8.7 Effect of novelty on food preferences. Dogs normally prefer diet P to diet R/CC, but will show preference for either R/CC or P if it is a novel diet. Preference for P is sustained (lower graph), but that for R/CC is reversed in a week (upper graph).[1379] (Copyright 1977, with permission of Monell Chemical Senses Center and Academic Press.)

Palatability does not depend on taste alone because elimination of olfaction (anosmia) eliminates preference for one meat over another, although anosmic dogs still preferred meat or a sucrose diet over a bland cereal diet.[871] Odor is important, but only for detecting minor differences between foods, as in distinguishing lamb from pork. Such major preferences as that for meat over nonmeat and for sucrose are not affected. Odor is most important for locating food;[1613] taste is most important for identifying food.

The food preferences are reflected in dogs' attraction to the odors of meats. The odor of cooked meat is preferred to that of raw meat, and that of fresh meat to that of 3-day-old meat. Despite their tendencies to roll on rotting organic matter, dogs showed little preference for aged dirty diapers or fish.[191]

Taste is important in a long-term sense as well. Dogs who have been adequately nourished but deprived of taste will overeat when food is again available, indicating that deprivation both of the taste of food as well as of calories is important.[1102] The practical application of this is that provision of a calorie-free, but tasty, food might be less stressful than fasting.

Environmental temperature

Food intake is believed to be controlled, in part, by the regulation of body temperature. Consequently, animals tend to eat more in the cold and less in the heat. This has been demonstrated in environments as diverse as Alaska and Florida and with breeds as different as huskies and beagles. Food intake doubled in the winter as temperatures fell from a summer high of 20°C (68°F) to a winter low of −17°C (1°F).[506] Indoor dogs eat less than those housed outside. This reduction in intake is probably due to the warmer indoor environment.[1070]

Gastrointestinal factors

Oropharyngeal factors alone are not sufficient to induce satiety. Dogs surgically prepared with esophageal fistulas can swallow food, but if the fistula is open, the food will drop from the esophagus and not reach the stomach (sham feeding). In this case, dogs will sham feed for hours, stopping only to rest. It is interesting that placing food into the stomach at the same time that the dog is eating and swallowing food does inhibit further sham feeding.[943] It has also been found that gastric loading immediately before a meal does not markedly inhibit food intake unless more than half of the normal meal is placed in the stomach. Apparently, in dogs at least, both oropharyngeal and gastric stimuli are necessary to induce satiety.

Food placed in the stomach just prior to a meal does not inhibit food intake, but a gastric load given 20 minutes before a meal does.[943] The delayed effect of a gastric load indicates that food must either be absorbed or some humoral factor must be released by the presence of the food in the upper gastrointestinal tract to inhibit food intake. There is evidence in various domestic animals that both the products of digestion and humoral factors inhibit food intake. Glucoreceptors in the liver or portal system also may be involved in satiety.

Food intake of dogs is suppressed by CCK and glucagon and is markedly depressed by the opiate blocker naloxone.[1122] Neither intraduodenal fat nor peripherally administered CCK suppresses sham feeding in dogs, although intracerebroventricularly administered CCK does.[1474] The difference in the effect of CCK on sham feeding and normally feeding dogs indicates the importance of integration of gastrointestinal and humoral events for satiety. Recently, another humoral factor, peptide YY, has been identified, which is released when fat accumulates in the intestinal cells. This may happen naturally when a dog eats a fatty meal, and the phenomenon can

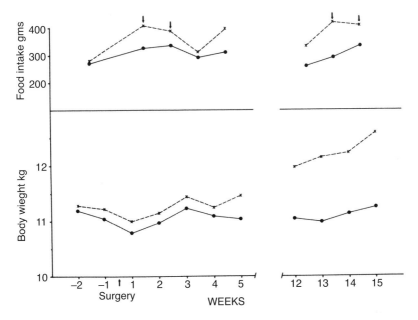

Fig. 8.8 Effect of ovariohysterectomy on food intake and body weight of beagle bitches. Solid lines = intact. Dashes = spayed bitches.[868] (Copyright 1979, with permission of J. Am. Vet. Med. Assoc.)

be used as a weight reduction strategy. The drug dirlotapide (Slentrol R$^{\circledR}$) is a selective microsomal triglyceride transfer protein inhibitor that blocks the assembly and release of lipoprotein chylomicrons into the blood stream, thus triggering peptide YY release and a decreased appetite.

Hormonal effect

During estrus, bitches tend to eat less; conversely, removing the source of estrogen stimulates food intake. Both cats and dogs have a lower metabolic rate following castration or spaying, which also accounts for their tendency to gain weight.[1625] Therefore, one of the side effects of ovariohysterectomy is a tendency for the spayed bitch to eat more and gain weight (Fig. 8.8). Presumably, this is due to the removal of the estrogen source. When a dry diet is available to dogs for only an hour a day, neutered dogs do not gain weight—a strategy owners could use.

Glucose utilization

Glucoprivic eating is seen in dogs. Dogs treated chronically with insulin eat more and gain weight,[719] and eating in response to glucoprivation produced by an inhibitor of glucose utilization has been demonstrated in dogs.[891] A lack of glucose stimulates intake, and an excess usually does not inhibit feeding. Neither intraportal nor intrajugular glucose suppresses intake.[208,209]

Defense of body weight

Dogs can defend their body weight against both decreases and increases. Dogs neither gain weight when force-fed nor lose weight when placed on calorically dilute diets. When dogs were given additional food each day through gastric fistulas, they decreased their oral intake, but not enough to prevent weight gain.[1739] The lack of caloric compensation may be due to the intragastric route of force-feeding; oropharyngeal signals, that is, taste and texture, were not elicited by the food, so satiety was not achieved.

Dogs can increase their volume of intake when their diet is diluted.[944] Dogs deprived of food will eat more when food is again available and, thereby, defend their body weight. Different breeds of dogs defend different body weights and different degrees of adiposity. A casual comparison of bulldogs and salukis makes this clear. The problem of overeating and obesity in dogs is discussed in the section about abnormalities of ingestive behavior (see the "Clinical Problems" section coming up). Dogs can also select some dietary components to obtain sufficient nutrition. For example, dogs can regulate their protein and energy intake when offered diets differing in protein content. When offered such a choice, they chose a 30% protein diet.[1620]

Integration of factors that stimulate and inhibit intake in the central nervous system

The effect of central nervous system depressants on food intake in dogs has not been systematically studied, but there is anecdotal evidence that dogs recovering from anesthesia will eat ravenously before they are fully conscious. Because of the danger of choking in dogs recovering from anesthesia, food should not be available to them. There is also anecdotal evidence that treatment with progestational agents increases food intake. This side effect of progestins used to prevent ovulation should be investigated further.

Dogs lesioned in the ventromedial hypothalamus show hyperphagia and weight gain.[1648] They also show hypersecretion of gastric acid.[1394] The excess production of hydrochloric acid might be related to the increase in food intake that has been noted in laboratory rats and dogs with lateral hypothalamic or dorsomedial amygdala lesions.[598]

Clinical problems

Obesity

Obesity is the most common behavioral problem involving ingestion. The cause is, most simply, an intake of energy that exceeds the output of energy. Therefore, obesity is most often observed in a nonworking animal fed a highly palatable diet. Clinical reports[57,436,1232] indicate evidence of obesity in 20–30% of dogs. These studies and a considerable body of anecdotal information indicate that twice as many spayed as unspayed bitches are obese. The reasons for this have just been discussed in the section on controls of feeding in dogs. There are differences in breed susceptibility to obesity. When a palatable food is made freely available to beagles, some get very obese; in a similar situation, terriers do not become obese[1379] (Fig. 8.9).

High dosages of amphetamines have been shown to depress food intake in dogs.[387] Their use as a treatment for canine obesity has not been evaluated carefully. Fortunately, obesity in animals is easily controlled by food restriction, use of commercially available low-caloric dog foods, and possibly the PYY stimulating drug dirlotapide. Owners may be concerned that their dogs will develop behavior problems if their food is restricted, but laboratory dogs on restricted intake did not become more aggressive, nor were they coprophagic. At first they are more active, but after a week or two, they are less active than they were before food restriction, apparently in an effort to conserve energy.[405]

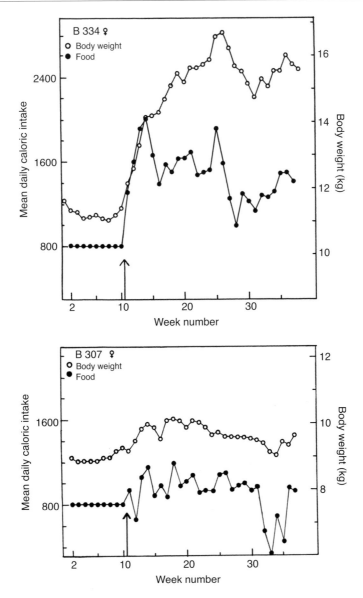

Fig. 8.9 Food intake and body weight of two beagles. Ad libitum feeding began at arrow. Lower graph is of a dog whose intake and body weight remained normal. Upper graph is of a dog that overate and became obese.[1379] (Copyright 1977, with permission of Monell Chemical Senses Center and Academic Press.)

Anorexia

A much more difficult clinical problem is anorexia, which can occur in dogs. An example was a Siberian husky that would not eat. The dog's owner cooked steak, eggs, stews, almost anything, but the dog was chronically underweight and ate intermittently. The dog was examined thoroughly, and no organic cause for the ingestion problem was found. Discussion with the owner revealed that she had simply taught the dog not to eat, and that this was the principal way in which the dog secured the attention of its owner, who led a very busy life. This was the finicky eater gone to the extreme. Starting when the dog was 8 weeks old, the owner adopted the habit of sitting with the dog while it ate and coaxing it along. The owner, a nursing home nutritionist, was very concerned with eating. The first time the pup did not eat, it was whisked off to the veterinarian. The owner did not believe the advice she got from this veterinarian or several others, and instead of just waiting for the pup to get hungry, she went home and cooked a large meal of eggs for it. This pattern persisted, and finally, not even steak excited the dog; it lived on dog biscuits that were always available and ice cream once a day. The treatment was to put the dog on regularly scheduled meals with no treats and to wait. Within 3 weeks and after a 5-day stretch of not eating, the dog was eating one good meal a day and gaining weight.

Pica

Another type of abnormal ingestive behavior is pica, or eating materials that are not normally food. Puppies are notorious swallowers of inappropriate objects that must be surgically removed from the gastrointestinal tract. Occasionally, pica may be the sign of a nutritional deficiency, but more frequently, it is simply an extreme form of attention seeking, because the owner will chase the dog to take the object from the animal. Muzzling the dog can prevent ingestion until the dog learns that the owners ignore his actions.

Grass eating

This behavior is so common that it should not be considered a true pica. Young dogs are more likely to eat grass than older ones, but[1828] dogs are no more likely to vomit after eating grass.[227] Puppies of grass-eating bitches eat more grass than those of bitches that do not eat grass. It may be a means of obtaining roughage. Grass eating in some situations may not be ingestion, but rather tasting and smelling substances left on the grass. This mouthing of grass is particularly common after a rain.

Coprophagia

One of the most common and most disturbing forms of pica is coprophagia in dogs. Dogs adopted as strays are more likely to be coprophagic.[1733] Unless the feces contain viable parasite ova or other infectious agents, coprophagia affects the owner's aesthetic values more than the dog's health. Sprinkling pepper or some noxious substance on feces may inhibit the vice. A better approach is to inject hot sauce into the center of several fecal masses so that the dog cannot tell that they have been adulterated. A much more effective treatment is to orally administer pancreatic enzyme tablets or commercial products. This probably imparts an objectionable taste to the dog's feces, but all the dogs whose feces are consumed must be treated. This is effective in about 25% of dogs treated. A more drastic treatment would be to treat the animal with apomorphine (0.04 mg/kg [0.02 mg/lb]) immediately after it ingests the feces. The taste aversion that may result from associating the eating of feces with vomiting and nausea could break the habit.[730] In rare cases, coprophagia can be an obsessive problem and, therefore, can be treated with clomipramine (See Chapter 9, "Miscellaneous Behavioral Disorders," for dose).

Psychogenic polyphagia and psychogenic polydipsia

Both psychogenic polyphagia and psychogenic polydipsia have been reported in dogs.[615] Psychogenic polyphagia is frequently noted when a rival pet is introduced into a household. Feeding the animals in separate places sometimes alleviates the problem, as does extra attention to the original pet. Psychogenic polydipsia may occur especially in young dogs, but care must be taken to differentiate it from the polydipsia secondary to polyuria. Water intake may be restricted in the case of psychogenic polydipsia but would be dangerous in the case of primary polyuria.

Adipsia and hypernatremia

This syndrome is rarely encountered but has been found in Miniature Schnauzer dogs[392] and in cats. It is interesting because it demonstrates two principles of ingestive behavior: (1) that there are multiple controls of thirst and (2) that animals will increase their intake of a diluted diet in order to keep their caloric intake constant. These animals do not drink in response to the osmotic stimuli, so they present with hypernatremia. They will, however, respond to hypovolemia, so they drink when furosemide, a diuretic that lowers blood volume, is administered. To ensure that the animals consume enough water, they can be maintained on a slurry of canned food and water. The controls of food intake are normal, so they inadvertently ingest water while eating.

CONTROL OF FOOD INTAKE IN CATS

Meal patterns

As do dogs, cats eat many small meals (12) per day when given free access to food, but unlike dogs, cats eat both in the light and in the dark.[1379] One might argue that this intake pattern is not natural, yet the caloric intake per meal is approximately equal to that contained in one mouse. A feral cat with good hunting skills might easily catch 12 mice (or 3 rats) per day.

Social facilitation

Cats have not been shown to increase their food intake when housed in groups rather than individually, nor does the sight of one cat eating stimulate other cats to eat when food is freely available. Nevertheless, many owners report that their cats eat only when they are nearby and that provision of food in the bedroom can prevent 5:00 a.m. meowing. Even when food is available in the kitchen, the hungry cat seems to need the owner's presence in order to eat. Perhaps the cat feels the need to be protected from predators.

Palatability

Cats are notoriously finicky. This reflects the strong influence of palatability on food intake in cats. There is one striking peculiarity of cats: They do not prefer sucrose as most animals do. Cats do not show a sucrose preference for aqueous solutions of sugar, but they do prefer sucrose in salt solutions. The taste of water may block the expression of a sweet preference in cats.[161] The feline preference for sucrose in saline solutions soon turns to aversion because vomiting and diarrhea result in the sucrase-deficient adult cat.

Cats will not eat diets containing medium-chain triglycerides or hydrogenated coconut oil. This may be because they break the triglycerides down to fatty acids in their mouths (cats possess lingual lipase) and are peculiarly sensitive to bitter tastes. They will avoid as little as 0.1% caprylic acid or 0.000005 M quinine. In comparison, rabbits and hamsters avoid quinine only at 0.002 M.

Cats prefer fish to meat and, as do dogs, prefer novel diets to familiar ones.[803] Cat-food manufacturers no doubt take advantage of both of these feline preferences. If the new diet is not more palatable than the familiar one, the cat will, after a few days, begin to choose the familiar food.[1379] While cats are drinking milk, their EEG is synchronized as it is when they are drowsy.[337,357] Observation of cats' behavior can be an indication of palatability. Cats lick their noses after encountering unpalatable food, but groom their faces (licked paw over ear) after eating palatable food.[1921]

When presented with a choice between a food frequently made available to them and one that is rarely offered, cats will choose the scarcer one, even if both foods are dry commercial cat food. Experience may modify the choice of a novel food. Farm cats avoid dry food, which is difficult to ingest, whereas pet cats avoid raw beef.[274]

Environmental temperature

There has not been a complete study of the effect of temperature on food intake in cats, but one demonstration showed that cold environmental temperature, rather than changes in brain or body temperature, affects feeding. This study found that cats drinking milk not only show a decline in brain temperature but also cease to eat.[13] If brain temperature was the factor affecting feeding, one would expect the cat to eat even more as its brain temperature fell.

Gastrointestinal factors

Gastrointestinal depressants of feeding have been studied to some extent. Glucoreceptors that suppress feeding in cats appear to be present in the liver.[1666] CCK and bombesin, a peptide related to CCK, suppress food intake of cats.[109,110]

Hormonal effects

As do dogs, cats increase their food intake when treated with oral progestins. The same hormone might be used to stimulate feeding in anorexic cats, but there are dangerous side effects.

Ovariohysterectomized and castrated cats have a lower metabolic rate,[1625] and if the cat is fed all it wants of a very palatable food and is not very active, obesity can result.[1690]

Glucose utilization

In contrast to most other species, cats have not been shown to respond to glucoprivation with an increase in intake. The glucose analogue, 2-deoxy-D-glucose, failed to stimulate feeding in cats,[940] but the failure to stimulate may have been a result of species differences in the effective dose of the drug rather than to species differences in the control of food intake.

Defense of body weight

The most important determinant of body weight in cats appears to be cyclical in nature. Cats lose and gain body weight in cycles of several months' duration.[1576] For this reason, it has been difficult to demonstrate defense of body weight. There have been two studies in which it appeared that when their diet was diluted, cats did not eat more and, therefore, lost weight.[845,978]

In both studies, the diet, a dry food, was diluted with a dry diluent, either kaolin or cellulose. The cats actually ate a smaller volume than they ate of the undiluted food, indicating that it was unpalatable. In contrast, when cats' food is diluted with water, they do compensate by increasing the volume of intake and maintaining a constant caloric intake.[334,1379] Because the cats were consuming more of a diet when it was diluted with water, their water intake was increased. A watery cat food may be used to increase water intake when clinically indicated, that is, in cats with urolithiasis or hypernatremia.[330]

Opiates

The role of endogenous opiates in feeding has not been well investigated, but the opiate blocker naloxone suppresses intake in cats.[608]

Clinical problems

Obesity

The incidence of obesity in cats has increased in the past 20 years from 10%–29%.[1690] Some of the risk factors for obesity in cats are neutering, confinement in an apartment, and free-choice feeding of a prescription diet.[1690]

Anorexia

Anorexia is seen more often in cats than other domestic animals. A moderately sick cat may further compromise its health by refusing to eat.

Although an otherwise healthy cat may fast for several days and will then be willing to eat large amounts or even hunt prey,[6] anorexia can be a serious clinical problem. Anorexia is most commonly encountered in hospitalized cats or in cats that are initially healthy but are then placed in a boarding kennel. Although an animal can be maintained by intragastric feeding, it is far more beneficial to the animal to reinstate voluntary eating because food taken by mouth stimulates gastric and intestinal secretions much more than does food given by stomach tube.

Advantage can be taken of the fact that depressants stimulate intake. The benzodiazepines, in particular diazepam, have been used to stimulate intake in anorexic patients. A common approach to this form of anorexia is treatment with benzodiazepine tranquilizers, which stimulate food intake in laboratory animals[2050] and in horses.[293]

Plant eating

Cats frequently eat grass. This is observed in free-ranging, prey-killing cats as well as in those eating canned or dry diets. It is not surprising, therefore, that cats may eat houseplants. Plant eating can have serious consequences to the cat because so many houseplants are poisonous, but regardless of whether the plant or the cat is at risk, the behavior is undesirable. If owners observe their cat eating a plant, they can punish the cat or frighten it away, but the cat is, like the destructive dog, most apt to misbehave in the owner's absence. The best solution is to provide the green plants that the cat apparently needs and certainly desires. Plants that are safe for cats can be purchased at pet suppliers. Although the cat is learning that it is permitted access to one plant, the decorative plants can be moved out of its reach. Later, the cat should be taught to discriminate the plants it must not eat from those that it may. A water gun can be used to punish the cat and aid in the discrimination process, but such a method, of course, depends on the owner's presence. The cat would have to be separated from the plants in the owner's absence. Another method is to spray the leaves of the plant with a hot-pepper solution. Still another method that would prevent elimination in the pots of large plants, as well as eating or climbing the plants, is to place mousetraps in the pot upside down so that if the cat jostles the pot or the soil, the traps will snap shut, scaring the cat.

Wool chewing and other picas

Wool chewing is a behavior problem that occurs with greater frequency in Siamese or Burmese cats than in other breeds.[275] It should be differentiated from nonnutritive suckling that many early-weaned kittens will perform. Wool chewing might be related to early weaning. In comparison to the age at which free-ranging cats are weaned (6 months), most domestic kittens are weaned early, but wool sucking is usually not presented as a clinical problem until the cat is an adult.

The behavior is usually characterized by chewing with the molars rather than sucking. The material chewed is usually wool, but in the absence of wool, the cat will generalize to other materials, including upholstery. The cats do not chew on raw wool but prefer knitted or loosely woven material. The behavior is sporadic, but large holes can be produced in a matter of minutes. The behavior seems to be related to feeding because (1) fasting stimulates the behavior and (2) access to plants or bones or even dry (as opposed to moist) food decreases the incidence of the behavior. There is no evidence of a nutritional deficiency, but it appears to be caused by a craving for fiber or indigestible roughage. For that reason, treatment should be aimed at supplying fiber. A higher-fiber diet should be fed, and safe plants should be made available. Offering scraps of sheepskin with the wool has been effective in some cats. If that does not eliminate the problem, give the cat woolen material, such as an old sweater or sock that it may eat. In order to teach the cat to differentiate between things it is allowed to eat and those it is not, treat a variety of other wool objects with a cologne and a solution of hot-pepper sauce. The principle is that the cat will learn to associate the smell of the cologne with the unpleasant taste of the hot-pepper sauce and will avoid objects that smell of the cologne. Articles of clothing, blankets, and so forth can then simply be sprayed with the cologne to deter the cat.

In severe cases in which the owner is considering euthanasia, feeding the cat a chicken wing each week is recommended as a source of chewable material. The danger of injury to the gastrointestinal tract from the bones is less than the danger of euthanasia (particularly considering that many cats kill and eat birds with impunity). Finally, the cat may be treated with a tricyclic antidepressant, such as clomipramine, which will help if the problem is a compulsive one, but the pattern of the behavior—sporadic and hunger related—does not resemble most compulsive behaviors (repetitive and anxiety related).

Some cats suck and tread on fabric, which can also destroy the material. This behavior may be more closely related to suckling deprivation as discussed in Chapter 5, "Maternal Behavior," but can persist for a lifetime, rather than taper off at 1 year. This behavior does not seem to be more common in Oriental breeds.

Cats may chew a variety of other materials. Plastics, especially telephone or computer cords, plastic bags, articles of clothing, or wood may be chewed. Oral pathology must be eliminated as a cause. In one case, the serotonin blocker and appetite stimulant cyproheptadine has been successful in inhibiting plastic eating (Dr. E. Schull, personal communication).

CONTROL OF FOOD INTAKE IN HORSES

Meal patterns

The normal feeding pattern of horses, as detailed in Chapter 3, "Biological Rhythms and Sleep," is to graze continuously for several hours and then to rest for longer or shorter periods depending on the weather conditions and distances that must be traveled to obtain water and sufficient forage. When offered a pelleted complete diet, a similar feeding pattern emerges: many long meals. It is interesting that whether the horse is grazing or eating pellets, the statistical definition of a meal (feeding with breaks of no more than 10 minutes' duration) is the same.[1099,1236] When fed free choice hay horses chew 40,000 times per day.[531] The domesticated horse is rarely on pasture and is given only limited amounts of hay. When given no long-stem roughage, horses will work to obtain it.[531] In short-term tests, horses offered six different forages were not as restless and did not sift through their bedding.[701]

Social facilitation

Horses eat when other horses eat, and eat more if they can see another horse eating.[1836] This is important when creep feeding a foal and when encouraging an anorexic horse to eat. Horses appear to prefer to eat from the floor and from shallow buckets or mangers. This enables the horse to see in all directions between its legs and may have evolved as an antipredator strategy. Grazing is, of course, from the ground rather than from the usual chest height of a manger. The problem that arises when feeding confined horses is to prevent ingestion of parasite ova or sand while still encouraging intake. Horses fight less and spend more time eating from tractor tire feeders where several horse can eat at once than from single feeders or from a long manager where horses can eat side by side.[1373]

Palatability

Randall et al.[1575] have reported the basic taste preferences of immature horses. They show a strong preference for sucrose, but no preferences for sour (hydrochloric acid), bitter (quinine), or even salt solutions. At high concentrations, all the solutions except sucrose were rejected. In a study of adult ponies, 9 of 10 showed a strong preference for sucrose.[789] Salt intake varies from 19 to 143 g per day.[1704] The interest in adding fat to equine diets has led to a comparison of various oils. Corn oil is the most preferred of the vegetable oils, which are preferred to tallows.[850] Horses prefer pelleted feed to hay and will work harder in an operant conditioning test to obtain the former.[1420] Timothy hay is preferred to reed canary grass and has a better calcium to phosphorus ratio.[1450]

Sensory-specific satiety exits in that horses spend longer eating flavored foods when several flavors are available simultaneously.[700] Variety itself is important.

Grazing

Grazing behavior is selective; that is, unless the pasture is composed of only one species of plant, the animal has the opportunity to be selective as to the species ingested. For example, in the Mediterranean climate of the Camargue, horses consume graminoids in the marshy areas, moving to the less preferred long grasses in the winter.[1236] Similarly, meadow and shrub land were the vegetation types grazed by feral horses in the Great Basin of Nevada, but food preferences and nutritional needs had to be weighed against the dangers of exposure in the winter and the irritation of insects in the summer.[214]

There have been several studies of the plants that ponies and horses choose to eat on pasture. Tyler[1909] found that the New Forest Ponies of England eat eight different species of plants but avoid the poisonous Senecio. These ponies will eat acorns, an over-consumption of which leads to acorn poisoning. Archer[70] found that of 29 species of grass, horses and ponies preferred timothy, white clover (but not red clover), and perennial rye grass. Dandelions were the most preferred herbs. Horses also avoid fecally contaminated grass and long grass.[596]

Pastures are not homogenous, so there are patches of varying nutritive value. Horses show dynamic averaging in which they return to the last patch they grazed after a short absence but a different one after a long absence—matching the long-term average of the patches.[460]

Horses prehend at a rate of 25 bites per minute (prehending bites should be differentiated from chewing). Intake rate depends on bite size and rate. The larger the horse, the larger the bite size, but intake also depends on the handling rate, that is, the time to chew each bite. Ponies may be constrained in intake when the grass is fibrous and requires more handling time. The intake rate of grass is 36 g dry matter/min for ponies and 76 g dry matter/min for horses.[596]

The grazing horse chews at a rate of 30–50 bites per minute for 8–12 hours per day. The frequency of oral stereotypies in stalled horses on low-roughage diets is probably a reflection of the oral activity seen in a natural environment.

Horses, sheep, and cattle each have different modes of prehending grass: horses use their lips; cattle, their tongues; and sheep, their teeth. Presumably, the ability to be selective varies with the method of prehension as well as with the size of the muzzle. Sheep should be more selective than horses. The reason selectivity is important is that the grazer can choose a more nutritious plant or plant part or can avoid a toxic one.

Horses vary considerably in their selectivity, which may account for deaths of only a few horses on a pasture where poisonous plants grow.[1219] Horses evolved to graze, spending the majority of their time with their heads down, moving slowly from patch of grass to patch of grass. Horse spend more time grazing and take more bites from swards with taller grass.[1401]

Gastrointestinal factors

The horse appears to depend more on pregastric signals to satiety than other species. When horses sham feed—that is, when most of what they have swallowed falls out of an esophageal fistula—they do not eat more than they do when the food reaches their stomachs.[1566] This is in contrast to dogs, which will eat very large meals under the same circumstances. Eventually, the sham-fed horses compensate for the lost feed by eating sooner than normal, but apparently the signal for satiety is some form of oropharyngeal metering; that is, 25 swallows means enough has been eaten. The importance of pregastric (oral) factors to horses is confirmed by the finding that prolactin levels increase after a meal is consumed, but not after the constituents are administered intragastrically.[458]

Another indication that chemoreceptors in the gastrointestinal tract are not important controls is that when administered either intragastrically or intracecally, neither glucose nor cellulose, the main digestible constituent of grass, and its breakdown products, the volatile fatty acids solutions, depress intake until they have been absorbed. Intake is suppressed, but only after a long latency. There is a mechanism for controlling caloric intake, but it appears to be postabsorptive.[1567,1568]

The first sign of colic in most horses is anorexia. This clinical observation, as well as controlled studies, indicates that pathological distention of the gastrointestinal tract inhibits feeding in the horse as in other species. This anorexia is probably mediated through pain receptors that travel in the sympathetic nerves. Analgesics intended for use in horses are often tested by determining whether a horse with a dilated cecum will eat when treated with the drug. In this case, the drug is probably working peripherally, so pain signals are not relayed to the brain, whereas naloxone inhibits feeding centrally.

Central nervous system depressants

Brown et al.[293] in a preliminary study found that the central nervous system depressant, diazepam, stimulates food intake in horses and that the commonly used tranquilizer, promazine, had a similar effect. Horses, in common with other more thoroughly studied species, increase their food intake when the brain, presumably the areas involved in satiety, is depressed (Fig. 8.10).

Defense of body weight

Horses can regulate their energy balance by controlling the amount they ingest. In other words, horses do not eat a fixed amount or eat until they are ill, but they increase or decrease the amount

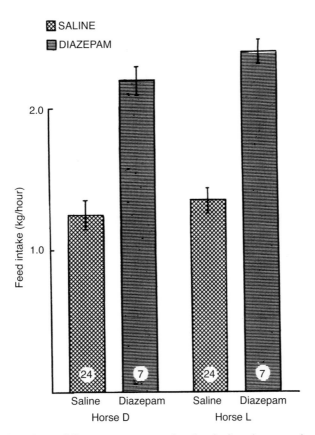

Fig. 8.10   Intake of two horses following intravenous saline (hatched) or diazepam (lined).

they eat to compensate for caloric dilution or enrichment.[1099] The pony gradually shifted to ad libitum feeding does not colic but does gain weight and is, therefore, in danger of laminitis; but the body weight reaches a plateau.

Geophagia

Horses sometimes exhibit pica, including geophagia. When soil from the site where the horse was eating is compared to soil from other areas of the same farm, it is found to be higher in iron and copper. This indicates an attraction to those elements.[1279] A more serious problem is ingestion of stones, the cause of which is unknown.

Polydipsia

Psychogenic polydipsia is also seen clinically in horses. The owner's main complaint is that the horse urinates frequently and copiously, so its stall is wet; in this case, the polyuria is secondary to the polydipsia. In horses, as in small animals, the condition must be differentiated from diabetes insipidus and other causes of secondary polydipsia.

CONTROL OF FOOD INTAKE IN CATTLE

Meal patterns

The time cattle spend grazing on pasture and eating in feedlots or loose housing has been reviewed in Chapter 3. Defining the difference between an intrameal and intermeal interval requires measuring many feeding bouts. Rook et al.[1621] define an intermeal interval as more than 5 minutes without eating. Cattle kept in the confinement of a feedlot or barn eat approximately a dozen meals a day.[342] Cattle show individual cyclic patterns of intake.[1824] Eating rate varies with the physical form of the feed. Cattle can eat 2.72 kg (6 lb) of hay in an hour.[234] Meal is eaten more slowly than pellets, which, in turn, is eaten more slowly than a slurry. Dilution of the meal with water actually increases the amount consumed per minute. Silage is eaten more slowly than hay, probably because of illness produced by consuming the fermented product too quickly.

In some dairy parlors, the cows are fed grain only while they are being milked. An important consideration for dairy farmers, therefore, is the speed with which cows can consume concentrates. It takes a cow 1–2 minutes to eat 0.5 kg (1 lb) of grain; slightly less time is required if the grain is cubed.[966] If a high-producing cow is milked in too short a time, she will not have time to consume the grain that she needs; another arrangement must be made to feed her. If cows are not fed grain in the milking parlor, however, they will not be as eager to enter. All these factors must be considered when planning a milking parlor and feeding system.

Rate of chewing in cattle has been studied by direct observation or by recording jaw movement using either a balloon under the jaw or a strain gauge on the halter.[183,459] These studies have led to the conclusion that cattle that eat fast also chew fast; by so doing, they eat more and therefore produce more. Cows should be selected for rapid intake both to solve the problem of eating enough while being milked and to help reduce negative energy balance during early lactation.

Feeder design is important. Cattle that have to reach under a horizontal bar to obtain feed may injure their necks. In other designs such as a post and rail, wastage of feed may occur.[1498]

Social facilitation

Cattle will also eat more in groups than they will individually, and first-calf heifers will eat more if grouped with older cows, but production may not be increased, because these increases must be balanced against the negative effects of dominance disputes. The more agonistic encounters, the more hay is wasted. Feeder design is important in reducing waste; a ring or cone is better than a trailer or a cradle for offering round bales to cattle.[308]

Another effect of the social hierarchy during group feeding of grain is that subordinate cows eat faster than dominant ones, probably because they have less time to eat before they are displaced by a dominant cow[601] and must compensate. Transponder-activated feeding devices are, theoretically, an excellent way to feed group-housed animals and still record individual intake, but several problems arise. Intake decreases as the number of cattle per feeding station increases, especially when there are more than five animals per station. When limited amounts of concentrates are fed in that manner, the cows' activities are disrupted as they test the station to determine whether they will be fed. Dominant cows can displace subordinate ones after the door has opened for the subordinate.

Palatability

Ruminants appear to have a definite sweet preference, but what tastes sweet to people may not taste sweet to cattle. On the basis of electrophysiological recording from the chorda tympani and glossopharyngeal nerves, cattle can taste saccharin but do not respond to aspartamate.[813,1722]

Cattle reject 20% sucrose, 0.08% acetic acid, and 2.5% quinine.[694] Twin cattle show similar rejection responses, as well as similar sweet preferences responses.[207] With regard to the more usual feed substances, factors in addition to taste and odor must be considered. Texture and ease of prehension may explain why cattle prefer pelleted to unpelleted feed. Unchopped silage is preferred to chopped silage,[489] in part because more bites are necessary to collect the chopped silage.

Palatability is affected by secondary plant compounds—those chemicals produced by the plant to reduce predation, that is, eating of the plants by herbivores. A common secondary plant compound is tannin, which browsers, such as deer but not domestic ruminants, have evolved to tolerate. Tannins reduce palatability because of their astringent properties;[1086] they also cause illness. There is, however, interest in adapting cattle to diets containing tannins to take advantage of many tannin-containing tropical forages.

A good example of the complexities of preference testing is that dairy heifers will choose a mean ratio of 40% grass silage and 60% corn silage, but the individual preferences ranged from a 34% to a 75% preference for the corn silage.[1994]

Grazing and selectivity

The preferences of ruminants for plant species vary and depend on a number of factors. These include (1) the growth stage of the plant—most ruminants prefer fast-growing, succulent species; (2) the mixture of species-clover, for example, may not be eaten if it is growing in a pure stand but will be eaten if grasses are growing with it; (3) the season of the year—ruminants will consume species that are green during the winter, although the same species will be rejected in the summer when other species are green; and (4) the relative abundance of herbage. These factors are particularly important in determining when a ruminant will ingest a poisonous plant. Many poisonous plants are bitter in taste or harsh in texture and are, therefore, avoided by ruminants; but when the poisonous plant is the first green plant to appear in the spring (hemlock or skunk cabbage) or the only forage available on a pasture, it will be. In addition to these factors, the location of the plant, in particular its distance from water (in arid regions) or shelter, will influence the amount of it consumed.[81] Cattle avoid fecally contaminated areas.

Various methods have been devised for determining preferences of grazing animals. The most accurate and most direct is to collect the food eaten by sheep or cattle through open esophageal fistulas. Another method is to observe the animals closely. This method is more accurate if the forages are planted in narrow pure stands from which the ruminants may choose. A third method is to sample the plant species and heights of the plants before and after the pasture has been grazed. A fourth method is to measure the alkanes in the feces, which will differ depending on the plant species ingested and which appear in the feces 24 hours after consumption. Studies using these methods have revealed that cattle graze selectively; that is, they do not necessarily eat plants in proportion to the number of each plant species in a pasture.[830] For example, Cowlishaw and Alder[390] found that cattle most preferred meadow fescue and timothy; perennial rye grass and cocksfoot were the next most preferred plants; and Agnotis and red fescue, the least preferred. Ruminants are less likely to graze on plants that contain old growth or cured material. Rapidly growing plants are the most palatable, provided that they are high enough in fiber.[670]

Cattle wrap their tongues around grass and pull to prehend it. This method of forage limits them to plants higher than 10 mm. On a fresh rye grass pasture, dairy cattle graze at a rate of 50–60 bites and 14–20 chews/min. Although they prefer longer swards, they will graze shorter swards at a higher bite rate of 70/min.[743] They are the least selective of the domestic ruminants. Sheep can graze much closer to the ground because they use their teeth to prehend, a fact that may have led to antagonism between cattle and sheep producers on a shared range.

Cattle eat most of their meals during daylight but may graze at night if short days or hot weather preclude obtaining the nutrient requirements during the day. Grazing time is 400–650 minutes per day at a bite (prehension) rate of 60 per minute.[542] Cattle prehend a gram or two at a time, taking in 30–50 g in a minute. As bite size increases, the cattle are both prehending and chewing with the same jaw movement.[1082] Stems interfere with the process of grasping leaves and, therefore, decrease bit size and rate. Clustered leaves can be prehended more efficiently.[487] Fasted cattle spend more time grazing than nonfasted ones, and although bite size was unaffected, they chewed less, swallowing larger particles.

Do animals forage optimally? Do they increase the time spent at patches of high-density food and spend longer at patches that were hard to obtain, that is, a longer walk from water or resting areas? These questions are only partially answered. Cattle apparently graze those patches that give them the largest bite weight and instantaneous intake. For example, cattle will select short, dense patches over short, sparse ones but will select against short, dense patches when tall, dense patches are available. Selecting for maximum bite weight and rate of intake seems to occur.[469] At the pasture level, cattle will avoid grazing in wet areas where plants have lower protein and higher fiber concentration.[838]

Cattle can be taught to eat or at least eat more of a novel forage by first associating a visual cue—an orange traffic—cone with a palatable feed and then placing that cone on the patch containing the novel plants.[1597]

One must consider the effect of adding concentrates to supplement cattle on pasture or range. Supplemental food blocks are used frequently for delivering extra calories, vitamins, minerals, or medication for cattle. Placement of these blocks is important because cattle will not use blocks placed close to the watering site as much as those placed in grazing areas.[333] Neophobia is also a problem. Short-term food deprivation does not decrease the latency to eat a novel feed.[835]

Environmental temperature

Cattle eat less when environmental temperatures are high. In addition to the direct effects of heat on intake, there are also effects on plant growth that may render them less palatable. One of the problems of raising cattle in the tropics or other hot environments is that food intake, and therefore production, falls. The use of tropical breeds and crosses with tropical breeds of ruminants helps alleviate the problem because these cattle eat more in the heat or eat more at night when the temperatures are lower.

Cold ambient temperature increases food intake in ruminants as in simple-stomached animals. This can be observed not only when environmental temperature falls but also when the animals' heat loss is increased. (See Baile and Forbes[113] and Forbes[601] for reviews of all aspects of the controls of food intake in ruminants, including thermostatic factors.)

Flies can also influence feeding. Cattle actually eat more when face flies are present in large numbers.[482]

Estrogen level

Food intake falls in estrous cattle.[911] The decrease in intake can be used to identify cows that are ready for breeding (see Chapter 4, Fig. 4.4). Stilbestrol is an estrogenic drug that has been used to fatten steers. In the doses given, it does not suppress intake and the anabolic effect of stilbestrol leads to weight gain.[809] Since stilbestrol was banned, other estrogenic compounds have been used to improve weight gain in feedlot cattle.

Rumen fill and the products of rumen fermentation

The anterior gastrointestinal tract of the ruminant (the rumen) is an anaerobic fermentation chamber in which bacteria—that produce cellulose—can release the energy that is utilized by the animal. This energy is otherwise unavailable to the animals and enables cattle, sheep, and other ruminants to survive on grass and roughage diets. In the case of grazing ruminants, the time necessary to collect food and fill the rumen is probably the limiting factor in food intake. For example, when cattle are grazing on the open range, they spend 56% of their time grazing and another 21% of the time ruminating[735] (see Chapter 3). In the case of cattle fed diets high in grain for fattening, and in the case of lactating dairy cattle eating concentrates, other factors inhibit food intake. For example, cattle fed a 75% concentrate diet spend only 2.5 hours a day eating. The motivation for oral activity is independent of gastrointestinal fill because hungry, rumen-fistulated cattle given rumen content infusions still engage in oral behaviors such as tongue rolling.[1162]

The end products of bacterial digestion in the rumen are the volatile fatty acids: acetic, butyric, and propionic. When acetic acid is added to the rumen, food intake is depressed; similar amounts injected via the jugular vein have no effect on food intake.[115] It therefore seems likely that acetic acid may stimulate receptors located in the rumen epithelium or in the portal circulation, or the effect may be osmotic. These receptors may, through central nervous system connections, inhibit food intake. Above and below approximately 50% forage in the diet, intake is reduced. On low-roughage, high-energy diets, production of volatile fatty acids is probably the most important satiety factor. On low-energy, high-roughage diets, rumen fill or abdominal fill is probably a satiety factor (Fig. 8.11). Intake falls in pregnant or fat cattle, presumably because of the increase in abdominal fill by the fetus or fat[224,967] (Fig. 8.12).

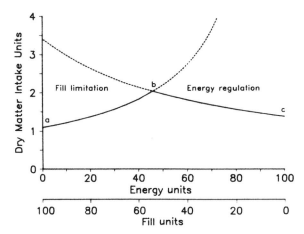

Fig. 8.11   Reciprocal relationship between dietary characteristics and dry matter intake. Line a to b represents intake limited by the fill effect of the diet. Line b to c represents intake limited by the energy demand of the animal. Dashed lines represent unattained intake predicted by extrapolating the theoretical equations.[1312] (With permission of J. Anim. Sci.)

Humoral and central neural factors

Few of the humoral or neurotransmitters have been studied in cattle. Most of the studies are performed on smaller ruminants and are discussed below in the section "Sheep and Goats." Intraportal propionate suppresses intake in cattle.[532] CCK may have a paracrine function, acting locally on the vagus nerve to suppress intake, although blood levels of CCK do not vary when the

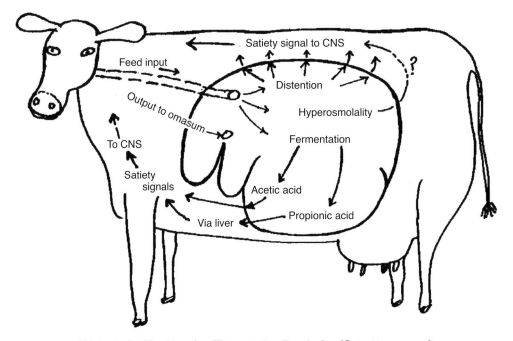

[Distention] = [Feed input] − [Fermentative digestion] − [Output to omasum]

Fig. 8.12   Controls of feeding in a ruminant. (Drawing by T.R. Houpt.)

cow eats meals of concentrate or roughage.[655] Ghrelin, produced in the abomasums, stimulates intake in cattle.[2116]

Corticosteroids increase food intake in cattle, but increase fat deposition, whereas ß-adrenergic agonists such as clenbuterol decrease fat deposition and increase muscle growth without increasing food intake.[600]

Defense of body weight

When dry cows are allowed to eat ad libitum, intake reaches a plateau in Jerseys, indicating a set point of body weight, but Holsteins under similar conditions continue to gain for a longer period, probably indicating that a breed selected for high production has less inhibition of intake.[1351]

Although cattle can vary their intake with availability of feed, there are constraints. When concentrates are available 24 hours per day, cows eat 80% more than when they are available for only 5 hours. Hay intake increases only 20%. This is strong evidence that rumen fill is not the only influence on satiety.

Cattle can, within limits, decrease their food intake as caloric density increases. Even young calves demonstrate this ability by decreasing their intake of milk replacer as the percentage of water in the replacer falls.[1503] The ability of cattle and other ruminants to respond to dietary dilution, that is, to increase their volume of intake as the nutrient density decreases, has been reviewed by Baile and Forbes.[112]

Low protein content of the diet suppresses food intake in ruminants as well as in simple-stomached animals, but because of the rumen microbial production of protein, the level of protein in the diet can be much lower before anorexia occurs. Furthermore, nonprotein nitrogen, particularly urea, can substitute for protein if enough carbohydrate is available to the bacteria for protein synthesis. Offering concentrates can decrease forage intake, but the decrease varies with quality of the forage. Intake of low-quality hay will be less affected than intake of good-quality hay (refer to Fig. 8.11).

Parasitism

Ruminants must weigh the cost benefit of grazing nutritious, but parasite-infected, that is, fecally contaminated forage; generally, they will avoid fecally contaminated sites and deplete the noncontaminated sites.[911] Gastrointestinal helminths stimulate the release of their host's gut hormones, including cholecystokinin. Therefore, the heavily parasitized ruminant loses weight not only because the parasites consume some of the food that their host ingests but also because the host ingests less.[1841] There are two possible explanations for the survival value of anorexia in parasitized animals: an effective immune response is stimulated by anorexia and later allows the hungry animal to select foods that will minimize the risks of infection or select foods that are high in antiparasitic compounds.[1078]

Clinical problems

The fat cow syndrome

An abnormality of feeding behavior that is being seen with increasing frequency is the fat cow syndrome.[1368,1369] Under some types of management, dairy cows may be fed in a group that includes both lactating and dry cows. The dry cows may overeat, gain weight—consisting mostly of fat—and later at calving or during lactation become ill or even die. The pathogenesis of the syndrome remains unclear, but the initial problem is that the cow overeats. High-producing dairy cattle have been bred to eat large amounts in order to supply the metabolic fuel for lactation. When lactation ceases, the increased food intake may persist and the fat cow syndrome may result. It is interesting that lacating cows respond more precisely to food deprivation by walking farther to obtain food than dry cows.[1706]

CONTROL OF FOOD INTAKE IN SHEEP

Although more studies have been conducted on the effects of rumen manipulations in cattle than in sheep, most of the other physiological studies of ruminant intake have been conducted on sheep, probably because of their size.

Meal patterns

Sheep eat approximately a dozen meals a day in a laboratory. Sheep can eat at a rate of 15–30 g of pelleted feed per minute, but only 9 g of hay per minute. Sheep eat a kilogram more if feed is available free choice rather than for a limited period of 3 hours per day.

Light stimulates growth and increased food intake in lambs. Even a flash of light at midnight—a skeleton day—can increase intake.

Social facilitation

Confined, isolated lambs eat less than grouped ones.[1985] Sheep eat less when in metabolism cages, which may be due to a lack of social facilitation in a gregarious species, as well as to confinement itself.[599]

Palatability can affect flocking behavior. When grazing sheep remain within 30 m of one another, but an individual sheep will move 60 m away to obtain pellets.[1762]

Palatability

Sheep do not appear to have a very marked sweet preference. Nevertheless, only 5% sucrose and glucose were preferred; higher concentrations produced no preferences or aversion. Lactose was rejected at a concentration of 2.5%. Sheep also showed no preference for molasses, for which cattle show a strong preference.[693] Although a supplement such as urea and molasses may be provided and will increase intake, 19% of sheep will not consume it.[488] In fact, sheep seem to avoid strong flavors even if the strong flavors predict a more nutritious food.[102] Sheep will learn to prefer flavored straw that is associated with nutrients, whether the nutrients are consumed or delivered intraruminally.[1944] Similarly, lambs will gradually eat more hay with added sucrose, apparently because of the postingestive consequences of the sugar, not the taste.[304]

Sheep are particularly neophobic, so it is best to present novel foods in a familiar environment and familiar foods in a novel environment for optimum intake.[306] Offering novel foods with a familiar flavor and frequently introducing novel foods can reduce neophobia.[1097] Similarly, offering lambs low-quality roughage early in life will stimulate them to eat low-quality roughage as adults.[468] Lambs will avoid poisonous foods better if an alternative food is available, particularly if the alternative is nutritious.[1025] Lambs prefer flavors paired with nutrients to flavored saccharin solutions, a form of nutritional wisdom.[306]

Lambs prefer soybean meal to commercial pellets, both of which were strongly preferred over fishmeal, flocked maize, or whole oats. Rolled barley and sugar beet pulp were moderately well accepted.[436] Sheep prefer pelleted feeds to chopped feeds.[1924]

Sheep are much more sensitive to unpleasant taste than other ruminants. They reject sour solutions of hydrochloric acid, acetic acid, lactic acid, or butyric acid at concentrations lower than those found in the rumen, yet the volatile fatty acids must surely be tasted when the sheep ruminates. A bitter solution of quinine (0.004 M) was rejected, but not one of urea, even at concentrations high enough to produce fatal toxicity.[692] Experience also plays a role in that sheep that initially rejected quinine-treated hay eventually accepted it even when nonbitter hay was available.[600]

When given a choice of two feeds, one with a level of protein content above their requirements and one below, the sheep ate enough of each to maintain their requirements. Even when straw is fed, the sheep can select the most nutritious portion and leave the less-digestible parts behind. Sheep are more likely to consume poisonous plants while food restricted.[147] Lambs will more readily eat food their dam has eaten, but the influences can begin prenatally. Feeding oregano essential oil to the pregnant ewe will result in acceptance of oregano flavored food in her lamb after weaning.[1770]

Defense of body weight

Blaxter et al.[234] found that intake in ad libitum-feeding sheep remained relatively constant from 1 year of age onward. Sheep can compensate for considerable dilution of their diet with straw or even inert diluents.

Not surprisingly, fasted sheep eat faster, taking larger bites than those who have been grazing at will, but it is interesting that their food preferences change, tending toward higher roughage feeds, such as grass, rather than the higher protein plant, clover. Within 24 hours of being fed a fiber-free diet, sheep will pseudoruminate (regurgitate without cud chewing) and ingest plastic fiber. Placing a pompom of fiber in the reflexogenic areas of the reticulorumen reduces this fiber hunger.[319]

Rumen factors

Fiber decreases intake, and the smaller the particle size, the greater the intake of those diets in which rumen distention limits intake. There is additivity of rumenal acetate and intraportal propionate in suppressing intake of sheep, indicating that several factors acting in concert could be necessary for satiety. This is the more natural situation than an increase or decrease in a single metabolite or hormone. When given a choice, sheep do not eat the most calorically dense food but choose sufficient long fiber to optimize rumen function.

Intestinal receptors

Gastrointestinal factors are as important in ruminants as in nonruminants. A high osmolality in the duodenum will suppress feeding and stimulate drinking by sheep.[329] Factors such as CCK and propionate act additively in suppressing ruminant intake,[566] but immunizing lambs against endogenous CCK did not result in a significant increase in intake.[1793,1901] If digesta enters the duodenum more rapidly, the sheep eats more, which suggests that abomasal fill may produce satiety.[1210]

Grazing and selectivity

Sheep graze up to 12 hours per day, and 90% of that time is spent biting.[1761,1764] A sheep takes 0.34 seconds to open and close its mouth in a prehension bite; therefore, it prehends at a rate of 60–80 bites per minute.[341] Sheep masticate (chew) 60–70 times per minute. Sheep prehend grass by breaking it between their lower incisors and upper dental pad. That and their narrow muzzle enable them to be more selective than cattle. They select leaves rather than stems. When the protein content of a diet is insufficient, food intake may be depressed. This may occur on poor-quality pastures. The rate of food intake depends on the plants grazed. For example, sheep can prehend and masticate clover faster than grass.[1490] Sheep expend energy moving from place to place while grazing, and they increase their food intake 20–50% over that in confinement to compensate for the extra energy expended. Sheep have peaks of grazing activity every 8 hours. They graze most intensely just before sunset.

The factors affecting grazing are bite rate, bite size, time spent grazing, and species of food selected. All of the following are important: learning, especially learning from the dam's food choice; motivation to be close to another sheep, social facilitation of the beginning, but not of the end, of a grazing bout; and physiological state. Sheep forage optimally, initially eating mostly a preferred species and later as the height of those plants decreases, switching more frequently to the less preferred, but more easily obtained plants.[1535] In general, the preferences are correlated with the dry matter and carbohydrate content of the grasses. Sheep select a diet higher in protein and lower in fiber content than that obtained from clipped pasture samples, indicating the advantage to the animal of selective grazing.[799,1821,1989]

Sheep will walk 3 or 6 meters to obtain clover, but are less likely to travel 20 m, the point at which the energy they would expend reaching the clover would exceed that provided by the clover.[340]

A practical consideration in pasture management is that sheep, as well as horses, avoid fecally contaminated grasses, although they seem to prefer grass subjected to urine contamination.[1222] Sheep do not select against parasite larvae; it is the feces themselves they avoid.[380] Sheep learn to avoid diets that exacerbate the effects of secondary plant metabolites. For example, lambs' intake decreases with increasing concentration of the terpenes found in sagebrush.[519] See "Taste Aversion" in Chapter 7. The effects are worse if the animal eats a high-carbohydrate, low-nitrogen diet.[147] There are interactions between the diet and the secondary compound in that lambs innately prefer grain (barley) to sugar beets, but reverse that preference if the diets also contain terpenes.[1947] Sheep will consume more shrub if a variety of shrubs, presumably with a variety of secondary compounds are offered. Activated charcoal that adsorbs terpenoids—the common toxin in shrubs—can be fed to encourage consumption.[1614]

It is unclear what senses are involved in forage preferences. Anosmic sheep do not avoid fecally contaminated feed as normal sheep do.[1899] Anosmic sheep and sheep with impaired vision (hooded with translucent eye coverings), however, showed preferences very similar to those of intact sheep, although the visually impaired sheep tended to graze at one level rather than grazing higher or lower on the plant to select the most succulent portions.[79] Even cutting of the gustatory nerves had little influence on forage preferences.[77] In the laboratory, anosmic sheep are no different than intact sheep in their meal patterns.[134]

Both food preferences and social factors influence food choices in sheep. Sheep in larger flocks graze for longer periods than sheep in smaller flocks.[1489] The satiety state of the grazer also influences plant selection. Previously fasted sheep eat more, as compared with nonfasted sheep, because the former take larger bites and choose fewer legumes than nonlegumes.[1412] When a fungus such as endophyte infests fescue, the sheep avoid it, apparently because they are nauseated.[23]

Environmental temperature

Sheep eat more when they are cold and less when they are hot. For example, sheared sheep eat 50% more after shearing as a result of the loss of insulation of their wool.[1863] At very low temperatures ($\sim 10°C$, or $14°F$), intake may be inhibited and the consequences of greater losses of energy of heat will be compounded by a decrease in energy intake.

Hormonal factors

Ewes eat less during estrus. Infusion of the amount of estrogen equivalent to that which occurs at estrus also suppresses intake.[601] Food intake decreases during late pregnancy in ewes carrying more than one lamb. The decrease can be as large as 40% if the only available forage is low-quality roughage. This can result in ketosis or pregnancy toxemia of sheep. During lactation, thin sheep eat more than fat ones—a phenomenon seen in all ruminants studied thus far.

Glucose utilization

Cross-circulation from hungry to satiated sheep stimulates intake of the satiated animal (and depresses intake of the hungry one), indicating the existence of humoral factors that influence feeding.[1732] Glucose or insulin levels may be among the humoral factors. Because virtually everything that the ruminant eats is exposed to rumen bacteria before reaching the intestine, very little dietary glucose becomes available to the animal. Instead, the ruminant depends on the volatile fatty acids for energy and produces glucose by the process of gluconeogenesis. Plasma glucose is low, approximately half that of simple-stomached animals. For these reasons, ruminants were assumed to be fairly independent of glucose utilization and not expected to eat in response to glucoprivation. As has been demonstrated in both sheep and goats, however, food intake can be markedly increased by insulin and the glucose analogue 2-deoxy-D-glucose.[888]

Central neural mechanisms

The easiest generalization that can be made about central stimulants of intake is that factors that depress activity, such as anesthetics and opiates, increase feeding. For example, central nervous system depressants, such as calcium, barbiturates, and benzodiazepines, also stimulate intake in ruminants.[167,467,1056,1223,1730,1731]

As the number of known neurotransmitters and neuromodulators grows, the hope of gaining a complete understanding of the pharmacology of central neural controls of feeding and other behaviors grows dimmer. CCK, discussed earlier here as a peripheral satiety factor, also exists in the brain, where it can act to produce satiety in sheep.[115]

The opioid peptides are also involved in feeding behavior. The mu and kappa receptor agonists given intracranially appear to stimulate intake in sheep; gamma agonists depress intake.[114] A mu opoid receptor ligand syndyphalin stimulates food intake over 48 hours.[1436]

Although sheep increase their food intake when norepinephrine is injected via the cerebral ventricles, cattle do not show the same response, nor does a clear picture emerge when adrenergic agonists or antagonists are injected.[116] Cerebrospinal fluid from hungry sheep stimulates intake by satiated sheep, indicating that humoral factors within the brain (or the ventricles) influence feeding.[1229] The serotonin antagonist cyproheptadine increases food intake in sheep.[504]

There has not yet been any practical application of these findings to increase the food intake of fattening cattle or lactating dairy cattle. It is not yet clear whether these drugs, which stimulate intake over the short term, would, if administered chronically, produce a long-term increase in food intake or meat and milk production.[1772] The problem of the effects of barbiturates and tranquilizers on human consumers also remains unknown. The latest approach is to stimulate production with bovine growth hormone or somatotropin and rely on the animal to increase intake to match the increased production (output).

Obesity can be produced in sheep by offering a pelleted diet free choice. The sheep will consume three to six times their maintenance requirements. After the sheep have gained weight, their intake falls and they actually eat more slowly than lean sheep. This indicates that the feedback from fat, presumably leptin (ob protein), is inhibiting intake. These sheep are more sensitive to the anorexic effects of opiate blockers.[17]

CONTROL OF FOOD INTAKE IN GOATS

Meal patterns and grazing

Goats eat 12 meals a day (remarkably similar to cattle and sheep), 8 of them during the day. Goats are more selective feeders than sheep and have a longer vertical reach than sheep of the same weight.[601] Browsing behavior is a skill that must be learned. Goats learn to break twigs off the plants rather than to chew them off.[1454] Attempts to increase consumption of goats with plentiful, but not particularly palatable, foods such as sagebrush have not been successful,[1604] but goats will consume more shrubs than sheep.[1614] Goat selectivity is strongly influenced by their dam and peers and by the plants to which they were exposed in their first year of life.[225] When fed as a group, food intake and time spent eating decline when feeding space is restricted. The dominant goat shows less reduction in intake.[971]

Goats readily consume glucose and sucrose solutions at concentrations as high as 40%.[206] Goats do not prefer bitter substances but will accept quinine-adulterated water at nearly 10 times the concentration that a rat will.[204,206] Field studies confirm that goats have a high tolerance for bitter taste.[388] Castrated male angora goats are in danger of urolithiasis. It is possible to increase their water intake, and thereby decrease their risk of urethral blockage, by adding vinegar or orange flavor to the water.[383] Increasing the crude protein of concentrates fed to goats increases their food intake and their milk production.[108] Propionate and lactate suppress intake in goats, but the site of action is beyond the rumen, presumably in the liver. Food intake falls during estrus.[539] Vasopressin suppresses intake in goats and may be the mechanism by which stress suppresses intake.

WATER INTAKE

At least three types of stimuli elicit thirst: a dry mouth, an increase in the osmotic pressure of the blood, and a decrease in the blood volume. In addition to these internal signals. Taste preferences influence water intake. For example, high concentration of magnesium (4 g/L), but not sodium sulfate found in some natural water sources, suppresses water intake.[720]

Increase in osmotic pressure

Hypertonic sodium chloride infused intravenously causes thirst in pigs,[929] horses,[1829] and dogs.[2058] An increase in the osmotic pressure of the blood is believed to stimulate osmoreceptors located in the brain.[2051] Goats drink copiously when hypertonic saline solutions (2% NaCl) are injected into the brain through a cannula.[60] Similarly, a mare whose water intake is restricted to half her normal intake will exhibit thirst as a result of an increase in the osmotic pressure of her blood and consequent stimulation of osmoreceptors.[869] Free-ranging cattle drink once a day. Under these conditions, lactating cattle drink larger amounts but drink no more frequently.[1644] Thirty kg pigs drink about 6 L per day. Feeding excessive protein increases water intake. In general, the ratio of gram of water consumed to gram of feed is 2.5 to 3.

Decrease in blood volume

Decrease in blood volume, for instance as a result of hemorrhage or peritoneal dialysis,[358] may stimulate thirst. A decrease in the blood volume would also be expected in a cow that produces 36 kg (80 lb) of milk (95% water) per day. A lactating cow drinks 45 kg (100 lb) more water a day than a dry cow for this reason.[735] The drug furosemide, frequently administered to race horses shortly before they perform, causes a decrease in plasma volume and thus stimulates thirst in horses[1829] and sheep.[2084] Water is lost when animals are heat stressed, whether they cool themselves primarily by panting (dogs), saliva spreading (cats), or sweating (horses). Therefore, water intake obviously increases with environmental temperature.

Angiotensin

Another type of drinking occurs in response to the hormone angiotensin. Angiotensinogen is acted upon by the kidney hormone, renin, and then by a pulmonary converting enzyme to form the octapeptide angiotensin II, which has several actions. It releases another hormone, aldosterone, which is involved in sodium reabsorption by the kidney. As its name implies, high doses of angiotensin II can increase blood pressure. Most interesting is its action on water intake; angiotensin II is the most potent dipsogen known. Angiotensin II, or procedures known to release the hormone, stimulate water intake in a wide variety of animals, including dogs,[592] cats,[378,1827] sheep,[3] goats,[59] pigs,[143] and horses.[58] The role that angiotensin release may play in normal thirst remains to be determined.

Situations in which blood supply to the kidneys is compromised stimulate renin release and, therefore, angiotensin release that could be expected to lead to thirst. Indeed, dogs in congestive heart failure show increased water intake.[1573]

Dry mouth

A desalivate animal takes frequent small draughts of water in order to swallow dry food. This type of drinking, prandial drinking, is also seen in intact pigs that take a small quantity of water into their mouths before swallowing a mouthful of grain.[833]

Multiple causes of thirst

Just as most food intake appears to occur without a major change in body energy balance, most drinking occurs without a change in body fluid balance. The osmotic and volume depletion stimuli to drinking are emergency mechanisms to restore body water under life-threatening conditions.

Most drinking in domestic animals is prandial, that is, in association with meals. For example, 75% of water intake in pigs is in association with meals. About 20% of the drinking occurs after feeding (within 10 minutes); 30%, as pauses in feeding; and 25% precedes meals. The drinking occurs before any changes take place in blood volume or osmolality. The animals appear to be drinking in anticipation of their needs, and the physiological mechanisms are the same as those that control the cephalic phase of gastric secretion.[893]

Thirst produced by overnight water deprivation is a combination of osmotic thirst and hypovolemic thirst. In contrast to the osmoreceptors that stimulate vasopressin secretion, those that stimulate thirst in the dog appear to be located on the blood side of the blood–brain barrier.[1873] Water intake of thirsty dogs is reduced to 80% if water is injected intracarotidly so that the osmoreceptors of the brain are no longer stimulated. Intravenous administration of an equal volume of water has no effect. If thirsty dogs are injected with isotonic saline so that peripheral blood volume is returned to normal, their water intake is reduced by 20%. If both intravenous isotonic saline and intracarotid water are administered, water-deprived dogs do not drink.[1572] Despite this evidence that thirst is inhibited when blood volume and osmotic pressure return to normal, dogs cease drinking before these parameters return to normal.[2058] There may be signals from the gastrointestinal tract that inhibit water intake, as there appear to be signals that inhibit food intake. The stomach has been implicated,[1898] but gastric fill alone does not suppress drinking in dogs;[1784] duodenal osmoreceptors are more likely candidates for the source of inhibition.

Water intake falls with environmental temperature, and this may account for the increased incidence of impaction colic during the winter when horses eat more and drink less. Providing warm water with meals increases water intake 40%.[1063] Horses drink more water from a bucket than from automatic waterers, and float-valve automatic waterers, in particular, may result in negative fluid balance.[1434] Horse prefer float valve to push lever drinkers.[1060]

Cattle fed silage—a somewhat wet feed—and limited amounts of concentrates drink four times a day. The drinks ranged 1–13 L (1–14 quarts).[601] Dairy cows spend 25 seconds drinking per bout, consuming 9 L in 15 sips.[1857] There may be central sodium receptors in cattle that when stimulated by an increase in NaCl in the cerebrospinal fluid increase water intake. Water intake increases in the heat and decreases in the cold, but when the environmental temperature falls below 0°C (32°F), water intake increases with the increased food intake necessary to control body temperature. Dogs may not be as thirsty in the cold. Their threshold for osmotic stimuli is higher, and their blood volume is elevated.[1784]

If given access to water, veal calves will drink a large quantity (3–8 L per day) in addition to milk replacer and will exhibit less nonnutritive oral behavior.[705] Early weaned (18 days) piglets may both over-drink and waste water, particularly when provided with a nipple drinker. They may associate the nipple with suckling. Provision of a push lever drinker reduces both water intake wastage and belly nosing of penmates.[1890]

SPECIFIC HUNGERS AND SALT APPETITE

The concept of the nutritional wisdom of animals has not been validated. Animals apparently cannot innately choose a diet containing a vitamin or other nutrient in which the animal is deficient.[1647] Horses fed a diet deficient in calcium will not eat more of a calcium supplement to correct the deficiency.[1705] There is better evidence for a phosphorus-specific hunger. Cattle and other ruminants chew on bones, and some will consume phosphorus supplements. Animals, at least laboratory animals, can learn to associate a particular diet with improvement in health. Conversely, animals can learn to avoid a diet they associate with a feeling of malaise. Given proper clues, such as a distinctive flavor, most domestic animals could probably learn to choose a diet that would correct a deficiency rather than choose a deficient diet. Examples of this ability are that lambs fed a diet high in energy but low in protein would preferentially eat feed that was high in protein and low in energy, and lambs fed a diet high in protein but low in energy would also choose a diet that rectified their imbalances.[1716]

There is, however, one nutrient that nearly all species select innately when they are deficient: sodium.[852] Salt hunger is a well-recognized phenomenon, especially in herbivores, whose diet tends to be low in sodium. In most species, removal of the adrenal glands and the consequent hyponatremia are followed by life-saving ingestion of sodium chloride. Pigs, for instance, drink sodium chloride solutions and survive, following experimental adrenalectomy.[1188] Ruminants can be made experimentally sodium deficient by creating a salivary fistula. The large loss of sodium bicarbonate in saliva produces a deficiency that sheep can correct by drinking precisely the quantity of sodium solution they need to bring their sodium levels up to normal. Treatment with a diuretic also stimulates sodium appetite in sheep.[2084]

Salt appetite is not stimulated during pregnancy and lactation in sheep despite the extra sodium demands.[1319] Sheep can be divided into those who excrete sodium predominantly in the feces, that is, who do not absorb excess sodium, and those who excrete sodium predominantly in the urine. The fecal excretors have a greater sodium preference.[1318] Although sodium is usually in low concentrations in the herbivore diet, in some environments, it may be in high concentrations, which results in decreased intake and digestibility. When consuming a high-salt diet, sheep will select a supplemental diet for energy rather than protein.[1866]

Cattle will travel farther for water than for salt.[660] Sodium-deficient cattle and sheep are able to learn an operant response to obtain a sodium reward.[2,1778] Sodium status is apparently assessed in the brain, where changes in the concentration of intracellular sodium act to initiate transcription and translation processes. The protein synthesized alters the ionic or membrane characteristics or increases the neurotransmitter capacity of the neurons.[456] The hormones that mediate salt hunger are angiotensin and aldosterone acting in synchrony. Because of the hormonal involvement, there is a latency for the appearance of the salt appetite.

Furosemide causes a loss of sodium as well as water in the urine. Sodium appetite as well as thirst is stimulated in horses treated with furosemide.[880] This phenomenon may be important because of the widespread use of furosemide in race horses.

The preference for sodium is innate, but animals can learn to associate a given mineral with postingestive consequences. For example, phosphorus- or calcium-deficient sheep will prefer a flavor associated with a feed containing the deficient mineral or even with ruminal infusion of phosphorus.[1945,1946]

9 Miscellaneous Behavioral Disorders

DOGS

Jumping up on owners or visitors, failing to come when called, and running away are minor behavior problems that nevertheless may strain the owner–dog bond. Tail chasing, light chasing, circling, and digging for imaginary prey appear to be compulsive problems. Phobias, especially fear of storms, are often a serious problem. Destructive chewing behavior caused by oral exploration, escape attempts, or separation anxiety are common complaints of owners. All these problems are dealt with in the veterinary clinical behavior textbooks.

Separation anxiety

Separation anxiety is a major problem for dogs and their owners. The dogs may bark, urinate, defecate, salivate, chew, or claw at the walls or doors that restrain the animal. The risk factors for separation anxiety are being a male, especially an intact male, having a single female owner or several females in the household, acquisition from a shelter, playing with the dog within 30 minutes of the owner's return. Dogs that yawn or stretch when their owners return are at lower risk for separation anxiety, presumably they have been sleeping while the owner was away.[594, 1280, 1845] Psychoactive medication and behavior modification can be used to treat the problem.[773, 863, 1088]

CATS

Destructiveness

In general, cats develop behavior problems much less frequently than dogs. Feline destructive behavior appears to fall into three categories: (1) clawing (discussed in Chapter 2); (2) wool sucking (a vice of Siamese cats in particular), which is sometimes transferred to synthetics, to the great detriment of sweaters and upholstery (wool sucking may or may not be related to early weaning); and (3) plant eating. Wool sucking and plant eating are discussed in Chapter 8, "Ingestive Behavior: Food and Water Intake."

Self-mutilation

This is sometimes referred to as feline hyeraesthesia. The cat's skin ripples and then it bites its own tail. After musculoskeletal and allergic causes have been eliminated, it may be treated as

Domestic Animal Behavior for Veterinarians and Animal Scientists, *Fifth Edition* by Katherine Albro Houpt
© 2011 John Wiley & Sons, Inc.

a form of psychomotor epilepsy. It does not meet the criteria for obsessive–compulsive disease and is usually treated with antiseizure medication. In many cases, the cat will not attack its tail if it cannot see it. Bandaging the tail or otherwise hiding it can be effective.

Withdrawal

A change in the cat's environment is not always followed by inappropriate urination. Another response can be withdrawal from the owner. In one case, the cat was taken from a suburban setting, where it was free to go out of doors, to a high-rise apartment. This formerly affectionate cat ignored its owner for weeks after the move. The owner then boarded the cat for two weeks; on its return to the apartment, it was again affectionate. The stress of boarding probably was responsible for the cat's adaptation to the less stressful apartment. Even more upsetting are the cases in which the cat withdraws from a wheelchair-bound person, just when that person needs more comforting. Not forcing contact and hand feeding can be effective.

HORSES

These large, powerful animals, which are trained to work closely with humans, may develop a wide range of irritating or even dangerous behaviors. These abnormal behaviors are commonly referred to as vices, but this term implies that the horse is making a moral decision. The term problem is used here. More roughage, straw bedding, more contact with other horses, and more time out of the stall prevent or attenuate these problems.

Behavior problems in the stable

Predisposing factors

The prevalence of stereotypic behaviors varies from 5 to 16% in the United Kingdom and appears to be higher in Canada.[1185] Among thoroughbreds, most stereotypic behavior was seen in mares and two-year-olds. A horse with one stereotypy is more likely to exhibit another.[1334] McGreevy and his colleagues found that lack of a variety of roughage, nonstraw (wood shavings or paper) bedding, three meals per day, and few horses in the immediate environment were all risk factors.[1277, 1278] The use of the horse was also important. Dressage and three-day event horses and racing Thoroughbreds had a greater prevalence than did endurance horses and racing standardbreds.[1278, 1587]

Locomotion problems

Stall walking and weaving. This behavior may often occur as part of a herd-rejoining behavior, in which case more visual contact with other horses or a stall companion will help. In other cases, it is claustrophobia, in that the confinement itself, with or without other horses, is a problem. Finally, stall walking may occur as a stereotypy, a repetitive, functionless behavior. This form of stall walking is usually slower than the others but is more difficult to interrupt. Horses that constantly circle their stalls may lose condition or fail to obtain it because they expend more energy walking than they ingest. Their performance is usually affected as well. Restraining the horse by tying it often converts a stall-walking horse into a weaver. Weaving is a behavior in which the horse stands in one spot but shifts its weight and its head from side to side and it may involve lifting each hoof in turn and walking in place. The cause of the behavior appears to be confinement. The treatment is to maintain the animal on pasture with a run-out shed for shelter. Other treatments are stall toys and more work. The size of the stall does not seem to influence the stall-walking behavior; a horse given access to an entire barn still circled in one corner. Stress appears to aggravate the problem; horses circle more frequently the evening before a hunt or show. Bagshaw et al.[112] did not find any calming effect of a small dose of tryptophan.

Weaving may be similar in etiology to stall walking. It is a stereotypy that appears in many zoo animals as well. Confinement and frustration are causes, and horses in pain may also weave. The form of self-stimulation probably offers the horse some comfort, as rocking does to humans. Tail rubbing is also probably a form of comforting self-stimulation, but medical causes must be eliminated. There is some evidence that stall walking and weaving may be inherited and possibly related to endogenous opiate production.[472, 1933] Providing a horse with more opportunity to look out of its stall, or providing a mirror, can decrease weaving.[382, 1237] It is interesting that a view of another horse reduces weaving, but horses that face one another in a stable are more likely to weave than those who do not face another horse.[1422] The stall door may be the critical factor as an obstacle between one horse and its companion. Weaving occurs before feeding and is negatively correlated with the amount of hay fed.[1422]

Pawing. Pawing has been described by Ödberg[1441] as a response to frustration, a displacement activity that originated from the activity of uncovering food buried under snow. Horses have been noted to paw in a variety of situations: when restrained from moving, when eating grain, when expecting feed, at a recumbent foal that does not stand, and in order to reach another horse. The most extreme forms of pawing occur in horses that have barrier frustration, that is, they are seeking to escape from their stalls. A typical case is that of a standardbred that had spent most of its life on pasture with a run-out shed for shelter. When confined in a box stall for training, it dug a hole measuring 1.5 m (4 ft) in depth in his stall. Some horses habituate to stall confinement eventually; others may do extensive damage to themselves and the stalls as they try to escape by jumping over the walls. Pawing is a less dangerous activity, but it damages dirt or clay floors. Pawing is exhibited by standardbreds but in many cases, the horses stand in the hole they created, taking pressure off their hind limbs in the case where the behavior has a function—comfort or pain relief. The second cause of pawing is an attempt to reach another horse. Horses are herd animals, and stallions, in particular, try to reach one another to play if they are young or to fight if they are mature. If dirt floors are replaced with concrete, the horses will stop pawing, but their motivation has not changed. The stallions may rear up to reach one another over stall walls that do not reach the ceiling or lean out the front of the stalls to make contact if that is possible. A concrete floor can be hazardous when slippery and is more stressful to the horses' limbs and feet because it is a rigid surface.

Pawing in anticipation of food is similar to kicking in anticipation of food and is discussed in the next section, "Stall Kicking." Pawing at recumbent foals may serve to stimulate the foal but can injure a foal, especially if the foal is unable to rise and the pawing continues for some time. The reason horses paw when eating grain is unknown. One hypothesis is that they may be responding to the highly palatable food that can be prehended quickly, which are too unnatural, and therefore frustrating, qualities.

Stall kicking. Aggressive kicking is discussed in Chapter 2. Only kicking directed against stall walls is considered here. Most horses kick stall walls with their hooves; a few knock their hocks against the wall. Both activities produce unwanted concussion on the horses' bones and joints. Kicking can damage the walls as well. A small hole made by kicking is often enlarged by wood-chewing. Stall kicking may also be a form of self-stimulation. The horse kicks to hear the sound its hoof makes as it strikes the wood. Sometimes, stabling a horse on a wooden floor that makes a similar sound (hoof on wood) as the horse walks on it will eliminate the kicking.

The most common form of pawing and kicking is that which the owner has operantly conditioned. The horse will tend to paw or kick at feeding time because it is frustrated to see or smell food (or the giver of food) but not be able to eat. This is reflected physiologically in the increase in heart rate observed in horses that see feed. The horse is, of course, fed, so the animal's behavior has been positively reinforced. It has learned that kicking or pawing is followed by food. The horse paws, and food appears. It will begin to paw or kick earlier and earlier. In effect, it is increasing the fixed ratio of number of responses (paws or kicks) for every reward. The longer the horse kicks before feeding, the longer it will take to extinguish the behavior. In order to extinguish the behavior, the owner should feed the horse only when it does not kick. The process will go much more quickly if many small meals a day are given. The horse must at first refrain from kicking only for two seconds before it is given a half cup of feed. Gradually, the criterion is raised so that there must be no kicking for 5 and then 10 and then 30 seconds before food will be given. Only when the horse refrains from kicking for a short time for several feedings or trials should a longer time be demanded. The training will go faster if the horse is taught a counter command such as "stand" for a food reward at the same time.

Oral problems

Cribbing is an oral behavior in which the horse grasps a horizontal surface, such as the rim of a bucket or the rail of a fence, with its incisors, flexes its neck, and aspirates air into its pharynx. Some horses aspirate air without grasping an object. This is called aerophagia or windsucking; the latter term can also be used to refer to pneumovaginitis. It was thought that the horse swallows the air, but this does not usually occur unless the horse is swallowing between cribbing bouts.[1281]

Cribbing occurs in association with food, in particular, eating grain or other highly palatable food.[690, 1075] See Fig. 9.1 for an illustration. The relation of cribbing to eating is similar to that of nonnutritive suckling in calves that occurs after drinking milk. Cribbing rate is highest during the 8 hours following feeding.[362]

About 2.5–5% of thoroughbreds and 0–6% of other breeds crib.[18, 878, 1238, 1933] Cribbing occurs less frequently in endurance horses (3%) than in those used for dressage or eventing (8%), who are confined in their stall for much longer periods.[1278] Horses whose neighbors crib are also more likely to crib, although having an aggressive neighbor is more of a risk factor.[1395]

It is a clinical impression that cribbing occurs more frequently in confined horses, but once established, it may persist even when the horse is on pasture. It may be the result, rather than the cause, of gastrointestinal problems. Aspirating air or inflating the pharynx may be a pleasurable sensation to an animal experiencing gastrointestinal discomfort. An undeniable consequence of cribbing is excessive wear of the incisor teeth. Although the opiate blockers such as naloxone will inhibit cribbing,[473] opiates fall or do not change in the blood when horses crib.[690] In fact, horses that crib have lower or similar blood levels of opiates than those of noncribbing horses, but the blood levels may not reflect brain levels.[690, 1488] Horses are more, not less, sensitive to pain when they crib.[1338] Cribbers do seem to have less vagal tone— that is, their resting heart beat is higher than that of noncribbers. When horses are deprived of the opportunity to crib, gastrointestinal motility slows.[1276]

The simplest method used to prevent cribbing is to place a strap around the throat just behind the poll so that pressure is exerted when the horse arches its neck and even more pressure is

Times/15 minutes

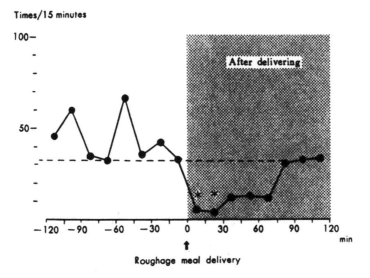

Roughage meal delivery

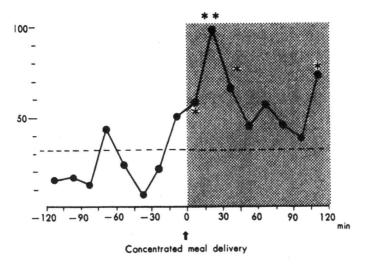

Concentrated meal delivery

Fig. 9.1   Mean frequency of cribbing before and after roughage meal (upper graph) and concentrated meal (lower graph) delivery. Dotted line indicates the mean level. *$P < .05$, **$P <. 01$.[1075] (With permission of Japan. J. Equine Sci.)

exerted when the animal attempts to swallow. The horse is, in effect, punished for cribbing. If a plain strap does not suffice, a spiked strap or metal collar, or one that is held in place with a head stall, can be used. A common observation of a horse wearing a cribbing strap is that it continues to grasp horizontal objects with its teeth but does not swallow as much air. Many stables are designed or modified so that few horizontal surfaces are available, but water and feed containers usually provide the horse some opportunity to crib. Shock has also been used to punish horses that crib.[122] Muzzles may also be used. These are wire baskets that permit the horse to eat and drink but not grasp a horizontal surface. Some horses learn to grasp a stick, pull it into the muzzle vertically, and crib on that. The muzzles seem more frustrating for the horse than the straps, and the horse will try to pull them off. When horses are prevented from cribbing by a cribbing collar, they show a postdeprivation rebound; that is, they crib more than they did before the collar was applied.[1276]

There have been a variety of surgical treatments for cribbing. These treatments include buccostomy; cutting the ventral branch of the spinal accessory nerve (9th cranial); myotomy of the ventral neck muscles; or a combination of partial myectomy of the omohyoideus, sternohyoideus, and sternothyrohyoideus and neurectomy of the ventral branch of the spinal accessory nerve.[584,606,714,749,982,1461,1703,1906] The success rates of these treatments vary from 0–70% and are no longer recommended. Cribbing "braces"—rings placed over the horses incisors so they cannot make contact with a surface—are initially effective, but can cause infections and frequently fall out or move out of place.

Beginning at 20 weeks of age, 10% of foals crib. Foals begin to crib when they are weaned into stalls and fed concentrate diet; those weaned on pasture do not begin to crib.[1977] One hypothetical result of cribbing is an increase in gastric acidity due to the oral stimulation (cephalic phase of digestion) of gastric acid output. Ulcers are more numerous and more severe in foals that crib.[1417] Dietary reduction of cribbing rate may be possible by feeding antacid.[1334,1417] Another—not necessarily contradictory—reason is that some component of concentrate diet stimulates cribbing. Gillham et al.[690] measured cribbing for 30 minutes before and after various feeds were given. The cribbing rate rose from 2/5 to 27/5 minutes when the horse was eating sweetened grain or pellets, but rose only to 8/5 minutes when alfalfa pellets were fed. Although it could be any of the grains—corn, oats, soybean—the most likely culprit is molasses. Oats are least likely to stimulate cribbing even when constituting 50% of the diet.[645] Although toys may not help with oral problems, provision of a simple foraging device that delivers food as the horse rolls it might help.[1213,2046] Increasing the frequency of meals appears to reduce cribbing but increase locomotor stereotypies.[379]

Is it necessary to prevent cribbing? The rate of epiploic foramen entrapment is higher in cribbing horses, possibly because air-filled viscera migrate around the abdominal cavity, especially when the horse exerts negative pressure while aspirating air.[69] Unless the otherwise healthy horse is losing weight or suffering from colic as a result of swallowing air or flatulent colic, the behavior is not interfering with the horse's well-being. The noise of cribbing often annoys the owner, but that is not a good reason to subject an animal to the risk of surgery and the possible side effects of infection and disfigurement that may interfere much more with the animal's function than cribbing did. Damage can be done to fences or to buckets because the horse exerts great pressure (~25 kg) when flexing its neck. Cribbing is considered an unsoundness, but this may not be justified. Cribbing is also considered to be contagious, and it has been shown that being stalled next to a cribbing horse increases the risk of cribbing; the same study showed that being stabled next to an aggressive horse increases the risk of cribbing much more. When owners of cribbing horses were surveyed, it was found that only 1% of horses exposed to a cribber began to crib.[18] The use to which a horse is put may also change the risk of cribbing[1277] Young horses may be more likely to learn the habit from an adult than are other adults.

Wood chewing. Both cribbing and wood-chewing (lignophagia) horses grasp horizontal surfaces with their teeth, but the wood-chewing horse actually ingests the wood, whereas the only damage the cribbing horse does is to mark the wood with its incisors. In contrast to cribbing, wood-chewing appears to have a definite cause: a lack of roughage in the diet. Wood-chewing is more common in dressage and eventing horses than in endurance horses that spend more time outside their stalls.[1278] Several investigators have noted that high-concentrate diets or pelleted diets increase the incidence of wood-chewing. Feral horses as well as well-fed pastured ponies have been observed to ingest trees and shrubs, so it would seem that there is some need or appetite for wood even when grasses are freely available. Farm managers are well aware that trees, especially young trees, must be protected from horses on pasture. Horses cannot digest wood; nevertheless, there may be some role for indigestible roughage in equine digestion. Jackson et al.[937] have found that wood-chewing increases in cold, wet weather.

Eliminating edges, covering edges with metal or wire, and painting the surface with taste repellents are the traditional methods for preventing horses from wood-chewing, but providing more roughage is a better practice both behaviorally and nutritionally. If roughage is provided, the horse's motivation to chew wood is reduced rather than thwarted. An increase in exercise reduces the rate of wood-chewing.[1069]

Trailering problems

Loading

Many horses exhibit undesirable behavior in relationship to ground transport. The most common undesirable response is failure to load. Both innate behaviors and learning contribute to loading problems. The properties of a trailer that release the horse's innate fears are (1) the dark interior of the trailer; (2) the hollow sound of hooves on the ramp, an indication of poor or insecure footing; and (3) the instability of the ramp and vehicle. In addition, horses are generally neophobic, that is, they are afraid of new or strange things.

Experience or learning plays a major part in loading problems. A horse that already has had unpleasant experiences with loading or riding in a trailer will also be understandably difficult to load. Hitting the horse may cause it to leap forward into a trailer, but the animal will associate pain with trailers and may be even more difficult to load on the next occasion. Learning to dislike loading is even more likely to occur if the horse injured itself while resisting loading. For example, the horse may rear back just as it reaches the entrance to the trailer and strike his head on the roof.

Far more common are less dramatic negative experiences. The horse may have been thrown against the side of the trailer many times. It may have lost its balance or may have struck its head. It may even have experienced motion sickness, which would be difficult to diagnose in an animal that does not vomit, such as the horse. The horse will have learned to associate one or more of these unpleasant experiences with trailers.

The first approach to solving a loading problem is to train the horse to move in response to a touch on its body. This procedure, if correctly done, takes only a few minutes. The handler, preferably a person who has not tried to load the horse, holds the horse with a lead rope and halter. A frightening but nonpainful stimulus, such as a lunge whip with a cloth tied to the end, is used to tap the horse. The horse should move away from the stimulus. The horse can be encouraged to walk forward, to stop, to move the hindquarters toward the handler, and to move the hindquarters away from the handler. After practicing these movements, the horse is walked to the trailer and urged to approach it but not allowed to enter. After a few repetitions, the horse is tapped on the hindquarters to encourage it to enter the trailer. The first entrance may be only partial, only the forefeet. Later, the horse can be allowed to enter the trailer with all four feet many times before the trip begins, and to back-off quietly. This method has been most successful but requires patience. Round pen training can be used to teach the horse to load; after the horse stops and starts in response to body movements, it can be "driven" into the trailer.

One could desensitize and counter condition the horse by rewarding it for loading itself. Desensitization takes time—days or weeks—and therefore is not a solution for the acute problem of how to load a horse as just covered here. Owners of horses with trailer problems should begin the desensitization program a month or more in advance of the proposed trailer trip. The horse and the trailer should be placed in a paddock. The trailer should be secured so that it does not tip, and the wheels should be blocked. The horse's food, all of it, should be put at the bottom of the trailer ramp. Each day the feed, hay and grain, should be placed a little farther up on the ramp. Next, the feed is placed on the floor of the trailer. Day by day, the feed should be placed farther and farther into the trailer, forcing the horse to load himself in order to eat. The horse should obtain no other feed except that in the trailer during the desensitization process. Very few horses will starve to death rather than enter a trailer. After the horse is loading itself into the trailer, it should be led onto the trailer for all its meals. Some horses will learn to load themselves but will still object to being led onto a trailer. The loading problem may not be completely solved even if the horse loads easily in its home paddock. The same horse may be reluctant to enter the same trailer when it is parked in a strange place. A few days of confining the horse in a paddock at another farm will help the horse generalize the lesson that getting on a trailer is safe and desirable. Another method to encourage a horse to enter a trailer is to put it in an unfamiliar place in such a way that entering the trailer is the only means of escape.

The rear-facing trailers sometimes offer a solution for horses that will not enter conventional trailers. The ramp of rear-facing trailers can be made into a horizontal platform. The horse can step onto the platform and be backed into the trailer. Riding in a rear-facing trailer is different and less stressful than riding in conventional trailers, so the horse will not associate riding in it with its previous experiences in conventional trailers and may therefore find loading easier. The horse should not refuse to back into the trailer on the second attempt if he does not dislike or fear the sensations of riding in the trailer.

There are some solutions to an acute trailer problem in which the horse must be loaded that do not cause the horse to associate pain with being loaded. If a horse must be forced onto a trailer, pushing is recommended over hitting. Long ropes tied to each side of the trailer held by two people can be crossed behind the horse and used to apply pressure to its rump. The ropes must be soft to avoid rope burns. The ends attached to the trailer should discourage the horse from leaping to either side of the ramp. The ropes should be held so that they can be dropped if the horse becomes entangled. Sometimes, two people can join hands behind the horse and use their arms to push against the horse's rump. This will encourage the horse that is only mildly reluctant to enter the trailer.

Horses are herd animals. Advantage can be taken of equine gregariousness to solve immediate trailer problems. A horse that is reluctant to enter a trailer may be willing to follow another. Naturally, this method—utilizing social facilitation is unlikely to be successful if the horse is already very excited. The same characteristic of horses—social facilitation of behavior—can be used to prevent trailer problems. A foal should be loaded beside its mother several times in its first few months because it will follow its dam onto the trailer as it follows her elsewhere. Of course, this method should not be used if the mare herself does not load. Bad behavior as well as good behavior can be learned by observation. If the foal's mother is reluctant to load, the foal can still be trained to load relatively easily after weaning is complete. With the foal correctly haltered and on a lead rope, gently encourage the foal to put one hoof on the ramp for a handful of grain. Gradually, encourage it to go farther and farther up the ramp. Talk softly and encouragingly, and immediately reward any progress with a rub or a little grain. Full loading may take several sessions. After the foal has moved onto the trailer the first time, feed it its daily grain ration in the trailer several times before traveling with it. Never use hitting, pushing, or pulling during these training sessions. Repeat the process in as many different vehicles and in as many different sites as possible to help the foal generalize. Before the foal goes on its first long trailer ride, it should take several short trips, one-half to one mile, ending with a grazing session. Gradually, take the foal on longer trips. The etiology of some horses' trailer problems may be a first trailer experience that consisted of four hours of fear and exhaustion while trying to balance on a strange surface. Several short trips help the horse to habituate to the trailer and the sensation of a moving vehicle while the animal is rested. The time involved can save much more time later; a foal properly introduced to trailering should load easily as an adult even when trailering episodes are years apart.

Horses are less stressed when traveling with a companion horse. In the absence of another horse, a mirror can be used because it decreases the behavioral (vocalizing, cessation of eating, head tossing) but not the physiological (increase in heart rate and body temperature) responses to trailering.[990]

Sedatives such as xylazine can be used in the acute situation. The sedative will be far more effective if the animal has not become excited or frightened before administration. It might also be possible to desensitize a horse to the loading procedure by repeatedly sedating it and loading it several times a day for a week or so, but in some experimental situations, animals cannot remember in the undrugged state what they learned in the drugged state; the phenomenon is called state-dependent learning. Sedatives have several disadvantages: a sedated horse cannot perform properly, and in some shows, cannot perform legally. Furthermore, a sedated horse is more at risk of losing its balance in a moving trailer. A way to avoid state-dependent learning is to decrease the dose of the sedative gradually over several sessions.

Moving trailer problems: scrambling

The next class of behavior problems involves horses that enter trailers without hesitating but misbehave when the trailer moves. The horse can be badly injured and the trailer can be damaged. There are several causes of struggling. Most are related to the horse's inability to keep its balance in the trailer. When given a choice of direction of travel in a stock trailer, horses are not uniform in their choice.[1779] Some horses stand facing backward, but more stand at an angle and change their position during travel. Thoroughbreds also orient away from the direction of travel but have no other preference for direction.[394, 1077]

The studies of the behavior and physiology of transported horses may indicate why they dislike trailers. Several investigators have found that heart rate increases and cortisol levels rise during trailering.[359, 1970] Horses stop eating and adopt a base-wide posture with their limbs abducted, indicating that they are trying to maintain their balance.

If the horse is struggling because it is losing its balance or is afraid of doing so, simple changes in the trailer may be all that is necessary. Removing the center partition of a two-horse trailer will allow the horse to plant its feet more widely. A layer of sand topped with wood chips on the floor of the trailer will prevent the horse from slipping. Alternative solutions are to transport the horse in a large horse van or a stock trailer. More horses travel well in stock trailers than in standard two-horse trailers. If a two-horse trailer must be used, there should be no bulkhead or compartment on which the horse can strike its head. A padded bar at the horse's chest level will restrain the animal but allow it to move its head without striking anything.

A horse may be reacting to erratic movements of the trailer. This can be ascertained if the horse scrambles only when a certain person is driving. A rarer cause of misbehavior is electric shock. If the horse struggles only when the brakes are applied, the wiring should be examined.

As already mentioned, horses may struggle in trailers because they are losing their balance, but some horses may be reacting in anticipation of the journey's end. Horses participating in such high-speed events as barrel racing or games are the most likely to scramble on the way to a competition. These horses could be desensitized by taking them on many trailer rides that end not with competing, but with grazing or a leisurely trail ride. Care must be taken to treat the horse in the same manner before a "therapeutic" trailer trip as before a ride to a show. The same tack and the same grooming routine should be used in both cases so that the horse cannot discriminate between trips that end in shows and those that end at less-exciting destinations. There are horses that do not scramble in trailers but do sweat or paw. These horses may be experiencing motion sickness. Although most horses travel better with another horse, a few are aggressive toward the other horse.

Horses that load and ride well but do not stand quietly in a stationary trailer are yet another problem. They will move, kick, and struggle when the trailer stops at a tollgate or a traffic light. Small food rewards for standing quietly during practice trailering sessions can be used to treat the problem. The reason horses fret in stationary trailers is unknown but may be the same as those for horses that struggle in the moving trailer. Better footing, driving ability, or a different type of trailer may be necessary to eliminate the problem. Many horses are both difficult to load and prone to misbehave in the moving trailer.[1114] Trailer problems can be solved if the horse ever loaded and trailered well.

A final problem is the horse that will not leave the trailer. Although horses can sometimes be backed where they will not walk, a horse that reaches back with a hind hoof and encounters nothing but air will be afraid to back off. Trailers with walk-through construction enabling the horse to enter from the back and exit from the front are helpful. To solve the immediate problem, the horse should be allowed to turn its head so that it can see where it is backing. It may be necessary to remove the center partition of a two-horse trailer so that the horse has room to do so. Horses are more reluctant to back off step-up trailers, those without a ramp. A loading dock of dirt can be made to give the animal a solid place to put its hind feet.

In summary, the best approach to the treatment of stable problems and trailer problems is to remove the cause of the problem, that is, to change the horse's motivation. This approach is more apt to be successful than punishment or physical restraint of the horse. Careful, early handling and optimal housing can prevent the emergence of these problems.

Behavior problems under saddle

Head shyness

The horse shown in Fig. 9.2 illustrates head shyness, a common equine behavior problem. Head shyness is usually, but not always, secondary to mismanagement of the horse when it was first handled. Occasionally, progressive desensitization may be used by a gentle and patient owner to overcome the vice, but while the horse is becoming accustomed to handling of its ears and poll, it will still be difficult to bridle, and attempting to do so will undo the desensitization. Horses will often tolerate handling of their head and ears best when they are hot, sweaty, and, apparently, itchy. Putting on the bridle with one check piece unfastened may be tolerated. Rubbing the bit with molasses rewards the horse for accepting the bit.

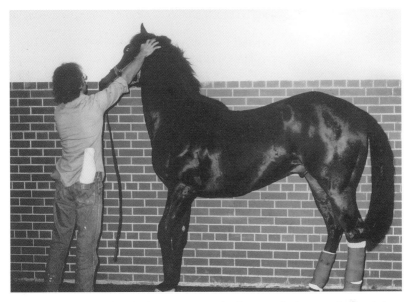

Fig. 9.2 A horse that kicks stall walls, thus aggravating hock injury. The horse is also head shy.

Head shaking

Head shaking is rarely a behavior problem.[1205] A lesion anywhere in the head or neck, especially in the nasal cavity, can cause head shakings. Some horses react to bright light with a reflexive sneeze. Goggles, essentially sun glasses, can help. Others are allergic and will head shake seasonally. These horses can be helped by a net over their noses.[1336] There have been many suggested drug treatments. Cyproheptadine and carbamazepine appear to be most helpful.

Bucking, shying, and grazing

Vices under saddle can vary from bucking and running away to grazing. The former habits are quite dangerous, but nothing discourages the child who is learning to ride more than the pony that puts its head down to graze at every opportunity. Muzzling the pony may discourage it from attempts to eat. The habit that is most apt to dislodge the rider is the simple fear response of shying. The good rider, who knows what objects are most likely to elicit a shying response in a particular horse, is prepared, and tries to distract the animal.

Phobias

Some horses have fears that might be classified as phobias. A horse that was badly stung by bees became uncontrollable whenever he heard any insect buzz. The horse could be desensitized by playing bee noises to him, in the same manner as dogs are desensitized to thunder. This technique may also be used to accustom horses to band music, applause, flash bulbs, and the other frightening aspects of parades and horse shows. The horse can be urged toward a frightening object and rewarded with both removal of the negative reinforcement (kicking) and a positive reinforcement, a pat.

Behavior-related problems

Many horses will move much more quickly toward their stable than away from it. These animals are called "barn rats." Other horses will trot smartly in a group of horses but must be pummeled into moving off by themselves. Such behavior is hardly surprising, as horses are herd animals and group, or allelomimetic, behavior is part of their evolutionary heritage. The horse racing back to the barn is rejoining its herd, if other horses are there, or is simply returning to its home range. Consideration of feral horse behavior indicates that many of the vices that appear to be spiteful, lazy, or stupid are in reality perfectly normal adaptive behaviors for an animal that must find food (graze while bridled), avoid predators (shy), and remain with its herd or rejoin it if separated (barn rat).

Physiologically based problems

Other common habits of horses may be explained on the basis of their physiology. Some horses are very hard to canter on the left lead but take the right easily. This is because some horses (70%) show definite handedness[724] even if they have been carefully schooled to canter both clockwise and counterclockwise.

The myriad other vices and training problems of horses are beyond the scope of this book.

CATTLE AND OTHER FARM ANIMALS

The behavior problems of farm animals have been reviewed by Fraser[629] and by Kiley-Worthington.[1014]

CATTLE

Problems related to changes in management

Dairy cattle present few behavior problems in general. This is probably due to selection on the part of the dairy farmer for tractable animals as well as high producers. The biggest problems that arise with dairy cattle concern changes in their management. When cattle that have formerly been milked and fed simultaneously in a stanchion barn are placed in free stalls and are not fed concentrates when they are milked, they may enter the milking parlor only reluctantly. Milking time can be prolonged for hours. Apparently, the milking procedure and the reward of relieving pressure on the udder is not enough to induce cattle to be milked. One solution is to feed grain during milking. Even if the cow requires more concentrates than she can consume while being milked, a portion of her grain can be fed at milking and the rest afterwards. Other management-related behavior problems have involved electrically operated squeeze gates that push the cattle closest to the gate when the cattle ahead balk. Time can be lost and injuries sustained if mechanical devices are not built with the behavior of the normal cow in mind.

Cattle that are always milked or handled from one side may become frightened or aggressive when handled from the other side. A veterinarian or stockperson should note the position of the milking machine outlet in stanchioned cattle and approach the cow from the same side. Milk production may be affected by milking from the "wrong" (the unfamiliar) side. Such obvious stresses as isolation and being chased by a dog can lower milk production,[2013] but the handler's attitude can also affect production either positively or negatively. If the handler is satisfied with the job, the cows will give more milk and will approach the milking area more quickly.[1719]

Feed throwing

This is a relatively new problem. The affected cattle throw their feed onto their own backs. It may be a response to the total mixed ration many cattle are fed or a consequence of tail docking.

Kicking

Beef cattle cause more problems for the average veterinarian because they have neither been selected for tractability nor handled often. A beef heifer brought from range or pasture and placed in a box stall is as dangerous as an ill-mannered horse. Such animals should be treated with caution because even when heavily tranquilized, they can and will kick. Cattle do not always "cowkick." They can place a well-aimed blow backward as well as forward. Such cattle should be fed only when they stand quietly. The food is the reward for nonkicking behavior.

Problems related to environment

Cattle not accustomed to stanchions, such as those living in loose-housing facilities, may find it difficult to lie down or arise when first stanchioned. Hospitalized cattle may be particularly affected because the illness for which they were hospitalized will be compounded by the stress of lack of rest.

Calves and adult bulls show a variety of oral "vices" such as bar licking and tongue rolling. Perhaps the most compelling evidence for the protective effect of stereotypies is the finding of Wiepkema et al.[2020] that veal calves that indulged in tongue rolling had a lower incidence of abomasal ulcers than calves that had no vices. Nonnutritive oral behavior, especially tongue play, occurs more frequently in penned than in pastured cattle. On pasture, there is more nonnutritive oral behavior if the pasture is low in plant height and density.[933]

PIGS

Few pigs, except sows in gestation crates are kept as individuals, so most of their behavior problems concern group interactions. Aggression has been discussed in Chapter 2 and sexual behavior in Chapter 4.

Other problems seen are rubbing the snout on the floor or on the flank of another pig. Bar biting by confined sows is believed to be a consequence of restraint or of food deprivation and may release endogenous opiates because treatment of the sow with the opiate blocker naloxone will halt the behavior.[399]

SHEEP AND GOATS

The only miscellaneous problem of sheep that has not been discussed elsewhere in this book is wool-chewing. This behavior is of unknown etiology.

Goats frequently become nuisances, especially if they are kept as pets and inadequately restrained. The behavior of the goat is not abnormal. It is an animal that browses normally, but it may browse on the ornamental flowerbeds or the crops. Goats are herd animals, and a solitary goat may seek human company if it has been kept as a pet since it was a kid. Normal caprine feeding, investigatory, and allelomimetic behavior may seem very abnormal to the naive goat owner.

10 Behavioral Genetics

Genetic determinants of behavior have made possible domestication and the varied uses to which we put animals, particularly dogs and horses. Of course, both nature (genetics) and nurture (environment) play a part in determining behavior, but it is only recently the mechanism of early environmental influences on behavior have been discovered. Rat pups that were licked a lot by their dams grew up to be less susceptible to stress and more reproductively competent.[621] This was true of foster pups as well as the mother's biological offspring. The mechanism of this effect is demethylation of the gene—a process that strongly influences the expression of genes. In this case, the affected gene was the one for glucocorticoid. This kind of nongenomic effect is of interest because it explains why, for example, a cloned animal does not have the same temperament as the original.

In this chapter, sex and breed differences in behavior, means of determining temperament, and the few examples in which a gene has been identified that is responsible, at least in part, for a given behavior will be presented.

DOGS

Sex differences

There are sex differences in many behaviors in addition to sexual behavior itself. Males are more reactive and more aggressive. Females are easier to housebreak, more obedient, and affectionate, but less active as indicated in surveys from several countries, whereas males are more aggressive, more active, more playful, and more likely to bark and be destructive.[774,1429]

Breed differences

In this well-investigated species, there are breed differences in behavioral neoteny, in temperament, in social signaling, in prevalence of behavior problems, and in opinions of dog experts on behavioral characteristics of various breeds.

At Berkeley, Jasper Rine and Elaine Ostrander crossed border collies and Newfoundland. The F2 generation was bred, and in the F3 generation it was found that the various behavior traits associated with each breed—retrieving and giving eyes for border collies and love of water and friendliness for Newfoundlands—were inherited separately. At the University of Arkansas, selection based on behavior resulted in two strains of pointers: a nervous and a normal strain. The former are much more difficult to train.

Coppinger and Schneider[385] compared breeds on both behavioral and physical characteristics, which they believe co-evolve. Some, like pugs, have puppy-like facial features—short nose and full cheeks—whereas German shepherds are fully adult. They ranked the breeds by developmental stages: heelers (huskies and corgis), headers-stalkers (collies), object players (hounds, retrievers, and poodles), and adolescents (St. Bernard, Komodors, and Great Pyrenees). The sheep-guarding dogs show juvenile behavior such as playing and lacking mature sexual behavior.

Most impressive is the effect of breed on the response to early isolation and handling. If puppies are completely isolated from the 3rd to the 20th week of life, they are markedly disturbed. Beagles react most fearfully, and Scottish terriers are more hyperactive and show an impaired (higher) threshold to pain.[1305] Partial isolation from 3 to 16 weeks has different effects on different breeds. Beagles become less active, and terriers become more active.[641,652] It was found that the early environment of puppies had no effect on the reaction of some breeds to mild punishment (saying "No" and hitting with a newspaper). Basenjis ignored the punishment; Shetland sheepdogs were always inhibited by the punishment. Beagles and wirehaired fox terriers were inhibited only if they had not been trained in early life.

Goodwin et al.[699] examined breed differences in signaling. They observed wolves and listed the signals they observed such as growl, stand over, stare, crouch, and submissive grin. Ten breeds of dogs were compared to wolves. Dogs of each breed lived in groups ranging in size from four to seven. They were observed for several hours and the behaviors they exhibited were compared to those of wolves. Siberian huskies were more like wolves than Labrador retrievers. The fewest behaviors were observed in the Cavalier King Charles spaniels, Norfolk terriers, and French bulldogs. The authors interpreted this as meaning that behaviors had been lost with domestication because of paedomorphosis.

The largest study of opinions of breed difference is that of Hart and Hart.[775] They surveyed 48 veterinarians and 48 obedience judges as to 13 traits in 56 breeds of dogs. Principle components analysis revealed three factors—reactivity, aggressiveness, and trainability—and a fourth factor that included playfulness and destructiveness. Cluster analysis of breeds with similar traits revealed seven clusters. It is interesting that snapping at children clusters with reactivity not with aggression.

The first studies on genetic differences in learning ability were carried out at Jackson Laboratory in Maine. Scott and Fuller[1714] reviewed the experiments, which compared learning ability in five breeds of dogs: cocker spaniels, beagles, wirehaired fox terriers, Shetland sheepdogs, and basenjis. These particular breeds were chosen because they did not differ much in body size, nor did any breed possess a breed-specific anatomical peculiarity, such as the achondroplasia of basset hounds. The five breeds were tested for their ability to learn three types of tasks: forced training, reward training, and problem solving.

The forced method of training was used to teach the dogs to sit still on a scale, to heel on a leash, and to stay and jump on command. In all three types of tasks, the cocker spaniels ranked highest in correct performance. The trainability of cockers in these situations is probably the result of selection within the breed for dogs that would crouch in response to a hand signal. Although cockers are not often used for hunting now, the behavioral predisposition remains. All the dogs learned to heel within the 10-day training period, but marked differences appeared in the types of errors that dogs of the various breeds made in the early sessions. Basenjis fought the leash and often pulled ahead or lagged behind. Shetland sheepdogs interfered with the trainer, that is, tangled the leash around the trainer's legs. Beagles vocalized in protest (Fig. 10.1).

Reward training consisted in showing the puppy a piece of fish in a box and then restraining it behind a wire gate before allowing the puppy to run to the box and eat the fish. The position of the box was changed to measure goal orientation versus habit formation. Basenjis performed

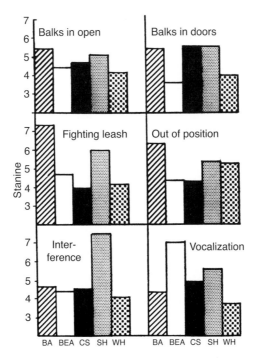

Fig. 10.1   Breed differences in response to leash training. BA, basenji; BEA, beagle; CS, cocker spaniel; WH, wirehaired fox terrier; SH, Shetland sheepdog. The higher the stanine score, the more often the dog exhibited the behavior.[1714] (With permission of University of Chicago Press.)

best on this test, probably because they could run the fastest. With the additional trials, all the dogs reduced the time they took to reach the reward. When motor skills of the five breeds were compared, the basenji was again the best.

Problem solving was also studied. The first type of problem the dogs were supposed to solve was a barrier or detour. The dogs were separated from a food reward by a wire barrier. When they learned to run around a short barrier, the barrier was extended and later formed into a U shape to increase the difficulty of the problem. The dogs were only 6 weeks of age and had considerable difficulty in solving the barrier problem that an adult dog could master easily. The puppies often yelped, and it was noted that they never solved the problem while yelping but instead engaged in stereotypic activity. Few puppies did well on the barrier test, but basenjis, which are already active at 6 weeks, did best. Puppies of other breeds still tend to be fat and clumsy at 6 weeks and would react to failure by going to sleep.

Another type of problem was a manipulation test in which the dogs were tested for their ability to pull a dish of food from under a box by pawing or pulling it out with their noses. Later, the dish was positioned in such a way that it could be maneuvered out from under the box only by pulling on a dowel and string attached to the dish. Again, the basenjis were the most successful. Most interesting was the effect of repeated failures on the dogs' performances. Although all puppies at first scratched and nosed at the box containing the food dish, those that had failed often took one look at the box and simply sat down to await the end of the trial, thus precluding any success.

When maze learning was tested in RLLRRR (right, left, left, and so on) or LRLL mazes, beagles did best. They completed the maze most quickly and made the fewest errors.

A final test of problem-solving behavior, when the dogs were 22 weeks old, was a delayed response test in which the dogs were shown a visual cue that indicated which side of a T-maze led to freedom. Before the dog was allowed to run the maze, a delay from 1 to 240 seconds was imposed. As in all problem solving, great individual differences emerged, but cocker spaniels could remember after the longest delay and Shetland sheepdogs had the poorest memory.

The extensive studies at Jackson indicate that care must be taken in comparing intelligence, even within a species, because breeds of dogs differ markedly in their relative performance depending on the task to be learned.

Behavior problems

The statistics on deaths caused by dogs allows one to determine breed differences in aggression. Between 1979 and 1998, pitbulls killed the greatest number of people followed by Rottweilers, German shepherds, huskies, malamutes, Dobermans, and chows. These are all large-breed dogs, but other popular large breeds such as Labradors and golden retrievers are not on the list. It is most interesting that Rottweilers have overtaken pitbulls and now kill more people per year. The number of Rottweilers registered had increased fivefold between 1979 and 1998, but the number of fatalities increased sevenfold. The statement is often made that popularity ruins the breed, but what probably happens is that while the percentage of aggressive dogs within a breed remains the same, the total numbers increase, so there are more aggressive dogs of that particular breed. Unfortunately, these statistics and the tendency of people to sue if bitten have led insurance companies to refuse policies to owners of pitbulls or Staffordshire terriers, German shepherd dogs, chow chows, and Dobermans. Breed-specific legislation has been enacted in only a few communities, but the insurance companies are essentially doing that nationwide.

Spaniel aggression

Canine aggression is the most common problem presented to clinical animal behaviorists and results in human injuries and canine euthanasia. One goal of canine behavioral geneticists is to eliminate aggressive dogs, or dogs carrying genes for aggression from the gene pool. Because aggression in hunting dogs, such as spaniels, is always undesirable and because the aggression displayed is impulsive, that is, unpredictable and extreme, the so-called "Springer Rage" syndrome has been identified and studied.

Borchelt[253] classified the types of aggression he treated in his urban consultations. Dominance aggression was most common in English springer spaniels (ESS), Doberman pinschers, toy poodles, and Lhasa apsos. Possessive aggression was most common in cocker spaniels. Protective aggression was most common in German shepherds, but fear aggression was also common in that breed as well as in cocker spaniels and miniature poodles.

When comparing a private practice in Ontario, a private practice in Kansas, and a university clinic in upstate New York, Landsberg et al.[1087] found that ESS were most often presented to the eastern clinics but not to the midwestern one. The geographical differences implicate genetic difference between the populations in the East and the Midwest. Two other behavior problems, separation anxiety and thunder phobia, revealed no breed differences.

Of course, breed differences in prevalence have to be compared with the numbers of dogs of each breed in the catchment area. Historically, ESS presents with dominance-related aggression more than would be predicted by regional breed distributions[189] and by national breed registration statistics.[1087] Reisner[1595] reported in a survey of over 2000 ESS owners that 65% of ESS with a history of biting (27% of total ESS) had bitten a familiar person.

The hunt for the gene involved in aggression is very difficult. For example, one may select one neurotransmitter, for example, serotonin. The difference between aggressive and nonaggressive dogs could be due to a gene controlling synthesis of the neurotransmitter, reuptake of the neurotransmitter, the enzymes that inactivate the neurotransmitter, or genes that control expression of any of the above genes.

There have been several promising candidate genes for canine aggression. These include the dopamine D4 receptor, the long form of which is associated with risk-seeking behavior in humans. Although Nimi and colleagues have shown that a usually gentle breed of dog, the golden retriever, has the short form of the dopamine D4 receptor and the territorially aggressive Shiba has the long form, this is not associated with behavior but rather with the genetic differences between an Asian and an Anglo-American breed.

Monoamine oxidase A is an enzyme that breaks down dopamine, and a mutation that lowers the amount of that enzyme is associated with incarceration of humans, if they had a bad childhood environment.[331] There is evidence in dogs that aggressive individuals have lower cerebrospinal levels of 5-hydroxyindole acetic acid and homovanillic acid, the major metabolites of serotonin and dopamine, respectively.[1595]

Takeuchi and her colleagues have identified polymorphisms in several genes in five breeds of dogs (golden retriever, Labrador retriever, Maltese, miniature schnauzer, and Shiba). Hashizume et al.[780] identified a single nucleotide polymorphism (T199C) located on the putative third exon of the canine monoamine oxidase B gene, which causes an amino acid substitution from cysteine to arginine. Takeuchi et al.[1844] found four single nucleotide polymorphisms (SNPs) in the tyrosine hydroxylase and dopamine beta hydroxylase genes. Ogata et al.[1447] found two SNPs in the glutamine transporter gene (GLT-1). The authors have related the polymorphisms with the breed behaviors as identified by Hart and Hart,[774] although there is no direct evidence that these could explain interbreed differences in behavioral problems.

Coat color is genetically determined and, because the precursor molecules of pigment are also the precursor molecules for neurotransmitters, it is not surprising that behavior differs with coat color. Yellow Labradors, as opposed to black or chocolate Labradors, are more likely to have backyard problems—barking, chewing, and digging[1043]—and to be more likely to present to a behavior clinic for aggression.[883]

There is high heritability of aggression, at least in golden retrievers, with heritability estimates of scores of 0.9 for aggression toward strangers and 0.88 for aggression to owners.[1919] Heritability of aggression toward other dogs is 0.91.[1152] Van den Berg[1919] investigated three genes involved in serotonin function: (1) serotonin receptor 1A (htr1A), (2) serotonin receptor 1B (htr1B) and serotonin receptor 2A (htr2A), and (3) serotonin transporter gene (slc6A4). Linkage analysis of pedigrees of golden retrievers did not demonstrate that any of these genes were linked with aggression.

A gene for aggression has been identified. A polymorphism of the neuronal/epithelial high-affinity glutamate transporter is associated with aggression toward strangers in Shiba inu.[1846] The neuronal/epithelium high-affinity glutamate transporter was also associated with activity in Labrador retrievers as was a polymorphism of the catecholamine methyl transferase gene.[1843]

HORSES

When quarter horses and thoroughbreds were compared on ability to learn a visual discrimination, the quarter horses did better, apparently because they were less distracted.[1204] Non-warmbloods learned more quickly than warmbloods (thoroughbreds, Arabian).[1155] There are breed differences in the incidence of behavior problems. Thoroughbreds are more likely to crib[18,1185,1278], whereas Arabians are more likely to stall walk and reject their foals.[973] Standardbreds are less likely to crib than thoroughbreds.[1587]

CATTLE

Breed differences

Social, sexual, and maternal behavior

Dominance is clearly influenced by heredity, for twin cattle are often of equal dominance.[550] Also, breed differences in dominance exist among dairy cattle. Among beef breeds, which do not differ markedly in weight, definite differences in temperament can also be found.[1962] Success (or failure) in dominance interactions is genetically determined in heifers.[1561]

Intraindividual and intrabreed differences in sexual behavior may be noted. For example, the Brown Swiss breed shows the least marked estrous activity of the dairy breeds. Black cattle show stronger signs of estrus than red, roan, or white cattle.[32] Male sexual behavior is definitely under genetic control as indicated by the nearly identical performance within pairs of twin bulls, but the marked difference between twin pairs (Fig 10.2). German Angus (Aberdeen Angus × German dual-purpose cattle) showed more maternal protectiveness than Simmental when their day-old calves were ear tagged.[855] There are marked genetic effects on maze learning ability of cattle.[68]

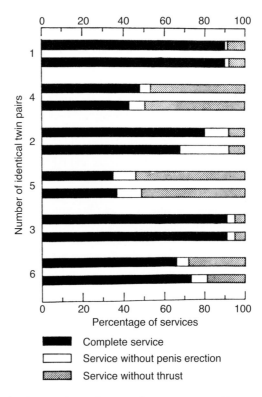

Fig. 10.2 Percentage distribution of complete copulations, mounts without penis erections, and mounts without thrust.[735] (Copyright 1975, with permission of W.B. Saunders Co.)

Feeding behavior

Cows sired by Piedmontese bulls were willing to graze farther from water than those sired by Angus.[1931] Piedmontese cattle were developed in mountainous regions, so they may make more uniform use of a rough-terrain environment. A high bite rate and low mastication rate are an adaption to maximize intake. Therefore, it is not surprising that Holsteins, a breed selected for high food intake, have a higher bite rate and slower mastication rate than Norwegian Reds.[1444]

SHEEP

Social behavior

Breed differences exist in the tendency to aggregate. For example, Clun Forest sheep gather in large groups, whereas Dalesbred and Jacob sheep are more dispersed and form smaller groups.[1749] Similarly, breed differences appear in the tendency to form separate subgroups within large flocks. Merinos rarely form subgroups, whereas Dorsets and Southdowns do. The grouping depends on the sheep's activity. Some sheep form subgroups only when grazing, whereas others form subgroups both when grazing and when camping.[87] Leadership in sheep is negatively correlated with the tendency to join the flock. In other words, independent sheep lead, and the others follow. There are breed differences, but these may be cultural in that lambs raised by blackface ewes have shorter interindividual distance and smaller group size than those raised by Suffolk ewes. There are breed differences in environmental preferences. Blackface sheep prefer uplands despite the poorer quality forage whereas Suffolk ewes prefer lowlands.

Maternal behavior

Signoret[1767] has shown that breed differences in the duration of estrus in sheep exist even in estrogen-induced estrus in ovariectomized ewes. Great breed differences appear in the frequency of abandonment of one of a pair of twin lambs. Merino sheep are much more likely to abandon one of their twin lambs than are Dorsets or Romney.[37] The more primitive breeds of sheep such as Romanov and those kept extensively such as Scottish blackface show stronger maternal behavior than Merinos or Suffolk.[510] Another example of genetic differences is that Targhee sheep do not show as strong maternal behavior as other breeds.[1783] An interesting study involved embryo transfer of lambs into ewes of another breed. This allows separation of genetic and learned components of behavior.[513] Lambs play a part in ewe–lamb proximity. Suffolk lambs stay closer to their mothers and vocalize more often than Blackface lambs. Blackface lambs also play more and female lambs stay closer than males. Lambs born to Blackface sheep were more active and Suffolk ewes nursed their lambs more often. Blackface lambs grazed more and Suffolk lambs raised by a Blackface ewe grazed more than Suffolk lambs raised by a Suffolk ewe—a breed and learning interaction.

PIGS

Breed differences

Breed differences appear in aggression, sexual behavior, and maternal behavior. Yorkshires are more aggressive than Berkshires.[1240] Breed differences appear in dominance by sex; more

Hampshire males are dominant over females than are Durocs.[196] Small pigs and newcomers to an established group are usually subordinate.[636] Yorkshires are easier to train to mount a dummy than Durocs[32], at least in the United Kingdom. Poor libido is seen more frequently in Landrace than in boars of the large white breed.[61] Playback of nursing calls decreased nursing intervals in one genotype of pigs (Meishan), but not another (Yorkshire and Landrace).[565]

TEMPERAMENT TESTS

Canine temperament

There have been many—at least 50 publications—on evaluation of canine temperament using a variety of methods from a battery of tests, experts' opinions, and ratings of individual dogs. A review of over 50 studies of canine temperament revealed seven traits: (1) reactivity, (2) fearfulness, (3) sociability, (4) activity, (5) responsiveness to training, (6) submissiveness, and (7) aggression.[965] Convergent validity is supported when a measure correlates with other measures to which it should be related. Discriminant validity is supported when a measure is empirically unrelated to other measures that are theoretically unrelated. Most of these tests had convergent, but no discriminative, validity.

The ratings of individual dogs are usually based on questionnaires filled out by owners. For example, Serpell and Hsu[1734] developed a questionnaire—CBARQ. The valid factors were stranger- or dog-directed fear/aggression, nonsocial fear, energy level, owner-directed aggression, chasing, trainability, and attachment.

Most temperament tests include response to a stranger, but the stranger must be trained because dogs give very different responses to a friendly stranger in comparison to a threatening stranger even when the stranger is the same person.[1932] The friendly stranger approaches at a normal speed while talking to the dog whereas the threatening stranger moves slowly and haltingly and stares at the dog silently. The dogs—Belgium shepherds—were consistent in their responses even a year later, but the owners' opinions of the dog's reaction did not agree with the dog's behavioral reactions.

Age affects the results of temperament test. Puppies that are exploratory at 6 weeks may not be so at 12 weeks, and vice versa. The same is true of social dominance.[2064] These findings indicate that tests of puppies at 7 weeks, popular as a means of predicting adult behavior, are unlikely to be valid. The tests involve scoring the puppies' reactions to handling and their willingness to approach or follow people.

The Campbell Test was conducted to assess dominant behavior in puppies.[318] The test consists of five parts and must be conducted at the age of 6–8 weeks. The test leader, not previously encountered by the puppy, should remain impassive and show no signs of emotion throughout the test. Puppies are subjected to the test individually with no other person, animal, or object present that could distract them. Activity is a better predictor of later behavior than is the puppy's response to handling at 7 weeks.[184]

Evaluation of temperament and prediction of performance of working dogs (guide and military dogs) are especially important to reduce investment in an unsuitable dog.[2036–2038] Each dog was evaluated for its response: to a stranger approaching the dog, and the handler, and attempting to play tug-of-war with the dog; to a paper figure and a rag doll that appeared suddenly and threatened it; to gunfire and to a threat to its handler. Using more than 1,000 dogs, the evaluators calculated four factors: (1) mental stability, (2) willingness to please, (3) affability, and (4) defense drive. Breed differences appeared between German shepherds and Labradors, which had little prey drive. They found that defense drive (attacks threatening people) and hardness (recovering quickly from startling stimuli) could be predicted by puppy weight. Heavier females scored better.

Slabbert and Odendaal[1776] used retrieval of objects at 8 weeks and aggression to a threatening stranger at 9 months to predict success in police dog training. Svartberg[1833,1834] identified five traits: (1) playfulness, (2) curiosity, (3) fear, (4) chase proneness, and (5) sociability, all of which could be explained as a shy/boldness trait and aggression. Another test revealed three factors: (1) exploration, (2) reaction to novelty, and (3) reaction to startling stimuli.[1028] The shyness/boldness could be used to predict success in working dogs. Weiss and Greenberg[1990] found that only the test for fear was valid in selecting working dogs from a shelter. German shepherd police dogs may show fearful, aggressive, or ambivalent response to the approach of a stranger wielding a stick. The fearful and ambivalent dogs are the passive coping animals who have greater activation of cortisol than the active coping ones who are aggressive.[861]

Hunting dogs are judged on their eagerness to hunt, speed, style, independence, seeking width, cooperation, and ability to work in the field. These traits are heritable.[281,883] When Labrador retrievers were rated for obedience, aggression to other dogs, concentration, affection demand, interest in the target, and anxiety, factor analysis revealed that a combination of those traits, which could be termed "willingness to work," was the key factor in determining success as a drug-detection dog.[1206]

Results of field trials revealed that Finnish Hounds were found to have the highest heritability scores for pursuit and tonguing (vocalization while in pursuit of a hare or fox).[1151] Reuterwall and Ryman calculated the heritability of temperament of Swedish army dogs to be low on the basis of eight traits: (1) affability (tested by having an unknown person approach the dog); (2) disposition for self-defense (an unknown person attacks the dog); (3) disposition for self-defense and defense of the handler (tested by having an unknown person attack the dog and the handler); (4) disposition for fighting in a playful manner (tested by asking the dog to fight for a sleeve or a stick); (5) courage (tested by having a man-shaped figure approach the dog); (6) ability to meet with sudden, strong auditory stimuli (tested by firing a gun at a distance and by making noise with tin cans just behind the dog); (7) disposition for forgetting unpleasant episodes (tested by scaring the dog at a certain location and then asking the dog to pass the location again); and (8) adaptiveness to different environments and situations (tested by observations throughout the test). The estimate of heritability of these traits was low.

The heritability of temperament was determined using[614] German shepherd dogs from the Division of Biosensor Research of the US Army. The specifics of the temperament test were not mentioned but were all determined by one person and were composite scores used to predict future performance and indicated the animal's ability to chase and attack a decoy. The hip dysplasia scores were also assigned by one person. There was a negative correlation between temperament and hip dysplasia.[1199]

Dog breeds are typically divided according to historical usage into Working, Hunting, Herding, Hound, and Terrier groups plus the Toy group, and in some countries, a separate Gun dog group. When the results of a temperament test involving reactions to strangers who attempt to play tug-of-war with the dog are compared to the historical use of the dog, there is little correlation, but there is a similarity in response within a breed. Most interesting is that of the two of the most popular breeds: the golden retriever is fearful, and the Labrador is bold. These results suggest that the present use of a dog differs from the historical use.[1832]

Dogs are used in animal-assisted therapy. These dogs must be able to interact with physically and/or mentally handicapped people, so the requirements are strict. A test was devised using a series of challenges, the first of which measured aggression to dogs and people. A dog that displayed aggression failed. Initiative was determined by the dog's approach to a person on the other side of the fence and its willingness to approach people in its enclosure. Jumping on fences or people was scored negatively because of the danger to handicapped people. Finally, the dog's response to food-lured commands such as sit and down and its willingness to go up and down stairs and walk on a leash were tested. Only 5 of 23 shelter dogs tested passed the test. The Delta Society has tests for service dogs and the Tuskegee temperament test measures suitability for pet visitations to hospital or nursing homes.[1692]

Some dogs are surrendered to shelters because they have behavior problems. Because the former owner may not have been forthright about the problem, a temperament test has been developed to identify behavior problems in adult dogs. A very extensive temperament test has been developed by Netto and Planta[1410] to evaluate dogs for aggressive tendencies. In another test, barking, separation anxiety, and aggression toward cats, joggers, or other dogs could be predicted, but aggression toward the owner—dominance aggression—was not.[1922] Temperament testers are not very reliable in that their evaluation of the dog on the basis of the same video tape of its behavior varies over time. Those testers with the most training and experience were most reliable.[464]

Two studies of a temperament test based loosely on the Sternberg test have attempted to validate its use in shelter dogs. Fifty percent of dogs that passed that temperament test lunged, growled, snapped or, rarely, bit but 90% were still in their adoptive home.[250,348]. Most of the aggression was in territorial situations. When the behavior problems identified by the relinquishing owner were compared with those identified by the adoptive owner, aggression to strange people, dogs, or veterinarians and anxiety when left alone were present in both homes, indicating that the dog did not change even when the environment did,[1808] but Paroz et al.[1475] found that aggressive dogs had played with a stranger much less as juveniles. No one has developed an adult canine temperament test that predicts success as a pet dog on the basis of positive qualities.

Porcine temperament test

Restraining a pig by placing it on its back—the back test or tonic immobility test—has been used to assess active (high resistance) and passive personality (low resistance) in pigs.[605,837] The pigs that resisted most at 3 days of age were more likely to approach people or venture out of their pens at 2 months of age,[1050] although some investigators did not find that correlation.[942] Lean growth is higher in pigs that resisted least.[332] When strange pigs are mixed, the high-resistance pigs are more aggressive both to one another and to low resistors if they are dominant.[1658] Although aggression over food appears to be a consistent characteristic of a pig, response to the back test and to novelty is not.[1659] By the time of puberty, most behavioral differences between these two groups have disappeared, but the low-resistance pigs have higher baseline cortisol[683] and gain more weight. Large white pigs are more easily immobilized in the back test than Landrace pigs.[445]

There appear to be three important traits, aggression, sociability, and exploration, as measured by aggression to an intruder, social dependence, and response to novelty. Aggression as an individual personality trait can be measured by adding a smaller "intruder" to a pig's home cage. The latency to attack is stable over time.[541]

Other important traits are activity (in an open field or other novel environment) and anxiety or fear.[51] Pigs raised in an enriched environment show more diverse behaviors and are more active in response to a novel object, and vocalize more in an open-field test, but they are less tractable.[182,2001] Pigs find an unpredictable intermittent sound more aversive than a continuous one and will avoid it.[1849] Another test of fear used a ball that rose from the trough from which the pigs had become accustomed to eat. A horn behind a curtain adjacent to the trough was the auditory stimulus and carbon dioxide in the trough the olfactory one. The pig's approach time, locomotion, and latency to eat were measured. Younger pigs were more frightened than older finishing pigs. The anxiolytic midazolam reduced fear in the younger pigs.[424] Elevated mazes in which the pig has a choice of open or closed arms and dark versus light tests have been used to measure fear in pigs.[604] Willingness to approach a human is another measure of temperament; nevertheless, pigs initially reluctant to approach people become less reluctant with repeated testing,[795] but the relative rank is consistent across time. Pigs that approach human are more likely to be subordinate in a feed competition test. The latency to approach novel objects (traffic cones, bucket, or basket ball) was not correlated with latency to approach a person; nevertheless, it was correlated with latency to leave the pen.[292]

Bovine temperament tests

Approach to a novel object and to familiar and unfamiliar humans has been used as a temperament test in cattle. Individual differences in the fearfulness of cattle are measured by their response to a novel object, a different environment, feed in an unfamiliar place, or a startling stimulus.[246] One cattle temperament test consists in leading, restraining in a corner, and stroking. There were genetic effects, a heritability factor of 0.22 for docility, and environmental effects as well. Cattle kept indoors were more docile than those kept outside.[1107]

When observed in an auction ring, sensitivity or temperament was based on whether the cattle stood still or walked, slowly trotted, or tried to escape the ring. Holsteins were more sound sensitive (sudden yell or air hose), than beef cattle but were no more sensitive to sudden movements (hand waving or children running).[1091]

The response of cattle in a chute is correlated with their behavior in a pen when the animals are ranked from 1 to 5 on temperament, where 1 is a calm animal and 5 is extremely agitated.[415] Speed of leaving (flight speed or exit velocity) is also used as a measure of temperament and is correlated with the animal's response to social separation. The animals that freeze when separated are probably more fearful. Those who move around when isolated have high rates of weight gain.[1380]

Ovine temperament tests

Temperament tests in sheep consist in isolating the sheep, measuring its approach to a novel object (usually, a red balloon dropping from the ceiling) and to a human. In some tests, the human sits in front of a partition separating the test sheep from its pen mates, so the sheep's desire to approach its flock competes with its desire to avoid a human. Sheep can be divided according to their response to isolation and to humans—one group that is very active and vocal (More Active) and the other that is Less Active. The more active sheep were less physiologically stressed and actually spent more time close to the human.[185] Most tests have been done on adults rather than lambs. Ewes are more fearful than rams, and ewes that are given testosterone are less fearful.[1928] Ewes that have lambed are less fearful than nulliparous ones.[1943] Sheep respond more to carnivores (stuffed, moving wolverine, lynx, bear, and a real dog) by fleeing and flocking together than they respond to novel objects such as a moving ball. Other signs of fear are alarm vocalizations, urinating, or defecating. Lighter weight sheep are more responsive than heavy sheep. The heritability of behaviors associated with an approach avoidance test in which the lamb must approach a human to approach its flock mates in a adjacent pen reveals low heritability: number of bleats (0.39), locomotion (0.29), and time near the human (0.22).[2052]

Caprine temperament

The response of goats to an arena is a repeatable and valid test. Vocalizations are the usual measure.[604] Kids can be divided into timid and bold animals on the basis of their approach to humans. The behavior of the mother and, in the case of timid kids, that of even strange goats, affected the willingness of the kids to approach humans.[1193] Goats would obtain plenty of long chain polyunsaturated acid when grazing, but a cereal and silage diet is deficient in linoleic acid, the precursor of docosahexanoic and arachadonic acid, so goat kids whose mother were supplemented with linoleic acid were less inhibited by a novel object.[507]

Feline temperament test

Several attempts have been made to categorize feline temperament in the following ways: (1) recording behavior in the home environment, whether that is the barnyard, the living room, or the laboratory; (2) recording behavior in a structured test situation, usually while exposing the cat to a familiar and/or a strange person and a novel stimulus; (3) rating various characteristics (active, aggressive, agile, curious, excitable, playful, solitary, tense, vocal, voracious, watchful), reactions to other cats (equable, hostile, fearful, or sociable), and reactions to people (equable, hostile, fearful, or sociable); or (4) accepting owner reports.[1306] The personality of cats seems to be composed of three characteristics: (1) alertness, (2) sociability, and (3) equability.[567]

A laboratory test of sociability is that of Adamec,[5] who showed that as early as 10 weeks, cats differed among themselves in their reactions to strange people, to rats, and to the aggressive vocalization of adult cats. The cats that demonstrated fearful behavior in those three situations were classified as defensive and represented 25% of the population. These cats are the ones least likely to accommodate to a multicat household. Another kitten temperament test[985] reveals that cats that are vocal as kittens are vocal as adults, that very active kittens were less likely to spend time with people as adults, and that some kittens were timid.

Although the genes involved in feline temperament have not been identified, a paternal influence on offspring has been identified. Because the sire never saw the kittens, his influence had to be genetic.[1594]

Equine temperament tests

Several equine temperament tests have been developed. Mackenzie's test involves leading a horse over a measured distance and then attempting to lead the horse after an umbrella has been snapped open in front of it, after a bunch of pots and pans have fallen from 10 feet, or when there is a piece of plastic on the ground.[1200] All these tests measure reaction to stimuli that are frightening. Anderson et al.[55] burst a balloon beside a horse, had a mechanical pig move in front of the horse, or opened an umbrella. The umbrella gave the most accurate results. Seaman et al.[1719] measured horses' responses to three stimuli on three occasions. The responses were to isolation in an arena, to a spray of water, and to a person. Only the response to isolation was consistent across time. Physiological responses to environmental changes vary with the type of changes. Horses are more likely to defecate when isolated, but more likely to walk when confronted with a novel object (a tricycle). The heart rate is the best physiological measure of emotionality when the horse's activity is controlled.[1245] The horses, cardiac responses to auditory (white noise) or visual (orange traffic cone) were similar, but their behavioral responses were different. They backed away from the visual stimulus.[350]

Visser et al.[1956] used the horse's response to an umbrella lowered from the ceiling when the horse was free in an arena, and measured the ease with which the horse could be led across a bridge. The horse's heart rate was correlated with its behavior. Flightiness and sensitivity were measured by the novel object (umbrella) test, and patience and willingness to perform by the handling (bridge) tests.[1953] There was some relationship between the reactions of an individual horse at 1 year and at 2 years of age to novel objects and between that reaction and its performance (number of jumps taken correctly at age 3), but there was no single test that consistently predicted performance.[1956] Kusunose used the horse's response—movement and heart rate—to a large rotating weather balloon and found that the horses' reactions were correlated with the handlers' assessment of their temperament.[1348] Momozawa et al.[1350] used a similar test; in this case, exposing a riding horse to two rotating balloons. The greater the number of defecations when exposed to the balloons, the more anxious the horse had been rated by its caretakers. Shaking a red and white garland in the horse's home stall and, in a separate test, covering its head for an hour revealed that jumpers are no more reactive than therapeutic riding horses.[1340]

The most extensive equine temperament testing has been performed by Hausberger and her associates.[783] Her test involved releasing the horse alone in an arena and measuring its behavior before and after a novel object—in this case, colored rails—were put in the arena. Included in the temperament tests was a learning task. The horse had to manipulate a lid with its muzzle for a food reward. Of the breeds tested, the Icelandic pony was the most successful. This breed has been genetically isolated for hundreds of years, which indicates that we have not been selecting for equine intelligence. (See Chapter 6 for more detail on early handling effects.)

Diet has an effect on temperament. Weaned foals fed a high-fat and high-fiber diet were more likely to investigate a novel object or person than those fed a high-starch, high-sugar diet.[1416] Adult horses fed a high-fat diet reacted as quickly to a startling stimulus (tiger head on a spring) than those fed a high-sugar diet, but they did not move as far or as long.[1588]

Most temperament tests are performed only once, so it is important to know how repeatable they are. Lansade and Bouissou[1093] found that reactivity to humans whether active or passive and whether familiar or strange was stable at least from 8 months to 2.5 years. The same group found that horse reaction to isolation was consistent over time. The number of neighs was particularly stable. The horse's attraction to other horses was not stable over time.[1094]

A more subjective term is personality, but there have been numerous attempts to describe horse personality, mostly using adjectives that handlers apply to the horse. In addition to an academic exercise the personality test is supposed to help assign the correct horse to the correct user, that is, riding for the handicapped and open jumping. Usually, the handlers are given a list of adjectives and asked to apply these to a horse. Those adjectives that are correlated with one another can be identified by factor analysis. The experimenter can then name the factors. When this method was used, there were following three factors:[1283]

(1) Agreeableness (obedience, nonaggression, kindness) and sociality
(2) Intelligence and curiosity
(3) Emotionality or nervousness

The easiest equine personality trait to identify[1349, 1350] is nervousness and this can be compared to the human personality trait neuroticism. Conscientiousness and extraversion also seem to be valid terms[1173,1333,1955] Trainability and affability, aggression to people or other horses are other important factors. In a large survey, in which over 1,000 people rated horses, thoroughbreds, Arabians and Welch ponies were rated not only most anxious and excitable but also most inquisitive.[1172]

There is a polymorphism in the horse—an A (adenine) to G guanine substitution—in the dopamine D4 receptor gene. This may code for an asparagine for aspartic acid amino acid substitution. Over a hundred 2-year-old thoroughbreds were genotyped and evaluated for temperament. Those horses who carried the G allele were more curious (examined novel objects) and less vigilant than horses carrying the A allele, according to their caretakers.[1349] This is one of the first examples of an allele in domestic animals associated with a given behavior. Because shying at novel objects is a frequent cause of injury to riders, this is particularly important. About 25% of horses are homozygous for the A allele.

LATERALITY OR HANDEDNESS IN ANIMALS

Handedness reflects which side of the brain is dominant. Therefore, differences between right- and left-handed humans and, probably most important, between ambidextrous people and the others have been related to various behavior patterns in humans. Recently, this has been extended to animals.

Horse

Horses show laterality. Colts are more often born with their left foreleg anterior to the right and retain this left bias.[1389] The left tendency increases with age, which may indicate a training effect.[1282] There are breed differences in laterality based on which leg is forward while grazing. Thoroughbreds are significantly left lateral, standardbred pacers slightly less so, and quarter horses used for cutting had no laterality. Horses turn their right ear toward a familiar whinny, indicating a left brain recognition.[162]

Cattle

When passing an object 40% of cattle pass to the right and 40% to the left.[1024]

Dog

There are several ways to test for laterality: the paw used to remove tape from the nose, to overturn a can under which a treat has been hidden, to remove a blanket placed over the dog's head or to hold a Kong toy and the paw raised when the dog is told to "Shake" or "Give paw".[1564,1996] Dogs display right and left paw preferences. Male and female showed paw preferences at the level of the population but in opposite directions. Female dogs had a greater preference for using their right paw for all tasks, while males were more inclined to use their left paw. Dogs inspected the left side of photographs of people's faces whether the photographs were right side up or upside down. They did not display similar laterality to dog faces.[727]

Brain laterality influences immunity through effects on cytokines. IL-2 and IL-6 gene expressions are higher in left-pawed dogs than in right-pawed and ambidextrous dogs. After rabies vaccine administration, decreasing levels of IL-2 and IL-6 gene expression are observed in left-pawed and right-pawed dogs, but not in ambidextrous dogs.[1563] Branson and Rogers[278] found that ambidextrous dogs were more likely to suffer from noise phobias such as storm phobia and fear of fireworks.

There is also a side bias in tail wagging. Dogs wag their tails to the right when facing the owner or an unfamiliar person, although the amplitude of the wag is smaller to an unfamiliar person. A cat also elicits a right-sided bias, but a strange dominant dog elicits a left-sided bias.[1564]

Hair whorls

Grandin and her colleagues[710,1090] have found a correlation of position of hair whorls in cattle and agitation in a chute. A whorl above the eyes may predict agitation.[709,710] Cattle with high whorls had higher crush scores, that is, were more agitated. Cattle with lower facial hair whorls had smaller flight distance and less interest in an unfamiliar human than those with whorls located higher on their faces.[1578] Olmos and Turner[1449] found that only crush scores (pushing, head tossing, and shaking) rather than flight speed or weight gain varied with hair whorl position.

References

1. Abitbol, M. L. and S. R. Inglis. 1997. Role of amniotic fluid in newborn acceptance and bonding in canines. *J. Matern. Fetal. Med.* 6:49–52.
2. Abraham, I., S. R. Baker, D. A. Denton, F. Kraintz, L. Kraintz and L. Purser. 1973. Components in the regulation of salt balance: Salt appetite studied by operant behaviour. *Aust. J. Exp. Biol. Med. Sci.* 51:5–81.
3. Abraham, S. F., R. M. Baker, E. H. Blaine, D. A. Denton and M. J. McKinley. 1975. Water drinking induced in sheep by angiotensin–a physiological or pharmacological effect? *J. Comp. Physiol. Psychol.* 88:503–518.
4. Adachi, I., H. Kuwahata and K. Fujita. 2007. Dogs recall their owner's face upon hearing the owner's voice. *Anim. Cogn.* 10:17–21.
5. Adamec, R. E. 1991. Anxious personality in the cat: Its ontogeny and physiology. In B. J. Carroll and J. E. Barrett (Eds.), *Psychopathology and the brain*, pp. 153–168. New York, NY: Raven Press.
6. Adamec, R. E. 1976. The interaction of hunger and preying in the domestic cat (*Felis catus*): An adaptive hierarchy? *Behav. Biol.* 18:263–272.
7. Adamec, R. E., C. Stark-Adamec and K. E. Livingston. 1983. The expression of an early developmentally emergent defensive bias in the adult domestic cat (*Felis catus*) in non-predatory situations. *Appl. Anim. Ethol.* 10:89–108.
8. Adams, D. K. 1929. Experimental studies of adaptive behavior in cats. *Comp. Psychol. Monogr.* 6:1–168.
9. Adams, G. J. and K. G. Johnson. 1995. Guard dogs: Sleep, work and the behavioural responses of people and other stimuli. *Appl. Anim. Behav. Sci.* 46:103–115.
10. Adams, G. J. and K. G. Johnson. 1994. Behavioural responses to barking and other auditory stimuli during night-time sleeping and waking in the domestic dog (*Canis familiaris*). *Appl. Anim. Behav. Sci.* 39:151–162.
11. Adams, G. J. and K. G. Johnson. 1994. Sleep work, and the effects of shift work in drug detector dogs *Canis familiaris*. *Appl. Anim. Behav. Sci.* 41:115–126.
12. Adams, G. J. and K. G. Johnson. 1993. Sleep-wake cycles and other night-time behaviours of the domestic dog (*Canis familiaris*). *Appl. Anim. Behav. Sci.* 36:233–248.
13. Adams, T. 1963. Hypothalamic temperature in the cat during feeding and sleep. *Science* 139:609–610.
14. Adkins-Regan, E., P. Orgeur and J. P. Signoret. 1989. Sexual differentiation of reproductive behavior in pigs: Defeminizing effects of prepubertal estradiol. *Horm. Behav.* 23:290–303.
15. Administratin, O. S. a. H. 1972. Federal regulation 37 (202), part II. In *Occupational safety and health standards*, pp. 102–122, 356. Washington, DC: Department of Labor.
16. Agrawal, H. C., M. W. Fox and W. A. Himwich. 1967. Neurochemical and behavioral effects of isolation-rearing in the dog. *Life Sci.* 6:71–78.
17. Alavi, F. K., J. P. McCann, A. Mauromoustakis and S. Sangiah. 1993. Feeding behavior and its responsiveness to naloxone differ in lean and obese sheep. *Physiol. Behav.* 53:317–323.
18. Albright, J. D., H. O. Mohammed, C. R. Heleski, C. L. Wickens and K. A. Houpt. 2009. Crib-biting in US horses: Breed predispositions and owner perceptions of aetiology. *Equine Vet. J.* 41:455–458.
19. Albright, J. L. 1969. Social environment and growth. In E. S. E. Hafez and I. A. Dyer (Eds.), *Animal growth and nutrition*, pp. 106–120. Philadelphia, PA: Lea & Febiger.
20. Albright, J. L., W. P. M. Gordon, W. C. Black, J. P. Dietrich, W. W. Snyder and C. E. Meadows. 1966. Behavioral responses of cows to auditory training. *J. Dairy Sci.* 49:104–106.
21. Aldinger, S. M., V. C. Speer, V. W. Hays and D. V. Catron. 1959. Effect of saccharin on consumption of starter rations by baby pigs. *J. Anim. Sci.* 18:1350–1355.

Domestic Animal Behavior for Veterinarians and Animal Scientists, Fifth Edition by Katherine Albro Houpt
© 2011 John Wiley & Sons, Inc.

22. Aldis, O. 1975. *Play fighting*. New York, NY: Academic Press.
23. Aldrich, C. G., M. T. Rhodes, J. L. Miner, M. S. Kerley and J. A. Paterson. 1993. The effects of endophyte-infected tall fescue consumption and use of a dopamine antagonist on intake, digestibility, body temperature, and blood constituents in sheep. *J. Anim. Sci.* 71:158–163.
24. Alexander, B. M., J. D. Rose, J. N. Stellflug, J. A. Fitzgerald and G. E. Moss. 2001. Low-sexually performing rams but not male-oriented rams can be discriminated by cell size in the amygdala and preoptic area: A morphometric study. *Behav. Brain Res.* 119:15–21.
25. Alexander, B. M., J. N. Stellflug, J. D. Rose, J. A. Fitzgerald and G. E. Moss. 1999. Behavior and endocrine changes in high-performing, low-performing, and male-oriented domestic rams following exposure to rams and ewes in estrus when copulation is precluded. *J. Anim. Sci.* 77:1869–1874.
26. Alexander, G. 1977. Role of auditory and visual cues in mutual recognition between ewes and lambs in Merino sheep. *Appl. Anim. Ethol.* 3:65–81.
27. Alexander, G. and L. R. Bradley. 1985. Fostering in sheep. IV. Use of restraint. *Appl. Anim. Behav. Sci.* 14:355–364.
28. Alexander, G. and E. E. Shillito. 1978. Maternal responses in Merino ewes to artificially coloured lambs. *Appl. Anim. Ethol.* 4:141–152.
29. Alexander, G. and E. E. Shillito. 1978. Visual discrimination between ewes by lambs. *Appl. Anim. Ethol.* 4:81–85.
30. Alexander, G. and E. E. Shillito. 1977. The importance of odour, apearance and voice in maternal recognition of the young in Merino sheep (*Ovis aries*). *Appl. Anim. Ethol.* 3:127–135.
31. Alexander, G. and E. E. Shillito. 1977. Importance of visual cues from various body regions in maternal recognition of the young in Merino sheep (*Ovis aries*). *Appl. Anim. Ethol.* 3:137–143.
32. Alexander, G., J.-P. Signoret and E. S. E. Hafez. 1974. Sexual and maternal behavior. In E. S. E. Hafez (Ed.), *Reproduction in farm animals*, pp. 222–254. Philadelphia, PA: Lea & Febiger.
33. Alexander, G. and D. Stevens. 1985. Fostering in sheep. III. Facilitation by the use of odorants. *Appl. Anim. Behav. Sci.* 14:345–354.
34. Alexander, G. and D. Stevens. 1981. Recognition of washed lambs by Merino ewes. *Appl. Anim. Ethol.* 7:77–86.
35. Alexander, G., D. Stevens and L. R. Bradley. 1988. Maternal behaviour in ewes following caesarian section. *Appl. Anim. Behav. Sci.* 19:273–277.
36. Alexander, G., D. Stevens and L. R. Bradley. 1983. Washing lambs and confinement as aids to fostering. *Appl. Anim. Ethol.* 10:251–261.
37. Alexander, G., D. Stevens, R. Kilgour, H. de Langen, B. E. Mottershead and J. J. Lynch. 1983. Separation of ewes from twin lambs: Incidence in several breeds. *Appl. Anim. Ethol.* 10:301–317.
38. Alexander, G., G. D. Stevens and L. R. Bradley. 1985. Fostering in sheep. I. Facilitation by use of textile lamb coats. *Appl. Anim. Ethol.* 14:315–334.
39. Alexander, G. and D. Williams. 1966. Teat-seeking activity in lambs during the first hours of life. *Anim. Behav.* 14:166–176.
40. Alexander, G. and D. Williams. 1964. Maternal facilitation of sucking drive in newborn lambs. *Science* 146:65–66.
41. Algers, B., P. Jensen and L. Steinwall. 1990. Behaviour and weight changes at weaning and regrouping of pigs in relation to teat quality. *Appl. Anim. Behav. Sci.* 26:143–155.
42. Algers, B., S. Rojanasthien and K. Uvnas-Moberg. 1990. The relationship between teat stimulation, oxytocin release and grunting rate in the sow during nursing. *Appl. Anim. Behav. Sci.* 26:267–276.
43. Algers, B. and K. Uvnas-Moberg. 2007. Maternal behavior in pigs. *Horm. Behav.* 52:78–85.
44. Allan, C. J., P. J. Holst and G. N. Hinch. 1991. Behaviour of parturient Australian bush goats. I. Doe behaviour and kid vigour. *Appl. Anim. Behav. Sci.* 32:55–64.
45. Allin, J. T. and E. M. Banks. 1972. Functional aspects of ultrasound production by infant albino rats (Rattus norvegicus). *Anim. Behav.* 20:175–185.
46. Allison, T. and D. V. Cicchetti. 1976. Sleep in mammals: Ecological and constitutional correlates. *Science* 194:732–734.
47. Altmann, M. 1941. Interrelations of the sex cycle and the behavior of the sow. *J. Comp. Psychol.* 31:481–498.
48. Ames, D. R. and L. A. Arehart. 1972. Physiological response of lambs to auditory stimuli. *J. Anim. Sci.* 34:994–998.
49. Andersen, I. L., K. E. Boe and A. L. Kristiansen. 1999. The influence of different feeding arrangements and food type on competition at feeding in pregnant sows. *Appl. Anim. Behav. Sci.* 65:91–104.

50. Andersen, I. L., S. Berg and K. E. Boe. 2005. Crushing of piglets by the mother sow (*Sus scrofa*)—purely accidental or a poor mother? *Appl. Anim. Behav. Sci.* 93:229–243.

51. Andersen, I. L., K. E. Boe, G. Foerevik, A. M. Janczak and M. Bakken. 2000. Behavioural evaluation of methods for assessing fear responses in weaned pigs. *Appl. Anim. Behav. Sci.* 69:227–240.

52. Anderson, D. M., C. V. Hulet, S. K. Hamadeh, J. N. Smith and L. W. Murray. 1990. Diet selection of bonded and non-bonded free-ranging sheep and cattle. *Appl. Anim. Behav. Sci.* 26:231–242.

53. Anderson, D. M., C. V. Hulet, J. N. Smith, W. L. Shupe and L. W. Murray. 1992. An attempt to bond weaned 3-month-old beef heifers to yearling ewes. *Appl. Anim. Behav. Sci.* 34:181–188.

54. Anderson, D. M., C. V. Hulet, J. N. Smith, W. L. Shupe and L. W. Murray. 1987. Heifer disposition and bonding of lambs to heifers. *Appl. Anim. Behav. Sci.* 19:27–30.

55. Anderson, D. M. and N. S. Urguhart. 1986. Using digital pedometers to monitor travel of cows grazing arid rangeland. *Appl. Anim. Behav. Sci.* 16:11–23.

56. Anderson, O. D. and R. Parmenter. 1941. A long-term study of the experimental neurosis in the sheep and dog. *Psychosom. Med.* 2:1–150.

57. Anderson, R. S. 1974. Obesity in the dog and cat. In C. S. G. Grunsell and F. W. G. Hill (Eds.), *The veterinary annual 1973*, pp. 182–186. Bristol, UK: John Wright and Sons.

58. Andersson, B., O. Augustinsson, E. Bademo, J. Junkergard, C. Kvart, G. Nyman and M. Wiberg. 1987. Systemic and centrally mediated angiotensin II effects in the horse. *Acta Physiol. Scand.* 129:143–149.

59. Andersson, B., L. Eriksson and R. Oltner. 1970. Further evidence for angiotensin-sodium interaction in central control of fluid balance. *Life Sci. I.* 9:1091–1096.

60. Andersson, B. and S. M. McCann. 1955. A further study of polydipsia evoked by hypothalamic stimulation in the goat. *Acta Physiol. Scand.* 33:333–346.

61. Anonymous. 1975. Behaviour of boars. *Vet. Rec.* 96:221.

62. Apley, M. D. and K. W. Kersting. 1999. The buller syndrome in feedlot steers. *Compendium Cont. Ed. Pract. Vet.* 21:S250–S256.

63. Apple, J. K. and J. V. Craig. 1992. The influence of pen size on toy preference in growing pigs. *Appl. Anim. Behav. Sci.* 35:149–155.

64. Appleby, M. C., E. A. Pajor and D. Fraser. 1992. Individual variation in feeding and growth of piglets: Effects of increased access to creep food. *Anim. Prod.* 55:147–152.

65. Appleby, M. C., E. A. Pajor and D. Fraser. 1991. Effects of management options on creep feeding by piglets. *Anim. Prod.* 53:361–366.

66. Appleby, M. C. and D. G. M. Wood-Gush. 1988. Effect of earth as an additional stimulus on the behaviour of confined piglets. *Behav. Proc.* 17:83–91.

67. Araba, B. D. and S. L. Crowell-Davis. 1994. Dominance relationships and aggression in foals (*Equus caballus*). *Appl. Anim. Behav. Sci.* 41:1–25.

68. Arave, C. W., R. C. Lamb, M. J. Arambel, D. Purcell and J. L. Walter. 1992. Behavior and maze learning ability of dairy calves as influenced by housing, sex and sire. *Appl. Anim. Behav. Sci.* 33:149–163.

69. Archer, D. C., G. K. Pinchbeck, N. P. French and C. J. Proudman. 2008. Risk factors for epiploic foramen entrapment colic: An international study. *Equine Vet. J.* 40:224–230.

70. Archer, M. 1973. The species preferences of grazing horses. *J. Br. Grassland Soc.* 28:123–128.

71. Archibald, J. 1974. *Canine surgery*. Santa Barbara, CA: American Veterinary Publications.

72. Arendt, J., A. M. Symons, C. A. Laud and S. J. Pryde. 1983. Melatonin can induce early onset of the breeding season in ewes. *J. Endocrinol.* 97:395–400.

73. Arey, D. S. 1999. Time course for the formation and disruption of social organisation in group-housed sows. *Appl. Anim. Behav. Sci.* 62:199–207.

74. Arey, D. S. and M. F. Franklin. 1995. Effects of straw and unfamiliarity on fighting between newly mixed growing pigs. *Appl. Anim. Behav. Sci.* 45:25–30.

75. Arey, D. S., A. M. Perchey and V. R. Fowler. 1991. The preparturient behaviour of sows in enriched pens and the effect of pre-formed nests. *Appl. Anim. Behav. Sci.* 31:61–68.

76. Arey, D. S., A. M. Petchey and V. R. Fowler. 1992. The peri-parturient behaviour of sows housed in pairs. *Appl. Anim. Behav. Sci.* 34:49–59.

77. Arnold, G. W. 1966. The special senses in grazing animals. II. Smell, taste, and touch and dietary habits in sheep. *Aust. J. Agric. Res.* 17:531–542.

78. Arnold, G. W. 1984. Comparison of the time budgets and circadian patterns of maintenance activities in sheep, cattle and horses grouped together. *Appl. Anim. Behav. Sci.* 13:19–30.

79. Arnold, G. W. 1966. The special senses in grazing animals. I. Sight and dietary habits in sheep. *Aust. J. Agric. Res.* 17:521–529.

80. Arnold, G. W., C. A. P. Boundy, P. D. Morgan and G. Bartle. 1975. The roles of sight and hearing in the lamb in the location and discrimination between ewes. *Appl. Anim. Ethol.* 1:167–176.

81. Arnold, G. W. and M. L. Dudzinski. 1978. *Ethology of free-ranging domestic animals.* Amsterdam, The Netherlands: Elsevier Scientific Publishing Co.

82. Arnold, G. W. and A. Grassia. 1982. Ethogram of agonistic behaviour for thoroughbred horses. *Appl. Anim. Ethol.* 8:5–25.

83. Arnold, G. W. and R. A. Maller. 1974. Some aspects of competition between sheep for supplementary feed. *Anim. Prod.* 19:309–319.

84. Arnold, G. W. and P. D. Morgan. 1975. Behaviour of the ewe and lamb at lambing and its relationship to lamb mortality. *Appl. Anim. Ethol.* 2:25–46.

85. Arnold, G. W. and P. J. Pahl. 1974. Some aspects of social behaviour in domestic sheep. *Anim. Behav.* 22:592–600.

86. Arnold, G. W., S. R. Wallace and R. A. Maller. 1979. Some factors involved in natural weaning processes in sheep. *Appl. Anim. Ethol.* 5:43–50.

87. Arnold, G. W., S. R. Wallace and W. A. Rea. 1981. Associations between individuals and home-range behaviour in natural flocks of three breeds of domestic sheep. *Appl. Anim. Ethol.* 7:239–257.

88. Arnold, N. A., K. T. Ng, E. C. Jongman and P. H. Hemsworth. 2007. The behavioural and physiological responses of dairy heifers milking facility noise with and without a pre-treatment adaptation phase. *Appl. Anim. Behav. Sci.* 106:13–25.

89. Arnold, N. A., K. T. Ng, E. C. Jongman and P. H. Hemsworth. 2007. Responses of dairy heifers to the visual cliff formed by a herringbone milking pit: Evidence of fear of heights in cows (*Bos taurus*). *J. Comp. Psychol.* 121:440–446.

90. Arnold, W., T. Ruf and R. Kuntz. 2006. Seasonal adjustment of energy budget in a large wild mammal, the Przewalski horse (*Equus ferus przewalskii*) II. Energy expenditure. *J. Exp. Biol.* 209:4566–4573.

91. Arnould, C., V. Piketty and F. Levy. 1991. Behaviour of ewes at parturition toward amniotic fluids from sheep, cows, and goats. *Appl. Anim. Behav. Sci.* 32:191–196.

92. Aronson, L. R. and M. L. Cooper. 1977. Central versus peripheral genital desensitization and mating behavior in male cats: Tonic and phasic effects. *Ann. N. Y. Acad. Sci.* 290:299–313.

93. Aronson, L. R. and M. L. Cooper. 1974. Olfactory deprivation and mating behavior in sexually experienced male cats. *Behav. Biol.* 11:459–480.

94. Aronson, L. R. and M. L. Cooper. 1966. Seasonal variation in mating behavior in cats after desensitization of glans penis. *Science* 152:226–230.

95. Asa, C. S. 1999. Male reproductive success in free-ranging feral horses. *Behav. Ecol. Sociobiol.* 47:93.

96. Asa, C. S., D. A. Goldfoot and O. J. Ginther. 1983. Assessment of the sexual behavior of pregnant mares. *Horm. Behav.* 17:405–413.

97. Asa, C. S., D. A. Goldfoot and O. J. Ginther. 1979. Sociosexual behavior and the ovulatory cycle of ponies (*Equus caaballus*) observed in harem groups. *Horm. Behav.* 13:46–65.

98. Aschoff, J. 1965. Circadian clocks. *Proceedings of the Feldafing Summer School,* Amsterdam, The Netherlands.

99. Ashmead, D. H., R. K. Clifton and E. P. Reese. 1986. Development of auditory localization in dogs: Single source and precedence effect sounds. *Dev. Psychobiol.* 19:91–103.

100. Askew, H. R. 1996. *Treatment of behavior problems in dogs and cats. A guide for the small animal veterinarian.* Oxford, UK: Blackwell Science.

101. Atkeson, F. W., A. O. Shaw and H. W. Cave. 1942. Grazing habits of dairy cattle. *J. Dairy. Sci.* 25:779–784.

102. Auffray, P. and J. C. Marcilloux. 1983. An analysis of feeding patterns in the adult pig. *Reprod. Nutr. Dev.* 23:517–524.

103. Aust, U., F. Range, M. Steurer and L. Huber. 2008. Inferential reasoning by exclusion in pigeons, dogs, and humans. *Anim. Cogn.* 11:587–597.

104. Awotwi, E. K., K. Oppong-Anane, P. C. Addae and E. O. Oddoye. 2000. Behavioural interactions between West African dwarf nanny goats and their twin-born kids during the first 48 h post-partum. *Appl. Anim. Behav. Sci.* 68:281–291.

105. Back, D. G., B. W. Pickett, J. L. Voss and G. E. Seidel Jr. 1974. Observations on the sexual behavior of nonlactating mares. *J. Am. Vet. Med. Assoc.* 165:717–720.

106. Bacon, W. E. 1973. Aversive conditioning in neonatal kittens. *J. Comp. Physiol. Psychol.* 83:306–313.

107. Bacon, W. E. and W. C. Stanley. 1963. Effect of deprivation level in puppies on performance maintained by a passive person reinforcer. *J. Comp. Physiol. Psychol.* 56:783–785.

108. Badamana, M. S., J. D. Sutton, J. D. Oldham and A. Mowlem. 1990. The effect of amount of protein in the concentrates on hay intake and rate of passage, diet digestibility and milk production in British Saanen goats. *Anim. Prod.* 51:333–342.

109. Bado, A., M. J. Lewin and M. Dubrasquet. 1989. Effects of bombesin on food intake and gastric acid secretion in cats. *Am. J. Physiol.* 256:R181–R186.

110. Bado, A., M. Rodriguez, M. J. Lewin, J. Martinez and M. Dubrasquet. 1988. Cholecystokinin suppresses food intake in cats: Structure-activity characterization. *Pharmacol. Biochem. Behav.* 31:297–303.

111. Baer, K. L., G. D. Potter, T. H. Friend and B. V. Beaver. 1983. Observation effect on learning in horses. *Appl. Anim. Ethol.* 11:123–129.

112. Bagshaw, C. S., S. L. Ralston and H. Fisher. 1994. Behavioral and physiological effect of orally administered tryptophan on horses subjected to acute isolation stress. *Appl. Anim. Behav. Sci.* 40:12.

113. Baile, C. A. and J. M. Forbes. 1974. Control of feed intake and regulation of energy balance in ruminants. *Physiol. Rev.* 54:160–214.

114. Baile, C. A., C. L. McLaughlin, F. C. Buonomo, T. J. Lauterio, L. Marson and M. A. Della-Fera. 1987. Opioid peptides and the control of feeding in sheep. *Fed. Proc.* 46:173–177.

115. Baile, C. A., C. L. McLaughlin and M. A. Della-Fera. 1986. Role of cholecystokinin and opioid peptides in control of food intake. *Physiol. Rev.* 66:172–234.

116. Baile, C. A., C. W. Simpson, L. F. Krabill and F. H. Martin. 1972. Adrenergic agonists and antagonists and feeding in sheep and cattle. *Life Sci. I.* 11:661–668.

117. Bailey, C. J. and L. W. Porter. 1955. Relevant cues in drive discrimination in cats. *J. Comp. Physiol. Psychol.* 48:180–182.

118. Bailey, J. D., L. H. Anderson and K. K. Schillo. 2005. Effects of novel females and stage of the estrous cycle on sexual behavior in mature beef bulls. *J. Anim. Sci.* 83:613–624.

119. Bain, M. J., B. L. Hart, K. D. Cliff and W. W. Ruehl. 2001. Predicting behavioral changes associated with age-related cognitive impairment in dogs. *J. Am. Vet. Med. Assoc.* 218:1792–1795.

120. Baker, A. E. M. and B. H. Crawford. 1986. Observational learning in horses. *Appl. Anim. Behav. Sci.* 15:7–13.

121. Baker, A. E. M. and G. E. Seidel. 1985. Why do cows mount other cows? *Appl. Anim. Behav. Sci.* 13:237–241.

122. Baker, G. J. and J. Kear-Colwell. 1974. Aerophagia (windsucking) and aversion therapy in the horse. *Proc. Am. Assoc. Eq. Pract.* 20:127–130.

123. Balch, C. C. 1955. Sleep in ruminants. *Nature* 175:940–941.

124. Baldwin, B. A. 1981. Shape discrimination in sheep and calves. *Anim. Behav.* 29:830–834.

125. Baldwin, B. A. 1979. Operant studies on shape discrimination in goats. *Physiol. Behav.* 23:455–459.

126. Baldwin, B. A. 1977. Ability of goats and calves to distinguish between conspecific urine samples using olfaction. *Appl. Anim. Ethol.* 3:145–150.

127. Baldwin, B. A. 1969. The study of behaviour in pigs. *Br. Vet. J.* 125:281–288.

128. Baldwin, B. A., D. J. Conner and G. B. Meese. 1974. Proceedings: Sensory reinforcement in the pig. *J. Physiol.* 242:27P.

129. Baldwin, B. A. and T. R. Cooper. 1979. The effects of olfactory bulbectomy on feeding behaviour in pigs. *Appl. Anim. Ethol.* 5:153–159.

130. Baldwin, B. A. and C. de la Riva. 1995. Effects of the 5-HT1A agonist 8-OH-DPAT on operant feeding in pigs. *Physiol. Behav.* 58:611–613.

131. Baldwin, B. A., C. de la Riva and I. S. Ebenezer. 1990. Effects of intracerebroventricular injection of dynorphin, leumorphin and alpha neo-endorphin on operant feeding in pigs. *Physiol. Behav.* 48:821–824.

132. Baldwin, B. A., I. S. Ebenezer and C. De La Riva. 1990. Effects of intracerebroventricular injection of muscimol or GABA on operant feeding in pigs. *Physiol. Behav.* 48:417–421.

133. Baldwin, B. A. and D. L. Ingram. 1968. Factors influencing behavioral thermoregulation in the pig. *Physiol. Behav.* 3:409–415.

134. Baldwin, B. A., C. L. McLaughlin and C. A. Baile. 1977. The effect of ablation of the olfactory bulbs on feeding behaviour in sheep. *Appl. Anim. Ethol.* 3:151–161.

135. Baldwin, B. A. and G. B. Meese. 1979. Social behaviour in pigs studied by means of operant conditioning. *Anim. Behav.* 27:947–957.

136. Baldwin, B. A. and G. B. Meese. 1977. The ability of sheep to distinguish between conspecifics by means of olfaction. *Physiol. Behav.* 18:803–808.

137. Baldwin, B. A. and G. B. Meese. 1977. Sensory reinforcement and illumination preference in the domesticated pig. *Anim. Behav.* 25:497–507.

138. Baldwin, B. A. and R. F. Parrott. 1985. Effects of intracerebroventricular injection of naloxone on operant feeding and drinking in pigs. *Pharmacol. Biochem. Behav.* 22:37–40.

139. Baldwin, B. A. and R. F. Parrott. 1979. Studies on intracranial electrical self-stimulation in pigs in relation to ingestive and exploratory behaviour. *Physiol. Behav.* 22:723–730.

140. Baldwin, B. A. and E. E. Shillito. 1974. The effects of ablation of the olfactory bulbs on parturition and maternal behaviour in Soay sheep. *Anim. Behav.* 22:220–223.

141. Baldwin, B. A. and D. B. Stephens. 1973. The effects of conditioned behaviour and environmental factors on plasma corticosteroid levels in pigs. *Physiol. Behav.* 10:267–274.

142. Baldwin, B. A. and D. B. Stephens. 1970. Operant conditioning procedures for producing emotional responses in pigs. *J. Physiol.* 210:127P–128P.

143. Baldwin, B. A. and S. N. Thornton. 1986. Operant drinking in pigs following intracerebroventricular injections of hypertonic solutions and angiotensin II. *Physiol. Behav.* 36:325–328.

144. Baldwin, B. A. and J. O. Yates. 1977. The effects of hypothalamic temperature variation and intracarotid cooling on behavioural thermoregulation in sheep. *J. Physiol.* 265:705–720.

145. Banks, E. M. 1964. Some aspects of sexual behavior in domestic sheep, *Ovis aries. Behaviour* 23:249–279.

146. Baranyiova, E., A. H. M. Martinikova, A. Necas and J. Zatloukal. 2003. Epidemiology of intraspecies bite wounds in dogs in the Czech Republic. *Acta Vet. Brno.* 72:55–62.

147. Baraza, E., J. J. Villalba and F. D. Provenza. 2005. Nutritional context influences preferences of lambs for foods with plant secondary metabolites. *Appl. Anim. Behav. Sci.* 92:293–305.

148. Barber, J. A. and S. L. Crowell-Davis. 1994. Maternal behavior of Belgian (*Equus caballus*) mares. *Appl. Anim. Behav. Sci.* 41:161–168.

149. Bareham, J. R. 1976. The behaviour of lambs on the first day after birth. *Br. Vet. J.* 132:152–162.

150. Bareham, J. R. 1975. The effect of lack of vision on suckling behaviour of lambs. *Appl. Anim. Ethol.* 1:245–250.

151. Barnes, R. H., A. U. Moore and W. G. Pond. 1970. Behavioral abnormalities in young adult pigs caused by malnutrition in early life. *J. Nutr.* 100:149–155.

152. Barnett, J. L., G. M. Cronin, T. H. McCallum and E. A. Newman. 1994. Effects of food and time of day on aggression when grouping unfamiliar adult pigs. *Appl. Anim. Behav. Sci.* 39:339–347.

153. Barnett, J. L., G. M. Cronin, T. H. McCallum and E. A. Newman. 1993. Effects of 'chemical intervention' techniques on aggression and injuries when grouping unfamiliar adult pigs. *Appl. Anim. Behav. Sci.* 16:249–257.

154. Barnett, J. L., G. M. Cronin, T. H. McCallum and E. A. Newman. 1993. Effects of pen size/shape and design on aggression when grouping unfamiliar adult pigs. *Appl. Anim. Behav. Sci.* 36:111–122.

155. Barnett, J. L., P. H. Hemsworth, C. G. Winfield and C. Hansen. 1986. Effects of social environment on welfare status and sexual behaviour of female pigs. I. Effects of group size. *Appl. Anim. Behav. Sci.* 16:249–257.

156. Baron, A., C. N. Stewart and J. M. Warren. 1957. Patterns of social interaction in cats (*Felis domestica*). *Behaviour* 11:56–66.

157. Barrett, P. and P. Bateson. 1978. The development of play in cats. *Behaviour* 66:106–120.

158. Barroso, F. G., C. L. Alados and J. Boza. 2000. Social hierarchy in the domestic goat: Effect on food habits and production. *Appl. Anim. Behav. Sci.* 69:35–53.

159. Barry, K. J. and S. L. Crowell-Davis. 1999. Gender differences in the social behavior of the neutered indoor-only domestic cat. *Appl. Anim. Behav. Sci.* 64:193–211.

160. Bartos, L., J. Bartosova and L. Starostova. 2008. Position of the head is not associated with changes in horse vision. *Equine Vet. J.* 40:599–601.

161. Bartoshuk, L. M., M. A. Harned and L. H. Parks. 1971. Taste of water in the cat: Effects on sucrose preference. *Science* 171:699–701.

162. Basile, M., S. Boivin, A. Boutin, C. Blois-Heulin, M. Hausberger and A. Lemasson. 2009. Socially dependent auditory laterality in domestic horses (*Equus caballus*). *Anim. Cogn.* 12:611–619.

163. Bateson, P. 1979. How do sensitive periods arise and what are they for? *Anim. Behav.* 27:470–486.

164. Bateson, P. 1978. Sexual imprinting and optimal outbreeding. *Nature* 273:659–660.

165. Bateson, P., M. Mendl and J. Feaver. 1990. Play in the domestic cat is enhanced by rationing of the mother during lactation. *Anim. Behav.* 40:514–525.

166. Bauer, E., C. Ward and B. Smits. 2009. Play like a puppy, play like a dog. *J. Vet. Behav.* 4:68–69.

167. Baumgardt, B. R. and A. D. Peterson. 1970. Hyperphagia in sheep induced by infusion of the ventriculo cisternal system with a depressant. *Fed. Proc.* 29:760.

168. Beach, F. A. 1974. Effects of gonadal hormones on urinary behavior in dogs. *Physiol. Behav.* 12:1005–1013.
169. Beach, F. A. 1970. Coital behavior in dogs. VI. Long-term effects of castration upon mating in the male. *J. Comp. Physiol. Psychol.* 70:1–32.
170. Beach, F. A. 1970. Coital behaviour in dogs. VIII. Social affinity, dominance and sexual preference in the bitch. *Behaviour* 36:131–148.
171. Beach, F. A. 1968. Coital behavior in dogs. III. Effects of early isolation on mating in males. *Behaviour* 30:218–238.
172. Beach, F. A., M. G. Buehler and I. F. Dunbar. 1983. Development of attraction to estrous females in male dogs. *Physiol. Behav.* 31:293–297.
173. Beach, F. A., I. F. Dunbar and M. G. Buehler. 1982. Sexual characteristics of female dogs during successive phases of the ovarian cycle. *Horm. Behav.* 16:414–442.
174. Beach, F. A. and R. W. Gilmore. 1949. Response of male dogs to urine from females in heat. *J. Mammal.* 30:391–392.
175. Beach, F. A., A. I. Johnson, J. J. Anisko and I. F. Dunbar. 1977. Hormonal control of sexual attraction in pseudohermaphroditic female dogs. *J. Comp. Physiol. Psychol.* 91:711–715.
176. Beach, F. A. and R. E. Kuehn. 1970. Coital behavior in dogs. X. Effects of androgenic stimulation during development of feminine mating responses in females and males. *Horm. Behav.* 1:347–367.
177. Beach, F. A., R. E. Kuehn, R. H. Sprague and J. J. Anisko. 1972. Coital behavior in dogs. XI. Effects of androgenic stimulation during development on masculine mating responses in females. *Horm. Behav.* 3:143–168.
178. Beach, F. A. and B. J. Leboeuf. 1967. Coital behavior in dogs. I. Preferential mating in the bitch. *Anim. Behav.* 15:546–558.
179. Beach, F. A. and A. Merari. 1968. Coital behavior in dogs. IV. Effects of progesterone in the bitch. *Proc. Natl. Acad. Sci. U. S. A.* 61:442–446.
180. Beamer, W., G. Bermant and M. T. Clegg. 1969. Copulatory behaviour of the ram, *Ovis aries*. II: Factors affecting copulatory satiation. *Anim. Behav.* 17:706–711.
181. Beattie, V. E. and N. E. O. O'Connell. 2002. Relationship between rooting behaviour and foraging in growing pigs. *Anim. Welfare* 11:295–303.
182. Beattie, V. E., N. Walker and I. A. Sneddon. 1995. Effect of rearing environment and change of environment on the behaviour of gilts. *Appl. Anim. Behav. Sci.* 46:57–65.
183. Beauchemin, K. A., S. Zelin, D. Genner and J. G. Buchanan-Smith. 1989. An automatic system for quantification of eating and ruminating activities of dairy cattle housed in stalls. *J. Dairy. Sci.* 72:2746–2759.
184. Beaudet, R. A., A. Chalifoux and A. Dallaire. 1994. Predictive value of activity level and behavioral evaluation on future dominance in puppies. *Appl. Anim. Behav. Sci.* 40:273–284.
185. Beausoleil, N. J., D. Blache, K. J. Stafford, D. J. Mellor and A. D. L. Noble. 2008. Exploring the basis of divergent selection for 'temperament' in domestic sheep. *Appl. Anim. Behav. Sci.* 109:261–274.
186. Beausoleil, N. J., K. J. Stafford and D. J. Mellor. 2006. Does direct human eye contact function as a warning cue for domestic sheep (*Ovis aries*)? *J. Comp. Psychol.* 120:269–279.
187. Beaver, B. 1980. *Veterinary aspects of feline behavior*. St. Louis, MO: C.V. Mosby.
188. Beaver, B. V. 1999. *Canine behavior: A guide for veterinarians*. Philadelphia, PA: W.B. Saunders Company.
189. Beaver, B. V. 1993. Profiles of dogs presented for aggression. *J. Am. Anim. Hosp. Assoc.* 29:564–569.
190. Beaver, B. V. 1983. Clinical classification of canine aggression. *Appl. Anim. Ethol.* 10:35–43.
191. Beaver, B. V., M. Fischer and C. E. Atkinson. 1992. Determination of favorite components of garbage by dogs. *Appl. Anim. Behav. Sci.* 34:129–136.
192. Beck, A. M. 1973. *The ecology of stray dogs. A study of free-ranging urban animals*. Baltimore, MD: York Press.
193. Becker, B. A., J. J. Ford, R. K. Christenson, R. C. Manak, G. L. Hahn and J. A. DeShazer. 1985. Cortisol response of gilts in tether stalls. *J. Anim. Sci.* 60:264–270.
194. Becker, R. F., J. E. King and J. E. Markee. 1962. Studies on olfactory discrimination in dogs. II. Discriminatory behavior in a free environment. *J. Comp. Physiol. Psychol.* 55:773–780.
195. Beckett, S. D., R. S. Hudson and D. F. Walker. 1978. Effect of local anesthesia of the penis and dorsal penile neurectomy on the mating ability of bulls. *J. Am. Vet. Med. Assoc.* 173:838–839.
196. Beilharz, R. G. and D. F. Cox. 1967. Social dominance in swine. *Anim. Behav.* 15:117–122.
197. Beilharz, R. G. and P. J. Mylrea. 1963. Social position and behaviour of dairy heifers in yards. *Anim. Behav.* 11:522–528.

198. Beilharz, R. G. and P. J. Mylrea. 1963. Social position and movement orders of dairy heifers. *Anim. Behav.* 11:529–533.
199. Beilharz, R. G. and K. Zeeb. 1982. Social dominance in dairy cattle. *Appl. Anim. Ethol.* 8:79–97.
200. Bekoff, M. 1977. Social communication in canids: Evidence for the evolution of a stereotyped mammalian display. *Science* 197:1097–1099.
201. Bekoff, M. 1974. Social play and play-soliciting by infant canids. *Am. Zool.* 14:323–340.
202. Bekoff, M., H. L. Hill and J. B. Mitton. 1975. Behavioural taxonomy in canids by discriminant function analyses. *Science* 190:1223–1225.
203. Belkin, M., U. Yinon, L. Rose and I. Reisert. 1977. Effect of visual environment on refractive error of cats. *Doc. Ophthalmol.* 42:433–437.
204. Bell, F. R. 1963. Alkaline taste in goats assessed by the preference test technique. *J. Comp. Physiol. Psychol.* 56:174–178.
205. Bell, F. R. 1960. The electoencephalogram of goats during somnolence and rumination. *Anim. Behav.* 8:39–42.
206. Bell, F. R. 1959. Preference thresholds for taste discrimination in goats. *J. Agric. Sci.* 52:125–128.
207. Bell, F. R. and H. L. Williams. 1959. Threshold values for taste in monozygotic twin calves. *Nature* 183:345–346.
208. Bellinger, L. L., G. J. Trietley and L. L. Bernardis. 1976. Failure of portal glucose and adrenaline infusions or liver denervation to affect food intake in dogs. *Physiol. Behav.* 16:299–304.
209. Bellinger, L. L. and F. E. Williams. 1990. The effect of portal infusions of epinephrine on ingestion, plasma glucose and insulin in dogs. *Physiol. Behav.* 48:479–483.
210. Bench, C. J. and H. W. Gonyou. 2006. Effect of environmental enrichment at two stages of development on belly nosing in piglets weaned at fourteen days. *J. Anim. Sci.* 84:3397–3403.
211. Bennett, M., K. A. Houpt and H. N. Erb. 1988. Effects of declawing on feline behavior. *Companion Anim. Pract.* 2:7–12.
212. Berg, I. A. 1944. Development of behavior: The micturition pattern in the dog. *J. Exp. Psychol.* 34:343–368.
213. Berger, A., K.-M. Scheibe, K. Eichhorn, A. Scheibe and J. Streich. 1999. Diurnal and ultradian rhythms of behaviour in a mare group of Przewalski horse (*Equus ferus przewalskii*), measured through one year under semi-reserve conditions. *Appl. Anim. Behav. Sci.* 64:1–17.
214. Berger, J. 1986. *Wild horses of the grand basin*. Chicago, IL: The University of Chicago Press.
215. Berger, J. 1977. Organizational systems and dominance in feral horses in the grand canyon. *Behav. Ecol. Sociobiol.* 2:131–146.
216. Berggren-Thomas, B. and W. D. Hohenboken. 1986. The effects of sire-breed, forage availability and weather on the grazing behavior of crossbred ewes. *Appl. Anim. Behav. Sci.* 15:217–228.
217. Berkson, G. 1968. Maturation defects in kittens. *Am. J. Ment. Defic.* 72:757–777.
218. Berman, M. and I. Dunbar. 1983. The social behavior of free-ranging urban dogs. *Appl. Anim. Ethol.* 10:5–17.
219. Bermant, G., M. T. Clegg and W. Beamer. 1969. Copulatory behaviour of the ram, Ovis aries. I. A normative study. *Anim. Behav.* 17:700–705.
220. Bielanski, W. and S. Wierzbowski. 1961. Depletion test in stallions. *Proceedings of the 4th International Congress on Animal Reproduction*, pp. 279–282.
221. Bigelow, J. A. and T. R. Houpt. 1988. Feeding and drinking patterns in young pigs. *Physiol. Behav.* 43:99–109.
222. Billing, A. E. and M. A. Vince. 1987. Teat-seeking behaviour in newborn lambs. I. Evidence for the influence of material skin temperature. *Appl. Anim. Behav. Sci.* 18:301–313.
223. Billings, A. E. and M. A. Vince. 1987. Teat-seeking behaviour in newborn lambs. II. Evidence for the influence of the dam's surface textures and degree of surface yield. *Appl. Anim. Behav. Sci.* 18:315–325.
224. Billings, H. J. and L. S. Katz. 1999. Facilitation of sexual behavior in French-Alpine goats treated with intravaginal progesterone-releasing devices and estradiol during the breeding and nonbreeding seasons. *J. Anim. Sci.* 77:2073–2078.
225. Biquand, S. and V. Biquand-Guyot. 1992. The influence of peers, lineage and environment on food selection of the criollo goat (*Capra hircus*). *Appl. Anim. Behav. Sci.* 34:231–245.
226. Bitterman, M. E. 1965. Phyletic differences in learning. *Am. Psychol.* 20:396–410.
227. Bjone, S. J., W. Y. Brown and I. R. Price. 2009. Maternal influence on grass-eating behaviour in puppies. *J. Vet. Behav.* 4:97–98.

228. Bjork, A., N. G. Olsson, E. Christensson, K. Martinsson and O. Olsson. 1988. Effects of amperozide on biting behavior and performance in restricted-fed pigs following regrouping. *J. Anim. Sci.* 66:669–675.

229. Blackshaw, J. K., A. W. Blackshaw and J. J. McGlone. 1997. Buller steer syndrome review. *Appl. Anim. Behav. Sci.* 54:97–108.

230. Blackshaw, J. K., A. J. Swain, A. W. Blackshaw, F. J. M. Thomas and K. J. Gillies. 1997. The development of playful behaviour in piglets from birth to weaning in three farrowing environments. *Appl. Anim. Behav. Sci.* 55:37–49.

231. Blair, R. and J. FitzSimons. 1970. A note on the voluntary feed intake and growth of pigs given diets containing an extremely bitter compound. *Anim. Prod.* 12:529–530.

232. Blakemore, C. and R. C. Van Sluyters. 1975. Innate and environmental factors in the development of the kitten's visual cortex. *J. Physiol.* 248:663–716.

233. Bland, K. P. and B. M. Jubilan. 1987. Correlation of flehmen by male sheep with female behaviour and oestrus. *Anim. Behav.* 35:735–738.

234. Blaxter, K. L. 1944. Food preferences and habits in dairy cows. *Br. Soc. Anim Prod.* Second Meeting, 85–94.

235. Bleicher, N. 1962. Behavior of the bitch during parturition. *J. Am. Vet. Med. Assoc.* 140:1076–1082.

236. Blissitt, M. J., K. P. Bland and D. F. Cottrell. 1990. Olfactory and vomeronasal chemoreception and the discrimination of oestrous and non-oestrous ewe urine odours by the ram. *Appl. Anim. Behav. Sci.* 27:325–335.

237. Blockey, M. A. B. 1981. Development of a serving capacity test for beef bulls. *Appl. Anim. Ethol.* 7:307–319.

238. Blockey, M. A. B. 1981. Further studies on the serving capacity test for beef bulls. *Appl. Anim. Ethol.* 7:337–350.

239. Blockey, M. A. B. 1981. Modification of a serving capacity test for beef bulls. *Appl. Anim. Ethol.* 7:336.

240. Blom, A. K., K. Halse and K. Hove. 1976. Growth hormone, insulin and sugar in the blood plasma of bulls. Interrelated diurnal variations. *Acta Endocrinol. (Copenh)* 82:758–766.

241. Boe, K. E. 1993. Maternal behaviour of lactating sows in a loose-housing system. *Appl. Anim. Behav. Sci.* 35:327–338.

242. Boe, K. E. 1991. The process of weaning in pigs: When the sow decides. *Appl. Anim. Behav. Sci.* 30:47–59.

243. Boe, K. E. 1994. Variation in maternal behaviour and production of sows in integrated loose housing systems in Norway. *Appl. Anim. Behav. Sci.* 41:53–62.

244. Boe, K. E., S. Berg and I. L. Andersen. 2006. Resting behaviour and displacements in ewes—effects of reduced lying space and pen shape. *Appl. Anim. Behav. Sci.* 98:249–259.

245. Boe, K. E. and P. Jensen. 1995. Individual differences in suckling and solid food intake by piglets. *Appl. Anim. Behav. Sci.* 42:183–192.

246. Boissy, A. and M.-F. Bouissou. 1995. Assessment of individual differences in behavioural reactions of heifers exposed to various fear-eliciting situations. *Appl. Anim. Behav. Sci.* 46:17–31.

247. Boivin, X., P. Le Neindre and J. M. Chupin. 1992. Establishment of cattle-human relationship. *Appl. Anim. Behav. Sci.* 32:325–335.

248. Boivin, X., P. Le Neindre, J. M. Chupin, J. P. Garel and G. Trillat. 1992. Influence of breed and early management on ease of handling and open-field behaviour of cattle. *Appl. Anim. Behav. Sci.* 32:313–323.

249. Boivin, X., R. Nowak, G. Despres, H. Tournadre and P. Le Neindre. 1997. Discrimination between shepherds by lambs reared under artificial conditions. *J. Anim. Sci.* 75:2892–2898.

250. Bollen, K. S. and J. Horowitz. 2008. Behavioral evaluation and demographic information in the assessment of aggressiveness in shelter dogs. *Appl. Anim. Behav. Sci.* 112:120–135.

251. Booth, W. D. and B. A. Baldwin. 1980. Lack of effect on sexual behaviour or the development of testicular function after removal of olfactory bulbs in prepubertal boars. *J. Reprod. Fertil.* 58:173–182.

252. Borchelt, P. L. 1991. Cat elimination behavior problems. *Vet. Clin. N. Am. Small Anim. Pract.* 21:257–264.

253. Borchelt, P. L. 1983. Aggressive behavior of dogs kept as companion animals: Classification and influence of sex, reproductive status and breed. *Appl. Anim. Ethol.* 10:45–61.

254. Borchelt, P. L., R. Lockwood, A. M. Beck and V. L. Voith. 1983. Attacks by packs of dogs involving predation on human beings. *Public Health Rep.* 98:57–66.

255. Borchelt, P. L. and V. L. Voith. 1996. Aggressive behavior in cats. In V. L. Voith and P. L. Borchelt (Eds.), *Readings in companion animal*, pp. 208–216. Trenton, NJ: Veterinary Learning Systems.

256. Borchelt, P. L. and V. L. Voith. 1996. Dominance aggression in the dog. In V. L. Voith and P. L. Borchelt (Eds.), *Readings in companion animal behavior*, pp. 230–246. Trenton, NJ: Veterinary Learning Systems.

257. Borchelt, P. L. and V. L. Voith. 1985. Aggressive behavior in dogs and cats. *Comp. Contin. Ed.* 11:949–957.

258. Borchelt, P. L. and V. L. Voith. 1985. Punishment. *Comp. Contin. Ed.* 9:780–791.

259. Borchelt, P. L. and V. L. Voith. 1981. Elimination behavior problems in cats. *Comp. Contin. Ed.* 3:730–737.

260. Bordi, A., G. DeRosa, F. Napolitano, M. Litterio, V. Marino and R. Rubino. 1994. Postpartum development of the mother-young relationship in goats. *Appl. Anim. Behav. Sci.* 42:145–152.

261. Borg, K. E., K. L. Esbenshade and B. H. Johnson. 1993. Effects of the peri-pubertal rearing environment on endocrine and behavioural responses in oestrous female exposure in the mature bull. *Appl. Anim. Behav. Sci.* 35:245–253.

262. Bottoms, G. D., O. F. Roesel, F. D. Rausch and E. L. Akins. 1972. Circadian variation in plasma cortisol and corticosterone in pigs and mares. *Am. J. Vet. Res.* 33:785–790.

263. Bouissou, M.-F. 1978. Effect of injections of testosterone propionate on dominance relationships in a group of cows. *Horm. Behav.* 11:388–400.

264. Bouissou, M.-F. 1971. Effet de l'absence d'informations optiques et de contact physique sur la manifestation des relations hierarchiques chez les bovine domestiques. *Ann. Biol. Anim. Biochem. Biophys.* 11:191–198.

265. Bouissou, M.-F. 1965. Observations sur la hierarchie social chez les bovins domestiques. *Ann. Biol. Anim. Biochem. Biophys.* 5:327–339.

266. Bouissou, M.-F. and V. Gaudioso. 1982. Effect of early androgen treatment on subsequent social behavior in heifers. *Horm. Behav.* 16:132–146.

267. Bowersox, S. S., T. L. Baker and W. C. Dement. 1984. Sleep-wakefulness patterns in the aged cat. *Electroencephalogr. Clin. Neurophysiol.* 58:240–252.

268. Bowling, A. T. and R. W. Touchberry. 1990. Parentage of great-basin feral horses. *J. Wildl. Manag.* 54:424–429.

269. Boy, V. and P. Duncan. 1979. Time budgets of camargue horses. I. Development changes in the time budgets of foals. *Behaviour* 71:187–202.

270. Boyd, L. 1998. The 24-h time budget of a takh harem stallion (*Equus ferus przewalskii*) pre- and post-reintroduction. *Appl. Anim. Behav. Sci.* 60:291–299.

271. Boyd, L. and N. Bandi. 2002. Reintroduction of takhi, *Equus ferus przewalskii*, to Hustai National Park, Mongolia: Time budget and synchrony of activity pre- and post-release. *Appl. Anim. Behav. Sci.* 78:87–102.

272. Boyd, L. E. 1980. *The nationality, foal suvivorship, and mare-foal behavior of feral horses in Wyoming's Red Desert*. Laramie, WY: University of Wyoming.

273. Bracke, M. B. M., J. J. Zonderland, P. Lenskens, W. G. P. Schouten, H. Vermeer, H. A. M. Spoolder, H. J. M. Hendriks and H. Hopster. 2006. Formalised review of environmental enrichment for pigs in relation to political decision making. *Appl. Anim. Behav. Sci.* 98:165–182.

274. Bradshaw, J. and C. Cameron-Beaumont. 2000. The signaling repertoire of the domestic cat and its undomesticated relatives. In D. C. Turner and P. Bateson (Eds.), *The domestic cat: The biology of its behaviour*, pp. 68–93. Cambridge, UK: Cambridge University Press.

275. Bradshaw, J. W. S. 1992. *The behaviour of the domestic cat*. Wallingford, UK: CAB International.

276. Bradshaw, J. W. S., E. J. Blackwell and R. A. Casey. 2009. Dominance in domestic dogs—useful construct or bad habit? *J. Vet. Behav.* 4:135–144.

277. Brakel, W. J. and R. A. Leis. 1976. Impact of social disorganization on behavior, milk yield, and body weight of dairy cows. *J. Dairy Sci.* 59:716–721.

278. Branson, N. J. and L. J. Rogers. 2006. Relationship between paw preference strength and noise phobia in Canis familiaris. *J. Comp. Psychol.* 120:176–183.

279. Bray, A. R. and M. Wodzicka-Tomaszewska. 1974. Perinatal behaviour and progesterone and corticosteroid levels in sheep. *Proc. Aust. Soc. Anim. Prod.* 10:318–321.

280. Breland, K. and M. Breland. 1966. *Animal behavior*. New York, NY: Macmillan.

281. Brenoe, U. T., A. G. Larsgard, K.-R. Johannessen and S. H. Uldal. 2002. Estimates of genetic parameters for hunting performance traits in three breeds of gun hunting dogs in Norway. *Appl. Anim. Behav. Sci.* 77:209–215.

282. Bressers, H. P. M., J. H. A. Te Brake, B. Engel and J. P. T. M. Noordhuizen. 1993. Feeding order of sows at an individual electronic feed station in a dynamic group-housing system. *Appl. Anim. Behav. Sci.* 36:123–134.

283. Brindley, E. L., D. J. Bullock and F. Maisels. 1989. Effects of rain and fly harassment on feeding behaviour of free-ranging feral goats. *Appl. Anim. Behav. Sci.* 24:31–41.

284. Brisbin, I. L. Jr and S. N. Austad. 1991. Testing the individual odour theory of canine olfaction. *Appl. Anim. Behav. Sci.* 42:63–69.

285. Bristol, F. 1982. Breeding behaviour of a stallion at pasture with 20 mares in synchronized oestrus. *J. Reprod. Fertil. Suppl.* 32:71–77.

286. Brobeck, J. R. 1955. Neural regulation of food intake. *Ann. N. Y. Acad. Sci.* 63:44–55.

287. Bronson, F. H. and W. K. Whitten. 1968. Oestrus-accelerating pheromone of mice: Assay, androgen-dependency and presence in bladder urine. *J. Reprod. Fertil.* 15:131–134.

288. Bronson, R. T. 1979. Brain weight:body weight scaling in breeds of dogs and cats. *Brain Behav. Evol.* 16:227–236.

289. Broom, D. M. and J. D. Leaver. 1978. Effects of group-rearing or partial isolation on later social behaviour of calves. *Anim. Behav.* 26:1255–1263.

290. Brouns, F. and S. A. Edwards. 1994. Social rank and feeding behaviour of group-housed sows fed competitively or ad libitum. *Appl. Anim. Behav. Sci.* 39:225–235.

291. Brouns, F., S. A. Edwards and P. R. English. 1994. Effect of dietary fibre and feeding system on activity and oral behaviour of group housed gilts. *Appl. Anim. Behav. Sci.* 39:215–223.

292. Brown, J. A., C. Dewey, C. F. M. Delange, I. B. Mandell, P. P. Purslow, J. A. Robinson, E. J. Squires and T. M. Widowski. 2009. Reliability of temperament tests on finishing pigs in group-housing and comparison to social tests. *Appl. Anim. Behav. Sci.* 118:28–35.

293. Brown, R. F., K. A. Houpt and H. F. Schryver. 1976. Stimulation of food intake in horses by diazepam and promazine. *Pharmacol. Biochem. Behav.* 5:495–497.

294. Brownlee, A. 1954. Play in domestic cattle in Britain: An analysis of its nature. *Br. Vet. J.* 110:48–68.

295. Bryant, M. J. 1975. A note on the effect of rearing experience upon the development of sexual behaviour in ram lambs. *Anim. Prod.* 21:97–99.

296. Bryant, M. J. and R. Ewbank. 1972. Some effects of stocking rate and group size upon agonistic behaviour in groups of growing pigs. *Br. Vet. J.* 128:64–70.

297. Bryant, M. J. and T. Tompkins. 1973. Sexual behaviour of sheep. *Vet. Rec.* 93:253.

298. Buchenauer, V. D. and B. Fritsch. 1980. Zum farbsehvermogen von hausziegen (*Capra bircus* L.). *Z. Tierpsychol.* 53:225–230.

299. Buckner, L. J., S. A. Edwards and J. M. Bruce. 1998. Behaviour and shelter use by outdoor sows. *Appl. Anim. Behav. Sci.* 57:69–80.

300. Budzynska, M. and D. M. Weary. 2008. Weaning distress in dairy calves: Effects of alternative weaning procedures. *Appl. Anim. Behav. Sci.* 112:33–39.

301. Burger, J. F. 1952. Sex physiology of pigs. *Onderstepoort J. Vet. Res. Suppl.* 2:1–218.

302. Burne, T. H., P. J. Murfitt and C. L. Gilbert. 2001. Influence of environmental temperature on PGF(2alpha)-induced nest building in female pigs. *Appl. Anim. Behav. Sci.* 71:293–304.

303. Burne, T. H., P. J. Murfitt and C. L. Gilbert. 2000. Deprivation of straw bedding alters PGF(2alpha)-induced nesting behaviour in female pigs. *Appl. Anim. Behav. Sci.* 69:215–225.

304. Burritt, E. A., H. F. Mayland, F. D. Provenza, R. L. Miller and J. C. Burns. 2005. Effect of added sugar on preference and intake by sheep of hay cut in the morning versus the afternoon. *Appl. Anim. Behav. Sci.* 94:245–254.

305. Burritt, E. A. and F. D. Provenza. 1997. Effect of an unfamiliar location on the consumption of novel and familiar foods by sheep. *Appl. Anim. Behav. Sci.* 54:317–325.

306. Burritt, E. A. and F. D. Provenza. 1992. Lambs form preferences for nonnutritive flavors paired with glucose. *J. Anim. Sci.* 70:1133–1136.

307. Burritt, E. A. and F. D. Provenza. 1991. Ability of lambs to learn with a delay between food ingestion and consequences given meals containing novel and familiar foods. *Appl. Anim. Behav. Sci.* 32:179–189.

308. Buskirk, D. D., A. J. Zanella, T. M. Harrigan, J. L. Van Lente, L. M. Gnagey and M. J. Kaercher. 2003. Large round bale feeder design affects hay utilization and beef cow behavior. *J. Anim. Sci.* 81:109–115.

309. Busnel, R.-G. 1963. *Acoustic behaviour of animals.* Amsterdam, The Netherlands: Elsevier Publishing Co.

310. Cairns, R. B. and D. L. Johnson. 1965. The development of interspecies social attachments. *Psychonom. Sci.* 2:337–338.

311. Cameron, E. Z. and W. L. Linklater. 2000. Individual mares bias investment in sons and daughters in relation to their condition. *Anim. Behav.* 60:359–367.

312. Cameron, E. Z., W. L. Linklater, K. J. Stafford and E. O. Minot. 2008. Maternal investment results in better foal condition through increased play behaviour in horses. *Anim. Behav.* 76:1511–1518.

313. Cameron, E. Z., K. J. Stafford, W. L. Linklater and C. J. Veltman. 1999. Suckling behaviour does not measure milk intake in horses, Equus caballus. *Anim. Behav.* 57:673–678.

314. Campbell, K. J., G. S. Baxter, P. J. Murray, B. E. Coblentz and C. J. Donlan. 2007. Development of a prolonged estrus effect for use in Judas goats. *Appl. Anim. Behav. Sci.* 102:12–23.

315. Campbell, R. G. 1976. A note on the use of a feed flabour to stimulate the feed intake of weaner pigs. *Anim. Prod.* 23:417–419.

316. Campbell, S. S. and I. Tobler. 1984. Animal sleep: A review of sleep duration across phylogeny. *Neurosci. Biobehav. Rev.* 8:269–300.

317. Campbell, W. E. 1989. *Better behavior in dogs and cats.* Loveland, CO: Alpine Publications, Inc.

318. Campbell, W. E. and A. Campbell. 1972. A behavior test for puppy selection. *Mod. Vet. Pract.* 12:29–33.

319. Campion, D. P. and B. F. Leek. 1997. Investigation of a "fibre appetite" in sheep fed a "long fibre-free" diet. *Appl. Anim. Behav. Sci.* 52:79–86.

320. Campitelli, S., C. Carenzi and M. Verga. 1982. Factors which influence parturition in the mare and development of the foal. *Appl. Anim. Ethol.* 9:7–14.

321. Canali, E., M. Varga, M. Montagna and A. Baldi. 1986. Social interactions and induced behavioural reactions in milk-fed female calves. *Appl. Anim. Behav. Sci.* 16:207–215.

322. Candland, D. K. and D. Milne. 1966. Species differences in approach-behaviour as a function of developmental environment. *Anim. Behav.* 14:539–545.

323. Carlstead, K. 1986. Predictability of feeding: Its effect on agonistic behaviour and growth in grower pigs. *Appl. Anim. Behav. Sci.* 16:25–38.

324. Caro, T. M. 1980. Effects of the mother, object play, and adult experience on predation in cats. *Behav. Neural Biol.* 29:29–51.

325. Caro, T. M. 1980. Predatory behaviour and social play in kittens. *Behaviour* 76:1–24.

326. Caro, T. M. 1980. Predatory behaviour in domestic cat mothers. *Behaviour* 74:128–148.

327. Carroll, J., C. J. Murphy, M. Neitz, J. N. Hoeve and J. Neitz. 2001. Photopigment basis for dichromatic color vision in the horse. *J. Vis.* 1:80–87.

328. Carson, K. and D. G. Wood-Gush. 1983. Behaviour of thoroughbred foals during nursing. *Equine Vet. J.* 15:257–262.

329. Carson, K. and D. G. M. Wood-Gush. 1983. Equine behaviour: I. A review of the literature on social and dam foal behaviour. *Appl. Anim. Ethol.* 10:165–178.

330. Carver, D. S. and H. N. Waterhouse. 1962. The variation in the water consumption of cats. *Proc. Anim. Care. Panel* 12:267–270.

331. Caspi, A., J. McClay, T. E. Moffitt, J. Mill, J. Martin, I. W. Craig, A. Taylor and R. Poulton. 2002. Role of genotype in the cycle of violence in maltreated children. *Science* 297:851–854.

332. Cassady, J. P. 2007. Evidence of phenotypic relationships among behavioral characteristics of individual pigs and performance. *J. Anim. Sci.* 85:218–224.

333. Cassini, M. H. and H. N. Hermitte. 1962. Patterns of environmental use by cattle and consumption of supplemental food blocks. *Appl. Anim. Behav. Sci.* 32:297–312.

334. Castonguay, T. W. 1981. Dietary dilution and intake in the cat. *Physiol. Behav.* 27:547–549.

335. Castren, H., B. Algers, A. M. DePassille, J. Rushen and K. Uvnas-Moberg. 1993. Preparturient variation in progesterone, prolactin, oxytocin and somatostatin in relation to nest building in sows. *Appl. Anim. Behav. Sci.* 38:91–102.

336. Cerny, V. A. 1977. Failure of dihydrotestosterone to elicit sexual behaviour in the female cat. *J. Endocrinol.* 75:173–174.

337. Cervantes, M., R. Ruelas and C. Beyer. 1983. Serotonergic influences on EEG synchronization induced by milk drinking in the cat. *Pharmacol. Biochem. Behav.* 18:851–855.

338. Chakraborty, P. K., W. B. Panko and W. S. Fletcher. 1980. Serum hormone concentrations and their relationships to sexual behavior at the first and second estrous cycles of the labrador bitch. *Biol. Reprod.* 22:227–232.

339. Chamberlain, B., F. R. Ervin, R. O. Pihl and S. N. Young. 1987. The effect of raising or lowering tryptophan levels on aggression in vervet monkeys. *Pharmacol. Biochem. Behav.* 28:503–510.

340. Champion, R. A., N. A. Lagstrom and A. J. Rook. 2007. Motivation of sheep to eat clover offered in a short-term closed economy test. *Appl. Anim. Behav. Sci.* 108:263–275.

341. Champion, R. A., S. M. Rutter, P. D. Penning and A. J. Rook. 1994. Temporal variation in grazing behavior of sheep and the reliability of sampling periods. *Appl. Anim. Behav. Sci.* 42:99–108.

342. Chase, L. E., P. J. Wangsness and B. R. Baumgardt. 1976. Feeding behavior of steers fed a complete mixed ration. *J. Dairy Sci.* 59:1923–1928.

343. Chaya, L., E. Cowan and B. Mcguire. 2006. A note on the relationship between time spent in turnout and behaviour during turnout in horses (*Equus caballus*). *Appl. Anim. Behav. Sci.* 98:155–160.

344. Chemineau, P. 1986. Sexual behavior and gonadal activity during the year in the tropical creole meat goat. I. Female estrous behavior and ovarian activity. *Reprod. Nutr. Develop.* 26:441–442.

345. Chen, J., Q. Weng, J. Chao, D. Hu and K. Taya. 2008. Reproduction and development of the released Przewalski's horses (*∗Equus przewalskii* in Xinjiang, China). *J. Equine Sci.* 19:1–7.

346. Chepko, B. D. 1971. A preliminary study of the effects of play deprivation on young goats. *Z. Tierpsychol.* 28:517–526.

347. Chesler, P. 1969. Maternal influence in learning by observation in kittens. *Science* 166:901–903.

348. Christensen, E., J. Scarlett, M. Campagna and K. A. Houpt. 2007. Aggressive behavior in adopted dogs that passed a temperament test. *Appl. Anim. Behav. Sci.* 106:85–95.

349. Christensen, H. R., G. W. Seifert and T. B. Post. 1982. The relationship between a serving capacity test and fertility of beef bulls. *Aust. Vet. J.* 58:241–244.

350. Christensen, J. W., L. J. Keeling and B. L. Nielsen. 2005. Responses of horses to novel visual, olfactory an auditory stimuli. *Appl. Anim. Behav. Sci.* 93:53–65.

351. Christensen, J. W., J. Ladewig, E. Sondergaard and J. Malmkvist. 2002. Effects of individual versus group stabling on social behaviour in domestic stallions. *Appl. Anim. Behav. Sci.* 75:233–248.

352. Christensen, J. W. and M. Rundgren. 2008. Predator odour *per se* does not frighten domestic horses. *Appl. Anim. Behav. Sci.* 112:136–145.

353. Christensen, J. W., T. Zharkikh and J. Ladwig. 2008. Do horses generalise between objects during habituation? *Appl. Anim. Behav. Sci.* 114:509–520.

354. Christiansen, F. O., M. Bakken and B. O. Braastad. 2001. Behavioural changes and aversive conditioning in hunting dogs by the second-year confrontation with domestic sheep. *Appl. Anim. Behav. Sci.* 72:131–143.

355. Christiansen, F. O., M. Bakken and B. O. Braastad. 2001. Social facilitation of predatory, sheep-chasing behaviour in Norwegian elkhounds, grey. *Appl. Anim. Behav. Sci.* 72:105–114.

356. Christie, D. W. and E. T. Bell. 1972. Studies on canine reproductive behaviour during the normal oestrous cycle. *Anim. Behav.* 20:621–631.

357. Church, S. C., J. A. Allen and J. W. S. Bradshaw. 1994. Anti-apostatic food selection by the domestic cat. *Anim. Behav.* 48:747–749.

358. Cizek, L. J., R. E. Semple, K. C. Huang and M. I. Gregersen. 1951. Effect of extracellular electrolyte depletion on water intake in dogs. *Am. J. Physiol.* 164:415–422.

359. Clark, D. K., T. H. Friend and G. Dellmeier. 1993. The effect of orientation during trailer transport on heart rate, cortisol and balance in horses. *Appl. Anim. Behav. Sci.* 38:179–189.

360. Clark, J. R., R. W. Bell, L. F. Tribble and A. M. Lennon. 1985. Effects of composition and density of the group on the performance, behaviour and age at puberty in swine. *Appl. Anim. Behav. Sci.* 14:127–135.

361. Clarke, I. J. and R. J. Scaramuzzi. 1978. Sexual behaviour and LH secretion in spayed androgenized ewes after a single injection of testosterone or oestradiol-17beta. *J. Reprod. Fertil.* 52:313–320.

362. Clegg, H. A., P. Buckley, M. A. Friend and P. D. McGreevy. 2008. The ethological and physiological characteristics of cribbing and weaving horses. *Appl. Anim. Behav. Sci.* 109:68–76.

363. Clegg, M. T., W. Beamer and G. Bermant. 1969. Copulatory behaviour of the ram, *Ovis aries*. III. Effects of pre- and postpubertal castration and androgen replacement therapy. *Anim. Behav.* 17:712–717.

364. Clutton-Brock, T. H., P. J. Greenwood and R. P. Powell. 1976. Ranks and relationships in highland ponies and highland cows. *Z. Tierpsychol.* 41:202–216.

365. Cohen-Tannoudji, J., J. Einhorn and J. P. Signoret. 1994. Ram sexual pheromone: First approach of chemical identification. *Physiol. Behav.* 56:955–961.

366. Cohen-Tannoudji, J., A. Locatelli and J. P. Signoret. 1986. Non-pheromonal stimulation by the male of LH release in the anoestrous ewe. *Physiol. Behav.* 36:921–924.

367. Cohn, R. 1956. A contribution to the study of color vision in cat. *J. Neurophysiol.* 19:416–423.

368. Coile, D. C., C. H. Pollitz and J. C. Smith. 1989. Behavioral determination of critical flicker fusion in dogs. *Physiol. Behav.* 45:1087–1092.

369. Cole, D. D. and J. N. Shafer. 1966. A study of social dominance in cats. *Behaviour* 27:39–53.

370. Cole, D. J. A., J. E. Duckworth and W. Holmes. 1967. Factors affecting voluntary feed intake in pigs. I. The effect of digestible energy content of the diet on the intake of castrated male pigs housed in holding pens and in metabolism crates. *Anim. Prod.* 9:141–148.

371. Collard, R. R. 1967. Fear of strangers and play behavior in kittens with varied social experience. *Child Dev.* 38:877–891.

372. Collias, N. E. 1956. The analysis of socialization in sheep and goats. *Ecology* 37:228–239.
373. Collins, J. P. and G. H. Rose. 1975. Light-dark discrimination and reversal learning in early postnatal kittens. *Dev. Psychobiol.* 8:511–518.
374. Collis, K. A. 1976. An investigation of factors related to the dominance order of a herd of dairy cows of similar age and breed. *Appl. Anim. Ethol.* 2:167–173.
375. Collis, K. A., S. J. Kay, A. J. Grant and A. J. Quick. 1979. The effect on social organization and milk production of minor group alterations in dairy cattle. *Appl. Anim. Ethol.* 5:103–111.
376. Colson, V., P. Orgeur, A. Foury and P. Mormède. 2006. Consequences of weaning piglets at 21 and 28 days on growth, behaviour and hormonal responses. *Appl. Anim. Behav. Sci.* 98:70–88.
377. Concannon, P. W., W. Hansel and W. J. Visek. 1975. The ovarian cycle of the bitch: Plasma estrogen, LH and progesterone. *Biol. Reprod.* 13:112–121.
378. Cooling, M. J. and M. D. Day. 1975. Drinking behaviour in the cat induced by renin, angiotensin I, II and isoprenaline. *J. Physiol.* 244:325–336.
379. Cooper, J. J., N. Mcall, S. Johnson and H. P. B. Davidson. 2005. The short-term effects of increasing meal frequency on stereotypic behaviour of stabled horses. *Appl. Anim. Behav. Sci.* 90:351–364.
380. Cooper, J., I. J. Gordon and A. W. Pike. 2000. Strategies for the avoidance of faeces by grazing sheep. *Appl. Anim. Behav. Sci.* 69:15–33.
381. Cooper, J. J., C. Ashton, S. Bishop, R. West, D. S. Mills and R. J. Young. 2003. Clever hounds: Social cognition in the domestic dog (*Canis familiaris*). *Appl. Anim. Behav. Sci.* 81:229–244.
382. Cooper, J. J., L. McDonald and D. S. Mills. 2000. The effect of increasing visual horizons on stereotypic weaving: Implications for the social housing of stabled horses. *Appl. Anim. Behav. Sci.* 69:67–83.
383. Cooper, R. A., S. Evans and J. A. Kirk. 1991. Effects of water additives on water consumption, urine output and urine mineral levels in Angora goats. *Anim. Prod.* 52:609.
384. Coppinger, R., J. Lorenz, J. Glendinning and P. Pinardi. 1983. Attentiveness of guarding dogs for reducing predation on domestic sheep. *J. Range Manag.* 36:275–279.
385. Coppinger, R. and R. Schneider. 2006. Evolution of working dogs. In J. Serpell (Ed.), *The domestic dog: Its evolution, behaviour and interactions with people*, pp. 21–47. Cambridge, UK: Cambridge University Press.
386. Corbett, J. L. 1953. Grazing behaviour in New Zealand. *Br. J. Anim. Behav.* 1:67–71.
387. Corson, S. A., E. L. Corson, V. Kirilcuk, J. Kirilcuk, W. Knopp and L. E. Arnold. 1972. Differential effects of amphetamines on several types of hyperkinetic and normal dogs and on learning disability. *Psychopharmacology* 26(Suppl.): 55.
388. Cory, V. L. 1927. Activities of livestock on the range. *Tex. Agric. Exp. Sta. Bull.* 367:5–47.
389. Coulon, M., B. L. Deputte, Y. Heyman, L. Delatouce, C. Richard and C. Baudoin. 2007. Visual discrimination by heifers (Bos taurus) of their own species. *J. Comp. Psychol.* 121:198–204.
390. Cowlishaw, S. J. and F. E. Alder. 1960. The grazing preferences of cattle and sheep. *J. Agric. Sci. (Camb.)* 54:257–265.
391. Cracknell, N. R., D. S. Mills and P. Kaulfuss. 2008. Can stimulus enhancement explain the apparent success of the model-rival technique in the domestic dog (*Canis familiaris*)? *Appl. Anim. Behav. Sci.* 114:461–472.
392. Crawford, M. A., M. D. Kittleson and G. D. Fink. 1984. Hypernatremia and adipsia in a dog. *J. Am. Vet. Med. Assoc.* 184:818–821.
393. Creel, S. R. and J. L. Albright. 1988. The effects of neonatal social isolation on the behavior and endocrine function of Holstein calves. *Appl. Anim. Behav. Sci.* 21:293–306.
394. Cregier, S. W. 1982. Reducing equine hauling stress: A review. *J. Eq. Vet. Sci.* 2:187–198.
395. Cresswell, E. 1960. Ranging behaviour studies with romney marsh and cheviot sheep in New Zealand. *Anim. Behav.* 8:32–38.
396. Cresswell, E. 1959. A cattle rangemeter. *Anim. Behav.* 7:244.
397. Cronin, G. M., B. N. Schirmer, T. H. McCallum, J. A. Smith and K. L. Butler. 1993. The effects of providing sawdust to pre-parturient sows in farrowing crates on sow behaviour, the duration of parturition and the occurrence of intra-partum stillborn piglets. *Appl. Anim. Behav. Sci.* 36:301–315.
398. Cronin, G. M. and J. A. Smith. 2002. Effects of accommodation type and straw bedding around parturition and during lactation on the behaviour of primiparous sows and survival and growth of piglets to weaning. *Appl. Anim. Behav. Sci.* 33:191–208.
399. Cronin, G. M., P. R. Wiepkema and J. M. van Ree. 1986. Endorphins implicated in stereotypies of tethered sows. *Experientia* 42:198–199.

400. Crowell-Davis, S. 2002. Social behaviour, communication and development of behaviour in the cat. In D. Horwitz, D. Mills and S. Heath (Eds.), *BSAVA canine and feline behavioural medicine*. Quidgeley, UK: British Small Animal Veterinary Society.

401. Crowell-Davis, S. L. 2007. Sexual behavior of mares. *Horm. Behav.* 52:12–17.

402. Crowell-Davis, S. L. 1994. Daytime rest behavior of the Welsh pony (*Equus caballus*) mare and foal. *Anim. Behav.* 40:197–210.

403. Crowell-Davis, S. L. 1986. Spatial relations between mares and foals of the Welsh pony (*Equus caballus*). *Anim. Behav.* 34:1007–1015.

404. Crowell-Davis, S. L. 1985. Nursing behaviour and maternal aggression among Welsh ponies (*Equus caballus*). *Anim. Behav.* 14:11–25.

405. Crowell-Davis, S. L., K. Barry, J. M. Ballam and D. P. Laflamme. 1995. The effect of caloric restriction on the behavior of pen-housed dogs: Transition from unrestricted to restricted diet. *Appl. Anim. Behav. Sci.* 43:27–41.

406. Crowell-Davis, S. L., K. Barry and R. Wolfe. 1997. Social behavior and aggressive problems of cats. *Vet. Clin. N. Am.: Small Anim. Pract.* 27:549–568.

407. Crowell-Davis, S. L. and A. B. Caudle. 1989. Coprophagy by foals: Recognition of maternal feces. *Appl. Anim. Behav. Sci.* 24:267–272.

408. Crowell-Davis, S. L. and K. A. Houpt. 1985. Coprophagy by foals: Effect of age and possible functions. *Equine Vet. J.* 17:17–19.

409. Crowell-Davis, S. L. and K. A. Houpt. 1985. The ontogeny of flehmen in horses. *Anim. Behav.* 33:739–774.

410. Crowell-Davis, S. L., K. A. Houpt and J. S. Burnham. 1985. Snapping by foals of Equus caballus. *Z. Tierpsychol.* 69:42–54.

411. Crowell-Davis, S. L., K. A. Houpt and C. M. Carini. 1986. Mutual grooming and nearest-neighbor relationships among foals of Equus caballus. *Appl. Anim. Behav. Sci.* 15:113–123.

412. Crowell-Davis, S. L., K. A. Houpt and J. Carnevale. 1985. Feeding and drinking behavior of mares and foals with free access to pasture and water. *J. Anim. Sci.* 60:883–889.

413. Crowell-Davis, S. L., K. A. Houpt and L. Kane. 1987. Play development in Welsh pony (*Equus caballus*) foal. *Appl. Anim. Behav. Sci.* 18:119–131.

414. Cummings, B. J., E. Head, W. Ruehl, N. W. Milgram and C. W. Cotman. 1996. The canine as an animal model of human aging and dementia. *Neurobiol. Aging* 17:259–268.

415. Curley, K. O. Jr, J. C. Paschal, T. H. Welsh Jr and R. D. Randel. 2006. Technical note: Exit velocity as a measure of cattle temperament is repeatable and associated with serum concentration of cortisol in Brahman bulls. *J. Anim. Sci.* 84:3100–3103.

416. Curtis, Q. F. 1937. Experimental neurosis in the pig. *Psychol. Bull.* 34:723.

417. Curtis, T. M., R. J. Knowles and S. L. Crowell-Davis. 2003. Influence of familiarity and relatedness on proximity and allogrooming in domestic cats (*Felis catus*). *Am. J. Vet. Res.* 64:1151–1154.

418. Czarkowska, J. 1983. Changes of some postural reflexes during the first postnatal weeks in the dog. *Acta Neurobiol. Exp. (Wars)* 43:27–35.

419. Dabrowska, B., W. Harmata, Z. Lenkiewicz, Z. Schiffer and R. J. Wojtusiak. 1981. Colour perception in cows. *Behav. Proc.* 6:1–10.

420. Daels, P. F. and J. P. Hughes. 1992. The abnormal estrous cycle. In A. O. McKinnon and J. L. Voss (Eds.), *Equine reproduction*, pp. 144–171. Malvern, PA: Lea & Febiger.

421. Dailey, J. W. and J. J. McGlone. 1997. Oral/nasal/facial and other behaviors of sows kept individually outdoors on pasture, soil or indoors in gestation crates. *Appl. Anim. Behav. Sci.* 52:25–43.

422. Dallaire, A. R. Y. 1974. Sleep and wakefulness in the housed pony under different dietary conditions. *Can. J. Comp. Med.* 38:65–71.

423. Dallaire, A. and Y. Ruckebusch. 1974. Sleep patterns in the pony with observations on partial perceptual deprivation. *Physiol. Behav.* 12:789–796.

424. Dalmau, A., E. Fabrega and A. Velarde. 2009. Fear assessment in pigs exposed to a novel object test. *Appl. Anim. Behav. Sci.* 117:173–180.

425. Dalton, D. C., M. E. Pearson and M. Sheard. 1967. The behaviour of dairy bulls kept in groups. *Anim. Prod.* 9:1–5.

426. Damm, B. I., B. Forkman and L. J. Pedersen. 2005. Lying down and rolling behaviour in sows in relation to piglet crushing. *Appl. Anim. Behav. Sci.* 9:3–20.

427. Damm, B. I., V. Moustsen, E. Jorgensen, L. J. Pedersen, T. Heiskanen and B. Forkman. 2006. Sow preferences for walls to lean against when lying down. *Appl. Anim. Behav. Sci.* 99:53–63.

428. Daniels, T. J. 1983. The social organization of free-ranging urban dogs. I. Non-estrus social behavior. *Appl. Anim. Ethol.* 10:341–363.
429. Daniels, T. J. 1983. The social organization of free-ranging urban dogs. II. Estrus groups and the mating system. *Appl. Anim. Ethol.* 10:365–373.
430. Dantzer, R. 1977. Effects of diazepam on conditioned suppression in pigs. *J. Pharmacol.* 8:405–414.
431. Dantzer, R. 1976. Effect of diazepam on performance of pigs in a progressive ratio schedule. *Physiol. Behav.* 17:161–163.
432. Dantzer, R. and B. A. Baldwin. 1974. Changes in heart rate during suppression of operant responding in pigs. *Physiol. Behav.* 12:385–391.
433. Dantzer, R. and B. A. Baldwin. 1974. Effects of chlordiazepoxide on heart rate and behavioural suppression in pigs subjected to operant conditioning procedures. *Psychopharmacologia* 37:169–177.
434. Dantzer, R., P. Mormede and B. Favre. 1976. Fear-dependent variations in continuous avoidance behavior of pigs. II. Effects of diazepam on acquisition and performance of Pavlovian fear conditioning and plasma corticosteroid levels. *Psychopharmacology (Berl)* 49:75–78.
435. Dards, J. L. 1983. The behaviour of dockyard cats: Interactions of adult males. *Appl. Anim. Behav. Sci.* 19:133–153.
436. Darke, P. G. 1978. Obesity in small animals. *Vet. Rec.* 102:545–546.
437. Davis, C. N., L. E. Davis and T. E. Powers. 1975. Comparative body compositions of the dog and goat. *Am. J. Vet. Res.* 36:309–311.
438. Davis, J. L. and R. A. Jensen. 1976. The development of passive and active avoidance learning in the cat. *Dev. Psychobiol.* 9:175–179.
439. Dawson, W. M. and R. L. Revens. 1946. Varying susceptibility in pigs to alarm. *J. Comp. Physiol. Psychol.* 39:297–305.
440. Day, J. E. L., I. Kyriazakis and A. B. Lawrence. 1995. The effect of food deprivation on the expression of foraging and exploratory behaviour in the growing pig. *Appl. Anim. Behav. Sci.* 42:193–206.
441. De Boer, J. 1977. The age of olfactory cues functioning in chemocommunication among male domestic cats. *Behav. Proc.* 2:209–225.
442. de Jong, I. C., I. T. Prelle, J. A. van de Burgwal, E. Lambooij, S. M. Korte, H. J. Blokhuis and J. M. Koolhaas. 2000. Effects of environmental enrichment on behavioral responses to novelty, learning, and memory, and the circadian rhythm in cortisol in growing pigs. *Physiol. Behav.* 68:571–578.
443. de Passille, A. M. and J. Rushen. 2006. What components of milk stimulate sucking in calves? *Appl. Anim. Behav. Sci.* 101:243–252.
444. De Paula Vieira, A., V. Guesdon, A. M. de Passille, M. A. G. von Keyserlingk and D. M. Weary. 2008. Behavioural indicators of hunger in dairy calves. *Appl. Anim. Behav. Sci.* 109:180–189.
445. de Sevilla, X. F., J. Casellas, J. Tibau and E. Fabrega. 2009. Consistency and influence on performance of behavioural differences in large white and landrace purebred pigs. *Appl. Anim. Behav. Sci.* 117: 13–19.
446. De Vuyst, A., G. Thines, L. Henriet and M. Soffie. 1964. Influence of auditory stimulations on the sexual behavior of the bull. *Experientia* 20:648–650.
447. D'Eath, R. B. 2005. Socialising piglets before weaning improves social hierarchy formation when pigs are mixed post-weaning. *Appl. Anim. Behav. Sci.* 93:199–211.
448. D'Eath, R. B. 2002. Individual aggressiveness measured in a resident-intruder test predicts the persistence of aggressive behaviour and weight gain of young pigs after mixing. *Appl. Anim. Behav. Sci.* 77:267–283.
449. deJonge, F. H., M. Ooms, W. W. Kuurman, J. H. R. Maes and B. M. Spruijt. 2008. Are pigs sensitive to variability in food rewards? *Appl. Anim. Behav. Sci.* 114:93–104.
450. deLahunta, A. 1977. *Veterinary neuroanatomy and clinical neurology*. Philadelphia, PA: W.B. Saunders Company.
451. Delgadillo, J. A., P. Poindron, D. Krehbiel, G. Duarte and E. Rosales. 1997. Nursing, suckling and postpartum anoestrus of creole goats kidding in January in subtropical Mexico. *Appl. Anim. Behav. Sci.* 55:91–101.
452. Deligeorgis, S. G., K. Karalis and G. Kanzouros. 2006. The influence of drinker location and colour on drinking behaviour and water intake of newborn pigs under hot environments. *Appl. Anim. Behav. Sci.* 96:233–244.
453. Delius, K., M. Gunderoth-Palmowski, I. Krause and W. Engelmann. 1984. Effects of lithium salts on the behaviour and the circadian system of *Mesocricetus auratus* W. *J. Interdiscipl. Cycle Res.* 15:299.
454. Delude, L. A. 1986. Activity patterns and behavior of sled dogs. *Appl. Anim. Behav. Sci.* 15:161–168.

455. DeNapoli, J. S., N. H. Dodman, L. Shuster, W. M. Rand and K. L. Gross. 2000. Effect of dietary protein content and tryptophan supplementation on dominance aggression, territorial aggression, and hyperactivity in dogs. *J. Am. Vet. Med. Assoc.* 217:504–508.

456. Denton, D. 1982. *The hunger for salt*. Berlin, Germany: Springer-Verlag.

457. DePassille, A. M. B., J. H. M. Metz, P. Mekking and P. R. Wiepkema. 1992. Does drinking milk stimulate sucking in young calves? *Appl. Anim. Behav. Sci.* 34:23–36.

458. DePew, C. L., D. L. Thompson Jr, J. M. Fernandez, L. L. Southern, L. S. Sticker and T. L. Ward. 1994. Plasma concentrations of prolactin, glucose, insulin, urea nitrogen, and total amino acids in stallions after ingestion of feed or gastric administration of feed components. *J. Anim. Sci.* 72:2345–2353.

459. Deswysen, A. G., W. C. Ellis and K. R. Pond. 1987. Interrelationships among voluntary intake, eating and ruminating behavior and ruminal motility of heifers fed corn silage. *J. Anim. Sci.* 64:835–841.

460. Devenport, J. A., M. R. Patterson and L. D. Devenport. 2005. Dynamic averaging and foraging decisions in horses (*Equus callabus*). *J. Comp. Psychol.* 119:352–358.

461. Devilat, J., W. G. Pond and P. D. Miller. 1970. Dietary amino acid balance in growing-finishing pigs: Effect of diet preference and performance. *J. Anim. Sci.* 30:536–543.

462. Diakow, C. 1971. Effects of genital desensitization on mating behavior and ovulation in the female cat. *Physiol. Behav.* 7:47–54.

463. Dickson, D. P., G. R. Barr and D. A. Wieckert. 1967. Social relationship of dairy cows in a feed lot. *Behaviour* 29:195–203.

464. Diesel, G., D. Brodbelt and D. U. Pfeiffer. 2008. Reliability of assessment of dogs' behavioural responses by staff working at a welfare charity in the UK. *Appl. Anim. Behav. Sci.* 115:171–181.

465. Dijkhuizen, T. J. and F. J. van Eerdenburg. 1997. Behavioural signs of oestrus during pregnancy in lactating dairy cows. *Vet. Q.* 19:194–196.

466. Dinger, J. E. and E. E. Noiles. 1986. Effect of controlled exercise on libido in 2-yr-old stallions. *J. Anim. Sci.* 62:1220–1223.

467. Dinius, D. A. and C. A. Baile. 1977. Beef cattle response to a feed intake stimulant given alone and in combination with a propionate enhancer and an anabolic agent. *J. Anim. Sci.* 45:147–153.

468. Distel, R. A., J. J. Villalba and H. E. Laborde. 1994. Effects of early experience on voluntary intake of low-quality roughage by sheep. *J. Anim. Sci.* 72:1191–1195.

469. Distel, R. A., J. J. Villalba, H. E. Laborde and M. A. Burgos. 1996. Persistence of the effects of early experience on consumption of low-quality roughage by sheep. *J. Anim. Sci.* 74:965–968.

470. Dodman, N. H., J. A. Normile, L. Shuster and W. Rand. 1994. Equine self-mutilation syndrome (57 cases). *J. Am. Vet. Med. Assoc.* 204:1219–1223.

471. Dodman, N. H., I. Reisner, L. Shuster, W. Rand, U. A. Luescher, I. Robinson and K. A. Houpt. 1996. Effect of dietary protein content on behavior in dogs. *J. Am. Vet. Med. Assoc.* 208:376–379.

472. Dodman, N. H., L. Shuster, M. H. Court and R. Dixon. 1987. Investigation into the use of narcotic antagonists in the treatment of a stereotypic behavior pattern (crib-biting) in the horse. *Am. J. Vet. Res.* 48:311–319.

473. Dodman, N. H., L. Shuster, M. H. Court and J. Patel. 1988. Use of a narcotic antagonist (nalmefene) to suppress self-mutilative behavior in a stallion. *J. Am. Vet. Med. Assoc.* 192:1585–1586.

474. Donaldson, L. E. and J. W. James. 1963. A connection between pregnancy and crush order in cows. *Anim. Behav.* 11:286.

475. Donovan, C. A. 1967. Some clinical observations on sexual attraction and deterrence in dogs and cattle. *Vet. Med. Small: Anim. Clin.* 62:1047–1051.

476. Donovan, C. A., L. Badinga, R. J. Collier, C. J. Wilcox and R. K. Braun. 1986. Factors influencing passive transfer in dairy calves. *J. Dairy Sci.* 69:754–759.

477. Doran, C. W. 1943. Activities and grazing habits of sheep on summer ranges. *J. Forestry* 41:253–258.

478. Dore, F. Y., S. Fiset, S. Goulet, M. C. Dumas and S. Gagnon. 1996. Search behavior in cats and dogs: Interspecific differences in working memory and spatial cognition. *Anim. Learn. Behav.* 24:142–149.

479. Dorries, K. M., E. Adkins-Regan and B. P. Halpern. 1995. Olfactory sensitivity to the pheromone, androstenone, is sexually dimorphic in the pig. *Physiol. Behav.* 57:255–259.

480. Dorries, K. M., E. Adkins-Regan and B. P. Halpern. 1991. Sex difference in olfactory sensitivity to the boar chemosignal, androstenone, and the domestic pig. *Anim. Behav.* 42:403–411.

481. Doty, R. L. and I. Dunbar. 1974. Attraction of beagles to conspecific urine, vaginal and anal sac secretion odors. *Physiol. Behav.* 12:825–833.

482. Dougherty, C. T., F. W. Knapp, P. B. Burrus, D. C. Willis and N. W. Bradley. 1993. Face flies (*Musca autumnalis* de geer) and the behavior of grazing beef cattle. *Appl. Anim. Behav. Sci.* 35:313–326.

483. Dougherty, D. M. and P. Lewis. 1993. Generalization of a tactile stimulus in horses. *J. Exp. Anal. Behav.* 59:521–528.

484. Dourmad, J. Y. 1993. Standing and feeding behaviour of the lactating sow: Effect of feeding level during pregnancy. *Appl. Anim. Behav. Sci.* 37:311–319.

485. Dove, H. R., R. G. Beilharz and J. L. Black. 1974. Dominance patterns and positional behaviour of sheep in yards. *Anim. Prod.* 19:157–168.

486. Dreschel, N. A. and D. A. Granger. 2005. Physiological and behavioral reactivity to stress in thunderstorm-phobic dogs and their caregivers. *Appl. Anim. Behav. Sci.* 95:153–168.

487. Dresher, M., I. M. A. Heitkonig, J. G. Raats and H. H. T. Prins. 2006. The role of grass stems as structural foraging deterrents and their effects on the foraging behaviour of cattle. *Appl. Anim. Behav. Sci.* 101:10–26.

488. Drickamer, L. C., R. D. Arthur and T. L. Rosenthal. 1999. Predictors of social dominance and aggression in gilts. *Appl. Anim. Behav. Sci.* 63:121–129.

489. Duckworth, J. E. and D. W. Shirlaw. 1958. A study of factors affecting feed intake and the eating behaviour of cattle. *Anim. Behav.* 6:147–154.

490. Dudink, S., H. Simonse, I. Marks, F. H. deJonge and B. M. Spruijt. 2006. Announcing the arrival of enrichment increases play behaviour and reduces weaning-stress-induced behaviours of piglets directly after weaning. *Appl. Anim. Behav. Sci.* 101:86–101.

491. Dufty, J. H. 1973. Clinical studies on bovine parturition–foetal aspects. *Aust. Vet. J.* 49:177–182.

492. Dufty, J. H. 1972. Clinical studies on bovine parturition. Maternal causes of dystocia and stillbirth in an experimental herd of Hereford cattle. *Aust. Vet. J.* 48:1–6.

493. Dufty, J. H. 1971. Determination of the onset of parturition in Hereford cattle. *Aust. Vet. J.* 47:77–82.

494. Dumas, C., B. St-Louis and L. Routhier. 2006. Decision making and interference in the domestic cat (*Felis catus*). *J. Comp. Psychol.* 120:367–377.

495. Dunbar, I. and M. Buehler. 1980. A masking effect of urine from male dogs. *Appl. Anim. Ethol.* 6:297–301.

496. Dunbar, I. F. 1978. Olfactory preferences in dogs: The response of male and female beagles to conspecific urine. *Biol. Behav.* 3:273–286.

497. Dunbar, I. F. and M. Carmichael. 1981. The response of male dogs to urine from other males. *Behav. Neural. Biol.* 31:465–470.

498. Dunbar, R. I. M., D. Buckland and D. Miller. 1990. Mating strategies of male feral goats: A problem in optimal foraging. *Anim. Behav.* 40:653–667.

499. Duncan, A. J. and S. A. Young. 2002. Can goats learn about foods through conditioned food aversions and preferences when multiple food options are simultaneously available? *J. Anim. Sci.* 80:2091–2098.

500. Duncan, P. 1985. Time-budgets of Camargue horses III. Environmental influences. *Behaviour* 92:188–208.

501. Duncan, P. 1980. Time-budgets of Camargue horses II. Time-budgets of adult horses and weaned sub-adults. *Behaviour* 72:26–49.

502. Duncan, P. and P. Cowtan. 1980. An unusual choice of habitat helps Camargue horses to avoid blood-sucking horse-flies. *Biol. Behav.* 5:55–60.

503. Duncan, P., P. H. Harvey and S. M. Wells. 1984. On lactation and associated behaviour in a natural herd of horses. *Anim. Behav.* 32:255–263.

504. Duquette, P. F. and L. A. Muir. 1979. Monitoring the effects of selected compounds on feeding behaviour of sheep. *J. Anim. Sci.* 49:1120–1124.

505. Durr, R. and C. Smith. 1997. Individual differences and their relation to social structure in domestic cats. *J. Comp. Psychol.* 111:412–418.

506. Durrer, J. L. and J. P. Hannon. 1962. Seasonal variations in caloric intake of dogs living in an arctic environment. *Am. J. Physiol.* 202:375–378.

507. Duvaux-Ponter, C., K. Rigalma, S. Roussel-Huchette, Y. Schawlb and A. A. Ponter. 2008. Effect of a supplement rich in linolenic acid, added to the diet of gestating and lactating goars, on the sensitivity to stress and learning ability of their offspring. *Appl. Anim. Behav. Sci.* 114:373–394.

508. Duxbury, M. M., J. A. Jackson, S. W. Line and R. K. Anderson. 2003. Evaluation of association between retention in the home and attendance at puppy socialization classes. *J. Am. Vet. Med. Assoc.* 223:61–66.

509. Dworkin, S. 1939. Conditioning neuroses in dog and cat. *Psychosom. Med.* 1:388–396.

510. Dwyer, C. M. 2008. Individual variation in the expression of maternal behaviour: A review of the neuroendocrine mechanisms in the sheep. *J. Neuroendocrinol.* 20:526–534.

511. Dwyer, C. M. 2003. Behavioural development in the neonatal lamb: Effect of maternal and birth-related factors. *Theriogenology* 59:1027–1050.

512. Dwyer, C. M., W. S. Dingwall and A. B. Lawrence. 1999. Physiological correlates of maternal-offspring behaviour in sheep: A factor analysis. *Physiol. Behav.* 67:443–454.
513. Dwyer, C. M. and A. B. Lawrence. 2000. Effects of maternal genotype and behaviour on the behavioural development of their offspring in sheep. *Behaviour* 137:1629–1654.
514. Dwyer, C. M. and A. B. Lawrence. 1999. Ewe-ewe and ewe-lamb behaviour in a hill and a lowland breed of sheep: A study using embryo transfer. *Appl. Anim. Behav. Sci.* 61:319–334.
515. Dwyer, C. M., K. A. McLean, L. A. Deans, J. Chirnside, S. K. Calvert and A. B. Lawrence. 1998. Vocalisations between mother and young in sheep: Effects of breed and maternal experience. *Appl. Anim. Behav. Sci.* 58:105–119.
516. Dwyer, C. M. and L. A. Smith. 2008. Parity effects on maternal behaviour are not related to circulating oestradiol concentrations in two breeds of sheep. *Physiol. Behav.* 93:148–154.
517. Dybkjaer, L., A. P. Jacobsen, F. A. Togersen and H. D. Poulsen. 2006. Eating and drinking activity of newly weaned piglets: Effects of individual characteristics, social mixing, and addition of extra zinc to the feed. *J. Anim. Sci.* 84:702–711.
518. Dyck, G. W., E. E. Swierstra, R. M. McKay and K. Mount. 1987. Effect of location of the teat suckled, breed and parity on piglet growth. *Can. J. Anim. Sci.* 67:929–939.
519. Dziba, L. E. and F. D. Provenza. 2008. Dietary monoterpene concentrations influence feeding patterns of lambs. *Appl. Anim. Behav. Sci.* 109:49–57.
520. Ebenezer, I. S., R. F. Parrott and S. V. Vellucci. 1999. Effects of the 5-HT1A receptor agonist 8-OH-DPAT on operant food intake in food-deprived pigs. *Physiol. Behav.* 67:213–217.
521. Eccles, R. 1982. Autonomic innervation of the vomeronasal organ of the cat. *Physiol. Behav.* 28:1011–1015.
522. Echeverri, A. C., H. W. Gonyou and A. W. Ghent. 1992. Preparturient behavior of confined ewes: Time budgets, frequencies, spatial distribution and sequential analysis. *Appl. Anim. Behav. Sci.* 34:329–344.
523. Eckstein, P. and S. Zuckerman. 1956. The oestrous cycle in the mammalia. In A. S. Parkes (Ed.), *Marshall's physiology of reproduction*, pp. 226–396. London, UK: Longmans, Green and Co.
524. Eckstein, R. A. and B. L. Hart. 2000. The organization and control of grooming in cats. *Appl. Anim. Behav. Sci.* 68:131–140.
525. Edwards, S. A. 1982. Factors affecting time to first suckling in dairy calves. *Anim. Prod.* 34:339–346.
526. Edwards, S. A. and D. M. Broom. 1982. Behavioural interactions of dairy cows with their newborn calves and the effects of parity. *Anim. Behav.* 30:525–535.
527. Ehrenlechner, S. and J. Unshelm. 1997. Whisker trimming by mother cats. *Appl. Anim. Behav. Sci.* 52:181–185.
528. Ehret, C. F., V. R. Potter and K. W. Dobra. 1975. Chronotypic action of theophylline and of pentobarbital as circadian zeitgebers in the rat. *Science* 188:1212–1215.
529. Ekkel, E. D., B. Savenije, W. G. Schouten, V. M. Wiegant and M. J. Tielen. 1997. The effects of mixing on behavior and circadian parameters of salivary cortisol in pigs. *Physiol. Behav.* 62:181–184.
530. Eldridge, F. and Y. Suzuki. 1976. A mare mule–dam or foster mother? *J. Hered.* 67:353–360.
531. Elia, J. B. 2002. *The effects of diets differing in fiber content on equine behavior and motivation for fiber.* Ithaca, NY: Cornell University Press.
532. Ellendorff, F., N. Parvizi, D. K. Pomerantz, A. Hartjen, A. Konig, D. Smidt and F. Elsaesser. 1975. Plasma luteinizing hormone and testosterone in the adult male pig: 24 hour fluctuations and the effect of copulation. *J. Endocrinol.* 67:403–410.
533. Elliot, O. and J. A. King. 1960. Effect of early food deprivation upon later consummatory behavior in puppies. *Psychol. Rep.* 6:391–400.
534. Elliot, O. and J. P. Scott. 1961. The development of emotional distress reactions to separation, in puppies. *J. Genet. Psychol.* 99:3–22.
535. Elliott, J. A., M. H. Stetson and M. Menaker. 1972. Regulation of testis function in golden hamsters: A circadian clock measures photoperiodic time. *Science* 178:771–773.
536. Ellis, S. L. H. and D. L. Wells. 2008. The influence of visual stimulation on the behaviour of cats housed in a rescue shelter. *Appl. Anim. Behav. Sci.* 113:166–174.
537. Ely, F. and W. E. Petersen. 1941. Factors involved in the ejection of milk. *J. Dairy Sci.* 24:211–223.
538. England, G. J. 1954. Observations on the grazing behaviour of different breeds of sheep at Pantryhuad Farm, Carmarthenshire. *Br. J. Anim. Behav.* 2:56–60.
539. Entsu, S., H. Dohi and A. Yamada. 1992. Visual acuity of cattle determined by the method of discrimination learning. *Appl. Anim. Behav. Sci.* 34:1–10.

540. Erhard, H. W., D. A. Elston and G. C. Davidson. 2006. Habituation and extinction in an approach-avoidance test: An example with sheep. *Appl. Anim. Behav. Sci.* 99:132–144.

541. Erhard, H. W. and M. Mendl. 1997. Measuring aggressiveness in growing pigs in a resident-intruder situation. *Appl. Anim. Behav. Sci.* 54:123–136.

542. Erlinger, L. L., D. R. Tolleson and C. J. Brown. 1990. Comparison of bite size, biting rate and grazing time of beef heifers from herds distinguished by mature size and rate of maturity. *J. Anim. Sci.* 68:3578–3587.

543. Escobar, J., W. G. Van Alstine, D. H. Baker and R. W. Johnson. 2007. Behaviour of pigs with viral and bacterial pneumonia. *Appl. Anim. Behav. Sci.* 105:42–50.

544. Escos, J., C. L. Alados and J. Boza. 1993. Leadership in a domestic goat herd. *Appl. Anim. Behav. Sci.* 38:41–47.

545. Esselmont, R. J., R. G. Glencross, M. J. Bryant and G. S. Pope. 1980. A quantitative study of pre-ovulatory behaviour in cattle (British Friesian heifers). *Appl. Anim. Ethol.* 6:1–17.

546. Estep, D. Q., S. L. Crowell-Davis, S.-A. Earl-Costello and S. A. Beatey. 1993. Changes in the social behaviour of drafthorse (*Equus caballus*) mares coincident with foaling. *Appl. Anim. Behav. Sci.* 35:199–213.

547. Evans, J. W., C. M. Winget, C. De Roshia and D. C. Holley. 1976. Ovulation and equine body temperature and heart rate circadian rhythms. *J. Interdiscip. Cycle Res.* 7:25–37.

548. Everitt, G. C. and D. S. M. Phillips. 1971. Calf rearing by multiple suckling and the effects of lactation performance of the cow. *Proc. N. Z. Soc. Anim. Prod.* 31:22–40.

549. Ewbank, R. 1973. Abnormal behaviour and pig nutrition. An unsuccessful attempt to induce tail biting by feeding a high energy, low fibre vegetable protein ration. *Br. Vet. J.* 129:366–369.

550. Ewbank, R. 1967. Behavior of twin cattle. *J. Dairy Sci.* 50:1510–1512.

551. Ewbank, R. 1967. Nursing and suckling behaviour amongst clun forest ewes and lambs. *Anim. Behav.* 15:251–258.

552. Ewbank, R. 1964. Observations on the suckling habits of twin lambs. *Anim. Behav.* 12:34–37.

553. Ewbank, R. 1963. Predicting the time of parturition in the normal cows: A study of the precalving drop in body temperature in relation to the external signs of imminent calving. *Vet. Rec.* 75:367–370.

554. Ewbank, R. and M. J. Bryant. 1972. Aggressive behaviour amongst groups of domesticated pigs kept at various stocking rates. *Anim. Behav.* 20:21–28.

555. Ewbank, R. and A. C. Mason. 1967. A note on the sucking behaviour of twin lambs reared as singles. *Anim. Prod.* 9:417–420.

556. Ewbank, R., G. B. Meese and J. E. Cox. 1974. Individual recognition and the dominance hierarchy in the domesticated pig. The role of sight. *Anim. Behav.* 22:473–480.

557. Ewer, R. F. 1959. Suckling behaviour in kittens. *Behaviour* 15:146–162.

558. Ewer, R. F. 1973. *The carnivores.* Ithaca, NY: Cornell University Press.

559. Ezeh, P. I., L. J. Myers, L. A. Hanrahan, R. J. Kemppainen and K. A. Cummins. 1992. Effects of steroids on the olfactory function of the dog. *Physiol. Behav.* 51:1183–1187.

560. Fabre-Nys, C. and H. Gelez. 2007. Sexual behavior in ewes and other domestic ruminants. *Horm. Behav.* 52:18–25.

561. Faerevik, G., I. L. Andersen and K. E. Boe. 2005. Preferences of sheep for different types of pen flooring. *Appl. Anim. Behav. Sci.* 90:265–276.

562. Fagen, R. M. and T. K. George. 1977. Play behavior and exercise in young ponies (*Equus caballus*). *Behav. Ecol. Sociobiol.* 2:267–269.

563. Falewee, C., E. Gaultier, C. Lafont, L. Bougrat and P. Pageat. 2006. Effect of a synthetic equine maternal pheromone during a controlled fear-eliciting situation. *Appl. Anim. Behav. Sci.* 101:144–153.

564. Farley, G. R., S. M. Barlow, R. Netsell and J. V. Chmelka. 1992. Vocalizations in the cat: Behavioral methodology and spectrographic analysis. *Exp. Brain Res.* 89:333–340.

565. Farmer, C. and S. Robert. 2006. Behavioural responses of sows and piglets from two genotypes to recorded nursing grunts played throughout lactation. *Appl. Anim. Behav. Sci.* 96:33–42.

566. Farner, D. S. 1961. Comparative physiology: Photoperiodicity. *Annu. Rev. Physiol.* 23:71–96.

567. Feaver, J., M. Mendl and P. Bateson. 1986. A method for rating the individual distinctiveness of domestic cats. *Anim. Behav.* 34:1016–1025.

568. Feddess, J. J. R., B. A. Young and J. A. DeShazor. 1989. Influence of temperature and light on feeding behaviour in pigs. *Appl. Anim. Behav. Sci.* 23:215–222.

569. Feh, C. 1999. Alliances and reproductive success in Camargue stallions. *Anim. Behav.* 57:705–713.

570. Feh, C. 1990. Long-term paternity data in relation to different aspects of rank for Camargue stallions, Equus caballus. *Anim. Behav.* 40:995–996.

571. Feh, C. and J. de Mazieres. 1993. Grooming at a preferred site reduces heart rate in horses. *Anim. Behav.* 46:1191–1194.

572. Feh, C. and B. Munkhtuya. 2008. Male infanticide and paternity analyses in a socially natural herd of Przewalski's horses: Sexual selection? *Behav. Proc.* 78:335–339.

573. Feist, J. D. and D. R. McCullough. 1976. Behavior patterns and communication in feral horses. *Z. Tierpsychol.* 41:337–371.

574. Feist, J. D. and D. R. McCullough. 1975. Reproduction in feral horses. *J. Reprod. Fertil. Suppl.* 23:13–18.

575. Feldman, H. N. 1994. Domestic cats and passive submission. *Anim. Behav.* 47:457–459.

576. Feldman, H. N. 1993. Maternal care and differences in the use of nests in the domestic cat. *Anim. Behav.* 45:13–23.

577. Feldmann, B. M. 1974. The problem of urban dogs. *Science* 185:903.

578. Feldmann, B. M. and T. H. Carding. 1973. Free-roaming urban pets. *Health Serv. Rep.* 88:956–962.

579. Ferreira, A., A. Carrau, E. Rodas, E. Rubianes and A. Benech. 1992. Diazepam facilitates acceptance of alien lambs by postparturient ewes. *Physiol. Behav.* 51:1117–1121.

580. Ferreira, G., A. Terrazas, P. Poindron, R. Nowak, P. Orgeur and F. Levy. 2000. Learning of olfactory cues is not necessary for early lamb recognition by the mother. *Physiol. Behav.* 69:405–412.

581. Ferrell, F. 1984. Preference for sugars and nonnutritive sweeteners in young beagles. *Neurosci. Biobehav. Rev.* 8:199–203.

582. Feuerstein, N. and J. Terkel. 2008. Interrelationships of dogs (*Canis familiaris*) and cats (*Felis catus L.*) living under the same roof. *Appl. Anim. Behav. Sci.* 113:150–165.

583. Finger, K. H. and H. Brummer. 1969. Suckling habits of calves reared without cows. *Dtsch. Tierarztl. Wochenschr.* 76:665–667.

584. Firth, E. C. 1980. Bilateral ventral accessory neurectomy in windsucking horses. *Vet. Rec.* 106:30–32.

585. Fiset, S. and F. Y. Dore. 2006. Duration of cats' (*Felis catus*) working memory for disappearing objects. *Anim. Cogn.* 9:62–70.

586. Fiset, S., S. Gagnon and C. Beaulieu. 2000. Spatial encoding of hidden objects in dogs (*Canis familiaris*). *J. Comp. Psychol.* 114:315–324.

587. Fiset, S., F. Landry and M. Ouellette. 2006. Egocentric search for disappearing objects in domestic dogs: Evidence for a geometric hypothesis of direction. *Anim. Cogn.* 9:1–12.

588. Fisher, A. D., M. Stewart, G. A. Verkerk, C. J. Morrow and L. R. Matthews. 2003. The effects of surface type on lying behaviour and stress responses in dairy cows during periodic weather-induced removal from pasture. *Appl. Anim. Behav. Sci.* 81:1–11.

589. Fisher, R. B. and M. L. Gardner. 1976. A diurnal rhythm in the absorption of glucose and water by isolated rat small intestine. *J. Physiol.* 254:821–825.

590. Fiske, J. C. and G. D. Potter. 1979. Discrimination reversal learning in yearling horses. *J. Anim. Sci.* 49:583–588.

591. Fitzgerald, J. A., A. Perkins and K. Hemenway. 1993. Relationship of sex and number of siblings in utero with sexual behavior of mature rams. *Appl. Anim. Behav. Sci.* 38:283–290.

592. Fitzsimons, J. T. and E. Szczepanska-Sadowska. 1974. Drinking and antidiuresis elicited by isoprenaline in the dog. *J. Physiol.* 239:251–267.

593. Flannery, B. 1997. Relational discrimination learning in horses. *Appl. Anim. Behav. Sci.* 54:267–280.

594. Flannigan, G. and N. H. Dodman. 2001. Risk factors and behaviors associated with separation anxiety in dogs. *J. Am. Vet. Med. Assoc.* 219:460–466.

595. Fletcher, I. C. and D. R. Lindsay. 1968. Sensory involvement in the mating behaviour of domestic sheep. *Anim. Behav.* 16:410–414.

596. Fleurance, G., H. Fritz, P. Duncan, I. J. Gordon, N. Edouard and C. Vial. 2009. Instantaneous intake rate in horses of different body sizes: Influence of sward biomass and fibrousness. *Appl. Anim. Behav. Sci.* 117:84–92.

597. Folman, Y. and R. Volcani. 1966. Copulatory behaviour of the prepubertally castrated bull. *Anim. Behav.* 14:572–573.

598. Fonberg, E. 1976. The relation between alimentary and emotional amygdalar regulation. In D. Novin, W. Wyrwicka and G. A. Bray (Eds.), *Hunger: Basic mechanisms and clinical implications*, pp. 61–75. New York, NY: Raven Press.

599. Fontenot, J. P. and R. E. Blaser. 1965. Symposium on factors influencing the voluntary intake of herbage by ruminants: Selection and intake by grazing animals. *J. Anim. Sci.* 24:1202–1208.

600. Foot, J. Z. and A. J. F. Russel. 1978. Pattern of intake of three roughage diets by nonpregnant, nonlactating Scottish blackface ewes over a long period and the effects of previous nutritional history on current intake. *Anim. Prod.* 26:203–215.

601. Forbes, J. M. 1995. *Voluntary food intake and diet selection in farm animals.* Wallingford, UK: CAB International.

602. Ford, J. J. and R. K. Christenson. 1981. Glucocorticoid inhibition of estrus in ovariectomized pigs: Relationship to progesterone action. *Horm. Behav.* 15:427–435.

603. Ford, J. J. and H. S. Teague. 1978. Effect of floor space restriction on age at puberty in gilts and on performance of barrows and gilts. *J. Anim. Sci.* 47:828–832.

604. Forkman, B., A. Boissy, M. C. Meunier-Salaun, E. Canali and R. B. Jones. 2007. A critical review of fear tests used on cattle, pigs, sheep, poultry and horses. *Physiol. Behav.* 92:340–374.

605. Forkman, B., I. L. Furuhaug and P. Jensen. 1995. Personality, coping patterns, and aggression in piglets. *Appl. Anim. Behav. Sci.* 45:31–42.

606. Forssell, G. 1926. The new surgical treatment against crib-biting. *Vet. J.* 82:538–548.

607. Foss, I. and G. Flottorp. 1974. A comparative study of the development of hearing and vision in various species commonly used in experiments. *Acta Otolaryngol.* 77:202–214.

608. Foster, J. A., M. Morrison, S. J. Dean, M. Hill and H. Frenk. 1981. Naloxone suppresses food/water consumption in the deprived cat. *Pharmacol. Biochem. Behav.* 14:419–421.

609. Foutz, A. S., M. M. Mitler and W. C. Dement. 1980. Narcolepsy. *Vet. Clin. N. Am.: Small Anim. Pract.* 10:65–80.

610. Fowler, D. G. and L. D. Jenkins. 1976. The effects of dominance and infertility of rams on reproductive performance. *Appl. Anim. Ethol.* 2:327–337.

611. Fox, M. W. 1975. The behaviour of cats. In E. S. E. Hafez (Ed.), *The behaviour of domestic animals*, pp. 410–436. Baltimore, MD: Williams & Wilkins.

612. Fox, M. W. 1972. *Understanding your dog.* New York, NY: Coward, McCann and Geoghegan.

613. Fox, M. W. 1971. *Integrative development of brain and behavior in the dog.* Chicago, IL: University of Chicago Press.

614. Fox, M. W. 1970. Reflex development and behavioral organization. In W. A. Himwich (Ed.), *Developmental neurobiology*, pp. 553–580. Springfield, IL: Charles C. Thomas.

615. Fox, M. W. 1968. *Abnormal behavior in animals.* Philadelphia, PA: W.B. Saunders Company.

616. Fox, M. W. and M. Bekoff. 1975. The behaviour of dogs. In E. S. E. Hafez (Ed.), *The behaviour of domestic animals*, pp. 370–409. Baltimore, MD: Williams & Wilkins.

617. Fox, M. W. and J. W. Spencer. 1967. Development of the delayed response in the dog. *Anim. Behav.* 15:162–168.

618. Fox, M. W. and G. Stanton. 1967. A developmental study of sleep and wakefulness in the dog. *J. Small Anim. Pract.* 8:605–611.

619. Fox, M. W. and D. Stelzner. 1966. Approach/withdrawal variables in the development of social behaviour in the dog. *Anim. Behav.* 14:362–366.

620. Fox, M. W. and D. Stelzner. 1966. Behavioural effects of differential early experience in the dog. *Anim. Behav.* 14:273–281.

621. Francis, D., J. Diorio, D. Liu and M. J. Meaney. 1999. Nongenomic transmission across generations of maternal behavior and stress responses in the rat. *Science* 286:1155–1158.

622. Francis-Smith, K. and D. G. Wood-Gush. 1977. Coprophagia as seen in thoroughbred foals. *Equine Vet. J.* 9:155–157.

623. Frank, D., M. Minero, S. Cannas and C. Palestrini. 2007. Puppy behaviours when left home alone: A pilot study. *Appl. Anim. Behav. Sci.* 104:61–70.

624. Frank, D. F., H. N. Erb and K. A. Houpt. 1999. Urine spraying in cats: Presence of concurrent disease and effects of a pheromone treatment. *Appl. Anim. Behav. Sci.* 61:263–272.

625. Frank, H. and M. G. Frank. 1983. Inhibition training in wolves and dogs. *Behav. Proc.* 8:363–377.

626. Franke Stevens, E. 1990. Instability of harems of feral horses in relation to season and presence of subordinate stallions. *Behaviour* 112:149–161.

627. Fraser, A. F. 1974. *Farm animal behaviour.* Baltimore, MD: Williams & Wilkins.

628. Fraser, A. F. 1968. *Reproductive behaviour in ungulates.* New York, NY: Academic Press.

629. Fraser, A. F. 1963. Behavior disorders in domestic animals. *Cornell Vet.* 53:213–223.

630. Fraser, D. 1987. Attraction to blood as a factor in tail-biting by pigs. *Appl. Anim. Behav. Sci.* 17:61–68.

631. Fraser, D. 1987. Mineral-deficient diets and the pig's attraction to blood: Implications of tail biting. *Can. J. Anim. Sci.* 67:909–918.

632. Fraser, D. 1977. Some behavioural aspects of milk ejection failure by sows. *Br. Vet. J.* 133:126–133.
633. Fraser, D. 1975. The effect of straw on the behaviour of sows in tether stalls. *Anim. Prod.* 21:59–68.
634. Fraser, D. 1975. The nursing and suckling behaviour of pigs. III. Behaviour when milk ejection is elicited by manual stimulation of the udder. *Br. Vet. J.* 131:416–426.
635. Fraser, D. 1975. The nursing and suckling behaviour of pigs. IV. the effect of interrupting the sucking stimulus. *Br. Vet. J.* 131:549–559.
636. Fraser, D. 1974. The behaviour of growing pigs during experimental social encounters. *J. Agric. Sci. (Camb.)* 82:147–163.
637. Fraser, D. 1974. The vocalizations and other behaviour of growing pigs in and "open field" test. *Appl. Anim. Behav. Sci.* 1:3–16.
638. Fraser, D. 1973. The nursing and suckling behaviour of pigs. I. The importance of stimulation of the anterior teats. *Br. Vet. J.* 129:324–336.
639. Fraser, D. and J. Rushen. 1993. A colostrum feeder for newborn lambs. *Appl. Anim. Behav. Sci.* 35:267–276.
640. Frazer-Sissom, D. E., D. A. Rice and G. Peters. 1991. How cats purr. *J. Zool. (Lond.)* 223:67–78.
641. Freedman, D. G. 1958. Constitutional and environmental interactions in rearing of four breeds of dogs. *Science* 127:585–586.
642. Freedman, D. G., J. A. King and O. Elliot. 1961. Critical period in the social development of dogs. *Science* 133:1016–1017.
643. Freeman, N. C. and J. S. Rosenblatt. 1978. The interrelationship between thermal and olfactory stimulation in the development of home orientation in newborn kittens. *Dev. Psychobiol.* 11:437–457.
644. Freeman, N. C. and J. S. Rosenblatt. 1978. Specificity of litter odors in the control of home orientation among kittens. *Dev. Psychobiol.* 11:459–468.
645. Freire, R., H. A. Clegg, P. Buckley, M. A. Friend and P. D. McGreevy. 2009. The effects of two different amounts of dietary grain on the digestibility of the diet and behaviour of intensively managed horses. *Appl. Anim. Behav. Sci.* 117:69–73.
646. Friend, D. W. 1973. Self-selection of feeds and water by unbred gilts. *J. Anim. Sci.* 37:1137–1141.
647. Friend, T. H., L. O'Connor, D. Knabe and G. Dellmeier. 1989. Preliminary trails of a sound-activated device to reduce crushing of piglets by sows. *Appl. Anim. Behav. Sci.* 24:23–29.
648. Froberg, S., E. Gratre, K. Svennersten-Sjaunja, I. Olsson, A. Orihuela, C. S. Galina, B. Garcia and L. Lidfors. 2008. Effect of suckling ('restricted suckling') on dairy cows' udder health and milk let-down and their calves' weight gain, feed intake and behaviour. *Appl. Anim. Behav. Sci.* 113:1–14.
649. Froberg, S. and L. Lidfors. 2009. Behaviour of dairy calves suckling the dam in a barn with automatic milking or being fed milk substitute from an automatic feeder in a group pen. *Appl. Anim. Behav. Sci.* 117:150–158.
650. Fuchs, T., C. Gaillard, S. Beghardt-Henrich, S. Ruefenacht and A. Steiger. 2005. External factors and reproducibility of the behaviour test in German shepherd dogs in Switzerland. *Appl. Anim. Behav. Sci.* 94:287–301.
651. Fuller, C. A., F. M. Sulzman and M. C. Moore-Ede. 1978. Thermoregulation is impaired in an environment without circadian time cues. *Science* 199:794–796.
652. Fuller, J. L. 1967. Experiential deprivation and later behavior. *Science* 158:1645–1652.
653. Fuller, J. L. 1956. Photoperiodic control of estrus in the Basenji. *J. Hered.* 47:179–180.
654. Fuller, J. L., C. A. Easler and E. M. Banks. 1950. Formation of conditioned avoidance responses in young puppies. *Am. J. Physiol.* 160:462–466.
655. Funston, R. N., D. D. Kress, K. M. Havstad and D. E. Doornbos. 1991. Grazing behavior of rangeland beef cattle differing in biological type. *J. Anim. Sci.* 69:1435–1442.
656. Gadbury, J. C. 1975. Some preliminary field observations on the order of entry of cows into herringbone parlours. *Appl. Anim. Ethol.* 1:275–281.
657. Gaebelein, C. J., R. A. Galosy, L. Botticelli, J. L. Howard and P. A. Obrist. 1977. Blood pressure and cardiac changes during signalled and unsignalled avoidance in dogs. *Physiol. Behav.* 19:69–74.
658. Gagnon, S. and F. Y. Dore. 1994. Cross-sectional study of object permanence in domestic puppies (Canis familiaris). *J. Comp. Psychol.* 108:220–232.
659. Ganjam, V. K. and R. M. Kenney. 1975. Androgens and oestrogens in normal and cryptorchid stallions. *J. Reprod. Fertil. Suppl.* 23: 67–73.
660. Ganskopp, D. 2001. Manipulating cattle distribution with salt and water in large arid-land pastures: A GPS/GIS assessment. *Appl. Anim. Behav. Sci.* 73:251–262.

661. Ganskopp, D., R. Cruz and D. E. Johnson. 2000. Least-effort pathways?: A GIS analysis of livestock trails in rugged terrain. *Appl. Anim. Behav. Sci.* 68:179–190.
662. Garbarg, M., C. Julien and J. C. Schwartz. 1974. Circadian rhythm of histamine in the pineal gland. *Life Sci.* 14:539–543.
663. Garcia, J., W. G. Hankins and K. W. Rusiniak. 1974. Behavioral regulation of the milieu interne in man and rat. *Science* 185:824–831.
664. Garcia, M. C., S. M. McDonnell, R. M. Kenney and H. G. Osborne. 1986. Bull sexual behavior tests: Stimulus cow affects performance. *Appl. Anim. Behav. Sci.* 16:1–10.
665. Gardner, L. P. 1945. Responses of sheep in a discrimination problem with variations of the position of the signal. *J. Comp. Physiol. Psychol.* 38:343–351.
666. Gardner, L. P. 1937. The responses of cows in a discrimination problem. *J. Comp. Psychol.* 23:35–57.
667. Gardner, L. P. 1937. The responses of cows to the same signal in different positions. *J. Comp. Psychol.* 23:333–350.
668. Gardner, L. P. 1937. The responses of horses in a discrimination problem. *J. Comp. Psychol.* 23:13–34.
669. Gardner, L. P. 1937. Responses of horses to the same signal in different positions. *J. Comp. Psychol.* 23:305–332.
670. Garner, R. H. 1963. The palatability of herbage plants. *J. Br. Grassland Soc.* 18:79–89.
671. Gary, L. A., G. W. Sherritt and E. B. Hale. 1970. Behavior of Charolais cattle on pasture. *J. Anim. Sci.* 30:203–206.
672. Gastal, M. O., E. L. Gastal, M. A. Beg and O. J. Ginther. 2007. Elevated plasma testosterone concentrations during stallion-like sexual behavior in mares (*Equus caballus*). *Horm. Behav.* 52:205–210.
673. Gaultier, E., L. Bonnafous, L. Bougrat, C. Lafont and P. Pageat. 2005. Comparison of the efficacy of a synthetic dog-appeasing pheromone with clomipramine for the treatment of separation-related disorders in dogs. *Vet. Rec.* 156:533–538.
674. Gaultier, E., L. Bonnafous, D. Vienet-Legue, C. Falewee, L. Bougrat, C. Lafont-Lecuelle and P. Pageat. 2008. Efficacy of dog-appeasing pheromone in reducing stress associated with social isolation in newly adopted puppies. *Vet. Rec.* 163:73–80.
675. Gaunet, F. 2008. How do guide dogs of blind owners and pet dogs of sighted owners (*Canis familiaris*) ask their owners for food? *Anim. Cogn.* 11:475–483.
676. Gazit, I., A. Goldblatt and J. Terkel. 2005. The role of context specificity in learning: The effects of training context on explosives detection in dogs. *Anim. Cogn.* 8:143–150.
677. Gazit, I. and J. Terkel. 2003. Explosives detection by sniffer dogs following strenuous physical activity. *Appl. Anim. Behav. Sci.* 81:149–161.
678. Geary, T. W. and J. J. Reeves. 1992. Relative importance of vision and olfaction for detection of estrus by bulls. *J. Anim. Sci.* 70:2726–2731.
679. Geist, V. 1971. *Mountain sheep. A study of behavior and evolution.* Chicago, IL: University of Chicago Press.
680. George, J. M. and I. A. Barger. 1974. Observations of bovine parturition. *Proc. Aust. Soc. Anim. Prod.* 10:314–317.
681. Georgsson, L. and J. Svendsen. 2002. Degree of competition at feeding differentially affects behavior and performance of group-housed growing-finishing pigs of different relative weights. *J. Anim. Sci.* 80:376–383.
682. Gerritsen, R., P. Langendijk, N. Soede and B. Kemp. 2005. Effects of artificial boar stimuli on the expression of oestrus in sows. *Appl. Anim. Behav. Sci.* 92:37–43.
683. Geverink, N. A., W. G. P. Schouten, G. Gort and V. M. Wiegant. 2002. Individual differences in aggression and physiology in peri-pubertal breeding gilts. *Appl. Anim. Behav. Sci.* 77:43–52.
684. Ghosh, B., D. K. Choudhuri and B. Pal. 1984. Some aspects of the sexual behaviour of stray dogs, *Canis familiaris*. *Appl. Anim. Behav. Sci.* 13:113–127.
685. Gibbs, J., R. C. Young and G. P. Smith. 1973. Cholecystokinin decreases food intake in rats. *J. Comp. Physiol. Psychol.* 84:488–495.
686. Giebel, H.-D. 1958. Visuelles lernvermogen bei einhufern. *Zool. Jahrb.* 67:487–520.
687. Gifford, A. K., S. Cloutier and R. C. Newberry. 2007. Objects as enrichment: Effects of object exposure time and delay interval on object recognition memory of the domestic pig. *Appl. Anim. Behav. Sci.* 107:206–217.
688. Gilbert, B. J. Jr and C. W. Arave. 1986. Ability of cattle to distinguish among different wavelengths of light. *J. Dairy Sci.* 69:825–832.

689. Gill, J., K. Skwarlo and A. Flisinska-Bojanowska. 1974. Diurnal and seasonal changes in carbohydrate metabolism in the blood of thoroughbred horses. *J. Interdiscipl.* 5:355–361.
690. Gillham, S. B., N. H. Dodman, L. Shuster, R. Kream and W. Rand. 1994. The effect of diet on cribbing behavior and plasma β-endorphin in horses. *Appl. Anim. Behav. Sci.* 41:147–153.
691. Gleitman, H. 1974. Getting animals to understand the experimenter's instructions. *Anim. Learn. Behav.* 2:1–5.
692. Glencross, R. G., R. J. Esselmont, M. J. Bryant and G. S. Pope. 1981. Relationships between the incidence of pre-ovulatory behavior and the concentrations of oestradiol-17β and progesterone in bovine plasma. *Appl. Anim. Ethol.* 7:141–148.
693. Goatcher, W. D. and D. C. Church. 1970. Taste responses in ruminants. II. Reactions of sheep to acids, quinine, urea and sodium hydroxide. *J. Anim. Sci.* 30:784–790.
694. Goatcher, W. D. and D. C. Church. 1970. Taste responses in ruminants. III. Reactions of pygmy goats, normal goats, sheep and cattle to sucrose and sodium chloride. *J. Anim. Sci.* 31:364–372.
695. Goddard, M. E. and R. G. Beilharz. 1982. Genetics of traits which determine the suitability of dogs as guide-dogs for the blind. *Appl. Anim. Ethol.* 9:299–315.
696. Gonyou, H. W., R. P. Chapple and G. R. Frank. 1992. Productivity, time budgets and social aspects of eating in pigs penned in groups of five or individually. *Appl. Anim. Behav. Sci.* 34:291–301.
697. Gonyou, H. W. and J. M. Stookey. 1985. Behavior of parturient ewes in group-lambing pens with and without cubicles. *Appl. Anim. Behav. Sci.* 14:163–171.
698. Gonyou, H. W. and W. R. Stricklin. 1984. Diurnal behavior of feedlot bulls during winter and spring in northern latitudes. *J. Anim. Sci.* 58:1075–1083.
699. Goodwin, D., J. W. S. Bradshaw and S. Wickens. 1997. Paedomorphosis affects agonistic visual signals of domestic dogs. *Anim. Behav.* 53:297–304.
700. Goodwin, D., H. P. B. Davidson and P. Harris. 2005. Sensory varieties in concentrate diets for stabled horses: Effects on behaviour and selection. *Appl. Anim. Behav. Sci.* 90:337–349.
701. Goodwin, D., H. P. Davidson and P. Harris. 2002. Foraging enrichment for stabled horses: Effects on behaviour and selection. *Equine Vet. J.* 34:686–691.
702. Goodwin, M., K. M. Gooding and F. Regnier. 1979. Sex pheromone in the dog. *Science* 203:559–561.
703. Gorecka, A., M. Golonka, M. Chruszczewski and T. Jezierski. 2007. A note on behaviour and heart rate in horses differing in facial hair whorl. *Appl. Anim. Behav. Sci.* 105:244–248.
704. Gorniak, S. L., J. A. Pfister, E. C. Lanzonia and E. R. Raspantini. 2008. A note on averting goats to a toxic but palatable plant, *Leucaena leucocephala. Appl. Anim. Behav. Sci.* 111:396–401.
705. Gottardo, F., S. Mattiello, G. Cozzi, E. Canali, E. Scanziani, L. Ravarotto, V. Ferrante, M. Verga and I. Andrighetto. 2002. The provision of drinking water to veal calves for welfare purposes. *J. Anim. Sci.* 80:2362–2372.
706. Goursaud, A. P. and R. Nowak. 1999. Colostrum mediates the development of mother preference by newborn lambs. *Physiol. Behav.* 67:49–56.
707. Grace, J. and M. Russek. 1969. The influence of previous experience on the taste behavior of dogs toward sucrose and saccharin. *Physiol. Behav.* 4:553–558.
708. Grandage, J. 1972. The erect dog penis: A paradox of flexible rigidity. *Vet. Rec.* 91:141–147.
709. Grandin, T. 1993. Behavioral agitation during handling of cattle in persistent over time. *Appl. Anim. Behav. Sci.* 36:1–9.
710. Grandin, T., M. J. Deesing, J. J. Struthers and A. M. Swinker. 1995. Cattle with hair whorl patterns above the eyes are more behaviorally agitated during restraint. *Appl. Anim. Behav. Sci.* 46:117–123.
711. Graves, H. B. 1984. Behavior and ecology of wild and feral swine (Sus scrofa). *J. Anim. Sci.* 58:482–492.
712. Green, J. S., R. A. Woodruff and T. T. Tueller. 1984. Livestock-guarding dogs for predator control: Costs, benefits and practicality. *Wildl. Soc. Bull.* 12:44–50.
713. Greene, W. A., L. Mogil and R. H. Foote. 1978. Behavioral characteristics of freemartins administered estradiol, estrone, testosterone, and dihydrotestosterone. *Horm. Behav.* 10:71–84.
714. Greet, T. R. 1982. Windsucking treated by myectomy and neurectomy. *Equine Vet. J.* 14:299–301.
715. Gregory, P. C., M. McFadyen and D. V. Rayner. 1989. Relation between gastric emptying and short-term regulation of food intake in the pig. *Physiol. Behav.* 45:677–683.
716. Griffith, C. A., E. S. Steigerwald and C. A. Buffington. 2000. Effects of a synthetic facial pheromone on behavior of cats. *J. Am. Vet. Med. Assoc.* 217:1154–1156.
717. Griffith, M. K. and J. E. Minton. 1992. Effect of light intensity on circadian profiles of melatonin, prolactin, ACTH, and cortisol in pigs. *J. Anim. Sci.* 70:492–498.

718. Grignard, L., A. Boissy, X. Boivin, J. P. Garel and P. Le Neindre. 2000. The social environment influences the behavioural responses of beef cattle to handling. *Appl. Anim. Behav. Sci.* 68:1–11.

719. Grossman, M. I., G. M. Cummins and A. C. Ivy. 1947. The effect of insulin on food intake after vagotomy and sympathectomy. *Am. J. Physiol.* 149:100–102.

720. Grout, A. S., D. M. Veira, D. M. Weary, M. A. von Keyserlingk and D. Fraser. 2006. Differential effects of sodium and magnesium sulfate on water consumption by beef cattle. *J. Anim. Sci.* 84:1252–1258.

721. Grubb, P. 1974. The rut and behaviour of Soay rams. In P. A. Jewell, C. Milner and J. M. Boyd (Eds.), *Island survivors: The ecology of the Soay sheep of St. Kilda*, pp. 195–223. London, UK: The Athlone Press of the University of London.

722. Grubb, P. 1974. Social organization of Soay sheep and the behaviour of ewes and lambs. In P. A. Jewell, C. Milner and J. M. Boyd (Eds.), *Island survivors: The ecology of the Soay sheep of St. Kilda*, pp. 131–159. London, UK: The Athlone Press of the University of London.

723. Grzimek, B. 1952. Versuche uber das farbsehen von pflanzenessern. I. Das farbige sehen (und die sehscharfe) von pferden. *Z. Tierpsychol.* 9:23–39.

724. Grzimek, B. 1949. Rangordnungsversuche mit pferden. *Z. Tierpsychol.* 6:455–464.

725. Gubernick, D. J., K. C. Jones and P. H. Klopfer. 1979. Maternal imprinting in goats. *Anim. Behav.* 27:314–315.

726. Guillemet, R., S. Comyn, J. -. Dourmad and M.-C. Meunier-Salaun. 2007. Gestating sows prefer concentrate diets to high-fibre diet in two-choice tests. *Appl. Anim. Behav. Sci.* 108:251–262.

727. Guo, K., K. Meints, C. Hall, S. Hall and D. Mills. 2009. Left gaze bias in humans, rhesus monkeys and domestic dogs. *Anim. Cogn.* 12:409–418.

728. Gurr, M. I., J. Kirtland, M. Phillip and M. P. Robinson. 1977. The consequences of early overnutrition for fat cell size and number: The pig as an experimental model for human obesity. *Int. J. Obes.* 1:151–170.

729. Gustafsson, M., P. Jensen, F. H. de Jonge and T. Schuurman. 1999. Domestication effects on foraging strategies in pigs (*Sus scrofa*). *Appl. Anim. Behav. Sci.* 62:305–317.

730. Gustavson, C. R., R. J. Garcia, W. G. Hankins and K. W. Rusiniak. 1974. Coyote predation control by aversive conditioning. *Science* 184:581–583.

731. Guy, N. C., U. A. Luescher, S. E. Dohoo, E. Spangler, J. B. Miller, I. R. Dohoo and L. A. Bate. 2001. A case series of biting dogs: Characteristics of the dogs, their behaviour, and their victims. *Appl. Anim. Behav. Sci.* 74:43–57.

732. Gygax, L., R. Siegwart and B. Wechsler. 2007. Effects of space allowance on the behaviour and cleanliness of finishing bulls kept in pens with fully slatted rubber coated flooring. *Appl. Anim. Behav. Sci.* 107:1–12.

733. Haag, E. L., R. Rudman and K. A. Houpt. 1980. Avoidance, maze learning and social dominance in ponies. *J. Anim. Sci.* 50:329–335.

734. Hafez, E. S. and J. A. Lineweaver. 1968. Suckling behaviour in natural and artificially fed neonate calves. *Z. Tierpsychol.* 25:187–198.

735. Hafez, E. S. E. 1975. The behaviour of cattle. In E. S. E. Hafez (Ed.), *The behaviour of domestic animals*, pp. 203–245. Baltimore, MD: Williams & Wilkins.

736. Hafez, E. S. E. 1975. *The behaviour of domestic animals*. Baltimore, MD: Williams & Wilkins.

737. Hafez, E. S. E. 1974. *Reproduction in farm animals*. Philadelphia, PA: Lea & Febiger.

738. Hafez, E. S. E. and J.-P. Signoret. 1969. The behaviour of swine. In E. S. E. Hafez (Ed.), *The behaviour of domestic animals*, pp. 349–390. Baltimore, MD: Williams & Wilkins.

739. Hagen, K. and D. M. Broom. 2003. Cattle discriminate between individual familiar herd members in a learning experiment. *Appl. Anim. Behav. Sci.* 82:13–28.

740. Hale, L. A. and S. E. Huggins. 1980. The electroencephalogram of normal 'grade' pony in sleep and wakefulness. *Comp. Biochem. Physiol.* 66A:251–257.

741. Hale, E. B. 1966. Visual stimuli and reproductive behavior in bulls. *J. Anim. Sci.* 25(Suppl): 36–48.

742. Haley, D. B., J. Rushen, I. J. H. Duncan, T. M. Widowski and A. M. De passille. 1998. Butting by calves, Bos taurus, and rate of milk flow. *Anim. Behav.* 56:1545–1551.

743. Hall, S. J. G. 2002. Behaviour of cattle. In P. Jensen (Ed.), *The ethology of domestic animals: An introductory text*, pp. 131–146. Wallingford, UK: CABI Publishing.

744. Hall, S. J. G. 1986. Chillingham cattle: Dominance and affinities and access to supplementary food. *Ethology* 71:201–215.

745. Hall, C. A. and H. J. Cassaday. 2006. An investigation into the effect of floor colour on the behaviour of the horse. *Appl. Anim. Behav. Sci.* 99:301–314.

746. Hall, S. J. G. 1989. Chillingham cattle: Social and maintenance behaviour in an ungulate that breeds all year round. *Anim. Behav.* 38:215–225.

747. Hall, S. L., J. W. S. Bradshaw and I. H. Robinson. 2002. Object play in adult domestic cats: The roles of habituation and disinhibition. *Appl. Anim. Behav. Sci.* 79:263–271.

748. Hamilton, G. V. 1911. A study of trial and error reactions in mammals. *J. Anim. Behav.* 1:33–66.

749. Hamm, D. 1977. A new surgical procedure to control crib-biting. *Proceedings of the 23rd Annual Meeting of the American Association of Equine Practice*, pp. 301–302.

750. Hammell, D. L., D. D. Kratzer and W. J. Bramble. 1975. Avoidance and maze learning in pigs. *J. Anim. Sci.* 40:573–579.

751. Hancock, J. 1950. Grazing habits of dairy cows in New Zealand. *Emp. J. Exp. Agric.* 18:249–263.

752. Hanggi, E. B. 1999. Categorization learning in horses (*Equus caballus*). *J. Comp. Psychol.* 3:243–252.

753. Hanggi, E. B. and J. F. Ingersoll. 2009. Long-term memory for categories and concepts in horses (Equus caballus). *Anim. Cogn.* 12:451–462.

754. Hanninen, L., H. Hepola, S. Raussi and H. Saloniemi. 2008. Effect of colostrum feeding method and presence of dam on the sleep, rest and sucking behaviour of newborn calves. *Appl. Anim. Behav. Sci.* 112:213–222.

755. Hansen, I. and V. Lind. 2008. Are double bunks used by indoor wintering sheep? Testing a proposal for organic farming in Norway. *Appl. Anim. Behav. Sci.* 115:37–43.

756. Hansen, K. E. and S. E. Curtis. 1980. Prepartal activity of sows in stall or pen. *J. Anim. Sci.* 51:456–460.

757. Hare, B., M. Brown, C. Williamson and M. Tomasello. 2002. The domestication of social cognition in dogs. *Science* 298:1634–1636.

758. Hare, B., J. Call and M. Tomasello. 1998. Communication of food location between human and dog (*Canis familiaris*). *Evol. Commun.* 2:137–159.

759. Hare, B. and M. Tomasello. 1999. Domestic dogs (*Canis familiaris*) use human and conspecific social cues to locate hidden food. *J. Comp. Psychol.* 11:173–177.

760. Harker, K. W., J. I. Taylor and D. H. L. Rollinson. 1956. Studies in the habits of Zebu cattle. V. Night paddocking and its effect on the animal. *J. Agric. Sci.* 47:44–49.

761. Harlow, H. F., M. K. Harlow and E. W. Hansen. 1963. The maternal affectional system of rhesus monkeys. In H. L. Rheingold (Ed.), *Maternal behavior in mammals*, pp. 254–281. New York, NY: John Wiley & Sons.

762. Harlow, H. F. and P. Settlage. 1939. The effect of curarization of the fore part of the body upon the retention of conditioned responses in cats. *J. Comp. Psychol.* 27:45–48.

763. Harman, A. M., S. Moore, R. Hoskins and P. Keller. 1999. Horse vision and an explanation for the visual behaviour originally explained by the 'ramp retina'. *Equine Vet. J.* 31:384–390.

764. Harrington, F. H. 1986. Timber wolf howling playback studies: Discrimination of pup from adult howls. *Anim. Behav.* 34:1575–1577.

765. Harrington, F. H. and L. D. Mech. 1978. Howling at two Minnesota wolf pack summer homesites. *Can. J. Zool.* 56:2024–2028.

766. Harrison, J. and J. Buchwald. 1983. Eyeblink conditioning deficits in the old cat. *Neurobiol. Aging* 4:45–51.

767. Hart, B. L. 2001. Effect of gonadectomy on subsequent development of age-related cognitive impairment in dogs. *J. Am. Vet. Med. Assoc.* 219:51–56.

768. Hart, B. L. 1978. *Feline behavior. A practitioner monograph*. Santa Barbara, CA: Veterinary Practice Publishing Co.

769. Hart, B. L. 1974. Environmental and hormonal influences on urine marking behavior in the adult male dog. *Behav. Biol.* 11:167–176.

770. Hart, B. L. 1970. Mating behavior in the female dog and the effects of estrogen on sexual reflexes. *Horm. Behav.* 1:93–104.

771. Hart, B. L. 1968. Role of prior experience in the effects of castration on sexual behavior of male dogs. *J. Comp. Physiol. Psychol.* 66:719–725.

772. Hart, B. L. and R. E. Barrett. 1973. Effects of castration on fighting, roaming, and urine spraying in adult male cats. *J. Am. Vet. Med. Assoc.* 163:290–292.

773. Hart, B. L., L. A. Hart and M. J. Bain. 2006. Canine and feline behavior therapy, 2nd Edn. Oxford, UK: Blackwell Publishing.

774. Hart, B. L. and L. A. Hart. 1988. *The perfect puppy: How to choose your dog by its behavior*. New York, NY: W.H. Freeman and Company.

775. Hart, B. L. and L. A. Hart. 1985. *Canine and feline behavioral therapy*. Philadelphia, PA: Lea & Febiger.

776. Hart, B. L. and C. M. Haugen. 1971. Scent marking and sexual behavior maintained in anosmic male dogs. *Commun. Behav. Biol.* 6:131–135.

777. Hart, B. L. and T. O. Jones. 1975. Effects of castration on sexual behavior of tropical male goats. *Horm. Behav.* 6:247–258.

778. Hart, B. L. and M. G. Leedy. 1985. Analysis of the catnip reaction: Mediation by olfactory system, not vomeronasal organ. *Behav. Neural Biol.* 44:38–46.

779. Hartman, B. L. and W. G. Pond. 1960. Design and use of a milking machine for sows. *J. Anim. Behav.* 19:780–785.

780. Hashizume, C., M. Suzuki, K. Masuda, Y. Momozawa, T. Kikusui, Y. Takeuchi and Y. Mori. 2003. Molecular cloning of canine monoamine oxidase subtypes A (MAOA) and B (MAOB) cDNAs and their expression in the brain. *J. Vet. Med. Sci.* 65:893–898.

781. Haskins, R. 1977. Effect of kitten vocalizations on maternal behavior. *J. Comp. Physiol. Psychol.* 91:830–838.

782. Hatch, R. C. 1972. Effect of drugs on catnip (Nepeta cataria)-induced pleasure behavior in cats. *Am. J. Vet. Res.* 33:143–155.

783. Haugse, C. N., W. E. Dinusson, D. L. Erickson, J. N. Johnson and M. L. Buchanan. 1965. A day in the life of a pig. *N. Dak. Farm Res.* 23:18–23.

784. Hausberger, M., E. Gautier, C. Muller and P. Jego. 2007. Lower learning abilities in stereotypic horses. *Appl. Anim. Behav. Sci.* 107:299–306.

785. Hausberger, M., S. Henry, C. Larose and M. A. Richard-Yris. 2007. First suckling: A crucial event for mother-young attachment? an experimental study in horses (Equus caballus). *J. Comp. Psychol.* 121:109–112.

786. Hausberger, M. and C. Muller. 2002. A brief note on some possible factors involved in the reactions of horses to humans. *Appl. Anim. Behav. Sci.* 76:339–344.

787. Haverbeke, A., A. De Smet, E. Depiereux, J.-M. Giffroy and C. Diederich. 2009. Assessing undesired aggression in military working dogs. *Appl. Anim. Behav. Sci.* 117:55–62.

788. Haverbeke, A., B. Laporte, E. Depiereux, J.-M. Giffroy and C. Diederich. 2008. Training methods of military dog handlers and their effects on the team's performances. *Appl. Anim. Behav. Sci.* 113:110–122.

789. Hawkes, J., M. Hedges, P. Daniluk, H. F. Hintz and H. F. Schryver. 1985. Feed preferences of ponies. *Equine Vet. J.* 17:20–22.

790. Hawking, F. 1971. Circadian rhythms in monkeys, dogs and other animals. *J. Interdiscipl. Cycle Res.* 2:153–156.

791. Hawking, F. 1971. Circadian rhythms of parasites. *J. Interdiscipl. Cycle Res.* 2:157–160.

792. Hay, M., M. C. Meunier-Salaun, F. Brulaud, M. Monnier and P. Mormede. 2000. Assessment of hypothalamic-pituitary-adrenal axis and sympathetic nervous system activity in pregnant sows through the measurement of glucocorticoids and catecholamines in urine. *J. Anim. Sci.* 78:420–428.

793. Hayes, K. E. N. and O. J. Ginther. 1989. Relationships between estrous behavior in pregnant mares and the presence of a female conceptus. *J. Eq. Vet. Sci.* 9:316–318.

794. Hayman, R. H. 1964. Exercise of mating preference by a Merino ram. *Nature* 203:160–162.

795. Hayne, S. M. and H. W. Gonyou. 2006. Behavioural uniformity or diversity? Effects on behaviour and performance following regrouping in pigs. *Appl. Anim. Behav. Sci.* 98:28–44.

796. Hayne, S. M. and H. W. Gonyou. 2003. Effects of regrouping on the individual behavioural characteristics of pigs. *Appl. Anim. Behav. Sci.* 82:267–278.

797. He, J., L. Ma, S. Kim, J. Nakai and C. R. Yu. 2008. Encoding gender and individual information in the mouse vomeronasal organ. *Science* 320:535–538.

798. Head, E., K. Moffat, P. Das, F. Sarsoza, W. W. Poon, G. Landsberg, C. W. Cotman and M. P. Murphy. 2005. Beta-amyloid deposition and tau phosphorylation in clinically characterized aged cats. *Neurobiol. Aging* 26:749–763.

799. Heady, H. F. 1964. Palatability of herbage and animal preference. *J. Range Manag.* 17:76–82.

800. Heath, S. E., S. Barabas and P. G. Craze. 2007. Nutritional supplementation in cases of canine cognitive dysfunction—A clinical trial. *Appl. Anim. Behav. Sci.* 105:296.

801. Hedlund, L., M. M. Lischko, M. D. Rollag and G. D. Niswender. 1977. Melatonin: Daily cycle in plasma and cerebrospinal fluid of calves. *Science* 195:686–687.

802. Heffner, H. E. 1983. Hearing in large and small dogs: Absolute thresholds and size of the tympanic membrane. *Behav. Neurosci.* 97:310–318.

803. Hegsted, D. M., S. N. Gershoff and E. Lentini. 1956. The development of palatability tests for cats. *Am. J. Vet. Res.* 17:733–737.

804. Heidenberger, E. 1997. Housing conditions and behavioural problems of indoor cats as assessed by their owners. *Appl. Anim. Behav. Sci.* 52:345–364.

805. Hein, A. and R. Held. 1967. Dissociation of the visual placing response into elicited and guided components. *Science* 158:390–392.
806. Heird, J. C., A. M. Lennon and R. W. Bell. 1981. Effects of early experience on the learning ability of yearling horses. *J. Anim. Sci.* 53:1204–1209.
807. Heird, J. C., D. D. Whitaker, R. W. Bell, C. B. Ramsey and C. E. Lokey. 1986. The effects of handling at different ages on the subsequent learning ability of 2-year-old horses. *Appl. Anim. Behav. Sci.* 15: 15–25.
808. Heitor, F. and L. Vicente. 2008. Maternal care and foal social relationships in a herd of Sorraia horses: Influence of maternal rank and experience. *Appl. Anim. Behav. Sci.* 113:189–205.
809. Heitzman, R. J. 1978. The use of hormones to regulate the utilization of nutrients in farm animals: Current farm practices. *Proc. Nutr. Soc.* 37:289–293.
810. Held, S., J. Baumgartner, A. Kilbride, R. W. Byrne and M. Mendl. 2005. Foraging behaviour in domestic pigs (*Sus scrofa*): Remembering and prioritizing food sites of different value. *Anim. Cogn.* 8:114–121.
811. Held, S., G. Mason and M. Mendl. 2006. Maternal responsiveness of outdoor sows from first to fourth parities. *Appl. Anim. Behav. Sci.* 98:216–233.
812. Held, S., M. Mendl, C. Devereux and R. W. Byrne. 2002. Foraging pigs alter their behaviour in response to exploitation. *Anim. Behav.* 64:156–166.
813. Hellekant, G., C. Hard af Segerstad and T. W. Roberts. 1994. Sweet taste in the calf: III. Behavioral responses to sweeteners. *Physiol. Behav.* 56:555–562.
814. Hemsworth, P. H. and J. L. Barnett. 1992. The effects of early contact with humans on the subsequent level of fear of humans in pigs. *Appl. Anim. Behav. Sci.* 35:83–90.
815. Hemsworth, P. H., J. L. Barnett and C. Hansen. 1987. The influence of inconsistent handling by humans on the behaviour, growth and corticosteroids of young pigs. *Act. Nerv. Super. (Praha)* 17:245–252.
816. Hemsworth, P. H., J. L. Barnett, C. Hansen and C. G. Winfield. 1986. Effects of social environment on welfare status and sexual behaviour of female pigs. II. Effects of space allowance. *Appl. Anim. Behav. Sci.* 16:259–267.
817. Hemsworth, P. H., J. L. Barnett, A. J. Tilbrook and C. Hansen. 1989. The effects of handling by humans at calving and during milking on the behaviour and milk cortisol concentrations of primiparous dairy cows. *Appl. Anim. Behav. Sci.* 22:313–326.
818. Hemsworth, P. H., R. G. Beilharz and D. B. Galloway. 1977. Influence of social conditions during rearing on the sexual behaviour of the domestic boar. *Anim. Prod.* 24:245–251.
819. Hemsworth, P. H., G. M. Cronin, C. Hansen and C. G. Winfield. 1984. The effects of two oestrus detection procedures and intense boar stimulation near the time of oestrus on mating efficiency of the female pig. *Appl. Anim. Behav. Sci.* 12:339–347.
820. Hemsworth, P. H., J. K. Findlay and R. G. Bielharz. 1978. The importance of physical contact with other pigs during rearing on the sexual behaviour of the male domestic pig. *Anim. Prod.* 27:201–207.
821. Hemsworth, P. H., E. O. Price and A. J. Tilbrook. 1992. Influence of the sexual motivation of the boar on the sexual partner preferences of oestrous gilts. *Appl. Anim. Behav. Sci.* 33:209–215.
822. Hemsworth, P. H. and A. J. Tilbrook. 2007. Sexual behavior of male pigs. *Horm. Behav.* 52:39–44.
823. Hemsworth, P. H., C. G. Winfield, J. L. Barnett, B. Schirmer and C. Hansen. 1986. A comparison of the effects of two estrus detection procedures and two housing systems on the oestrus detection rate of female pigs. *Appl. Anim. Behav. Sci.* 16:345–351.
824. Hemsworth, P. H., C. G. Winfield, R. G. Beilharz and D. B. Galloway. 1977. Influence of social conditions post-puberty on the sexual behaviour of the domestic male pig. *Anim. Prod.* 25:305–309.
825. Hemsworth, P. H., C. G. Winfield and P. D. Mullaney. 1976. A study of the development of the teat order in piglets. *Appl. Anim. Ethol.* 2:225–233.
826. Hendricks, J. C., A. R. Morrison, G. L. Farnbach, S. A. Steinberg and G. Mann. 1981. A disorder of rapid eye movement sleep in a cat. *J. Am. Vet. Med. Assoc.* 178:55–57.
827. Hendriks, W. H., M. F. Tarttelin and P. J. Moughan. 1995. Twenty-four hour feline excretion patterns in entire and castrated cats. *Physiol. Behav.* 58:467–469.
828. Henry, S., D. Hemery, M.-A. Richard and M. Hausberger. 2005. Human–mare relationships and behaviour of foals toward humans. *Appl. Anim. Behav. Sci.* 93:341–362.
829. Hepper, P. G. 1986. Sibling recognition in the domestic dog. *Anim. Behav.* 34:288–289.
830. Herbel, C. H. and A. B. Nelson. 1966. Species preference of Hereford and Santa Gertrudis cattle on a southern New Mexico range. *J. Range Manag.* 19:177–181.
831. Herd, R. M. 1988. A technique for cross-mothering beef calves which does not affect growth. *Appl. Anim. Behav. Sci.* 19:239–244.

832. Hernandez, L., H. Barral, G. Halffter and S. S. Colon. 1999. A note on the behavior of feral cattle in the Chihuahuan Desert of Mexico. *Appl. Anim. Behav. Sci.* 63:259–267.

833. Herring, S. W. and R. P. Scapino. 1973. Physiology of feeding in miniature pigs. *J. Morphol.* 141:427–460.

834. Hersher, L., J. B. Richmond and A. U. Moore. 1963. Maternal behavior in sheep and goats. In H. L. Rheingold (Ed.), *Maternal behavior in mammals*. New York, NY: John Wiley & Sons.

835. Herskin, M. S., L. Munksgaard and A. M. Kristensen. 2003. Behavioural and adrenocortical responses of dairy cows toward novel food: Effects of food deprivation, milking frequency and energy density in the daily ration. *Appl. Anim. Behav. Sci.* 82:251–265.

836. Hessel, E. F., K. Reiners and H. F. Van Den Weghe. 2006. Socializing piglets before weaning: Effects on behavior of lactating sows, pre- and postweaning behavior, and performance of piglets. *J. Anim. Sci.* 84:2847–2855.

837. Hessing, M. J. C., A. M. Hagels, J. A. M. van Beck, P. R. Wiepkema, G. P. Schouten and R. Krukow. 1993. Individual behavioural characteristics in pigs. *Appl. Anim. Behav. Sci.* 37:285–295.

838. Hessle, A., M. Rutter and K. Wallin. 2008. Effect of breed, season and pasture moisture gradient on foraging behaviour in cattle on semi-natural grasslands. *Appl. Anim. Behav. Sci.* 111:108–119.

839. Hetts, S. 1999. *Pet behaviour protocols*. Lakewood, CO: AAHA Press.

840. Hetts, S., J. Derrell Clark, J. P. Calin, C. E. Arnold and J. M. Mateo. 1992. Influence of housing conditions on beagle behaviour. *Appl. Anim. Behav. Sci.* 34:137–155.

841. Hetzer, H. O. and W. R. Harvey. 1967. Selection for high and low fatness in swine. *J. Anim. Sci.* 26:1244–1251.

842. Hill, C. T., P. D. Krawczel, H. M. Dann, C. S. Ballard, R. C. Hovey, W. A. Falls and R. J. Grant. 2009. Effect of stocking density on the short-term behavioural responses of dairy cows. *Appl. Anim. Behav. Sci.* 117:144–149.

843. Hill, J. O., E. J. Pavlik, G. L. Smith III, G. M. Burghardt and P. B. Coulson. 1976. Species-characteristic responses to catnip by undomesticated felids. *J. Chem. Ecol.* 2:239–253.

844. Hinch, G. N., J. J. Lynch and C. J. Thwaites. 1982. Patterns and frequency of social interactions in young grazing bulls and steers. *Appl. Anim. Ethol.* 9:15–30.

845. Hirsch, E., C. Dubose and H. L. Jacobs. 1978. Dietary control of food intake in cats. *Physiol. Behav.* 20:287–295.

846. Hite, M., H. M. Hanson, N. R. Bohidar, P. A. Conti and P. A. Mattis. 1977. Effect of cage size on patterns of activity and health of beagle dogs. *Lab. Anim. Sci.* 27:60–64.

847. Hoagland, T. A. and M. A. Diekman. 1982. Influence of supplemental lighting during increasing daylength on libido and reproductive hormones in prepubertal boars. *J. Anim. Sci.* 55:1483–1489.

848. Hoffman, R. 1985. On the development of social behavior in immature males of a feral horse population (*Equus przewalski* f. caballus). *Zeitschrift Saugetierkunde* 50:302–314.

849. Hoffman, R. M., D. S. Kronfeld, J. L. Holland and K. M. Greiwe-Crandell. 1995. Preweaning diet and stall weaning method influences on stress response in foals. *J. Anim. Sci.* 73:2922–2930.

850. Holland, J. L., D. S. Kronfeld, G. A. Rich, K. A. Kline, J. P. Fontenot, T. N. Meacham and P. A. Harris. 1998. Acceptance of fat and lecithin containing diets by horses. *Appl. Anim. Behav. Sci.* 56:91–96.

851. Holm, L., M. B. Jensen, L. J. Pedersen and J. Ladewig. 2008. The importance of a food feedback in rooting materials for pigs measured by double demand curves with and without a common scaling factor. *Appl. Anim. Behav. Sci.* 111:68–84.

852. Holmes, J. H. and L. J. Cizek. 1951. Observations on sodium chloride depletion in dog. *Am. J. Physiol.* 164:407–414.

853. Holmes, L. N., G. K. Song and E. O. Price. 1987. Head partitions facilitate feeding by subordinate horses in the presence of dominant pan-mates. *Appl. Anim. Behav. Sci.* 19:179–182.

854. Hopkins, S. G., T. A. Schubert and B. L. Hart. 1976. Castration of adult male dogs: Effects on roaming, aggression, urine marking, and mounting. *J. Am. Vet. Med. Assoc.* 168:1108–1110.

855. Hoppe, S., H. R. Brandt, G. Erhardt and M. Gauly. 2008. Maternal protective behaviour of German Angus and Simmental beef cattle after parturition and its relation to production traits. *Appl. Anim. Behav. Sci.* 114:297–306.

856. Hoppenbrouwers, T. and M. B. Sterman. 1975. Development of sleep state patterns in the kitten. *Exp. Neurol.* 49:822–838.

857. Horowitz, A. 2009. Attention to attention in domestic dog (*Canis familiaris*) dyadic play. *Anim. Cogn.* 12:107–118.

858. Horrell, I. and J. Hodgson. 1992. The bases of sow-piglet identification. 2. Cues used by piglets to identify their dame and home pen. *Appl. Anim. Behav. Sci.* 33:329–343.

859. Horrell, I. and J. Hodgson. 1992. The bases of sow-piglet identification. I. The identification by sows of their own piglets and the presence of intruders. *Appl. Anim. Behav. Sci.* 33:319–327.

860. Horrell, R. I. and M. Eaton. 1984. Recognition of maternal environment in piglets: Effects of age and some discrete complex stimuli. *Q. J. Exp. Psychol. B* 36:119–130.

861. Horvath, Z., B. Z. Igyarto, A. Magyar and A. Miklosi. 2007. Three different coping styles in police dogs exposed to a short-term challenge. *Horm. Behav.* 52:621–630.

862. Horwitz, D. F., D. S. Mills and S. Heath. 2002. In Horwitz D. F., Mills D. S. and Heath S. (Eds.), *BSAVMA manual of canine and feline behavioural medicine*. Gloucester, UK: British Small Animal Veterinary Association.

863. Horwitz, D. F. and J. C. Neilson. 2007. *Blackwell's five-minute veterinary consult clinical companion: Canine and feline behavior*. Oxford, UK: Blackwell Publishing.

864. Hosoi, E., L. R. Rittenhouse, D. M. Swift and R. W. Richards. 1995. Foraging strategies of cattle in a Y-maze: Influence of food availability. *Appl. Anim. Behav. Sci.* 43:189–196.

865. Houpt, K. A. 1983. Disruption of the human-companion animal bond: Aggressive behavior in dogs. In A. H. Katcher and A. M. Beck (Eds.), *New perspective on our lives with companion animals*, pp. 197–204. Philadelphia, PA: University of Pennsylvania Press.

866. Houpt, K. A. 1978. Palatability and canine food preferences. *Canine Pract.* 5:29–35.

867. Houpt, K. A. 1977. Horse behavior: Its relevancy to the equine practitioner. *J. Eq. Med. Surg.* 1:87–94.

868. Houpt, K. A., B. Coren, H. F. Hintz and J. E. Hilderbrant. 1979. Effect of sex and reproductive status on sucrose preference, food intake, and body weight of dogs. *J. Am. Vet. Med. Assoc.* 174:1083–1085.

869. Houpt, K. A., A. Eggleston, K. Kunkle and T. R. Houpt. 2000. Effect of water restriction on equine behaviour and physiology. *Equine Vet. J.* 32:341–344.

870. Houpt, K. A. and H. F. Hintz. 1982. Some effects of maternal deprivation and maintenance behavior, spatial relationships and responses to environmental novelty in foals. *Appl. Anim. Ethol.* 9:221–230.

871. Houpt, K. A., H. F. Hintz and P. Shepherd. 1978. The role of olfaction in canine food preferences. *Chem. Senses Flavor* 3:281–290.

872. Houpt, K. A. and T. R. Houpt. 1988. Social and illumination preferences of mares. *J. Anim. Sci.* 66:2159–2164.

873. Houpt, K. A. and T. R. Houpt. 1976. Comparative aspects of the ontogeny of taste. *Chem. Senses Flavor* 2:219–228.

874. Houpt, K. A., T. R. Houpt, J. L. Johnson, H. N. Erb and S. C. Yeon. 2001. The effect of exercise deprivation on the behaviour and physiology of straight stall confined pregnant mares. *Anim. Welfare* 10:257–267.

875. Houpt, K. A., T. R. Houpt and W. G. Pond. 1979. The pig as a model for the study of obesity and of control of food intake: A review. *Yale J. Biol. Med.* 52:307–329.

876. Houpt, K. A., T. R. Houpt and W. G. Pond. 1977. Food intake controls in the suckling pig: Glucoprivation and gastrointestinal factors. *Am. J. Physiol.* 232:E510–E514.

877. Houpt, K. A. and R. R. Keiper. 1982. The position of the stallion in the equine dominance hierarchy of feral and domestic ponies. *J. Anim. Sci.* 54:945–950.

878. Houpt, K. A. and R. Kusunose. 2000. Genetics of behaviour. In T. A. Bowling and A. Ruvinsky (Eds.), *The genetics of the horse*, pp. 281–306. Wallingford, UK: CABI Publishing.

879. Houpt, K. A., K. Law and V. Martinisi. 1978. Dominance hierarchies in domestic horses. *Appl. Anim. Ethol.* 4:273–283.

880. Houpt, K. A., N. Northrup, T. Wheatley and T. R. Houpt. 1991. Thirst and salt appetite in horses treated with furosemide. *J. Appl. Physiol.* 71:2380–2386.

881. Houpt, K. A., M. S. Parsons and H. F. Hintz. 1982. Learning ability of orphan foals, of normal foals and of their mothers. *J. Anim. Sci.* 55:1027–1032.

882. Houpt, K. A., W. Rivera and L. Glickstein. 1989. The flehmen response of bulls and cows. *Theriogenology* 32:343–350.

883. Houpt, K. A. and M. B. Willis. 2001. Genetics of behaviour. In A. Ruvinsky and J. Sampson (Eds.), *The genetics of the dog*, pp. 371–394. Wallingford, UK: CABI Publishing.

884. Houpt, K. A. and G. Wollney. 1989. Frequency of masturbation and time budgets of dairy bulls used for semen production. *Appl. Anim. Behav. Sci.* 24:217–225.

885. Houpt, K. A. and T. R. Wolski. 1980. Stability of equine hierarchies and the prevention of dominance related aggression. *Equine Vet. J.* 12:15–18.

886. Houpt, K. A. and T. R. Wolski. 1979. Equine maternal behavior and aberrations. *Equine Pract.* 1:7–20.

887. Houpt, T. R. 1984. Controls of feeding in pigs. *J. Anim. Sci.* 59:1345–1353.

888. Houpt, T. R. 1974. Stimulation of food intake in ruminants by 2-deoxy-D-glucose and insulin. *Am. J. Physiol.* 227:161–167.

889. Houpt, T. R., S. M. Anika and K. A. Houpt. 1979. Preabsorptive intestinal satiety controls of food intake in pigs. *Am. J. Physiol.* 236:R328–R337.

890. Houpt, T. R., B. A. Baldwin and K. A. Houpt. 1983. Effects of duodenal osmotic loads on spontaneous meals in pigs. *Physiol. Behav.* 30:787–795.

891. Houpt, T. R. and H. H. Hance. 1969. Effect of 2-deoxy-D-glucose on food intake by the goat, rabbit and dog. *Fed. Proc.* 28:648.

892. Houpt, T. R., K. A. Houpt and A. A. Swan. 1983. Duodenal osmoconcentration and food intake in pigs after ingestion of hypertonic nutrients. *Am. J. Physiol.* 245:R181–R189.

893. Houpt, T. R., L. C. Weixler and D. W. Troy. 1986. Water drinking induced by gastric secretagogues in pigs. *Am. J. Physiol.* 251:R157–R164.

894. Howery, L. D., F. D. Provenza, R. E. Banner and C. B. Scott. 1998. Social and environmental factors influence cattle distribution on rangeland. *Appl. Anim. Behav. Sci.* 55:231–244.

895. Hubrecht, R. C. 1993. A comparison of social and environmental enrichment methods for laboratory housed dogs. *Appl. Anim. Behav. Sci.* 37:345–361.

896. Hubrecht, R. C., J. A. Serpell and T. B. Poole. 1992. Correlates of pen size and housing conditions on the behaviour of kennelled dogs. *Appl. Anim. Behav. Sci.* 34:365–383.

897. Hudson, S. J. 1977. Multiple fostering of calves onto nurse cows at birth. *Appl. Anim. Behav. Sci.* 3:57–63.

898. Hudson, S. J. and M. M. Mullord. 1977. Investigations of maternal bonding in dairy cattle. *Appl. Anim. Ethol.* 3:271–276.

899. Hughes, G. P. and D. Reid. 1951. Studies on the behaviour of cattle and sheep in relation to the utilization of grass. *J. Agric. Sci.* 41:350–366.

900. Hughes, P. E., P. H. Hemsworth and C. Hansen. 1985. The effects of supplementary olfactory and auditory stimuli on the stimulus value and mating success of the young boar. *Appl. Anim. Behav. Sci.* 14:245–252.

901. Hulbert, L. E. and J. J. McGlone. 2006. Evaluation of drop versus trickle-feeding systems for crated or group-penned gestating sows. *J. Anim. Sci.* 84:1004–1014.

902. Hulet, C. V. 1966. Behavioral, social and psychological factors affecting mating time and breeding efficiency in sheep. *J. Anim. Sci.* 25(Suppl): 5–20.

903. Hulet, C. V., G. Alexander and E. S. E. Hafez. 1975. *The behaviour of sheep.* Baltimore, MD: Williams & Wilkins.

904. Hulet, C. V., D. M. Anderson, J. N. Smith and W. L. Shupe. 1989. Bonding of goats to sheep and cattle for protection from predators. *Appl. Anim. Behav. Sci.* 22:261–267.

905. Hulet, C. V., R. L. Balckwell and S. K. Ercanbrack. 1964. Observations on sexually inhibited rams. *J. Anim. Sci.* 23:1095–1097.

906. Hulet, C. V., R. L. Balckwell, S. K. Ercanbrack, D. A. Price and L. O. Wilson. 1962. Mating behavior of the ewe. *J. Anim. Sci.* 21:870–874.

907. Hunter, L. and K. A. Houpt. 1987. Bedding material preferences of ponies. *J. Anim. Sci.* 67:1986–1991.

908. Hunter, W. S. 1917. The delayed reaction in a child. *Psychol. Rev.* 24:74–87.

909. Hunthausen, W. 1997. Effects of aggressive behavior on canine welfare. *J. Am. Vet. Med. Assoc.* 210:1134–1136.

910. Hunthausen, W. and G. M. Landsberg. 1993. *Providing behavior services in veterinary practices.* Denver, CO: American Animal Hospital Association.

911. Hurnik, J. F., G. J. King and H. A. Robertson. 1975. Estrous and related behaviour in postpartum Holstein cows. *Appl. Anim. Ethol.* 2:55–68.

912. Hutson, G. D. 1985. The influence of barley food rewards on sheep movement through a handling system. *Appl. Anim. Behav. Sci.* 14:263–273.

913. Hutson, G. D. 1980. The effect of previous experience on sheep movement through yards. *Appl. Anim. Ethol.* 6:233–240.

914. Hutson, G. D., M. F. Argent, L. G. Dickenson and B. G. Luxford. 1992. Influence of parity and time since parturition on responsiveness of sows to a piglet distress call. *Appl. Anim. Behav. Sci.* 34:303–313.

915. Hutson, G. D. and M. J. Haskell. 1990. The behaviour of farrowing sows with free and operant access to an earth floor. *Appl. Anim. Behav. Sci.* 26:363–372.

916. Hutson, G. D., E. O. Price and L. G. Dickenson. 1993. The effect of playback volume and duration of the response of sows to piglet distress calls. *Appl. Anim. Behav. Sci.* 37:31–37.

917. Hutson, G. D., J. L. Wilkinson and B. G. Luxford. 1991. The response of lactating sows to tactile, visual and auditory stimuli associated with a model piglet. *Appl. Anim. Behav. Sci.* 32:129–137.

918. Huynh, T. T. T., A. J. A. Aarnink, W. J. J. Gerrits, M. J. H. Heetkamp, T. T. Canh, H. A. M. Spoodler, B. Kemp and M. W. A. Verstegen. 2005. Thermal behaviour of growing pigs in response to high temperature and humidity. *Appl. Anim. Behav. Sci.* 91:1–16.
919. Igel, G. J. and A. D. Calvin. 1960. The development of affectional responses in infant dogs. *J. Comp. Physiol. Psychol.* 53:302–305.
920. Illius, A. W., N. B. Haynes and G. E. Lamming. 1976. Effects of ewe proximity on peripheral plasma testosterone levels and behaviour in the ram. *J. Reprod. Fertil.* 48:25–32.
921. Illmann, G. and J. Madlafousek. 1995. Occurrence and characteristics of unsuccessful nursing in minipigs during the first week of life. *Appl. Anim. Behav. Sci.* 44:9–18.
922. Illmann, G., K. Neuhauserova, Z. Pokorna, H. Chaloupkova and M. Simeckova. 2008. Maternal responsiveness of sows towards piglet's screams during the first 24 h postpartum. *Appl. Anim. Behav. Sci.* 112:248–259.
923. Illmann, G. and M. Spinka. 1993. Maternal behaviour of dairy heifers and sucking of their newborn calves in group housing. *Appl. Anim. Behav. Sci.* 36:91–98.
924. Illmann, G., M. Spinka and Z. Stetkova. 1999. Predictability of nursings without milk ejection in domestic pigs. *Appl. Anim. Behav. Sci.* 61:303–311.
925. Ingolfsdottir, H. B. and H. Sigurjonsdottir. 2008. The benefits of high rank in the wintertime—A study of the Icelandic horse. *Appl. Anim. Behav. Sci.* 114:485–491.
926. Ingram, D. L. and M. J. Dauncy. 1985. Circadian rhythms in the pig. *Comp. Biochem. Physiol.* 82A:1–5.
927. Ingram, D. L., M. J. Dauncy and K. F. Legge. 1985. Synchronization of motor activity in young pigs to a non-circadian rhythm without affecting food intake and growth. *Comp. Biochem. Physiol.* 80A:363–368.
928. Ingram, D. L. and K. F. Legge. 1974. Effects of environmental temperature on food intake in growing pigs. *Comp. Biochem. Physiol.* 48A:573–581.
929. Ingram, D. L. and D. B. Stephens. 1979. The relative importance of thermal, osmotic and hypovolaemic factors in the control of drinking in the pig. *J. Physiol.* 293:501–512.
930. Innes, L. and S. McBride. 2008. Negative versus positive reinforcement: An evaluation of training strategies for rehabilitated horses. *Appl. Anim. Behav. Sci.* 112:357–368.
931. Inselman-Temkin, B. R. and J. P. Flynn. 1973. Sex-dependent effects of gonadal and gonadotropic hormones on centrally-elicited attack in cats. *Brain Res.* 60:393–410.
932. Irwin, M. R., D. R. Melendy, M. S. Amoss and D. P. Hutcheson. 1979. Roles of predisposing factors and gonadal hormones in the buller syndrome of feedlot steers. *J. Am. Vet. Med. Assoc.* 174:367–370.
933. Ishiwata, T., K. Uetake, R. J. Kilgour, Y. Eguchi and T. Tanaka. 2007. Oral behaviors of beef steers in pen and pasture environments. *J. Appl. Anim. Welfare Sci.* 10:185–192.
934. Izard, M. K. and J. G. Vandenbergh. 1982. Priming pheromones from oestrous cows increase synchronization of oestrus in dairy heifers after PGF-2 alpha injection. *J. Reprod. Fertil.* 66:189–196.
935. Jackson, B. and A. Reed. 1969. Catnip and the alteration of consciousness. *JAMA* 207:1349–1350.
936. Jackson, B. and D. W. Robinson. 1971. Evidence of hypothalamic a and b adrenergic receptors involved in the control of food intake of the pig. *Br. Vet. J.* 127:li–liii.
937. Jackson, S. A., R. A. Rich and S. L. Ralston. 1984. Feeding behavior and feed efficiency in groups of horses as a function of feeding frequency and use of alfafa hay cubes. *J. Anim. Sci.* 1:152–153.
938. Jago, J. G., N. R. Cox, J. J. Bass and L. R. Matthews. 1997. The effect of prepubertal immunization against gonadotropin-releasing hormone on the development of sexual and social behavior of bulls. *J. Anim. Sci.* 75:2609–2619.
939. Jago, J. G., C. C. Krohn and L. R. Matthews. 1999. The influence of feeding and handling on the development of the human-animal interactions in young cattle. *Appl. Anim. Behav. Sci.* 62:137–151.
940. Jalowiec, J. E., J. Panksepp, H. Shabshelowitz, A. J. Zolovick, W. Stern and P. J. Morgane. 1973. Suppression of feeding in cats following 2-deoxy-D-glucose. *Physiol. Behav.* 10:805–807.
941. James, W. T. and T. F. Gilbert. 1955. The effect of social facilitation on food intake of puppies fed separately and together for the first 90 days of life. *Br. J. Anim. Behav.* 3:131–133.
942. Janczak, A. M., L. J. Pederson and M. Bakken. 2003. Aggression, fearfullness and coping styles in female pigs. *Appl. Anim. Behav. Sci.* 81:13–28.
943. Janowitz, H. D. and M. I. Grossman. 1949. Effect of variations in nutritive density on intake of food of dogs and rats. *Am. J. Physiol.* 158:184–193.
944. Janowitz, H. D. and M. I. Grossman. 1949. Some factors affecting the food intake of normal dogs and dogs with esophagostomy and gastric fistula. *Am. J. Physiol.* 159:143–148.
945. Jarvis, A. M. and M. S. Cockram. 1995. Some factors affecting resting behaviour of sheep in slaughterhouse lairages after transport from farms. *Anim. Welfare* 4:53–60.

946. Jensen, M. B. 1999. Adaptation to tethering in yearling dairy heifers assessed by the use of lying down behaviour. *Appl. Anim. Behav. Sci.* 62:115–123.

947. Jensen, M. B., K. S. Vestergaard and C. C. Krohn. 1998. Play behaviour in dairy calves kept in pens: The effect of social contact and space allowance. *Appl. Anim. Behav. Sci.* 56:97–108.

948. Jensen, M. B., K. S. Vestergaard, C. C. Krohn and L. Munksgaard. 1997. Effect of single versus group housing and space allowance on responses of calves during open-field tests. *Appl. Anim. Behav. Sci.* 54:109–121.

949. Jensen, P. 1993. Nest building in domestic sows: The role of external stimuli. *Anim. Behav.* 45:351–358.

950. Jensen, P. 1986. Observations on the maternal behavior of freeranging domestic pigs. *Appl. Anim. Behav. Sci.* 16:131–142.

951. Jensen, P. 1984. Effects of confinement on social interaction patters in dry sows. *Appl. Anim. Behav. Sci.* 12:93–101.

952. Jensen, P. 1980. An ethogram of social interaction patterns in grouphoused dry sows. *Appl. Anim. Ethol.* 6:341–350.

953. Jensen, P., K. Floren and B. Hobroh. 1987. Peri-parturient changes in behaviour in free-ranging domestic pigs. *Appl. Anim. Behav. Sci.* 17:69–76.

954. Jensen, P., G. Stangel and B. Algers. 1991. Nursing and suckling behaviour of semi-naturally kept pigs during the first 10 days postpartum. *Appl. Anim. Behav. Sci.* 31:195–209.

955. Jensen, P. and J. Yngvesson. 1998. Aggression between unacquainted pigs—sequential assessment and effects of familiarity and weight. *Appl. Anim. Behav. Sci.* 58:49–61.

956. Jeppesen, L. E. 1982. Teat-order in groups of piglets reared on an artificial sow. I. Formation of teat-order and influence of milk yield on teat preference. *Appl. Anim. Ethol.* 8:335–345.

957. Jeppesen, L. E. 1982. Teat-order in groups of piglets reared on an artificial sow. II. Maintenance of teat-order with some evidence for the use of odour cues. *Appl. Anim. Ethol.* 8:347–355.

958. Jewell, P. A., S. J. Hall and M. M. Rosenberg. 1986. Multiple mating and siring success during natural oestrus in the ewe. *J. Reprod. Fertil.* 77:81–89.

959. Jezierski, T., Z. Jaworski and A. Gorecka. 1999. Effects of handling on behaviour and heart rate in Konik horses: Comparison of stable and forest reared youngstock. *Appl. Anim. Behav. Sci.* 62:1–11.

960. Jimenez-Severiano, H., J. Quintal-Franco, V. Vega-Murillo, E. Zanella, M. E. Wehrman, B. R. Lindsey, E. J. Melvin and J. E. Kinder. 2003. Season of the year influences testosterone secretion in bulls administered luteinizing hormone. *J. Anim. Sci.* 81:1023–1029.

961. John, E. R., P. Chesler, F. Bartlett and I. Victor. 1968. Observation learning in cats. *Science* 159:1489–1491.

962. Johnson, A., W. Engelmann, B. Pflug and W. Klemke. 1980. Influence of lithium ions on human circadian rhythms. *Z. Naturforsch.* 35:503–507.

963. Johnson, B. F. and C. Chura. 1974. Diurnal variation in the effect of tolbutamide. *Am. J. Med. Sci.* 268:93–96.

964. Johnstone-Wallace, D. B. and K. Kennedy. 1944. Grazing management practices and their relationship to the behaviour and grazing habits of cattle. *J. Agric. Sci.* 34:190–197.

965. Jones, A. C. and S. D. Gosling. 2005. Temperament and personality in dogs (*Canis familiaris*): A review and evaluation of past research. *Appl. Anim. Behav. Sci.* 95:1–53.

966. Jones, C. G., K. D. Maddever, D. L. Court and M. Phillips. 1966. The time taken by cows to eat concentrates. *Anim. Prod.* 8:489–497.

967. Jones, J. B., N. L. Carmichael, C. M. Wathes, R. P. White and R. B. Jones. 2000. The effects of acute simultaneous exposure to ammonia on the detection of buried odourized food by pigs. *Appl. Anim. Behav. Sci.* 65:305–319.

968. Jongman, E. C., I. Bidstrup and P. H. Hemsworth. 2005. Behavioural and physiological measures of welfare of pregnant mares fitted with a novel urine collection device. *Appl. Anim. Behav. Sci.* 93:147–163.

969. Jorgensen, G. and K. Boe. 2007. A note on the effect of daily exercise and paddock size on the behaviour of domestic horses (*Equus caballus*). *Appl. Anim. Behav. Sci.* 107:166–173.

970. Jorgensen, G. H. M., I. L. Andersen and K. E. Boe. 2009. The effect of different pen partition configurations on the behaviour of sheep. *Appl. Anim. Behav. Sci.* 119:66–70.

971. Jorgensen, G. H. M., I. L. Andersen and K. E. Boe. 2007. Feed intake and social interactions in dairy goats—The effects of feeding space and type of roughage. *Appl. Anim. Behav. Sci.* 107:239–251.

972. Juarbe-Diaz, S. V. and K. A. Houpt. 1996. Comparison of two antibarking collars for treatment of nuisance barking. *J. Am. Anim. Hosp. Assoc.* 32:231–235.

973. Juarbe-Diaz, S. V., K. A. Houpt and R. Kusunose. 1998. Prevalence and characteristics of foal rejection in Arabian mares. *Equine Vet. J.* 30:424–428.

974. Kalums, H. 1955. The discrimination by the nose of the dog of individual human odours and in particular of the odours of twins. *Br. J. Anim. Behav.* 3:25–31.

975. Kaminski, J., J. Call and J. Fischer. 2004. Word learning in a domestic dog: Evidence for "fast mapping". *Science* 304:1682–1683.

976. Kaminski, J., J. Fischer and J. Call. 2008. Prospective object search in dogs: Mixed evidence for knowledge of what and where. *Anim. Cogn.* 11:367–371.

977. Kaminski, J., J. Riedel, J. Call and M. Tomasello. 2005. Domestic goats, *Capra hircus*, follow gaze direction and use social cues in an object choice task. *Anim. Behav.* 69:11–18.

978. Kanarck, R. B. 1975. Availability and caloric density of the diet as determinants of meal patterns in cats. *Physiol. Behav.* 15:611–618.

979. Kanno, Y. 1977. Experimental studies on body temperature rhythm in dogs. I. Application of cosinor method to body temperature rhythm in dogs (author's transl). *Nippon Juigaku Zasshi* 39:69–76.

980. Karas, G. G., R. I. Willham and D. F. Cox. 1962. Avoidance learning in swine. *Psychol. Rep.* 11: 51–54.

981. Kare, M. R., W. C. Pond and J. Campbell. 1965. Observations on the taste reactions in pigs. *Anim. Behav.* 13:265–269.

982. Karlander, S., J. Mansson and G. Tufvesson. 1965. Buccostomy as a method of treatment for arcophagia (windsucking) in the horse. *Nordisk Vet. Med.* 17:455–458.

983. Karn, H. W. and H. R. Malamud. 1939. The behavior of dogs on the double alternation problem in the temporal maze. *J. Comp. Psychol.* 27:461–466.

984. Karn, J. F. and D. C. Clanton. 1974. Electronically controlled individual cattle feeding. *J. Anim. Sci.* 39:136.

985. Karsh, E. B. and D. C. Turner. 1988. The human-cat relationship. In D. C. Turner and P. Bateson (Eds.), *The domestic cat*, pp. 159–177. Cambridge, UK: Cambridge University Press.

986. Kaseda, Y. and A. M. Khalil. 1996. Harem size and reproductive success of stallions in Misaki feral horses. *Appl. Anim. Behav. Sci.* 47:163–174.

987. Kasper, M. and A. M. Beck. 1997. Effect of environmental temperature on the behavior of clydesdales during preparation time before athletic performances. *Equine Pract.* 19:25–28.

988. Katz, L. S., E. O. Price, S. J. Wallach and J. J. Zenchak. 1988. Sexual performance of rams reared with or without females after weaning. *J. Anim. Sci.* 66:1166–1173.

989. Kaulfuss, P. and D. S. Mills. 2008. Neophilia in domestic dogs (*Canis familiaris*) and its implication for studies of dog cognition. *Anim. Cogn.* 11:553–556.

990. Kay, R. and C. Hall. 2009. The use of a mirror reduces isolation stress in horses being transported by trailer. *Appl. Anim. Behav. Sci.* 116:237–243.

991. Keil, N. M. and W. Langhans. 2001. The development of intersucking in dairy calves around weaning. *Appl. Anim. Behav. Sci.* 72:295–308.

992. Keiper, R. R. 1985. *The assateague ponies*. Centreville, MD: Tidewater Press.

993. Keiper, R. R. 1976. Social organization of feral ponies. *Proc. Penn. Acad. Sci.* 50:69–70.

994. Keiper, R. R. and J. Berger. 1982. Refuge-seeking and pest avoidance by feral horses in desert and island environments. *Appl. Anim. Ethol.* 9:111–120.

995. Keiper, R. R. and K. A. Houpt. 1984. Reproduction in feral horses: An eight-year study. *Am. J. Vet. Res.* 45:991–995.

996. Keiper, R. R. and H. Receveur. 1992. Social interactions of free-ranging Przewalski horses in semi-reserves in The Netherlands. *Appl. Anim. Behav. Sci.* 33:303–318.

997. Keiper, R. R. and H. H. Sambraus. 1986. The stability of equine dominance hierarchies and the effects of kinship, proximity and foaling status on hierarchy rank. *Appl. Anim. Behav. Sci.* 16:121–130.

998. Kendrick, K. M., K. Atkins, M. R. Hinton, K. B. Broad, C. Fabre-Nys and E. B. Keverne. 1995. Facial an vocal discrimination in sheep. *Anim. Behav.* 49:1665–1676.

999. Kendrick, K. M., A. P. da Costa, A. E. Leigh, M. R. Hinton and J. W. Peirce. 2001. Sheep don't forget a face. *Nature* 414:165–166.

1000. Kendrick, K. M. and E. B. Keverne. 1991. Importance of progesterone and estrogen priming for the induction of maternal behavior by vaginocervical stimulation in sheep: Effects of maternal experience. *Physiol. Behav.* 49:745–750.

1001. Kendrick, K. M., E. B. Keverne and B. A. Baldwin. 1987. Intracerebroventricular oxytocin stimulates maternal behaviour in the sheep. *Neuroendocrinology* 46:56–61.

1002. Kendrick, K. M., E. B. Keverne, B. A. Baldwin and D. F. Sharman. 1986. Cerebrospinal fluid levels of acetylcholinesterase, monoamines and oxytocin during labour, parturition, vaginocervical stimulation, lamb separation and suckling in sheep. *Neuroendocrinology* 44:149–156.

1003. Kennedy, J. M. and B. A. Baldwin. 1972. Taste preferences in pigs for nutritive and non-nutritive sweet solutions. *Anim. Behav.* 20:706–718.

1004. Kenny, F. J. and P. V. Tarrant. 1987. The behaviour of young Friesian bulls during social re-grouping at an abattoir. influence of an overhead electrified wire grid. *Appl. Anim. Behav. Sci.* 18:233–246.

1005. Kent, J. P. 1984. A note on multiple fostering of calves onto nurse cows at a few days post-partum. *Appl. Anim. Behav. Sci.* 12:183–186.

1006. Kerruish, B. M. 1955. The effect of sexual stimulation prior to service on the behaviour and conception rate of bulls. *Br. J. Anim. Behav.* 3:125–130.

1007. Keverne, E. B., F. Levy, P. Poindron and D. R. Lindsay. 1983. Vaginal stimulation: An important determinant of maternal bonding in sheep. *Science* 219:81–83.

1008. Key, C. and R. M. MacIver. 1977. Factors affecting sexual preferences in sheep. *Appl. Anim. Ethol.* 3:291.

1009. Khalil, A. M. and Y. Kaseda. 1997. Behavioral patterns and proximate reason of young male separation in Misaki feral horses. *Appl. Anim. Behav. Sci.* 54:281–289.

1010. Khalil, A. M. and N. Murakami. 1999. Effect of natal dispersal on the reproductive strategies of the young Misaki feral stallions. *Appl. Anim. Behav. Sci.* 62:281–291.

1011. Kiddy, C. A., D. S. Mitchell, D. J. Bolt and H. W. Hawk. 1978. Detection of estrus-related odors in cows by trained dogs. *Biol. Reprod.* 19:389–395.

1012. Kiley, M. 1976. Fostering and adoption in beef cattle. *Br. Cattle Breeders Club Dig.* 31:42–55.

1013. Kiley, M. 1972. The vocalizations of ungulates, their causation and function. *Z. Tierpsychol.* 31:171–222.

1014. Kiley-Worthington, M. 1977. *Behavioural problems of farm animals.* Stocksfield, UK: Oriel Press.

1015. Kiley-Worthington, M. 1976. The tail movements of ungulates, canids and felids with particular reference to their causation and function as displays. *Behaviour* 56:69–115.

1016. Kiley-Worthington, M. and P. Savage. 1978. Learning in dairy cattle using a device for economical management of behaviour. *Appl. Anim. Ethol.* 4:119–124.

1017. Kilgour, R. 1981. Use of the Hebb-Williams closed-field test to study the learning ability of Jersey cows. *Anim. Behav.* 29:850–860.

1018. Kilgour, R. 1972. Some observations on the suckling activity of calves on nurse cows. *Proc. N. Z. Soc. Anim. Prod.* 32:132–136.

1019. Kilgour, R. and D. N. Campin. 1973. The behaviour of entire bulls of different ages at pasture. *Proc. N. Z. Soc. Anim. Prod.* 33:125–138.

1020. Kilgour, R. and T. H. Scott. 1959. Leadership in a herd of dairy cows. *Proc. N. Z. Soc. Anim. Prod.* 19:36–43.

1021. Kilgour, R., B. H. Skarsholt, J. F. Smith, K. J. Bremmer and M. C. L. Morrison. 1977. Observations on the behaviour and factors influencing the sexually-active group in cattle. *Proc. N. Z. Soc. Anim. Prod.* 37:128–135.

1022. Kilgour, R. and C. G. Winfield. 1977. Pen-mating of pedigree sheep. *N. Z. J. Agric.* 134:25–27.

1023. Kilgour, R., C. G. Winfield, K. J. Bremmer, M. M. Mullord, H. de Langen and S. J. Hudson. 1976. Behaviour of early-weaned calves in indoor individual cubicles and group pens. *N. Z. Vet. J.* 23:119–123.

1024. Kilgour, R. J., G. J. Melville and P. L. Greenwood. 2006. Individual differences in the reaction of beef cattle to situations involving social isolation, close proximity of humans, restraint and novelty. *Appl. Anim. Behav. Sci.* 99:21–40.

1025. Kim, F. B., R. E. Jackson, G. D. Gordon and M. S. Cockram. 1994. Resting behaviour of sheep in a slaughterhouse lairage. *Appl. Anim. Behav. Sci.* 40:45–54.

1026. Kimball, B. A., F. D. Provenza and E. A. Burritt. 2002. Importance of alternative foods on the persistence of flavor aversions: Implications for applied flavor avoidance learning. *Appl. Anim. Behav. Sci.* 76:249–258.

1027. King, J. E., B. A. Becker and J. E. Markee. 1964. Studies on olfactory discrimination in dogs: (3) ability to detect human odour trace. *Anim. Behav.* 12:311–315.

1028. King, T., P. H. Hemsworth and G. J. Coleman. 2003. Fear of novel and startling stimuli in domestic dogs. *Appl. Anim. Behav. Sci.* 82:45–64.

1029. Kirkpatrick, J. F., R. Vail, S. Devous, S. Schwend, C. B. Baker and L. Wiesner. 1976. Diurnal variation of plasma testosterone in wild stallions. *Biol. Reprod.* 15:98–101.

1030. Kirkwood, R. N., J. M. Forbes and P. E. Hughes. 1981. Influence of boar contact on attainment of puberty in gilts after removal of the olfactory bulbs. *J. Reprod. Fertil.* 61:193–196.

1031. Kitchell, R. L. 1972. Dogs know what they like. *Friskies Res. Dig.* 8:1–4.

1032. Klemm, W. R., C. J. Sherry, L. M. Schake and R. F. Sis. 1983. Homosexual behavior in feedlot steers: An aggression hypothesis. *Appl. Anim. Ethol.* 11:187–195.

1033. Kling, A. and D. Coustan. 1964. Electrical stimulation of the amygdala and hypothalamus in the kitten. *Exp. Neurol.* 10:81–89.

1034. Kling, A., J. K. Kovach and T. J. Tucker. 1969. The behaviour of cats. In E. S. E. Hafez (Ed.), *The behaviour of domestic animals*, pp. 482–512. Baltimore, MD: Williams & Wilkins.

1035. Klingel, H. 1974. A comparison of the social behaviour of the equidae. In V. Geist and F. Walther (Eds.), The behaviour of ungulates and its relation to management, pp. 124–132. Morges, Switzerland: International Union for Conservation of Nature and Natural Resources.

1036. Klopfer, F. D. 1966. Visual learning in swine. In L. K. Bustad, R. O. McClellan and M. P. Burns (Eds.), Swine in biomedical research, pp. 559–574. Richland, WA: Battelle Memorial Institute Pacific Northwest Laboratory.

1037. Klopfer, F. D. 1961. Early experience and discrimination learning in swine. *Am. Zool.* 1:366.

1038. Klopfer, F. D. and J. Gamble. 1966. Maternal "imprinting" on goats: The role of chemical senses. *Z. Tierpsychol.* 23:588–592.

1039. Knecht, C. D., J. E. Oliver, R. Redding, R. Selcer and G. Johnson. 1973. Narcolepsy in a dog and a cat. *J. Am. Vet. Med. Assoc.* 162:1052–1053.

1040. Knight, T. W. and P. R. Lynch. 1980. Source of ram pheromones that stimulate ovulation in the ewe. *Anim. Reprod. Sci.* 3:133–136.

1041. Knowles, R. J., T. M. Curtis and S. L. Crowell-Davis. 2004. Correlation of dominance as determined by agonistic interactions with feeding order in cats. *Am. J. Vet. Res.* 65:1548–1556.

1042. Koba, Y. and H. Tanida. 2001. How do miniature pigs discriminate between people? Discrimination between people wearing coveralls of the same colour. *Appl. Anim. Behav. Sci.* 73:45–58.

1043. Kobelt, A. J., P. H. Hemsworth, J. L. Barnett, G. J. Coleman and K. L. Butler. 2007. The behaviour of Labrador retrievers in suburban backyards: The relationships between the backyard environment and dog behaviour. *Appl. Anim. Behav. Sci.* 106:70–84.

1044. Koepke, J. E. and K. H. Pribram. 1971. Effect of milk on the maintenance of sucking behavior in kittens from birth to six months. *J. Comp. Physiol. Psychol.* 75:363–377.

1045. Kolb, B. and A. J. Nonneman. 1975. The development of social responsiveness in kittens. *Anim. Behav.* 23:368–374.

1046. Kondo, S. and J. F. Hurnik. 1990. Stabilization of social hierarchy in dairy cows. *Appl. Anim. Behav. Sci.* 57:287–297.

1047. Kondo, S., N. Kawakami, H. Kohama and S. Nishino. 1983. Changes in activity spatial pattern and social behavior in calves after grouping. *Appl. Anim. Ethol.* 11:217–228.

1048. Kongsted, A. G., J. E. Hermansen and T. Kristensen. 2007. Relation between parity and feed intake, fear of humans, and social behaviour in non-lactating sows group-housed under various on-farm conditions. *Anim. Welfare* 16:263–266.

1049. Konrad, K. W. and M. Bagshaw. 1970. Effect of novel stimuli on cats reared in a restricted environment. *J. Comp. Physiol. Psychol.* 70:157–164.

1050. Kooij, E.-v. E. d., A. H. Kuijpers, J. W. Schrama, F. J. C. M. van Eerdenburg, W. G. P. Schouten and M. J. M. Tielen. 2002. Can we predict behaviour in pigs? Searching for consistency in behaviour over time and across situations. *Appl. Anim. Behav. Sci.* 75:293–305.

1051. Koopmans, S. J., M. Ruis, R. Dekker, H. van Diepen, M. Korte and Z. Mroz. 2005. Surplus dietary tryptophan reduces plasma cortisol and noradrenaline concentrations and enhances recovery after social stress in pigs. *Physiol. Behav.* 85:469–478.

1052. Korda, K. W. and M. Bagshaw. 1977. Effect of stimuli emitted by sucklings on tactile contact of the bitches with sucklings and on number of licking cats. *Acta Neurobiol.* 37:99–115.

1053. Kouwenberg, A. -L., C. J. Walsh, B. E. Morgan and G. M. Martin. 2009. Episodic-like memory in crossbred Yucatan minipigs (*Sus scrofa*). *Appl. Anim. Behav. Sci.* 117:165–172.

1054. Kovach, J. K. and A. Kling. 1967. Mechanisms of neonate sucking behaviour in the kitten. *Anim. Behav.* 15:91–101.

1055. Kovalcik, K. and M. Kovalcik. 1986. Learning ability and memory testing in cattle of different ages. *Appl. Anim. Behav. Sci.* 15:27–29.

1056. Krabill, L. F., P. J. Wangsness and C. A. Baile. 1978. Effects of elfazepam on digestibility and feeding behavior in sheep. *J. Anim. Sci.* 46:1356–1359.

1057. Kranendonk, G., H. Van Der Mheen, M. Fillerup and H. Hopster. 2007. Social rank of pregnant sows affects their body weight gain and behavior and performance of the offspring. *J. Anim. Sci.* 85:420–429.

1058. Kratzer, D. D. 1969. Effects of age on avoidance learning in pigs. *J. Anim. Sci.* 28:175–179.

1059. Kratzer, D. D., W. M. Netherland, R. E. Pulse and J. P. Baker. 1977. Maze learning in quarter horses. *J. Anim. Sci.* 45:896–902.

1060. Krawczel, P. D., T. H. Friend and R. Johnson. 2006. A note on the preference of naive horses for different water bowls. *Appl. Anim. Behav. Sci.* 100:309–313.

1061. Krebs, J. R. and N. B. Davies. 1978. *Behavioural ecology: An evolutionary approach.* Sunderland, MA: Sinauer Associates.

1062. Kristal, M. B., A. C. Thompson, S. B. Heller and B. R. Komisaruk. 1986. Placenta ingestion enhances analgesia produced by vaginal/cervical stimulation in rats. *Physiol. Behav.* 36:1017–1020.

1063. Kristula, M. A. and S. M. McDonnell. 1994. Drinking water temperature affects consumption of water during cold weather in ponies. *Appl. Anim. Behav. Sci.* 41:155–160.

1064. Krohn, C. C., J. G. Jago and X. Boivin. 2001. The effect of early handling on the socialisation of young calves to humans. *Appl. Anim. Behav. Sci.* 74:121–133.

1065. Krohn, C. C. and L. Munksgaard. 1993. Behaviour of dairy cows kept in extensive (loose housing/pasture) or intensive (tie stall) environments. II. Lying and lying-down behaviour. *Appl. Anim. Behav. Sci.* 37:1–16.

1066. Kronberg, S. L., R. B. Muntifering and E. L. Ayers. 1993. Feed aversion learning in cattle with delayed negative consequences. *J. Anim. Sci.* 71:1767–1770.

1067. Krueger, K. 2007. Behaviour of horses in the "round pen technique". *Appl. Anim. Behav. Sci.* 104:162–170.

1068. Kry, K. and R. Casey. 2007. The effect of hiding enrichment on stress levels and behaviour of domestic cats (*Felis sylvestris catus*) in a shelter setting and the implications for adoption potential. *Anim. Welfare* 16:375–383.

1069. Krzak, W. E., H. W. Gonyou and L. M. Lawrence. 1991. Wood chewing by stabled horses: Diurnal pattern and effects of exercise. *J. Anim. Sci.* 69:1053–1058.

1070. Kuhn, G. and W. Hardegg. 1988. Effects of indoor and outdoor maintenance of dogs upon food intake, body weight, and different blood parameters. *Z. Versuchstierkd.* 31:205–214.

1071. Kuipers, M. and T. S. Whatson. 1979. Sleep in piglets: An observational study. *Appl. Anim. Ethol.* 5:145–151.

1072. Kuntz, R., C. Kubalek, T. Ruf, F. Tataruch and W. Arnold. 2006. Seasonal adjustment of energy budget in a large wild mammal, the Przewalski horse (*Equus ferus przewalskii*) I. Energy intake. *J. Exp. Biol.* 209:4557–4565.

1073. Kuo, Z. Y. 1930. The genesis of the cat's responses to the rat. *J. Comp. Psychol.* 11:1–35.

1074. Kurz, J. C. and R. L. Marchinton. 1972. Radiotelemetry studies of feral hogs in South Carolina. *J. Wildl. Manag.* 36:1240–1248.

1075. Kusunose, R. 1992. Diurnal pattern of cribbing in stabled horses. *Jpn. J. Equine Sci.* 3:173–176.

1076. Kusunose, R. and H. Sawazaki. 1984. The behavioral development of thoroughbred foals and the relationship between dams and foals. *Jap. J. Zootech.* 55:263–271.

1077. Kusunose, R. and K. Torikai. 1996. Behavior of untethered horses during vehicle transport. *J. Eq. Sci.* 7:21–26.

1078. Kusunose, R. and A. Yamanobe. 2002. The effect of training schedule on learned tasks in yearling horses. *Appl. Anim. Behav. Sci.* 78:225–233.

1079. Kusunose, R. H., H. Hatakeyama, F. Ichikawa, K. Kubo, A. Kiguchi, Y. Asai and K. Ito. 1986. Behavioural studies on yearling horses in field environments. 2. Effects of the group size on the behavior of horses. *Bull. Equine Res. Ins.* 23:1–6.

1080. Kusunose, R. H., H. Hatakeyama, F. Ichikawa, H. Oki, Y. Asai and K. Ito. 1987. Behavioral studies on yearling horses in field environments. 3. Effects of the pasture shape on the behavior of horses. *Bull. Equine Res. Ins.* 24:1–5.

1081. Kusunose, R. H., H. Hatakeyama, K. Kubo, A. Kiguchi, Y. Asai, Y. Fujii and K. Ito. 1985. Behavioral studies on yearling horses in field environments. 1. Effects of the field size on the behavior of horses. *Bull. Equine Res. Ins.* 22:1–7.

1082. Laca, E. A., E. D. Ungar and M. W. Demment. 1994. Mechanisms of handling time and intake rate of a large mammalian grazer. *Appl. Anim. Behav. Sci.* 39:3–19.

1083. Ladewig, J. and B. L. Hart. 1980. Flehmen and vomeronasal organ function in male goats. *Physiol. Behav.* 24:1067–1071.

1084. Lagerweij, E., P. C. Nelis, V. M. Wiegant and J. M. van Ree. 1984. The twitch in horses: A variant of acupuncture. *Science* 225:1172–1174.

1085. Lammers, G. J. and A. De Lange. 1986. Pre- and post-farrowing behaviour in primiparous domesticated pigs. *Appl. Anim. Behav. Sci.* 15:31–43.

1086. Landau, S., N. Silanikove, Z. Nitsan, D. Barkai, H. Baram, F. D. Provenza and A. Perevolotsky. 2000. Short-term changes in eating patterns explain the effects of condensed tannins on feed intake in heifers. *Appl. Anim. Behav. Sci.* 69:199–213.

1087. Landsberg, G. M. 1991. The distribution of canine behavior cases at three behavior referral practices. *Vet. Med.* 86:1011–1018.

1088. Landsberg, G. M., W. Hunthausen and L. Ackerman. 1997. *Handbook of behaviour problems of the dog and cat.* Woburn, MA: Butterworth-Heinemann.

1089. Langbein, J., K. Siebert, G. Nurnberg and G. Manteuffel. 2007. Learning to learn during visual discrimination in group housed dwarf goats (*Capra hircus*). *J. Comp. Psychol.* 121:447–456.

1090. Lanier, J. L., T. Grandin, R. Green, D. Avery and K. McGee. 2001. A note on hair whorl position and cattle temperament in the auction ring. *Appl. Anim. Behav. Sci.* 73:93–101.

1091. Lanier, J. L., T. Grandin, R. D. Green, D. Avery and K. McGee. 2000. The relationship between reaction to sudden, intermittent movements and sounds and temperament. *J. Anim. Sci.* 78:1467–1474.

1092. Lansade, L., M. Bertrand and M.-F. Bouissou. 2005. Effects of neonatal handling on subsequent manageability, reactivity and learning ability of foals. *Appl. Anim. Behav. Sci.* 92:143–158.

1093. Lansade, L. and M.-F. Bouissou. 2008. Reactivity to humans: A temperament trait of horses which is stable across time and situations. *Appl. Anim. Behav. Sci.* 114:492–508.

1094. Lansade, L., M.-F. Bouissou and H. W. Erhard. 2008. Fearfulness in horses: A temperament trait stable across time and situations. *Appl. Anim. Behav. Sci.* 115:182–200.

1095. Lansade, L., G. Pichard and M. Leconte. 2008. Sensory sensitivities: Components of a horse's temperament dimension. *Appl. Anim. Behav. Sci.* 114:534–553.

1096. Lauber, M. C. Y., P. H. Hemsworth and J. L. Barnett. 2006. The effects of age and experience on behavioural development in dairy calves. *Appl. Anim. Behav. Sci.* 99:41–52.

1097. Launchbaugh, K. L. and F. D. Provenza. 1994. The effect of flavor concentration and toxin dose on the formation and generalization of flavor aversions in lambs. *J. Anim. Sci.* 72:10–13.

1098. Laundre, J. 1977. The daytime behavior of domestic cats in a free-roaming population. *Anim. Behav.* 25:990–998.

1099. Laut, J. E., K. A. Houpt, H. F. Hintz and T. R. Houpt. 1985. The effects of caloric dilution on meal patterns and food intake of ponies. *Physiol. Behav.* 35:549–554.

1100. Lawrence, A. B. 1990. Mother-daughter and peer relationships of Scottish hill sheep. *Anim. Behav.* 39:481–486.

1101. Lawrence, A. B., J. C. Petherick, K. McLean, C. L. Gilbert, C. Chapman and J. A. Russell. 1992. Naloxone prevents interruption of parturition and increases plasma oxytocin following environmental disturbance in parturient sows. *Physiol. Behav.* 52:917–923.

1102. Lawson, D. C., S. S. Shiffman and T. N. Pappas. 1993. Short-term oral sensory deprivation: Possible cause of binge eating in sham-feeding dogs. *Physiol. Behav.* 53:1231–1234.

1103. Lay, D. C. Jr, M. F. Haussmann, H. S. Buchanan and M. J. Daniels. 1999. Danger to pigs due to crushing can be reduced by the use of a simulated udder. *J. Anim. Sci.* 77:2060–2064.

1104. Lazo, A. 1994. Social segregation and the maintenance of social stability in a feral cattle population. *Anim. Behav.* 48:1133–1141.

1105. Le Boeuf, B. J. 1970. Copulatory and aggressive behavior in the prepuberally castrated dog. *Horm. Behav.* 1:127–136.

1106. Le Boeuf, B. J. 1967. Interindividual associations in dogs. *Behaviour* 29:268–295.

1107. Le Neindre, P., G. Trillat, J. Sapa, F. Menissier, J. N. Bonnet and J. M. Chupin. 1995. Individual differences in docility in Limousin cattle. *J. Anim. Sci.* 73:2249–2253.

1108. Lee, C., S. Colegate and A. D. Fisher. 2006. Development of a maze test and its application to assess spatial learning and memory in Merino sheep. *Appl. Anim. Behav. Sci.* 96:43–51.

1109. Lee, C., A. D. Fisher, M. T. Reed and J. M. Henshell. 2008. The effect of low energy electric shock on cortisol, β-endorphin, heart rate and behaviour of cattle. *Appl. Anim. Behav. Sci.* 113:32–42.

1110. Lee, C., J. M. Henshall, T. J. Wark, C. C. Crossman, M. T. Reed, H. G. Brewer, J. O'Grady and A. D. Fisher. 2009. Associative learning by cattle to enable effective and ethical virtual fences. *Appl. Anim. Behav. Sci.* 119:15–22.

1111. Lee, C., K. Prayaga, M. Reed and J. Henshall. 2007. Methods of training cattle to avoid a location using electrical cues. *Appl. Anim. Behav. Sci.* 108:229–238.

1112. Lee, C., K. C. Prayaga, A. D. Fisher and J. M. Henshall. 2008. Behavioral aspects of electronic bull separation and mate allocation in multiple-sire mating paddocks. *J. Anim. Sci.* 86:1690–1696.

1113. Lee, J., T. Floyd and K. A. Houpt. 2001. Operant and two-choice preference applied to equine welfare. 35th International Congress of the ISAE. University of California, Davis.

1114. Lee, J., K. A. Houpt and O. Dogherty. 2001. A survey of trailering problems in horses. *J. Eq. Vet. Sci.* 21:23–26.

1115. Lees, J. L. and M. Weatherhead. 1970. A note on mating preferences of clun forest ewes. *Anim. Prod.* 12:173–175.

1116. Lefebvre, D., C. Diederich, M. Delcourt and J.-M. Giffroy. 2007. The quality of the relation between handler and military dogs influences efficiency and welfare of dogs. *Appl. Anim. Behav. Sci.* 104:49–60.

1117. Lehmann, K., E. Kallweit and F. Ellendorff. 2006. Social hierarchy in exercised and untrained group-house horses–a brief report. *Appl. Anim. Behav. Sci.* 96:343–347.

1118. Lehner, P. N., C. McCluggage, D. R. Mitchell and D. H. Neil. 1983. Selected parameters of the fort collins, colorado, dog population. *Appl. Anim. Ethol.* 10:19–25.

1119. Lenhardt, M. L. 1977. Vocal contour cues in maternal recognition of goat kids. *Appl. Anim. Ethol.* 3:211–219.

1120. Lensink, B. J., S. Raussi, X. Boivin, M. Pyykkonen and I. I. Veissier. 2001. Reactions of calves to handling depend on housing condition and previous experience with humans. *Appl. Anim. Behav. Sci.* 70:187–199.

1121. Lensink, J., I. Veissier and A. Boissy. 2006. Enhancement of performances in a learning task in suckler calves after weaning and relocation: Motivational versus cognitive control?: A pilot study. *Appl. Anim. Behav. Sci.* 100:171–181.

1122. Levine, A. S., C. E. Sievert, J. E. Morley, B. A. Gosnell and S. E. Silvis. 1984. Peptidergic regulation of feeding in the dog (*Canis familiaris*). *Peptides* 5:675–679.

1123. Levine, E., P. Perry, J. Scarlett and K. A. Houpt. 2005. Intercat aggression in households following the introduction of a new cat. *Appl. Anim. Behav. Sci.* 90:325–336.

1124. Levine, E. D., D. Ramos and D. S. Mills. 2007. A prospective study of two self-help CD based desensitization conditioning programmes with the use of dog appeasing pheromone for the treatment of firework fears in dogs (*Canis familiaris*). *Appl. Anim. Behav. Sci.* 105:311–329.

1125. Levis, D. G., J. L. Barnett, P. H. Hemsworth and E. Jongman. 1995. The effect of breeding facility and sexual stimulation on plasma cortisol in boars. *J. Anim. Sci.* 73:3705–3711.

1126. Levy, F., R. Gervais, U. Kindermann, M. Litterio, P. Poindron and R. Porter. 1991. Effects of early post-partum separation on maintenance of maternal responsiveness and selectivity in parturient ewes. *Appl. Anim. Behav. Sci.* 31:101–110.

1127. Levy, F., A. Locatelli, V. Piketty, Y. Tillet and P. Poindron. 1995. Involvement of the main but not the accessory olfactory system in maternal behavior of primiparous and multiparous ewes. *Physiol. Behav.* 57:97–104.

1128. Levy, F. and P. Poindron. 1987. The importance of amniotic fluids for the establishment of maternal behaviour in experienced and inexperienced ewes. *Anim. Behav.* 35:1188–1192.

1129. Levy, F., P. Poindron and P. Le Neindre. 1983. Attraction and repulsion by amniotic fluids and their olfactory control in the ewe around parturition. *Physiol. Behav.* 31:687–692.

1130. Lewis, E., L. A. Boyle, J. V. O'Doherty, P. B. Lynch and P. Brophy. 2006. The effect of providing shredded paper or ropes to piglets in farrowing crates on their behaviour and health and the behaviour and health of their dams. *Appl. Anim. Behav. Sci.* 96:1–17.

1131. Lewis, N. J. 1999. Frustration of goal-directed behaviour in swine. *Appl. Anim. Behav. Sci.* 64:19–29.

1132. Lewis, N. J. and J. F. Hurnik. 1985. The development of nursing behaviour in swine. *Appl. Anim. Behav. Sci.* 14:225–232.

1133. Leyhausen, P. 1979. *Cat behaviour*. New York, NY: Garland STPM Press.

1134. Leyhausen, P. 1975. *Verhaltensstudien an katzen*. Berlin, Germany: Paul Parey.

1135. Leyhausen, P. 1973. Addictive behavior in free-ranging animals. In L. Goldberg and F. Hoffmeister (Eds.), *Bayer symposium IV. Psychic dependence*. Berlin, Germany: Springer-Verlag.

1136. Li, Y. and H. W. Gonyou. 2002. Analysis of belly nosing and associated behaviour among pigs weaned at 12–14 days of age. *Appl. Anim. Behav. Sci.* 77:285–294.

1137. Liberg, O. 1983. Courtship behaviour and sexual selection in the domestic cat. *Appl. Anim. Ethol.* 10:117–132.

1138. Lickliter, R. E. 1987. Activity patterns and companion preferences of domestic goat kids. *Appl. Anim. Behav. Sci.* 19:137–145.

1139. Lickliter, R. E. 1985. Behavior associated with parturition in the domesticated goat. *Appl. Anim. Behav. Sci.* 13:335–345.

1140. Lickliter, R. E. 1984. Mother-infant spatial relationships in domestic goats. *Appl. Anim. Behav. Sci.* 13:93–100.

1141. Lickliter, R. E. and J. R. Heron. 1984. Recognition of mother by newborn goats. *Appl. Anim. Behav. Sci.* 12:187–192.

1142. Liddell, H. S. 1954. Conditioning and emotions. *Sci. Am.* 190:48–57.

1143. Liddell, H. S. 1926. The effect of thyroidectomy on some unconditioned responses of the sheep and goat. *Am. J. Physiol.* 75:579–590.

1144. Liddell, H. S. 1926. A laboratory for the study of conditioned motor reflexes. *Am. J. Psychol.* 37:418–419.

1145. Liddell, H. S. and O. D. Anderson. 1931. A comparative study of the conditioned motor reflex in the rabbit, sheep, goat, and pig. *Am. J. Physiol.* 97:539–540.

1146. Liddell, H. S., W. T. James and O. D. Anderson. 1934. The comparative physiology of the conditioned motor reflex based on experiments with the pig, dog, sheep, goat and rabbit. *Comp. Psychol. Monogr.* 11:1–89.

1147. Lidffors, L. M. 1993. Corss-sucking in group-housed dairy calves before and after weaning off milk. *Appl. Anim. Behav. Sci.* 38:15–24.

1148. Lidfors, L. and P. Jensen. 1988. Behaviour of free-ranging beef cows and calves. *Appl. Anim. Behav. Sci.* 20:237–247.

1149. Ligout, S., M.-F. Bouissou and X. Boivin. 2008. Comparison of the effects of two different handling methods on the subsequent behaviour of Anglo-Arabian foals toward humans and handling. *Appl. Anim. Behav. Sci.* 113:175–188.

1150. Ligout, S., R. H. Porter and R. Bon. 2002. Social discrimination in lambs: Persistence and scope. *Appl. Anim. Behav. Sci.* 76:239–248.

1151. Liinamo, A. E., L. Karjalainen, M. Ojala and V. Vilva. 1997. Estimates of genetic parameters and environmental effects for measures of hunting performance in Finnish hounds. *J. Anim. Sci.* 75:622–629.

1152. Liinamo, A.-E., L. Van Den Berg, P. A. J. Leegwater, M. B. H. Schilder, J. A. M. van Arendonk and B. A. van Oost. 2007. Genetic variation in aggression-related traits in Golden Retriever dogs. *Appl. Anim. Behav. Sci.* 104:95–106.

1153. Lin, L., J. Faraco, R. Li, H. Kadotani, W. Rogers, X. Lin, X. Qiu, P. J. de Jong, S. Nishino and E. Mignot. 1999. The sleep disorder canine narcolepsy is caused by a mutation in the hypocretin (orexin) receptor 2 gene. *Cell* 98:365–376.

1154. Lindahl, I. L. 1964. Time of parturition in ewes. *Anim. Behav.* 12:231–234.

1155. Lindberg, A. C., A. Kelland and C. J. Nicol. 1999. Effects of observational learning on acquisition of an operant response in horses. *Appl. Anim. Behav. Sci.* 61:187–199.

1156. Lindell, E. M., H. N. Erb and K. A. Houpt. 1997. Intercat aggression: A retrospective study examining types of aggression, sexes of fighting pairs, and effectiveness of treatment. *Appl. Anim. Behav. Sci.* 55:153–162.

1157. Lindsay, D. R. 1966. Mating behaviour of ewes and its effect on mating efficiency. *Anim. Behav.* 14:419–424.

1158. Lindsay, D. R. 1966. Modification of behavioural oestrus in the ewe by social and hormonal factors. *Anim. Behav.* 14:73–83.

1159. Lindsay, D. R. 1965. The importance of olfactory stimuli in the mating behaviour of the ram. *Anim. Behav.* 13:75–78.

1160. Lindsay, D. R. and I. C. Fletcher. 1972. Ram-seeking activity associated with oestrous behaviour in ewes. *Anim. Behav.* 20:452–456.

1161. Lindsay, D. R. and I. C. Fletcher. 1968. Sensory involvement in the recognition of lambs by their dams. *Anim. Behav.* 16:415–417.

1162. Lindsay, D. R. and T. J. Robinson. 1961. Studies on the efficiency of mating in the sheep. I. The effect of paddock size and number of rams. *J. Agric. Sci.* 57:137–140.

1163. Lindsay, D. R. and T. J. Robinson. 1961. Studies on the efficiency of mating in the sheep. II. The effect of freedom of rams, paddock size, and age of ewes. *J. Agric. Sci.* 57:141–145.

1164. Line, S. W., B. L. Hart and L. Sanders. 1985. Effect of prepubertal versus postpubertal castration on sexual and aggressive behavior in male horses. *J. Am. Vet. Med. Assoc.* 186:249–251.

1165. Linklater, W. L. 2000. Adaptive explanation in socio-ecology: Lessons from the equidae. *Biol. Rev. Camb. Philos. Soc.* 75:1–20.

1166. Linklater, W. L. and E. Z. Cameron. 2009. Social dispersal but with philopatry reveals incest avoidance in a polygynous ungulate. *Anim. Behav.* 77:1085–1093.

1167. Linklater, W. L., E. Z. Cameron, E. O. Minot and K. J. Stafford. 1999. Stallion harassment and the mating system of horses. *Anim. Behav.* 58:295–306.

1168. Linnane, M. I., A. J. Brereton and P. S. Giller. 2001. Seasonal changes in circadian grazing patterns of Kerry cows (Bos taurus) in semi-feral conditions in Killarney National Park, Co. Kerry, Ireland. *Appl. Anim. Behav. Sci.* 71:277–292.

1169. Liptrap, R. M. and J. I. Raeside. 1978. A relationship between plasma concentrations of testosterone and corticosteroids during sexual and aggressive behaviour in the boar. *J. Endocrinol.* 76:75–85.

1170. Lit, L. and C. A. Crawford. 2006. Effects of training paradigms on search dog performance. *Appl. Anim. Behav. Sci.* 98:277–292.

1171. Littlejohn, A. and R. Munro. 1972. Equine recumbency. *Vet. Rec.* 90:83–85.

1172. Lloyd, A. S., J. E. Martin, H. L. I. Bornett-Gauci and R. G. Wilkinson. 2008. Horse personality: Variation between breeds. *Appl. Anim. Behav. Sci.* 112:369–383.

1173. Lloyd, A. S., J. E. Martin, H. L. I. Bornett-Gauci and R. G. Wilkinson. 2007. Evaluation of a novel method of horse personality assessment: Rater-agreement and links to behaviour. *Appl. Anim. Behav. Sci.* 105:205–222.

1174. Loberg, J. and L. Lidfors. 2001. Effect of stage of lactation and breed on dairy cows' acceptance of foster calves. *Appl. Anim. Behav. Sci.* 74:97–108.

1175. Loberg, J. M., C. E. Hernandez, T. Thierfelder, M. B. Jensen, C. Berg and L. Lidfors. 2008. Weaning and separation in two steps—a way to decrease stress in dairy calves suckled by foster cows. *Appl. Anim. Behav. Sci.* 111:222–234.

1176. Loberg, J. M., C. E. Hernandez, T. Thierfelder, M. B. Jensen, C. Berg and L. Lidfors. 2007. Reaction of foster cows to prevention of suckling from and separation from four calves simultaneously or in two steps. *J. Anim. Sci.* 85:1522–1529.

1177. Lockwood, R. 1987. Pit bull terriers. *Arthrozoos* 1:193–194.

1178. Lohse, C. L. 1974. Preferences of dogs for various meats. *J. Am. Anim. Hosp. Assoc.* 10:187–192.

1179. Lorenz, K. Z. 1952. *King Solomon's ring: New light on animal ways.* New York, NY: Thomas Y. Crowell Co.

1180. Lorenz, K. Z. 1957. Companionship in bird life. In C. H. Schiller and K. S. Lashley (Eds.), *Instinctive behavior. The development of a modern concept*, pp. 82–128. New York, NY: International Universities Press.

1181. Lou, Z. and J. F. Hurnik. 1994. An ellipsoid farrowing crate: Its ergonomical design and effects on pig productivity. *J. Anim. Sci.* 72:2610–2616.

1182. Lowe, S. E. and J. W. Bradshaw. 2001. Ontogeny of individuality in the domestic cat in the home environment. *Anim. Behav.* 61:231–237.

1183. Lowman, B. G., M. S. Hankey, N. A. Scott, D. W. Deas and E. A. Hunter. 1981. Influence of time of feeding on time of parturition in beef cows. *Vet. Rec.* 109:557–559.

1184. Luescher, A. U. 1993. Hyperkinesis in dogs: Six case reports. *Can. Vet. J.* 34:368–370.

1185. Luescher, U. A., D. B. McKeown and H. Dean. 1998. A cross-sectional study on compulsive behaviour (stable vices) in horses. *Eq. Vet. J. Suppl.* 27:14–18.

1186. Lunn, D. P., P. A. Cuddon, S. Shaftoe and R. M. Archer. 1993. Familial occurrence of narcolepsy in miniature horses. *Equine Vet. J.* 25:483–487.

1187. Lunstra, D. D., G. W. Boyd and L. R. Corah. 1989. Effects of natural mating stimuli on serum luteinizing hormone, testosterone and estradiol-17 ß in yearling beef bulls. *J. Anim. Sci.* 67:3277–3288.

1188. Lustgarten, C., G. D. Bottoms and J. R. Shaskas. 1973. Experimental adrenalectomy of pigs. *Am. J. Vet. Res.* 34:279–282.

1189. Lyimo, Z. C., M. Nielen, W. Ouweltjes, T. A. Kruip and F. J. van Eerdenburg. 2000. Relationship among estradiol, cortisol and intensity of estrous behavior in dairy cattle. *Theriogenology* 53:1783–1795.

1190. Lynch, J. J. and G. Alexander. 1976. The effect of gramineous windbreaks on behaviour and lamb mortality among shorn and unshorn Merino sheep during lambing. *Appl. Anim. Ethol.* 2:305–325.

1191. Lynch, J. J., G. N. Hinch and D. B. Adams. 1992. *The behaviour of sheep: Biological principles and implications of production.* Oxon, UK: CAB International.

1192. Lynch, J. J. and J. F. McCarthy. 1967. The effect of petting on a classically conditioned emotional response. *Behav. Res. Ther.* 5:55–62.

1193. Lyons, D. M., E. O. Price and G. P. Moberg. 1988. Social modulation of pituitary-adrenal responsiveness and individual differences in behavior of young domestic goats. *Physiol. Behav.* 43:451–458.

1194. Maarschalkerweerd, R. J., N. Endenburg, J. Kirpensteijn and B. W. Knol. 1997. Influence of orchiectomy on canine behaviour. *Vet. Rec.* 140:617–619.

1195. Macaulay, A. S., G. L. Hahn, D. H. Clark and D. V. Sisson. 1995. Comparison of calf housing types and tympanic temperature rhythms in Holstein calves. *J. Dairy Sci.* 78:856–862.

1196. MacDonald, D. 1981. The behaviour and ecology of farm cats. *The ecology and control of feral cats*, pp. 23–29. Potters Bar, UK: Universities Federation for Animal Welfare.

1197. Macfarlane, J. S. 1974. The effect of two post-weaning management systems on the social and sexual behaviour of Zebu bulls. *Appl. Anim. Ethol.* 1:31–34.

1198. Mackenzie, S. A., E. A. Oltenacu and E. Leighton. 1985. Heritability estimate for temperament scores in German shepherd dogs and its genetic correlation with hip dysplasia. *Behav. Genet.* 15:475–482.

1199. Mackenzie, S. A., E. A. B. Oltenacu and K. A. Houpt. 1986. Canine behavioral genetics–a review. *Appl. Anim. Behav. Sci.* 15:365–393.

1200. Mackenzie, S. A. and E. Thiboutot. 1997. Stimulus reactivity tests for the domestic horse (*Equus caballus*). *Eq. Pract.* 19:21.

1201. Macpherson, K. and W. A. Roberts. 2006. Do dogs (*Canis familiaris*) seek help in an emergency? *J. Comp. Psychol.* 120:113–119.

1202. Macuda, T. and B. Timney. 1999. Luminance and chromatic discrimination in the horse (*Equus caballus*). *Behav. Proc.* 44:301–307.

1203. Mader, D. R. and E. O. Price. 1984. The effects of sexual stimulation on the sexual performance of Hereford bulls. *J. Anim. Sci.* 59:294–300.

1204. Mader, D. R. and E. O. Price. 1980. Discrimination learning in horses: Effects of breed, age and social dominance. *J. Anim. Sci.* 50:962–965.

1205. Madigan, J. E. and S. A. Bell. 2001. Owner survey of headshaking in horses. *J. Am. Vet. Med. Assoc.* 219:334–337.

1206. Maejima, M., M. Inoue-Murayama, K. Tonosaki, N. Matsuura, S. Kato, Y. Saito, A. Weiss, Y. Murayama and S. Ito. 2007. Traits and genotypes may predict the successful training of drug detection dogs. *Appl. Anim. Behav. Sci.* 107:287–298.

1207. Maier, N. R. F. and T. C. Schneirla. 1964. *Principles of animal psychology*. New York, NY: Dover Publications.

1208. Mal, M. E. and C. A. McCall. 1996. The influence of handling during different ages on a halter training test in foals. *Appl. Anim. Behav. Sci.* 50:115–120.

1209. Mal, M. E., C. A. McCall, K. A. Cummins and M. C. Newland. 1994. Influence of preweaning handling methods on post-weaning learning ability and manageability of foals. *Appl. Anim. Behav. Sci.* 40:187–195.

1210. Malbert, C. H. and Y. Ruckebusch. 1989. Hyperphagia induced by pylorectomy in sheep. *Physiol. Behav.* 45:495–499.

1211. Malm, K. 1995. Regurgitation in relations to weaning in the domestic dog: A questionnaire study. *Appl. Anim. Behav. Sci.* 43:111–122.

1212. Malm, K. and P. Jensen. 1993. Regurgitation as a weaning strategy–a selective review on an old subject in a new light. *Appl. Anim. Behav. Sci.* 36:47–64.

1213. Malpass, J. P. and B. J. Weigler. 1994. A simple and effective environmental enrichment device for ponies in long-term indoor confinement. *Contemp. Top. Lab. Anim. Sci.* 33:74–76.

1214. Manson, F. J. and M. C. Appleby. 1990. Spacing of dairy cows at a food trough. *Appl. Anim. Behav. Sci.* 26:69–81.

1215. Marcella, K. L. 1983. A note on canine aggression towards veterinarians. *Appl. Anim. Ethol.* 10:155–157.

1216. Marchant, J. N., X. Whittaker and D. M. Broom. 2001. Vocalisations of the adult female domestic pig during a standard human approach test and their relationships with behavioural and heart rate measures. *Appl. Anim. Behav. Sci.* 72:23–39.

1217. Marcuse, F. L. and A. U. Moore. 1946. Motor criteria of discrimination. *J. Comp. Psychol.* 39:25–27.

1218. Marcuse, F. L. and A. U. Moore. 1944. Tantrum behavior in the pig. *J. Comp. Psychol.* 37:235–241.

1219. Marinier, S. L. and A. J. Alexander. 1992. Use of field observations to measure individual grazing ability in horses. *Appl. Anim. Behav. Sci.* 33:1–10.

1220. Marinier, S. L., A. J. Alexander and G. H. Waring. 1988. Flehmen behaviour in the domestic horse: Discrimination of conspecific odours. *Appl. Anim. Behav. Sci.* 19:227–237.

1221. Maros, K., M. Gacsi and A. Miklosi. 2008. Comprehension of human pointing gestures in horses (*Equus caballus*). *Anim. Cogn.* 11:457–466.

1222. Marten, G. C. and J. E. Donker. 1964. Selective grazing induced by animal excreta. I. Evidence of occurrence and superficial remedy. *J. Dairy Sci.* 47:773–776.

1223. Martin, F. H., J. R. Seoane and C. A. Baile. 1973. Feeding in satiated sheep elicited by intraventricular injections of CSF from fasted sheep. *Life Sci.* 13:177–184.

1224. Martin, J. E. and S. A. Edwards. 1994. Feeding behaviour of outdoor sows: The effects of diet quantity and type. *Appl. Anim. Behav. Sci.* 41:63–74.

1225. Martin, J. T. 1975. Movement of feral pigs in North Canterbury, New Zealand. *J. Mammal.* 56:914–915.

1226. Martin, P. 1986. An experimental study of weaning in the domestic cat. *Behaviour* 99:221–249.

1227. Martin, P. 1984. The time and energy costs of play behaviour in the cat. *Z. Tierpsychol.* 64:298–312.

1228. Martin, P. and P. Bateson. 1985. The ontogeny of locomotor play behaviour in the domestic cat. *Anim. Behav.* 33:502–510.

1229. Martin, R. J., J. L. Gobble, T. H. Hartsock, H. B. Graves and J. H. Ziegler. 1973. Characterization of an obese syndrome in the pig. *Proc. Soc. Exp. Biol. Med.* 143:198–203.

1230. Martin, T. I., T. R. Zentall and L. Lawrence. 2006. Simple discrimination reversals in the domestic horse (*Equus caballus*): Effect of discriminative stimulus modality on learning to learn. *Appl. Anim. Behav. Sci.* 101:328–338.

1231. Martins, T. 1949. Disgorging of food to the puppies by the lactating dog. *Physiol. Zool.* 22:169–172.

1232. Mason, E. 1970. Obesity in pet dogs. *Vet. Rec.* 86:612–616.

1233. Mateo, J. M., D. Q. Estep and J. S. McCann. 1991. Effects of differential handling on the behaviour of domestic ewes (*Ovis aries*). *Appl. Anim. Behav. Sci.* 32:45–54.

1234. Mattner, P. E., A. W. H. Braden and K. E. Turnbill. 1967. Studies in flock mating of sheep. I. Mating behaviour. *Aust. J. Exp. Agric. Anim. Husb.* 7:103–109.

1235. May, R., J. van Dijk, J. M. Forland, R. Andersen and A. Landa. 2008. Behavioural patterns in ewe-lamb pairs and vulnerability to predation by wolverines. *Appl. Anim. Behav. Sci.* 112:58–67.

1236. Mayes, E. and P. Duncan. 1986. Temporal patterns of feeding in free-ranging horses. *Behaviour* 96:105–129.

1237. McAfee, L. M., D. S. Mills and J. J. Cooper. 2002. The use of mirrors for the control of stereotype weaving behaviour in the stabled horse. *Appl. Anim. Behav. Sci.* 78:159–173.

1238. McBane, S. 1987. *Behaviour problems of horses*. North Pomfret, VT: David and Charles.

1239. McBride, G. 1963. The "teat order" and communication in young pigs. *Anim. Behav.* 11:53–56.

1240. McBride, G., J. W. James and N. Hodgens. 1964. Social behaviour of domestic animals. IV. Growing pigs. *Anim. Prod.* 6:129–139.

1241. McBride, G., J. W. James and G. S. F. Wyeth. 1965. Social behaviour of domestic animals. VII. Variation in weaning weight in pigs. *Anim. Prod.* 7:67–74.

1242. McCall, C. A. 1991. Utilizing taped stallion vocalizations as a practical aid in estrus detection in mares. *Appl. Anim. Behav. Sci.* 28:305–310.

1243. McCall, C. A. 1989. *Behavior problems of horses*. North Pomfret, VT: David and Charles.

1244. McCall, C. A. and S. E. Burgin. 2002. Equine utilization of secondary reinforcement during response extinction and acquisition. *Appl. Anim. Behav. Sci.* 78:253–262.

1245. McCall, C. A., S. Hall, W. H. McElhenney and K. A. Cummins. 2006. Evaluation and comparison of four methods of ranking horses based on reactivity. *Appl. Anim. Behav. Sci.* 96:115–127.

1246. McCall, C. A., G. D. Potter, T. H. Friend and R. S. Ingram. 1981. Learning abilities in yearling horses using the Hebb-Williams closed field maze. *J. Anim. Sci.* 53:928–933.

1247. McCall, C. A., G. D. Potter and J. L. Kreider. 1985. Locomotor, vocal and other behavioural responses to varying methods of weaning foals. *Appl. Anim. Behav. Sci.* 14:27–35.

1248. McCall, C. A., A. M. A. Salters and S. M. Simpson. 1993. Relationship between number of conditioning trials per training session and avoidance learning in horses. *Appl. Anim. Behav. Sci.* 36:291–299.

1249. McClure, S. R., M. K. Chaffin and B. V. Beaver. 1992. Nonpharmacologic management of stereotypic self-mutilative behavior in a stallion. *J. Am. Vet. Med. Assoc.* 200:1975–1977.

1250. McConnell, P. B. 1990. Acoustic structure and receiver response in domestic dogs, *Canis familiaris*. *Anim. Behav.* 39:897–904.

1251. McConnell, P. B. and J. R. Baylis. 1985. Interspecific communication in cooperative herding: Acoustic and visual signals from human shepherds and herding dogs. *Z. Tierpsychol.* 67:302–328.

1252. McCowan, B., A. M. DiLorenzo, S. Abichandani, C. Borelli and J. S. Cullor. 2002. Bioacoustic tools for enhancing animal management and productivity: Effects of recorded calf vocalizations on milk production in dairy cows. *Appl. Anim. Behav. Sci.* 77:13–20.

1253. McCune, S. 1995. The impact of paternity and early socialisation on the development of cats' behaviour to people and novel objects. *Appl. Anim. Behav. Sci.* 45:109–124.

1254. McDonald, C. L., R. G. Beilharz and J. C. McCutchan. 1981. Training cattle to control by electric fences. *Appl. Anim. Ethol.* 7:113–121.

1255. McDonnell, S. 2003. *A practical field guide to horse behavior: The equid ethogram.* Lexington, KY: Eclipse Press.

1256. McDonnell, S. 1986. Reproductive behavior of the stallion. *Vet. Clin. N. Am.: Equine Pract.* 2:535–555.

1257. McDonnell, S. and S. C. Murray. 1995. Bachelor and harem stallion behavior and endocrinology. *Biol. Reprod. Mono.* 1:577–590.

1258. McDonnell, S. M. 2008. Practical review of self-mutilation in horses. *Anim. Reprod. Sci.* 107:219–228.

1259. McDonnell, S. M. 1992. Sexual behavior dysfunction in stallion. In N. E. Robinson (Ed.), *Current therapy in equine medicine*, pp. 668–671. Philadelphia, PA: W.B. Saunders Company.

1260. McDonnell, S. M., N. K. Diehl, M. C. Garcia and R. M. Kenney. 1989. Gonadotropin releasing hormone (GnRH) affects precopulatory behavior in testosterone-treated geldings. *Physiol. Behav.* 45:145–149.

1261. McDonnell, S. M. and J. C. S. Haviland. 1995. Agonistic ethogram of the equid bachelor band. *Appl. Anim. Behav. Sci.* 43:147–188.

1262. McDonnell, S. M., R. M. Kenney, P. E. Meckley and M. C. Garcia. 1986. Novel environment suppression of stallion sexual behavior and effects of diazepam. *Physiol. Behav.* 37:503–505.

1263. McDonnell, S. M., R. M. Kenney, P. E. Meckley and M. C. Garcia. 1985. Conditioned suppression of sexual behavior in stallions and reversal with diazepam. *Physiol. Behav.* 34:951–956.

1264. McDonnell, S. M. and A. Poulin. 2002. Equid play ethogram. *Appl. Anim. Behav. Sci.* 78:263–290.

1265. McDougall, K. D. and W. McDougal. 1931. Insight and foresight in various animals—monkey, raccoon, rat, and wasp. *J. Comp. Psychol.* 11:237–273.

1266. McEachron, D. L., D. F. Kripke, R. Hawkins, E. Haus, D. Pavlinac and L. Deftos. 1982. Lithium delays biochemical circadian rhythms in rats. *Neuropsychobiology* 8:12–29.

1267. McGeer, E. G. and P. L. McGeer. 1966. Circadian rhythm in pineal tyrosine hydroxylase. *Science* 153:73–74.

1268. McGinty, D. J., M. Stevenson, T. Hoppenbrouwers, R. M. Harper, M. B. Sterman and J. Hodgman. 1977. Polygraphic studies of kitten development: Sleep state patterns. *Dev. Psychobiol.* 10:455–469.

1269. McGlone, J. J. 1986. Influence of resources on pig aggression and dominance. *Behav. Proc.* 12:134–144.

1270. McGlone, J. J. 1985. Olfactory cues and pig agonistic behavior: Evidence for a submissive pheromone. *Physiol. Behav.* 34:195–198.

1271. McGlone, J. J. 1985. A quantitative ethogram of aggressive and submissive behaviors in recently re-grouped pigs. *J. Anim. Sci.* 61:559–565.

1272. McGlone, J. J. and D. L. Anderson. 2002. Synthetic maternal pheromone stimulates feeding behavior and weight gain in weaned pigs. *J. Anim. Sci.* 80:3179–3183.

1273. McGlone, J. J. and S. E. Curtis. 1985. Behavior and performance of weanling pigs in pens equipped with hide areas. *J. Anim. Sci.* 60:20–24.

1274. McGlone, J. J. and J. L. Morrow. 1987. Individual differences among mature boars in T-maze preference for estrous or non-estrous sows. *Appl. Anim. Behav. Sci.* 17:77–82.

1275. McGlone, J. J., R. I. Nicholson, J. M. Hellman and D. N. Herzog. 1993. The development of pain in young pigs associated with castration and attempts to prevent castration-induced behavioral changes. *J. Anim. Sci.* 71:1441–1446.

1276. McGreevy, P. and C. Nicol. 1998. Physiological and behavioral consequences associated with short-term prevention of crib-biting in horses. *Physiol. Behav.* 65:15–23.

1277. McGreevy, P. D., P. J. Cripps, N. P. French, L. E. Green and C. J. Nicol. 1995. Management factors associated with stereotypic and redirected behaviour in the thoroughbred horse. *Equine Vet. J.* 27:86–91.

1278. McGreevy, P. D., N. P. French and C. J. Nicol. 1995. The prevalence of abnormal behaviours in dressage, eventing and endurance horses in relation to stabling. *Vet. Rec.* 137:36–37.

1279. McGreevy, P. D., L. A. Hawson, T. C. Habermann and S. R. Cattle. 2001. Geophagia in horses: A short note on 13 cases. *Appl. Anim. Behav. Sci.* 71:119–125.

1280. McGreevy, P. D. and A. M. Masters. 2008. Risk factors for separation-related distress and feed-related aggression in dogs: Additional findings from a survey of Australian dog owners. *Appl. Anim. Behav. Sci.* 109:320–328.

1281. McGreevy, P. D., J. D. Richardson, C. J. Nicol and J. G. Lane. 1995. Radiographic and endoscopic study of horses performing an oral based stereotypy. *Equine Vet. J.* 27:92–95.

1282. McGreevy, P. D. and P. C. Thomson. 2006. Differences in motor laterality between breeds of performance horse. *Appl. Anim. Behav. Sci.* 99:183–190.

1283. McGrogan, C., M. D. Hutchison and J. E. King. 2008. Dimensions of horse personality based on owner and trainer supplied personality traits. *Appl. Anim. Behav. Sci.* 113:206–214.

1284. McGuire, R. A., W. M. Rand and R. J. Wurtman. 1973. Entrainment of the body temperature rhythm in rats: Effect of color and intensity of environmental light. *Science* 181:956–957.

1285. McKinley, J. and T. D. Sambrook. 2000. Use of human-given cues by domestic dogs (*Canis familiaris*) and horses (*Equus caballus*). *Anim. Cogn.* 3:13–22.

1286. McLaughlin, C. L., C. A. Baile, L. L. Buckholtz and S. K. Freeman. 1983. Preferred flavors and performance of weanling pigs. *J. Anim. Sci.* 56:1287–1293.

1287. McLaughlin, C. L., L. F. Krabill, G. C. Scott and C. A. Baile. 1976. Chemical stimulants of feeding animals. *Fed. Proc.* 35:579.

1288. McLeman, M. A., M. T. Mendl, R. B. Jones and C. M. Wathes. 2008. Social discrimination of familiar conspecifics by juvenile pigs, *Sus scrofa*: Development of a non-invasive method to study the transmission of unimodal and bimodal cues between live stimuli. *Appl. Anim. Behav. Sci.* 115:123–137.

1289. McPhee, C. P., G. McBride and J. W. James. 1964. Social behaviour of domestic animals. III. Steers in small yards. *Anim. Prod.* 6:9–15.

1290. Mech, L. D. 1975. Hunting behavior in two similar species of social canids. In M. W. Fox (Ed.), *The wild canids. their systematics, behavioral ecology and evolution*, pp. 363–368. New York, NY: Van Nostrand Reinhold Co.

1291. Meese, G. B. and B. A. Baldwin. 1975. The effects of ablation of the olfactory bulbs on aggressive behaviour in pigs. *Appl. Anim. Ethol.* 1:251–262.

1292. Meese, G. B. and B. A. Baldwin. 1975. Effects of olfactory bulb ablation and maternal behaviour in sows. *Appl. Anim. Ethol.* 1:379–386.

1293. Meese, G. B., D. J. Conner and B. A. Baldwin. 1975. Ability of the pig to distinguish between conspecific urine samples using olfaction. *Physiol. Behav.* 15:121–125.

1294. Meese, G. B. and R. Ewbank. 1973. The establishment of and nature of the dominance hierarchy in the domesticated pig. *Anim. Behav.* 21:326–334.

1295. Meese, G. B. and R. Ewbank. 1973. Exploratory behaviour and leadership in the domesticated pig. *Br. Vet. J.* 129:251–259.

1296. Meier, G. W. 1961. Infantile handling and development in Siamese kittens. *J. Comp. Physiol. Psychol.* 54:284–286.

1297. Meier, G. W. and J. L. Stuart. 1959. Effects of handling on the physical and behavioral development of Siamese kittens. *Psychol. Rep.* 5:497–501.

1298. Meikle, D. B., L. C. Drickamer, S. H. Vessey, T. L. Rosenthal and K. S. Fitzgerald. 1993. Maternal dominance rank and secondary sex ratio in domestic swine. *Anim. Behav.* 46:79–85.

1299. Melese-d'Hospital, P. 1996. Eliminating urine odors in the home. In V. L. Voith and P. L. Borchelt (Eds.), *Companion animal behavior*, pp. 191–197. Trenton, NJ: Veterinary Learning Systems.

1300. Melin, M., G. G. N. Hermans, G. Pettersson and H. Wiktorsson. 2006. Cow traffic in relation to social rank and motivation of cows in an automatic milking system with control gates and an open waiting area. *Appl. Anim. Behav. Sci.* 96:201–214.

1301. Melin, M., G. Pettersson, H. Svennersten-Sjaunja and H. Wiktorsson. 2007. The effects of restricted feed access and social rank on feeding behavior, ruminating and intake for cows managed in automated milking systems. *Appl. Anim. Behav. Sci.* 107:13–21.

1302. Melo, M. I., J. R. Sereno, M. Henry and G. D. Cassali. 1998. Peripuberal sexual development of pantaneiro stallions. *Theriogenology* 50:727–737.

1303. Melrose, D. R., H. C. Reed and R. L. Patterson. 1971. Androgen steroids associated with boar odour as an aid to the detection of oestrus in pig artificial insemination. *Br. Vet. J.* 127:497–502.

1304. Melzack, R. 1962. Effects of early perceptual restriction on simple visual discrimination. *Science* 137:978–979.

1305. Melzack, R. and T. H. Scott. 1957. The effects of early experience on the response to pain. *J. Comp. Physiol. Psychol.* 50:155–161.

1306. Mendl, M. and R. Harcourt. 1988. Individuality in the domestic cat. In D. C. Turner and P. Bateson (Eds.), *The domestic cat: The biology of its behaviour*, pp. 41–54. Cambridge, UK: Cambridge University Press.

1307. Mendl, M., K. Randle and S. Pope. 2002. Young female pigs can discriminate individual differences in odours from conspecific urine. *Anim. Behav.* 64:97–101.

1308. Mendl, M., A. J. Zanella and D. M. Broom. 1992. Physiological and reproductive correlates of behavioural strategies in female domestic pigs. *Anim. Behav.* 44:1107–1121.

1309. Mendl, M., A. J. Zanella, D. M. Broom and C. T. Whittemore. 1995. Maternal social status and birth sex ratio in domestic pigs: An analysis of mechanisms. *Anim. Behav.* 50:1361–1370.

1310. Merrick, A. W. and D. W. Scharp. 1971. Electroencephalography of resting behavior in cattle, with observations on the question of sleep. *Am. J. Vet. Res.* 32:1893–1897.

1311. Mersmann, H. J., M. D. MacNeil, S. C. Seiderman and W. G. Pond. 1987. Compensatory growth in finishing pigs after feed restriction. *J. Anim. Sci.* 64:752–764.

1312. Mertens, D. R. 1987. Predicting intake and digestibility using mathematical models of ruminal function. *J. Anim. Sci.* 64:1548–1558.

1313. Metz, J. H. M. 1985. The reaction of cows to a short-term deprivation of lying. *Appl. Anim. Behav. Sci.* 13:301–307.

1314. Metz, J. H. M. and H. W. Gonyou. 1990. Effect of age and housing conditions on the behavioural and haemolytic reaction of piglets to weaning. *Appl. Anim. Behav. Sci.* 27:299–309.

1315. Metz, J. H. M. and P. Mekking. 1984. Crowding phenomena in dairy cows as related to available idling space in a cubicle housing system. *Appl. Anim. Behav. Sci.* 12:63–78.

1316. Michael, R. P. 1973. The effects of hormones on sexual behavior in female cat and rhesus monkey. In R. O. Greep and E. B. Astwood (Eds.), *Handbook of physiology, section 7, endocrinology, volume II, female reproductive system, part 1*, pp. 187–221. Washington, DC: American Physiological Society.

1317. Michelena, P., J. Gautrais, J.-F. Gerard, R. Bon and J.-L. Deneubourg. 2008. Social cohesion in groups of sheep: Effect of activity level, sex composition and group size. *Appl. Anim. Behav. Sci.* 112:81–93.

1318. Michell, A. R. 1992. Sodium preference in sheep excreting sodium predominantly in urine or faeces. *Physiol. Behav.* 52:285–286.

1319. Michell, A. R. and P. Moss. 1988. Salt appetite during pregnancy in sheep. *Physiol. Behav.* 42:491–493.

1320. Miklosi, A. 2007. In Miklosi A. (Ed.), *Dog behaviour, evolution, and cognition*. New York, NY: Oxford University Press.

1321. Miklosi, A., R. Polgardi, J. Topal and V. Csanyi. 2000. Intentional behaviour in dog-human communication: An experimental analysis of "showing" behaviour in the dog. *Anim. Cogn.* 3:159–166.

1322. Miklosi, A., P. Pongracz, G. Lakatos, J. Topal and V. Csanyi. 2005. A comparative study of the use of visual communicative signals in interactions between dogs (*Canis familiaris*) and humans and cats (*Felis catus*) and humans. *J. Comp. Psychol.* 119:179–186.

1323. Miles, R. C. 1958. Learning in kittens with manipulatory, exploratory, and food incentives. *J. Comp. Physiol. Psychol.* 51:39–42.

1324. Milgram, N. W., B. Adams, H. Callahan, E. Head, B. Mackay, C. Thirlwell and C. W. Cotman. 1999. Landmark discrimination learning in the dog. *Learn. Mem.* 6:54–61.

1325. Milgram, N. W., E. Head, E. Weiner and E. Thomas. 1994. Cognitive functions and aging in the dog: Acquisition of nonspatial visual tasks. *Behav. Neurosci.* 108:57–68.

1326. Milgram, N. W., C. T. Siwak-Tapp, J. Araujo and E. Head. 2006. Neuroprotective effects of cognitive enrichment. *Ageing Res. Rev.* 5:354–369.

1327. Miller, E. R., S. Vathana, F. F. Green, J. R. Black, D. R. Romsos and D. E. Ullrey. 1974. Dietary caloric density and caloric intake in the pig. *J. Anim. Sci.* 39:980.

1328. Miller, P. E. and C. J. Murphy. 1995. Vision in dogs. *J. Am. Vet. Med. Assoc.* 207:1623–1634.

1329. Miller, R. M. 1991. *Imprint training of the newborn foal*. Colorado Springs, CO: The Western Horseman, Inc.

1330. Miller, R. R. 1981. Male aggression, dominance, and breeding behavior in red desert feral horses. *Z. Tierpsychol.* 57:340–351.

1331. Miller, R. R. and R. H. Denniston. 1979. Interband dominance in feral horses. *Z. Tierpsychol.* 51:41–47.

1332. Mills, D. and R. Ledger. 2001. The effects of oral selegiline hydrochloride on learning and training in the dog: A psychobiological interpretation. *Prog. Neuropsychopharmacol. Biol. Psychiatry* 25:1597–1613.

1333. Mills, D. S. 1998. Personality and individual differences in the horse, their significance, use and measurement. *Equine Vet. J. Suppl.* (27): 10–13.

1334. Mills, D. S., R. D. Alston, V. Rogers and N. T. Longford. 2002. Factors associated with the prevalence of stereotypic behaviour amongst thoroughbred horses passing through auctioneer sales. *Appl. Anim. Behav. Sci.* 78:115–124.

1335. Mills, D. S., D. Ramos, M. G. Estelles and C. Hargrave. 2006. A triple blind placebo-controlled investigation into the assessment of the effect of dog appeasing pheromone (DAP) on anxiety related behaviour of problem dogs in the veterinary clinic. *Appl. Anim. Behav. Sci.* 98:114–126.

1336. Mills, D. S. and K. Taylor. 2003. Field study of the efficacy of three types of nose net for the treatment of headshaking in horses. *Vet. Rec.* 152:41–44.

1337. Mills, D. S. and J. C. White. 2000. Long-term follow up of the effect of a pheromone therapy on feline spraying behaviour. *Vet. Rec.* 147:746–747.

1338. Minero, M., E. Canali, V. Ferrante, M. Verga and F. O. Odberg. 1999. Heart rate and behavioural responses of crib-biting horses to two acute stressors. *Vet. Rec.* 145:430–433.

1339. Minero, M., M. V. Tosi, E. Canali and F. Wemelsfelder. 2009. Quantitative and qualitative assessment of the response of foals to the presence of an unfamiliar human. *Appl. Anim. Behav. Sci.* 116:74–81.

1340. Minero, M., D. Zucca and E. Canali. 2006. A note on reaction to novel stimulus and restraint by therapeutic riding horses. *Appl. Anim. Behav. Sci.* 97:335–342.

1341. Mirza, S. N. and F. D. Provenza. 1994. Socially induced food avoidance in lambs: Direct or indirect maternal influence? *J. Anim. Sci.* 72:899–902.

1342. Mirza, S. N. and F. D. Provenza. 1992. Effects of age and conditions of exposure on maternally mediated food selection by lambs. *Appl. Anim. Behav. Sci.* 33:35–42.

1343. Mistlberger, R. E., T. A. Houpt and M. C. Moore-Ede. 1990. Food-anticipatory rhythms under 24-hour schedules of limited access to single macronutrients. *J. Biol. Rhythms* 5:35–46.

1344. Mitler, M. M., O. Soave and W. C. Dement. 1976. Narcolepsy in seven dogs. *J. Am. Vet. Med. Assoc.* 168:1036–1038.

1345. Mohan, R. A. B., W. J. McCaughey, W. McLauchlan, D. J. Kilpatrick and S. McGaughey. 1991. Behavioural response to mixing of entire bulls, vasectomised bulls and steers. *Appl. Anim. Behav. Sci.* 31:157–168.

1346. Mohr, E. and H. Krzywanek. 1990. Variations of core-temperature rhythms in unrestrained sheep. *Physiol. Behav.* 48:467–473.

1347. Molliver, M. E. 1963. Operant control of vocal behavior in the cat. *J. Exp. Anal. Behav.* 6:197–202.

1348. Moltz, H. 1960. Imprinting: Empirical basis and theoretical significance. *Psychol. Bull.* 57:291–314.

1349. Momozawa, Y., R. Kusunose, T. Kikusui, Y. Takeuchi and Y. Mori. 2005. Assessment of equine temperament questionnaire by comparing factor structure between two separate surveys. *Appl. Anim. Behav. Sci.* 92:77–84.

1350. Momozawa, Y., T. Ono, F. Sato, T. Kikusui, Y. Takeuchi, Y. Mori and R. Kusunose. 2003. Assessment of equine temperament by a questionnaire survey to caretakers and evaluation of its reliability by simultaneous behavior test. *Appl. Anim. Behav. Sci.* 84:127–138.

1351. Mondard, A.-M. and P. Duncan. 1996. Consequences of natal dispersal in female horses. *Anim. Behav.* 52:565–579.

1352. Montgomery, G. G. 1957. Some aspects of the sociality of the domestic horse. *Trans. Kans Acad. Sci.* 60:419–424.

1353. Moore, A. S., H. W. Gonyou and A. W. Ghent. 1993. Integration of newly introduced and resident sows following grouping. *Appl. Anim. Behav. Sci.* 38:257–267.

1354. Moore, A. S., H. W. Gonyou, J. M. Stookey and D. G. McLaren. 1994. Effect of group composition and pen size on behaviour, productivity and immune response of growing pigs. *Appl. Anim. Behav. Sci.* 40:13–30.

1355. Moore, A. U. and F. L. Marcuse. 1945. Salivary, cardiac and motor indices of conditioning in two sows. *J. Comp. Psychol.* 38:1–16.

1356. Moore, C. L., W. G. Whittlestone, M. Mullord, P. N. Priest, R. Kilgour and J. L. Albright. 1975. Behavior responses of dairy cows trained to activate a feeding device. *J. Dairy Sci.* 58:1531–1535.

1357. Moore, R. M. Jr, R. B. Zehmer, J. I. Moulthrop and R. L. Parker. 1977. Surveillance of animal-bite cases in the United States, 1971–1972. *Arch. Environ. Health* 32:267–270.

1358. Mooring, M. S., A. J. Gavazzi and B. L. Hart. 1998. Effects of castration on grooming in goats. *Physiol. Behav.* 64:707–713.

1359. Morag, M. 1967. Influence of diet on the behaviour pattern of sheep. *Nature* 213:110.

1360. Morgan, C. A., G. C. Emmans, B. J. Tolkamp and I. Kyriazakis. 2000. Analysis of the feeding behavior of pigs using different models. *Physiol. Behav.* 68:395–403.

1361. Morgan, C. A., B. J. Tolkamp, G. C. Emmans and I. Kyriazakis. 2000. The way in which the data are combined affects the interpretation of short-term feeding behavior. *Physiol. Behav.* 70:391–396.

1362. Morgan, M. and K. A. Houpt. 1989. Feline behavior problems: The influence of declawing. *Arthrozoos* 3:50–53.

1363. Morgan, P. D. and G. W. Arnold. 1974. Behavioural relationships between Merino ewes and lambs during the four weeks after birth. *Anim. Prod.* 19:169–176.

1364. Morgan, P. D., C. A. P. Boundy, G. W. Arnold and D. R. Lindsay. 1975. The roles played by the senses of the ewe in the location and recognition of lambs. *Appl. Anim. Ethol.* 1:139–150.

1365. Mormede, P. and R. Dantzer. 1977. Effects of dexamethasone on fear conditioning in pigs. *Behav. Biol.* 21:225–235.

1366. Mormede, P. and R. Dantzer. 1977. Experimental studies on avoidance behavior in pigs. *Appl. Anim. Ethol.* 3:173–185.

1367. Morrison, A. R. 1983. A window on the sleeping brain. *Sci. Am.* 248:94–102.

1368. Morrison, S. R., H. F. Hintz and R. L. Givens. 1968. A note on effect of exercise on behaviour and performance of confined swine. *Anim. Prod.* 10:341–344.

1369. Morrow, D. A. 1976. Fat cow syndrome. *J. Dairy Sci.* 59:1625–1629.

1370. Morrow-Tesch, J. and J. J. McGlone. 1990. Sensory systems and nipple attachment behavior in neonatal pigs. *Physiol. Behav.* 47:1–4.

1371. Morrow-Tesch, J. and J. J. McGlone. 1990. Sources of maternal odors and the development of odor preferences in baby pigs. *J. Anim. Sci.* 68:3563–3571.

1372. Morrow-Tesch, J. L., J. J. McGlone and J. L. Salak-Johnson. 1994. Heat and social stress effects on pig immune measures. *J. Anim. Sci.* 72:2599–2609.

1373. Motch, S. E., H. W. Harpster, S. Ralston, N. Ostiguy and N. K. Diehl. 2007. A note on yearling horse ingestive and agonistic behaviours in three concentrate feeding systems. *Appl. Anim. Behav. Sci.* 106:167–172.

1374. Moulton, D. G., E. H. Ashton and J. T. Eayrs. 1960. Studies in olfactory acuity. 4. Relative detectability of n-aliphatic acids by the dog. *Anim. Behav.* 8:117–128.

1375. Mounier, L., I. Veissier, S. Andanson, E. Delval and A. Boissy. 2006. Mixing at the beginning of fattening moderates social buffering in beef bulls. *Appl. Anim. Behav. Sci.* 96:185–200.

1376. Mount, N. C. 1979. *Adaptation to thermal environment: Man and his productive animals.* Baltimore, MD: University Park Press.

1377. Mount, N. C. and M. F. Seabrook. 1993. A study of aggression when group housed sows are mixed. *Appl. Anim. Behav. Sci.* 36:383.

1378. Moya, S. L., L. A. Boyle, P. B. Lynch and S. Arkins. 2008. Surgical castration of pigs affects the behavioural response to a low-dose lipopolysaccharide (LPS) challenge after weaning. *Appl. Anim. Behav. Sci.* 112:40–57.

1379. Mugford, R. A. 1977. External influences on the feeding of carnivores. In M. R. Kare and O. Maller (Eds.), *The chemical senses and nutrition,* pp. 25–50. New York, NY: Academic Press.

1380. Muller, R. and M. A. G. von Keyserlingk. 2006. Consistency of flight speed and its correlation to productivity and to personality in *Bos taurus* beef cattle. *Appl. Anim. Behav. Sci.* 99:193–204.

1381. Munkenbeck, N. 1983. *A test of color vision and a spectral sensitivity curve in the sheep (Ovis aries).* Ithaca, NY: Cornell University Press.

1382. Munksgaard, L., A. M. DePassille, J. Rushen, M. S. Herskin and A. M. Kristensen. 2001. Dairy cows' fear of people: Social learning, milk yield and behaviour at milking. *Appl. Anim. Behav. Sci.* 73:15–26.

1383. Munksgaard, L., A. M. dePassille, J. Rushen and J. Ladewig. 1999. Dairy cows' use of colour cues to discriminate between people. *Appl. Anim. Behav. Sci.* 65:1–11.

1384. Munksgaard, L., M. B. Jensen, L. J. Pedersen, S. W. Hansen and L. Matthews. 2005. Quantifying behavioural priorities—effects of time constraints on behaviour of dairy cows, *Bos taurus. Appl. Anim. Behav. Sci.* 92:3–14.

1385. Munro, J. 1956. Observations on the sucking behaviour of young lambs. *Br. J. Anim. Behav.* 4:34–36.

1386. Murphey, R. M., F. A. Duarte, W. C. Novaes and M. C. Penedo. 1981. Age group differences in bovine investigatory behavior. *Dev. Psychobiol.* 14:117–125.

1387. Murphey, R. M., C. R. Ruiz-Miranda and F. A. de Moura Duarte. 1990. Maternal recognition in Gyr (*Bos indicus*) calves. *Appl. Anim. Behav. Sci.* 27:183–191.

1388. Murphree, O. D., J. E. Peters and R. A. Dykman. 1969. Behavioral comparisons of nervous, stable, and crossbred pointers at ages, 2, 3, 6, 9, and 12 months. *Cond. Reflex* 4:20–23.

1389. Murphy, J., A. Sutherland and S. Arkins. 2005. Idiosyncratic motor laterality in the horse. *Appl. Anim. Behav. Sci.* 91:297–310.

1390. Myer, J. J., F. D. Martin and I. L. Brisbin. 2002. Characteristics of wild pig farrowing nests and beds in the upper coastal plain of South Carolina. *Appl. Anim. Behav. Sci.* 78:1–17.

1391. Myers, G. C. 1916. The importance of primacy in the learning of a pig. *J. Anim. Behav.* 6:64–69.

1392. Myers, R. D. and D. C. Mesker. 1960. Operant responding in a horse under several schedules of reinforcement. *J. Exp. Anal. Behav.* 3:161–164.

1393. Mylrea, P. J. and R. G. Beilharz. 1964. The manifestation and detection of oestrous in heifers. *Anim. Behav.* 12:25–30.

1394. Nagamachi, Y. 1972. Effect of satiety center damage on food intake, blood glucose and gastric secretion in dogs. *Am. J. Dig. Dis.* 17:139–148.

1395. Nagy, K., A. Schrott and P. Kabai. 2008. Possible influence of neighbours on stereotypic behaviour in horses. *Appl. Anim. Behav. Sci.* 111:321–328.

1396. Nagy, P., G. Duchamp, P. Chavatte-Palmer, P. F. Daels and D. Guillaume. 2002. Induction of lactation in mares with a dopamine antagonist needs ovarian hormones. *Theriogenology* 58:589–592.

1397. Napolitano, F., V. Marino, G. De Rosa, R. Capparelli and A. Bordi. 1995. Influence of artificial rearing on behavioral and immune response in lambs. *Appl. Anim. Behav. Sci.* 45:245–253.

1398. Natoli, E. 1990. Mating strategies in cats: A comparison of the role and importance of infanticide in domestic cats, *Felis catus* L. and lions, *Panthera leo* L. *Anim. Behav.* 40:183–186.

1399. Natoli, E. 1985. Spacing pattern in a colony of urban stray cats (*Felis catus* L.) in the historic centre of Rome. *Appl. Anim. Behav. Sci.* 14:289–304.

1400. Natoli, E. and E. De Vito. 1991. Agonistic behavior, dominance rank and copulatory success in a large multi-male feral cat, *Felis catus* L.; colony in central Rome. *Anim. Behav.* 42:227–241.

1401. Naujeck, A., J. Hill and M. J. Gibb. 2005. Influence of sward height on diet selection by horses. *Appl. Anim. Behav. Sci.* 9:49–63.

1402. Neathery, M. W. 1971. Acceptance of orphan lambs by tranquilized ewes (*Ovis aries*). *Anim. Behav.* 19:75–79.

1403. Neff, W. D. and I. T. Diamond. 1958. The neural basis of auditory discrimination. In H. F. Harlow and C. N. Woolsey (Eds.), *Biological and biochemical bases of behavior*, pp. 101–126. Madison, WI: University of Wisconsin Press.

1404. Neilson, J. C., R. A. Eckstein and B. L. Hart. 1997. Effects of castration on problem behaviors in male dogs with reference to age and duration of behavior. *J. Am. Vet. Med. Assoc.* 211:180–182.

1405. Neilson, J. C., B. L. Hart, K. D. Cliff and W. W. Ruehl. 2001. Prevalence of behavioral changes associated with age-related cognitive impairment in dogs. *J. Am. Vet. Med. Assoc.* 218:1787–1791.

1406. Neitz, J., T. Geist and G. H. Jacobs. 1989. Color vision in the dog. *Vis. Neurosci.* 3:119–125.

1407. Neitz, J. and G. H. Jacobs. 1989. Spectral sensitivity of cones in an ungulate. *Vis. Neurosci.* 2:97–100.

1408. Nelson, R. J. 2005. *An introduction to behavioral endocrinology* (3rd Edition). Sunderland, MA: Sinauer Associates.

1409. Nelson, S. H., A. D. Evans and R. B. Bradbury. 2005. The efficacy of collar-mounted devices in reducing the rate of predation of wildlife by domestic cats. *Appl. Anim. Behav. Sci.* 94:273–285.

1410. Netto, W. J. and D. J. U. Planta. 1997. Behavioural testing for aggression in the domestic dog. *Appl. Anim. Behav. Sci.* 52:243–263.

1411. Newberry, R. C. and D. G. M. Wood-Gush. 1986. Social relationships of piglets in a seminatural environment. *Anim. Behav.* 34:1311–1318.

1412. Newman, J. A., P. D. Penning, A. J. Parson, A. Harvey and R. J. Orr. 1994. Fasting affects intake behaviour and diet preference in grazing sheep. *Anim. Behav.* 47:185–193.

1413. Nicastro, N. 2004. Perceptual and acoustic evidence for species-level differences in meow vocalizations by domestic cats (Felis catus) and African wild cats (Felis silvestris lybica). *J. Comp. Psychol.* 118:287–296.

1414. Nicastro, N. and M. J. Owren. 2003. Classification of domestic cat (Felis catus) vocalizations by naive and experienced human listeners. *J. Comp. Psychol.* 117:44–52.

1415. Nicol, C. J. 2002. Equine learning: Progress and suggestions for future research. *Appl. Anim. Behav. Sci.* 78:193–208.

1416. Nicol, C. J., A. J. Badnell-Waters, R. Bice, A. Kelland, A. D. Wilson and P. A. Harris. 2005. The effects of diet and weaning method on the behaviour of young horses. *Appl. Anim. Behav. Sci.* 95:205–221.

1417. Nicol, C. J., H. P. Davidson, P. A. Harris, A. J. Waters and A. D. Wilson. 2002. Study of crib-biting and gastric inflammation and ulceration in young horses. *Vet. Rec.* 151:658–662.

1418. Nikitopoulou, G. and J. L. Crammer. 1976. Change in diurnal temperature rhythm in manic-depressive illness. *Br. Med. J.* 1:1311–1314.

1419. Ninomiya, S., M. Aoyama, Y. Ujiie, R. Kusunose and A. Kuwano. 2008. Effects of bedding material on the lying behavior in stabled horses. *J. Equine Sci.* 19:53–56.

1420. Ninomiya, S., T. Mitsumasu, M. Aoyama and R. Kusunose. 2007. A note on the effect of a palatable food reward on operant conditioning in horses. *Appl. Anim. Behav. Sci.* 108:342–347.

1421. Ninomiya, S., S. Sato, R. Kusunose, T. Mitumasu and Y. Obara. 2007. A note on a behavioural indicator of satisfaction in stabled horses. *Appl. Anim. Behav. Sci.* 106:184–189.

1422. Ninomiya, S., S. Sato and K. Sugawara. 2007. Weaving in stabled horses and its relationship to other behavioural traits. *Appl. Anim. Behav. Sci.* 106:134–143.

1423. Noble, G. K., E. Houghton, C. J. Roberts, J. Faustino-Kemp, S. S. de Kock, B. C. Swanepoel and M. N. Sillence. 2007. Effect of exercise, training, circadian rhythm, age, and sex on insulin-like growth factor-1 in the horse. *J. Anim. Sci.* 85:163–171.

1424. Noble, M. and C. K. Adams. 1963. Conditioning in pigs as a function of the interval between CS and US. *J. Comp. Physiol. Psychol.* 56:215–219.

1425. Noda, K. and K. Chikamori. 1976. Effect of ammonia via prepyriform cortex on regulation of food intake in the rat. *Am. J. Physiol.* 231:1263–1266.

1426. Nolte, D. L. and F. D. Provenza. 1992. Food preferences in lambs after exposure to flavors in solid foods. *Appl. Anim. Behav. Sci.* 32:337–347.

1427. Nonneman, A. J. and J. M. Warren. 1977. Two-cue learning by brain-damaged cats. *Physiol. Psychol.* 5:397–402.

1428. Normando, S., L. Corain, M. Salvadoretti, L. Meers and P. Valsecchi. 2009. Effects of an enhanced human interaction program on shelter dogs' behaviour analysed using a novel nonparametric test. *Appl. Anim. Behav. Sci.* 116:211–219.

1429. Notari, L. and D. Goodwin. 2007. A survey of behavioural characteristics of pure-bred dogs in Italy. *Appl. Anim. Behav. Sci.* 103:118–130.

1430. Nowak, R. 1991. Senses involved in discrimination of Merino ewes at close contact and from distance by their newborn lambs. *Anim. Behav.* 42:357–366.

1431. Nowak, R., M. Keller, D. Val-Laillet and F. Levy. 2007. Perinatal visceral events and brain mechanisms involved in the development of mother-young bonding in sheep. *Horm. Behav.* 52:92–98.

1432. Noyes, L. 1976. A behavioural comparison of gnotobiotic with normal neonate pigs, indicating stress in the former. *Appl. Anim. Ethol.* 2:113–121.

1433. Nunez, C. M. V., J. S. Adelman, C. Mason and D. I. Rubenstein. 2009. Immunocontraception decreases group fidelity in a feral horse population during the non-breeding season. *Appl. Anim. Behav. Sci.* 117:74–83.

1434. Nyman, S. and K. Dahlborn. 2001. Effect of water supply method and flow rate on drinking behavior and fluid balance in horses. *Physiol. Behav.* 73:1–8.

1435. Oberosler, R., C. Carenzi and M. Vega. 1982. Dominance hierarchies of cows on alpine pastures as related to phenotype. *Appl. Anim. Ethol.* 8:67–77.

1436. Obese, F. Y., B. K. Whitlock, B. P. Steele, F. C. Buonomo and J. L. Sartin. 2007. Long-term feed intake regulation in sheep is mediated by opioid receptors. *J. Anim. Sci.* 85:111–117.

1437. O'Brien, P. H. 1988. Feral goat organization: A review and comparative analysis. *Appl. Anim. Behav. Sci.* 21:209–221.

1438. O'Brien, P. H. 1984. Feral goat home range: Influence of social class and environmental variables. *Appl. Anim. Behav. Sci.* 12:373–385.

1439. O'Connell, J. M., P. S. Giller and W. J. Meaney. 1993. Weanling training and cubicle usage as heifers. *Appl. Anim. Behav. Sci.* 37:185–195.

1440. O'Connor, C. E., A. B. Lawrence and D. G. M. Wood-Gush. 1992. Influence of litter size and parity on maternal behaviour at parturition in Scottish Blackface sheep. *Appl. Anim. Behav. Sci.* 33:345–355.

1441. Odberg, F. O. 1973. An interpretation of pawing by the horse (*Equus caballus* Linnaeus), displacement activity and original functions. *Saugetierkund. Mitteil.* 21:1–12.

1442. Odberg, F. O. and K. Francis-Smith. 1977. Studies on the formation of ungrazed eliminative areas in fields used by horses. *Appl. Anim. Ethol.* 3:34.

1443. Odde, K. G., G. H. Hiracofe and R. R. Schalles. 1985. Suckling behavior in range beef calves. *J. Anim. Sci.* 61:307–309.

1444. O'Driscoll, K., L. Boyle and A. Hanlon. 2009. The effect of breed and housing system on dairy cow feeding and lying behaviour. *Appl. Anim. Behav. Sci.* 116:156–162.

1445. O'Farrell, V. and E. Peachey. 1990. Behavioural effects of ovariohysterectomy in bitches. *J. Small Anim. Pract.* 31:595–598.

1446. Offord, K. P., L. D. Satter and D. A. Weickert. 1969. Study of behavioral conditioning and feed intake in dairy heifers. *J. Dairy. Sci.* 52:918.

1447. Ogata, N., C. Hashizume, Y. Momozawa, K. Masuda, T. Kikusui, Y. Takeuchi and Y. Mori. 2006. Polymorphisms in the canine glutamate transporter-1 gene: Identification and variation among five dog breeds. *J. Vet. Med. Sci.* 68:157–159.

1448. Ogata, N. and Y. Takeuchi. 2001. Clinical trial of a feline pheromone analogue for feline urine marking. *J. Vet. Med. Sci.* 63:157–161.

1449. Olmos, G. and S. P. Turner. 2008. The relationships between temperament during routine handling tasts, weight gain and facial hair whorl position in frequenty handled beef cattle. *Appl. Anim. Behav. Sci.* 115:25–36.

1450. Ordakowski-Burk, A. L., R. W. Quinn, T. A. Shellem and L. R. Vough. 2006. Voluntary intake and digestibility of reed canarygrass and timothy hay fed to horses. *J. Anim. Sci.* 84:3104–3109.

1451. Orgeur, P. 1995. Sexual play behavior in lambs androgenized in utero. *Physiol. Behav.* 57:185–187.

1452. Orgeur, P., P. Mimouni and J.-P. Signoret. 1990. The influence of rearing conditions on the social relationships of young male goats (*Capra hircus*). *Appl. Anim. Behav. Sci.* 27:105–113.

1453. Orihuela, A. and C. S. Galina. 1997. Social order measured in pasture and pen conditions and its relationship to sexual behavior in Brahman (Bos indicus) cows. *Appl. Anim. Behav. Sci.* 52:3–11.

1454. Ortega-Reyes, L. and F. D. Provenza. 1993. Amount of experience and age affect the development of foraging skills of goats browsing blackbrus (*Coleogyne ramosissima*). *Appl. Anim. Behav. Sci.* 36:169–183.

1455. Osterman, S. and I. I. Redbo. 2001. Effects of milking frequency on lying down and getting up behaviour in dairy cows. *Appl. Anim. Behav. Sci.* 70:167–176.

1456. Osthaus, B., S. E. Lea and A. M. Slater. 2005. Dogs (*Canis lupus familiaris*) fail to show understanding of means-end connections in a string-pulling task. *Anim. Cogn.* 8:37–47.

1457. Otten, W., B. Puppe, E. Kanitz, P. C. Schon and B. Stabenow. 2002. Physiological and behavioral effects of different success during social confrontation in pigs with prior dominance experience. *Physiol. Behav.* 75:127–133.

1458. Over, R., J. Cohen-Tannoudji, M. Dehnhard, R. Claus and J. P. Signoret. 1990. Effect of pheromones from male goats on LH-secretion in anoestrous ewes. *Physiol. Behav.* 48:665–668.

1459. Overall, K. L. 1997. *Clinical behavioral medicine for small animals.* St. Louis, MO: C.V. Mosby.

1460. Owen, J. B. and W. J. Ridgman. 1967. The effect of dietary energy content on the voluntary intake of pigs. *Anim. Prod.* 9:107–113.

1461. Owen, R., F. J. McKeating and D. W. Jagger. 1980. Neurectomy in windsucking horses. *Vet. Rec.* 106:134–135.

1462. Owens, J. L., T. N. Edey, B. M. Bindon and L. R. Piper. 1984. Parturient behaviour and calf survival in a herd selected for twinning. *Appl. Anim. Behav. Sci.* 13:321–333.

1463. Packwood, J. and B. Gordon. 1975. Stereopsis in normal domestic cat, Siamese cat, and cat raised with alternating monocular occlusion. *J. Neurophysiol.* 38:1485–1499.

1464. Pageat, P. and E. Gaultier. 2003. Current research in canine and feline pheromones. *Vet. Clin. N. Am. Small Anim. Pract.* 33:187–211.

1465. Pajor, E. A., D. Fraser and D. L. Kramer. 1991. Consumption of solid food by suckling pigs: Individual variation and relation to weight gain. *Appl. Anim. Behav. Sci.* 32:139–155.

1466. Pajor, E. A., D. M. Weary, C. Caceres, D. Fraser and D. L. Kramer. 2002. Alternative housing for sows and litters: Part 3. Effects of piglet diet quality and sow-controlled housing on performance and behaviour. *Appl. Anim. Behav. Sci.* 76:267–277.

1467. Pal, S. K. 2008. Maturation and development of social behaviour during early ontogeny in free-ranging dog puppies in West Bengal, India. *Appl. Anim. Behav. Sci.* 111:95–107.

1468. Pal, S. K. 2005. Parental care in free-ranging dogs, *Canis familiaris. Appl. Anim. Behav. Sci.* 90:31–47.

1469. Pal, S. K. 2003. Urine marking by free-ranging dogs (*Canis familiaris*) in relation to sex, season, place and posture. *Appl. Anim. Behav. Sci.* 80:45–59.

1470. Palazzolo, D. L. and S. K. Quadri. 1987. The effects of aging on the circadian rhythm of serum cortisol in the dog. *Exp. Gerontol.* 22:379–387.

1471. Palen, G. F. and G. V. Goddard. 1966. Catnip and oestrous behaviour in the cat. *Anim. Behav.* 14:372–377.

1472. Palmer, A. C., G. F. Smith and S. J. Turner. 1980. Cataplexy in a Guernsey bull. *Vet. Rec.* 106:421.

1473. Panaman, R. 1981. Behaviour and ecology of free-ranging farm cats (Felis catus). *Z. Tierpsychol.* 56:59–73.

1474. Pappas, T. N., R. L. Melendez, K. M. Strah and H. T. Debas. 1985. Cholecystokinin is not a peripheral satiety signal in the dog. *Am. J. Physiol.* 249:G733–G738.

1475. Paroz, C., S. G. Gebhardt-Henrich and A. Steiger. 2008. Reliability and validity of behaviour tests in Hovawart dogs. *Appl. Anim. Behav. Sci.* 115:67–81.

1476. Parratt, C. A., K. J. Chapman, C. Turner, P. H. Jones, M. T. Mendl and B. G. Miller. 2006. The fighting behaviour of piglets mixed before and after weaning in the presence or absence of a sow. *Appl. Anim. Behav. Sci.* 101:54–67.

1477. Parrott, R. F. 1993. Peripheral and central effects of CCK receptor agonists on operant feeding in pigs. *Physiol. Behav.* 53:367–372.

1478. Parrott, R. F. and B. A. Baldwin. 1984. Olfactory stimuli and intermale aggression in androgen-treated castrated sheep. *Aggress. Behav.* 10:115–122.
1479. Parrott, R. F. and W. D. Booth. 1984. Behavioural and morphological effects of 5 alpha-dihydrotestosterone and oestradiol-17 beta in the prepubertally castrated boar. *J. Reprod. Fertil.* 71:453–461.
1480. Parsons, S. D. and G. L. Hunter. 1967. Effect of the ram on duration of oestrus in the ewe. *J. Reprod. Fertil.* 14:61–70.
1481. Pavlov, I. P. 1927. *Conditioned reflexes: An investigation of the physiological activity of the cerebral cortex*. London, UK: Oxford University Press.
1482. Pedersen, L. J. 2007. Sexual behaviour in female pigs. *Horm. Behav.* 52:64–69.
1483. Pedersen, L. J. and T. Jensen. 2008. Effects of late introduction of sows to two farrowing environments on the progress of farrowing and maternal behavior. *J. Anim. Sci.* 86:2730–2737.
1484. Pedersen, L. J., E. Jørgensen, T. Heiskanen and B. I. Damm. 2006. Early piglet mortality in loose-housed sows related to sow and piglet behaviour and to the progress of parturition. *Appl. Anim. Behav. Sci.* 96:215–232.
1485. Pedersen, L. J., T. Rojkittikhun, S. Einarsson and L.-E. Edqvist. 1993. Postweaning grouped sows: Effects of aggression on hormonal patterns and oestrous behaviour. *Appl. Anim. Behav. Sci.* 38:25–39.
1486. Pekas, J. C. 1985. Animal growth during liberation from appetite suppression. *Growth* 49:19–27.
1487. Pekas, J. C. and W. E. Trout. 1993. Cholecystokinin octapeptide immunization: Effect on growth of barrows and gilts. *J. Anim. Sci.* 71:2499–2505.
1488. Pell, S. M. and P. D. McGreevy. 1999. A study of cortisol and beta-endorphin levels in stereotypic and normal thoroughbreds. *Appl. Anim. Behav. Sci.* 64:81–90.
1489. Penning, P. D., A. J. Parsons, J. A. Newman, R. J. Orr and A. Harvey. 1993. The effects of group size on grazing time in sheep. *Appl. Anim. Behav. Sci.* 37:101–109.
1490. Penning, P. D., A. J. Parsons, R. J. Orr, A. Harvey and R. A. Champion. 1995. Intake and behaviour responses by sheep, in different physiological states, when grazing monocultures of grass or white clover. *Appl. Anim. Behav. Sci.* 45:63–78.
1491. Penning, P. D., A. J. Rook and R. J. Orr. 1991. Patterns of ingestive behaviour of sheep continuously stocked on monocultures of ryegrass or white clover. *Appl. Anim. Behav. Sci.* 31:237–250.
1492. Penny, R. H., F. W. Hill, J. E. Field and J. T. Plush. 1972. Tail-biting in pigs: A possible sex incidence. *Vet. Rec.* 91:482–483.
1493. Pepelko, W. E. and M. T. Clegg. 1965. Influence of season of the year upon patterns of sexual behavior in male sheep. *J. Anim. Sci.* 24:633–637.
1494. Pepelko, W. E. and M. T. Clegg. 1965. Studies of mating behaviour and some factors influencing the sexual response in the male sheep *Ovis aries*. *Anim. Behav.* 13:249–258.
1495. Perez-Leon, I., A. Orihuela, L. Lidfors and V. Aguirre. 2006. Reducing mother-young separation distress by inducing ewes into oestrus at the day of weaning. *Anim. Welfare* 15:383–389.
1496. Perkins, A. and J. A. Fitzgerald. 1994. The behavioral component of the ram effect: The influence of ram sexual behavior on the induction of estrus in anovulatory ewes. *J. Anim. Sci.* 72:51–55.
1497. Persson, N. 1962. Self-stimulation in the goat. *Acta Physiol. Scand.* 55:276–285.
1498. Petchey, A. M. and J. Abdulkader. 1991. Intake and behaviour of cattle at different food barriers. *Anim. Prod.* 52:576–577.
1499. Petersen, V. 1994. The development of feeding and investigatory behaviour in free-ranging domestic pigs during their first 18 weeks of life. *Appl. Anim. Behav. Sci.* 42:87–98.
1500. Petersen, H. V., K. Vestergaard and P. Jensen. 1989. Integration of piglets into social groups of free-ranging domestic pigs. *Appl. Anim. Behav. Sci.* 23:223–226.
1501. Petersen, V., H. B. Simonsen and L. G. Lawson. 1995. The effect of environmental stimulation on the development of behaviour in pigs. *Appl. Anim. Behav. Sci.* 45:215–224.
1502. Petit, M. 1972. Emploi du temps des troupeaux de vaches-meres et de leurs veaux sur les paturages d'altitude de l'aubrac. *Ann. Zootech.* 21:5–27.
1503. Pettijohn, T. F., T. W. Wong, P. D. Ebert and J. P. Scott. 1977. Alleviation of separation distress in 3 breeds of young dogs. *Dev. Psychobiol.* 10:373–381.
1504. Pfaffenberger, C. J. and J. P. Scott. 1959. The relationship between delayed socialization and trainability in guide dogs. *J. Genet. Psychol.* 95:145–155.
1505. Pfister, J. A., B. L. Stegelmeier, C. D. Cheney and D. R. Gardner. 2007. Effect of previous locoweed (*Astragalus* and *Oxytropis* species) intoxication on conditioned taste aversions in horses and sheep. *J. Anim. Sci.* 85:1836–1841.

1506. Pfister, J. A., B. L. Stegelmeier, C. D. Cheney, M. H. Ralphs and D. R. Gardner. 2002. Conditioning taste aversions to locoweed (Oxytropis sericea) in horses. *J. Anim. Sci.* 80:79–83.

1507. Phillips, C. 2002. *Cattle behaviour & welfare*. Oxford, UK: Blackwell Science.

1508. Phillips, C. J. and C. A. Lomas. 2001. The perception of color by cattle and its influence on behavior. *J. Dairy Sci.* 84:807–813.

1509. Phillips, C. J. C., D. Fraser and B. K. Thompson. 1991. Preference of sows for a partially enclosed farrowing crate. *Appl. Anim. Behav. Sci.* 32:35–43.

1510. Phillips, C. J. C. and S. A. Schofield. 1990. The effect of environment and stage of the oestrous cycle on the behaviour of dairy cows. *Appl. Anim. Behav. Sci.* 27:21–31.

1511. Phillips, C. J. C. and L. Weiguo. 1991. Brightness discrimination abilities of calves relative to those of humans. *Appl. Anim. Behav. Sci.* 31:25–33.

1512. Piccione, G., C. Bertolucci, G. Caola and A. Foa. 2007. Effects of restricted feeding on circadian activity rhythms of sheep—A brief report. *Appl. Anim. Behav. Sci.* 107:233–238.

1513. Pick, D. F., G. Lovell, S. Brown and D. Dail. 1994. Equine color perception revisited. *Appl. Anim. Behav. Sci.* 42:61–65.

1514. Pickerel, T. M., S. L. Crowell-Davis, A. B. Caudle and D. Q. Estep. 1993. Sexual preferences of mares (*Equus caballus*) for individual stallions. *Appl. Anim. Behav. Sci.* 38:1–13.

1515. Pickett, B. W., L. C. Faulkner and J. L. Voss. 1975. Effect of season on some characteristics of stallion semen. *J. Reprod. Fertil. Suppl.* 23: 25–28.

1516. Pickett, B. W., J. L. Voss and E. L. Squires. 1977. Impotence and abnormal sexual behavior in the stallion. *Theriogenology* 8:329–347.

1517. Pinckard, K. L., J. Stellflug and F. Stormshak. 2000. Influence of castration and estrogen replacement on sexual behavior of female-oriented, male-oriented, and asexual rams. *J. Anim. Sci.* 78:1947–1953.

1518. Pinheiro Machado Fo, L. C. 1997. Timing of the attraction towards the placenta and amniotic fluid by the parturient cow. *Appl. Anim. Behav. Sci.* 53:183–192.

1519. Pinheiro Machado, F. L. C., J. F. Hurnik and J. H. Burton. 1997. The effect of amniotic fluid ingestion on the nociception of cows. *Physiol. Behav.* 62:1339–1344.

1520. Pitts, A. D., D. M. Weary, D. Fraser, E. A. Pajor and D. L. Kramer. 2002. Alternative housing for sows and litters. Part 5. Individual differences in the maternal behaviour of sows. *Appl. Anim. Behav. Sci.* 76:291–306.

1521. Pitts, A. D., D. M. Weary, E. A. Pajor and D. Fraser. 2000. Mixing at young ages reduces fighting in unacquainted domestic pigs. *Appl. Anim. Behav. Sci.* 68:191–197.

1522. Podberscek, A. L., J. K. Blackshaw and A. W. Beattie. 1991. The behaviour of laboratory colony cats and their reactions to a familiar and unfamiliar person. *Appl. Anim. Behav. Sci.* 31:119–130.

1523. Podberscek, A. L. and J. A. Serpell. 1997. Aggressive behaviour in English cocker spaniels and the personality of their owners. *Vet. Rec.* 141:73–76.

1524. Podberscek, A. L. and J. A. Serpell. 1997. Environmental influences on the expression of aggressive behaviour in English cocker spaniels. *Appl. Anim. Behav. Sci.* 52:215–227.

1525. Poindron, P., A. Terrazas, L. Montes de Oca Mde, N. Serafin and H. Hernandez. 2007. Sensory and physiological determinants of maternal behavior in the goat (Capra hircus). *Horm. Behav.* 52:99–105.

1526. Pollard, J. C. 1992. Effects of litter size on the vocal behaviour of ewes. *Appl. Anim. Behav. Sci.* 34:75–84.

1527. Pollard, J. C., K. J. Shaw and R. P. Littlejohn. 1999. A note on sheltering behaviour of ewes before and after lambing. *Appl. Anim. Behav. Sci.* 61:313–318.

1528. Pollard, J. S., M. D. Baldock and R. F. Lewis. 1971. Learning rate and use of visual information on five animal species. *Aust. J. Psychol.* 23:29–34.

1529. Pond, W. G. and J. H. Maner. 1974. *Swine production in temperate and tropical environments*. San Francisco, CA: W.H. Freeman and Co.

1530. Pongracz, P., A. Miklosi, E. Kubinyi, K. Gurobi, J. Topal and V. Csanyi. 2001. Social learning in dogs: The effect of a human demonstrator on the performance of dogs in a detour task. *Anim. Behav.* 62:1109–1117.

1531. Pongracz, P., A. Miklósi, V. Vida and V. Csányi. 2005. The pet dogs ability for learning from a human demonstrator in a detour task is independent from the breed and age. *Appl. Anim. Behav. Sci.* 90:309–323.

1532. Pongracz, P., V. Vida, P. Banhegyi and A. Miklosi. 2008. How does dominance rank status affect individual and social learning performance in the dog (*Canis familiaris*)? *Anim. Cogn.* 11:75–82.

1533. Porter, R. H., R. Nowak and P. Orgeur. 1995. Influence of a conspecific agemate on distress bleating by lambs. *Appl. Anim. Behav. Sci.* 45:239–244.

1534. Porter, R. H., R. Nowak, P. Orgeur, F. Levy and B. Schaal. 1997. Twin/non-twin discrimination by lambs: An investigation of salient stimulus characteristics. *Behaviour* 134:463–475.

1535. Prache, S., G. Bechet and J. C. Damasceno. 2006. Diet choice in grazing sheep: A new approach to investigate the relationships between preferences and intake-rate on a daily time scale. *Appl. Anim. Behav. Sci.* 99:253–270.

1536. Prato-Previde, E., S. Marshall-Pescini and P. Valsecchi. 2008. Is your choice my choice? The owners' effect on pet dogs' (Canis lupus familiaris) performance in a food choice task. *Anim. Cogn.* 11:167–174.

1537. Prescott, C. W. 1973. Reproduction patterns in the domestic cat. *Aust. Vet. J.* 49:126–129.

1538. Presicce, G. A., C. C. Brockett, T. Cheng, R. H. Foote, G. F. Rivard and W. R. Klemm. 1993. Behavioral responses of bulls kept under artificial conditions to compounds presented for olfaction, taste or with topical nasal application. *Appl. Anim. Behav. Sci.* 37:273–284.

1539. Price, E. O., J. K. Blackhaw, A. Blackshaw, R. Borgwardt, M. R. Dally and R. H. Bondurant. 1994. Sexual responses of rams to ovariectomized and intact estrous ewes. *Appl. Anim. Behav. Sci.* 42:67–71.

1540. Price, E. O., R. Borgwardt and M. R. Dally. 1999. Effect of early fenceline exposure to estrous ewes on the sexual performance of yearling rams. *Appl. Anim. Behav. Sci.* 64:241–247.

1541. Price, E. O., R. Borgwardt and M. R. Dally. 1993. Effect of ewe restraint on the libido and serving capacity of rams. *Appl. Anim. Behav. Sci.* 35:339–345.

1542. Price, E. O., R. Borgwardt and A. Orihuela. 1998. Early sexual experience fails to enhance sexual performance in male goats. *J. Anim. Sci.* 76:718–720.

1543. Price, E. O., H. Erhard, R. Borgwardt and M. R. Dally. 1992. Measures of libido and their relation to serving capacity in the ram. *J. Anim. Sci.* 70:3376–3380.

1544. Price, E. O., G. D. Hutson, M. I. Price and R. Borgwardt. 1994. Fostering in swine as affected by age of offspring. *J. Anim. Sci.* 72:1697–1701.

1545. Price, E. O., L. S. Katz, S. J. R. Wallach and J. J. Zenchak. 1988. The relationship of male-male mounting to the sexual preferences of young rams. *Appl. Anim. Behav. Sci.* 21:347–355.

1546. Price, E. O., C. L. Martinez and B. L. Coe. 1984. The effects of twinning and mother-offspring behavior in range beef cattle. *Appl. Anim. Behav. Sci.* 13:309–320.

1547. Price, E. O., V. M. Smith and L. S. Katz. 1984. Sexual stimulation of male dairy goats. *Appl. Anim. Behav. Sci.* 13:83–92.

1548. Price, E. O., J. Thos and G. B. Anderson. 1981. Maternal responses of confined beef cattle to single versus twin calves. *J. Anim. Sci.* 53:934–939.

1549. Price, E. O. and S. J. Wallach. 1991. Development of sexual and aggressive behaviors in Hereford bulls. *J. Anim. Sci.* 69:1019–1027.

1550. Price, E. O. and S. J. Wallach. 1991. Effects of group size and the male-to-female ratio on the sexual performance and aggressive behavior of bulls in serving capacity tests. *J. Anim. Sci.* 69:1034–1040.

1551. Price, E. O. and S. J. R. Wallach. 1990. Rearing bulls with females fails to enhance sexual performance. *Appl. Anim. Behav. Sci.* 26:339–347.

1552. Price, E. O., S. J. R. Wallach and G. V. Silver. 1990. The effects of long-term individual vs. group housing on the sexual behavior of beef bulls. *Appl. Anim. Behav. Sci.* 27:277–285.

1553. Prince, J. H. 1977. The eye and vision. In M. J. Swenson (Ed.), *Duke's physiology of domestic animals.* Ithaca, NY: Cornell University Press.

1554. Proops, L., F. Burden and B. Osthaus. 2009. Mule cognition: A case of hybrid vigour? *Anim. Cogn.* 12:75–84.

1555. Provenza, F. D. and J. C. Malechek. 1986. A comparison of feed selection and foraging behavior in juvenile and adult goats. *Appl. Anim. Behav. Sci.* 16:49–61.

1556. Provenza, F. D., L. Ortega-Reyes, C. B. Scott, J. J. Lynch and E. A. Burritt. 1994. Antiemetic drugs attenuate food aversions in sheep. *J. Anim. Sci.* 72:1989–1994.

1557. Pryor, P. A., B. L. Hart, M. J. Bain and K. D. Cliff. 2001. Causes of urine marking in cats and effects of environmental management on frequency of marking. *J. Am. Vet. Med. Assoc.* 219:1709–1713.

1558. Puppe, B. 1998. Effects of familiarity and relatedness on agonistic pair relationships in newly mixed domestic pigs. *Appl. Anim. Behav. Sci.* 58:233–239.

1559. Puppe, B., K. Ernst, P. C. Schön and G. Manteuffel. 2007. Cognitive enrichment affects behavioural reactivity in domestic pigs. *Appl. Anim. Behav. Sci.* 105:75–86.

1560. Purcell, D., C. W. Arava and J. L. Walters. 1988. Relationship of three measures of behavior to milk production. *Appl. Anim. Behav. Sci.* 21:307–313.

1561. Purcell, D. and C. W. Arave. 1991. Isolation vs. group rearing in monozygous twin heifer calves. *Appl. Anim. Behav. Sci.* 31:147–156.

1562. Putnam, P. A. and R. E. Davis. 1963. Ration effects on drylot steer feeding patterns. *J. Anim. Sci.* 22:437–443.

1563. Quaranta, A., M. Siniscalchi, M. Albrizio, S. Volpe, C. Buonavoglia and G. Vallortigara. 2008. Influence of behavioural lateralization on interleukin-2 and interleukin-6 gene expression in dogs before and after immunization with rabies vaccine. *Behav. Brain Res.* 186:256–260.

1564. Quaranta, A., M. Siniscalchi and G. Vallortigara. 2007. Asymmetric tail-wagging responses by dogs to different emotive stimuli. *Curr. Biol.* 17:R199–R201.

1565. Ralphs, M. H. and C. D. Cheney. 1993. Influence of cattle age, lithium chloride dose level, and food type in the retention of food aversions. *J. Anim. Sci.* 71:373–379.

1566. Ralston, S. L. 1984. Controls of feeding in horses. *J. Anim. Sci.* 59:1354–1361.

1567. Ralston, S. L. and C. A. Baile. 1983. Effects of intragastric loads of xylose, sodium chloride and corn oil on feeding behavior of ponies. *J. Anim. Sci.* 56:302–308.

1568. Ralston, S. L., D. E. Freeman and C. A. Baile. 1983. Volatile fatty acids and the role of the large intestine in the control of feed intake in ponies. *J. Anim. Sci.* 57:815–825.

1569. Ramirez, A., A. Quiles, M. Hevia and F. Sotillo. 1995. Behavior of Murciano-Granadina goat in the hour before parturition. *Appl. Anim. Behav. Sci.* 44:29–35.

1570. Ramirez, A., A. Quiles, M. L. Hevia and F. Sotillo. 1998. Behaviour of the Murciano-Granadina goat during the first hour after parturition. *Appl. Anim. Behav. Sci.* 56:223–230.

1571. Ramonet, Y., J. Bolduc, R. Bergeron, S. Robert and M.-C. Meunier-Salaun. 2000. Feeding motivation in pregnant sows: Effects of fibrous diets on an operant conditioning procedure. *Appl. Anim. Behav. Sci.* 66:21–29.

1572. Ramsay, D. J., B. J. Rolls and R. J. Wood. 1977. Thirst following water deprivation in dogs. *Am. J. Physiol.* 232:R93–R100.

1573. Ramsay, D. J., B. J. Rolls and R. J. Wood. 1975. The relationship between elevated water intake and oedema associated with congestive cardiac failure in the dog. *J. Physiol.* 244:303–312.

1574. Randall, G. C. 1972. Observations on parturition in the sow. I. Factors associated with the delivery of the piglets and their subsequent behaviour. *Vet. Rec.* 90:178–182.

1575. Randall, R. P., W. A. Schurg and D. C. Church. 1978. Response of horses to sweet, salty, sour and bitter solutions. *J. Anim. Sci.* 47:51–55.

1576. Randall, W. and V. Lakso. 1968. Body weight and food intake rhythms and their relationship to the behavior of cats with brain stem lesions. *Psychonom. Sci.* 11:33–34.

1577. Randall, W., R. Swenson, V. Parsons, J. Elbin and M. Trulson. 1975. The influence of seasonal changes in light on hormones in normal cats and in cats with lesions of the superior colliculi and pretectum. *J. Interdiscip. Cycle Res.* 6:253–266.

1578. Randle, H. D. 1998. Facial hair whorl position and temperament in cattle. *Appl. Anim. Behav. Sci.* 56:139–147.

1579. Range, F., U. Aust, M. Steurer and L. Huber. 2008. Visual categorization of natural stimuli by domestic dogs. *Anim. Cogn.* 11:339–347.

1580. Range, F., L. Horn, T. Bugnyar, G. K. Gajdon and L. Huber. 2009. Social attention in keas, dogs, and human children. *Anim. Cogn.* 12:181–192.

1581. Rashotte, M. E., J. C. Smith, T. Austin, C. Pollitz, T. W. Castonguay and L. Jonsson. 1984. Twenty-four-hour free-feeding patterns of dogs eating dry food. *Neurosci. Biobehav. Rev.* 8:205–210.

1582. Rasmussen, D. K., R. Weber and B. Wechsler. 2006. Effects of animal/feeding-place ratio on the behaviour and performance of fattening pigs fed via sensor-controlled liquid feeding. *Appl. Anim. Behav. Sci.* 98:45–53.

1583. Rasmussen, O. G., E. M. Banks, T. H. Berry and D. E. Becker. 1962. Social dominance in gilts. *J. Anim. Sci.* 21:520–522.

1584. Raussi, S., A. Boissy, E. Delval, P. Pradel, J. Kaihilahti and I. Veissier. 2005. Does repeated regrouping alter the social behaviour of heifers? *Appl. Anim. Behav. Sci.* 93:1–12.

1585. Ray, D. E. and C. B. Roubicek. 1971. Behavior of feedlot cattle during two seasons. *J. Anim. Sci.* 33:72–76.

1586. Rayner, D. V. and S. Miller. 1993. Voluntary intake and gastric emptying in pigs: Effects of fat and a CCK inhibitor. *Physiol. Behav.* 54:917–922.

1587. Redbo, I., P. Redbo-Torstensson, F. O. Odberg, A. Hadendahl and J. Holm. 1998. Factors affecting behavioural disturbances in race-horses. *Anim. Sci.* 66:475–481.

1588. Redondo, A. J., J. Carranza and P. Trigo. 2009. Fat diet reduces stress and intensity of startle reaction in horses. *Appl. Anim. Behav. Sci.* 118:69–75.

1589. Reed, H. C., D. R. Melrose and R. L. Patterson. 1974. Androgen steroids as an aid to the detection of oestrus in pig artificial insemination. *Br. Vet. J.* 130:61–67.

1590. Rehkamper, G. and A. Gorlach. 1998. Visual identification of small sizes by adult dairy bulls. *J. Dairy Sci.* 81:1574–1580.

1591. Reinhardt, V., F. M. Mutiso and A. Reinhardt. 1978. Resting habits of Zebu cattle in a nocturnal enclosure. *Appl. Anim. Ethol.* 4:261.

1592. Reinhardt, V., F. M. Mutiso and A. Reinhardt. 1978. Social behaviour and social relationships between female and male prepubertal bovine calves (*Bos indicus*). *Appl. Anim. Ethol.* 4:43–54.

1593. Reisner, I. 1991. The pathophysiologic basis of behavior problems. *Vet. Clin. North Am. Small Anim. Pract.* 21:207–224.

1594. Reisner, I. R., K. A. Houpt, H. N. Erb and F. W. Quimby. 1994. Friendliness to humans and defensive aggression in cats: The influence of handling and paternity. *Physiol. Behav.* 55:1119–1124.

1595. Reisner, I. R., J. J. Mann, M. Stanley, Y. Y. Huang and K. A. Houpt. 1996. Comparison of cerebrospinal fluid monoamine metabolite levels in dominant-aggressive and non-aggressive dogs. *Brain Res.* 714:57–64.

1596. Remmers, J. E. and H. Gautier. 1972. Neural and mechanical mechanisms of feline purring. *Respir. Physiol.* 16:351–361.

1597. Renken, W. J., L. D. Howery, G. B. Ruyle and R. M. Enns. 2008. Cattle generalise visual cues from the pen to the field to select initial feeding patches. *Appl. Anim. Behav. Sci.* 109:128–140.

1598. Rensch, B. 1956. Increase of learning capability with increase of brain-size. *Am. Natur.* 90:81–95.

1599. Reppert, S. M., H. G. Artman, S. Swaminathan and D. A. Fisher. 1981. Vasopressin exhibits a rhythmic daily pattern in cerebrospinal fluid but not in blood. *Science* 213:1256–1257.

1600. Rheingold, H. L. 1963. Maternal behavior in the dog. In H. L. Rheingold (Ed.), *Maternal behavior in mammals*, pp. 169–202. New York, NY: John Wiley & Sons.

1601. Rheingold, H. L. and C. O. Eckerman. 1971. Familiar social and nonsocial stimuli and the kitten's response to a strange environment. *Dev. Psychobiol.* 4:71–89.

1602. Rhind, S. M., S. R. McMillen, E. Duff, C. E. Kyle and S. Wright. 2000. Effect of long-term feed restriction on seasonal endocrine changes in Soay sheep. *Physiol. Behav.* 71:343–351.

1603. Riches, J. H. and R. H. Watson. 1954. The influence of the introduction of rams on the incidence of oestrus in Merino ewes. *Aust. J. Agric. Res.* 5:141–147.

1604. Richman, L. M., D. E. Johnson and R. F. Angel. 1994. Evaluation of a positive conditioning technique for influencing big sagebrush (*Artemisia tridentata* subspp. *wyomingensis*) consumption by goats. *Appl. Anim. Behav. Sci.* 40:229–240.

1605. Ringo, J., M. L. Wolbarsht, H. G. Wagner, R. Crocker and F. Amthor. 1977. Trichromatic vision in the cat. *Science* 198:753–755.

1606. Rioja-Lang, F. C., D. J. Roberts, S. D. Healy, A. B. Lawrence and M. J. Haskell. 2009. Dairy cows trade-off feed quality with proximity to a dominant individual in Y-maze choice tests. *Appl. Anim. Behav. Sci.* 117:159–164.

1607. Riol, J. A., J. M. Sanchez, V. G. Eguren and V. R. Gaudioso. 1989. Colour perception in fighting cattle. *Appl. Anim. Behav. Sci.* 23:199–206.

1608. Rivas-Munoz, R., G. Fitz-Rodriguez, P. Poindron, B. Malpaux and J. A. Delgadillo. 2007. Stimulation of estrous behavior in grazing female goats by continuous or discontinuous exposure to males. *J. Anim. Sci.* 85:1257–1263.

1609. Rivera, E., S. Benjamin, B. Nielsen, J. Shelle and A. J. Zanella. 2002. Behavioral and physiological responses of horses to initial training: The comparison between pastured versus stalled horses. *Appl. Anim. Behav. Sci.* 78:235–252.

1610. Robert, S. J., J. J. Matte, C. Farmer, C. L. Girard and G. P. Martineau. 1993. High-fibre diets for sows: Effects of stereotypies and adjunctive drinking. *Appl. Anim. Behav. Sci.* 37:297–309.

1611. Roberts, S. J. 1971. *Veterinary obstetrics and genital diseases (theriogenology)*. Ithaca, NY: Stehen J. Roberts.

1612. Robinson, D. W. 1975. Food intake regulation in pigs. IV. The influence of dietary threonine imbalance on food intake, dietary choice and plasma acid patterns. *Br. Vet. J.* 131:595–600.

1613. Rogers, V. P., G. T. Hartke and R. L. Kitchell. 1967. Behavioral technique to analyze a dog's ability to discriminate flavors in commercial food products. In Y. Hayashi (Ed.), *Olfaction and taste*, pp. 353–359. Oxford, UK: Pergamon Press.

1614. Rogosic, J., J. A. Pfister, F. D. Provenza and D. Grbesa. 2006. The effect of activated charcoal and number of species offered on intake of Mediterranean shrubs by sheep and goats. *Appl. Anim. Behav. Sci.* 101:305–317.

1615. Rohde, K. A. and H. W. Gonyou. 1987. Strategies of teat-seeking behavior in neonatal pigs. *Appl. Anim. Behav. Sci.* 19:57–72.

1616. Romano, J. E., C. J. Christians and B. G. Crabo. 2000. Continuous presence of rams hastens the onset of estrus in ewes synchronized during the breeding season. *Appl. Anim. Behav. Sci.* 66:65–70.

1617. Romeyer, A., P. Poindron and P. Orgeur. 1994. Olfaction mediates the establishment of selective bonding in goats. *Physiol. Behav.* 56:693–700.

1618. Romeyer, A., P. Poindron, R. H. Porter, F. Levy and P. Orgeur. 1994. Establishment of maternal bonding and its mediation by vaginocervical stimulation in goats. *Physiol. Behav.* 55:395–400.

1619. Romeyer, A., R. H. Porter, F. Levy, R. Nowak, P. Orgeur and P. Poindron. 1993. Maternal labelling is not necessary for the establishment of discrimination between kids by recently parturient goats. *Anim. Behav.* 46:705–712.

1620. Romsos, D. R. and D. Ferguson. 1983. Regulation of protein intake in adult dogs. *J. Am. Vet. Med. Assoc.* 182:41–43.

1621. Rook, A. J. and C. A. Huckle. 1997. Activity bout criteria for grazing dairy cows. *Appl. Anim. Behav. Sci.* 54:89–96.

1622. Rook, A. J. and P. D. Penning. 1991. Synchronisation of eating, ruminating and idling activity by grazing sheep. *Appl. Anim. Behav. Sci.* 32:157–166.

1623. Rook, A. J., S. J. Rodway-Dyer and J. E. Cook. 2005. Effects of resource density on spatial memory and learning by foraging sheep. *Appl. Anim. Behav. Sci.* 95:143–151.

1624. Rooney, N. J., J. W. S. Bradshaw and I. H. Robinson. 2001. Do dogs respond to play signals given by humans? *Anim. Behav.* 61:715–722.

1625. Root, M. V., S. D. Johnston and P. N. Olson. 1996. Effect of prepuberal and postpuberal gonadectomy on heat production measured by indirect calorimetry in male and female domestic cats. *Am. J. Vet. Res.* 57:371–374.

1626. Rosa, H. J., D. T. Juniper and M. J. Bryant. 2000. The effect of exposure to oestrous ewes on rams' sexual behaviour, plasma testosterone concentration and ability to stimulate ovulation in seasonally anoestrous ewes. *Appl. Anim. Behav. Sci.* 67:293–305.

1627. Rose, J. E. 1968. Discussion following paper, cortical representation by E. F. evans. In A. V. S. de Reuck and J. Knight (Eds.), *Hearing mechanisms in vertebrates. Ciba Foundation symposium*, pp. 287–295. London, UK: Churchill Ltd.

1628. Roselli, C. E., K. Larkin, J. M. Schrunk and F. Stormshak. 2004. Sexual partner preference, hypothalamic morphology and aromatase in rams. *Physiol. Behav.* 83:233–245.

1629. Roselli, C. E. and F. Stormshak. 2009. The neurobiology of sexual partner preferences in rams. *Horm. Behav.* 55:611–620.

1630. Rosenblatt, J. S. 1971. Suckling and home orientation in the kitten. A comparative developmental study. In E. Tobach, L. R. Aronson and E. Shaw (Eds.), *The biopsychology of development*, pp. 345–410. New York, NY: Academic Press.

1631. Rosenblatt, J. S. 1965. The basis of synchrony in the behavioral interaction between the mother and her offspring in the laboratory rat. In B. M. Foss (Ed.), *Determinants of infant behaviour*, pp. 3–45. New York, NY: John Wiley & Sons.

1632. Rosenblatt, J. S. 1965. Effects of experience on sexual behavior in male cats. In F. A. Beach (Ed.), *Sex and behavior*, pp. 416–439. New York, NY: John Wiley & Sons.

1633. Rosenblatt, J. S. and L. R. Aronson. 1958. The decline of sexual behavior in male cats after castration with special reference to the role of prior sexual experience. *Behaviour* 12:285–338.

1634. Rosenblatt, J. S. and L. R. Aronson. 1958. The influence of experience on the behavioural effects of androgen in prepuberally castrated male cats. *Anim. Behav.* 6:171–182.

1635. Rosenblatt, J. S. and T. C. Schneirla. 1962. The behaviour of cats. In E. S. E. Hafez (Ed.), *The behaviour of domestic animals*, pp. 453–488. Baltimore, MD: Williams & Wilkins.

1636. Ross, S. 1951. Sucking behavior in neonate dogs. *J. Abnorm. Psychol.* 46:142–149.

1637. Ross, S. and J. Berg. 1956. Stability of food dominance relationships in a flock of goats. *J. Mammal.* 37:129–131.

1638. Ross, S. and J. P. Scott. 1949. Relationship between dominance and control of movement in goats. *J. Comp. Physiol. Psychol.* 42:75–80.

1639. Ross, S., J. P. Scott, M. Cherner and V. H. Denenberg. 1960. Effects of restraint and isolation on yelping in puppies. *Anim. Behav.* 8:1–5.

1640. Rossdale, P. D. 1967. Clinical studies on the newborn thoroughbred foal. I. Perinatal behaviour. *Br. Vet. J.* 123:470–481.

1641. Rossi, A. P. and C. Ades. 2008. A dog at the keyboard: Using arbitrary signs to communicate requests. *Anim. Cogn.* 11:329–338.

1642. Rossi, R., E. Del Prete, J. Rokitzky and E. Scharrer. 1999. Circadian drinking during ad libitum and restricted feeding in pygmy goats. *Appl. Anim. Behav. Sci.* 61:253–261.

1643. Roth, B. A., E. Hillmann, M. Stauffacher and N. M. Keil. 2008. Improved weaning reduces cross-sucking and may improve weight gain in dairy calves. *Appl. Anim. Behav. Sci.* 111:251–261.

1644. Rouda, R. R., D. M. Anderson, J. D. Wallace and L. W. Murray. 1994. Free-ranging cattle water consumption in southcentral New Mexico. *Appl. Anim. Behav. Sci.* 39:29–38.

1645. Rowell, T. E. 1991. Till death do us part: Long-lasting bonds between ewes and their daughters. *Anim. Behav.* 42:681–682.

1646. Roy, J. H. B., K. W. G. Shillam and J. Palmer. 1955. The outdoor rearing of calves on grass with special reference to growth rate and grazing behaviour. *J. Dairy Res.* 22:252–269.

1647. Rozin, P. 1967. Thiamine specific hunger. In C. F. Code and W. Heidel (Eds.), *Handbook of physiology. Section 6. Alimentary canal, volume I. Control of food and water intake*, pp. 411–431. Washington, DC: American Physiological Society.

1648. Rozkowska, E. and E. Fonberg. 1973. Salivary reactions after ventromedial hypothalamic lesions in dogs. *Acta Neurobiol. Exp. (Wars)* 33:553–562.

1649. Rubenstein, D. I. and M. A. Hack. 1992. Horse signals: The sounds and scents of fury. *Evol. Ecol.* 6:254–260.

1650. Rubin, L., C. Oppegard and H. F. Hindz. 1980. The effect of varying the temporal distribution of conditioning trials on equine learning behavior. *J. Anim. Sci.* 50:1184–1187.

1651. Ruckebusch, Y. 1975. The hypnogram as an index of adaptation of farm animals to changes in their environment. *Appl. Anim. Ethol.* 2:3–18.

1652. Ruckebusch, Y. 1974. Sleep deprivation in cattle. *Brain Res.* 78:495–499.

1653. Ruckebusch, Y. 1972. The relevance of drowsiness in the circadian cycle of farm animals. *Anim. Behav.* 20:637–643.

1654. Ruckebusch, Y., R. W. Dougherty and H. M. Cook. 1974. Jaw movements and rumen motility as criteria for measurement of deep sleep in cattle. *Am. J. Vet. Res.* 35:1309–1312.

1655. Ruckebusch Y., Gaujoux. 1976. Sleep patterns of the laboratory cat. *Electroencephalogr. Clin. Neurophysiol.* 41:483–490.

1656. Ruckebusch, Y., M. Gaujoux and B. Eghbali. 1977. Sleep cycles and kinesis in the foetal lamb. *Electroencephalogr. Clin. Neurophysiol.* 42:226–237.

1657. Rudge, M. R. 1970. Mother and kid behaviour in feral goats (*Capra hircus* L.). *Z. Tierpsychol.* 27:687–692.

1658. Ruis, M. A. W., J. H. A. Te Brake, B. Engel, W. G. Buist, H. J. Blokhuis and J. M. Koolhaas. 2002. Implications of coping characteristics and social status for welfare and production of paired growing gilts. *Appl. Anim. Behav. Sci.* 75:207–231.

1659. Ruis, M. A. W., J. H. A. Te Brake, J. A. van de Burgwal, I. C. de Jong, H. J. Blokhuis and J. M. Koolhaas. 2000. Personalities in female domesticated pigs: Behavioural and physiological indications. *Appl. Anim. Behav. Sci.* 66:31–47.

1660. Ruiz-Miranda, C. R. 1993. Use of pelage pigmentation in the recognition of mothers in a group by 2- to 4-month-old domestic goat kids. *Appl. Anim. Behav. Sci.* 36:317–326.

1661. Rushen, J. 1984. Stereotyped behaviour, adjunctive drinking and the feeding periods of tethered sows. *Anim. Behav.* 32:1059–1067.

1662. Rushen, J. and A. M. de Passille. 1995. The motivation of non-nutritive sucking in calves, *Bos taurus*. *Anim. Behav.* 49:1503–1510.

1663. Rushen, J., A. M. De Passille and W. Schouten. 1990. Stereotypic behavior, endogenous opioids, and postfeeding hypoalgesia in pigs. *Physiol. Behav.* 48:91–96.

1664. Rushen, J., G. Foxcroft and A. M. De Passille. 1993. Nursing-induced changes in pain sensitivity, prolactin, and somatotropin in the pig. *Physiol. Behav.* 53:265–270.

1665. Rushen, J., J. Ladewig and A. M. de Passille. 1995. A novel environment inhibits milk ejection in the pig but not through HPA activity. *Appl. Anim. Behav. Sci.* 45:53–61.

1666. Russek, M. and P. J. Morgane. 1963. Anorexic effect of intraperitoneal glucose in the hypothalamic hyperphagic cat. *Nature* 199:1004–1005.

1667. Rutberg, A. T. 1990. Inter-group transfer in Assateague pony mares. *Anim. Behav.* 40:945–952.

1668. Rutberg, A. T. and S. A. Greenbrg. 1990. Dominance, aggression frequencies and modes of aggressive competition in feral pony mares. *Anim. Behav.* 40:322–331.

1669. Rutberg, A. T. and R. R. Keiper. 1993. Proximate causes of natal dispersal in feral ponies: Some sex differences. *Anim. Behav.* 46:969–975.

1670. Rutter, S. M., V. Tainton, R. A. Champion and P. Le Grice. 2002. The effect of a total solar eclipse on the grazing behaviour of dairy cattle. *Appl. Anim. Behav. Sci.* 79:273–283.

1671. Rybarczyk, P., Y. Koba, J. Rushen, H. Tanida and A. M. de Passille. 2001. Can cows discriminate people by their faces? *Appl. Anim. Behav. Sci.* 74:175–189.

1672. Ryder, M. L. 1976. Seasonal changes in the coat of the cat. *Res. Vet. Sci.* 21:280–283.

1673. Sacks, J. J., L. Sinclair, J. Gilchrist, G. C. Golab and R. Lockwood. 2000. Breeds of dogs involved in fatal human attacks in the United States between 1979 and 1998. *J. Am. Vet. Med. Assoc.* 217:836–840.

1674. Sacks, J. J., R. W. Smith and S. E. Bonzo. 1989. Dog bite-related fatalities from 1979 to 1988. *JAVMA* 262:1489–1492.

1675. Salzinger, K. and M. B. Waller. 1962. The operant control of vocalization in the dog. *J. Exp. Anal. Behav.* 5:383–389.

1676. Sambraus, H. H. and D. Sambraus. 1975. Pragung von nutztieren auf menschen. *Z. Tierpsychol.* 38: 1–17.

1677. Sandem, A.-I. and B. O. Braastad. 2005. Effects of cow–calf separation on visible eye white and behaviour in dairy cows—A brief report. *Appl. Anim. Behav. Sci.* 95:233–239.

1678. Sandem, A.-I., B. O. Braastad and M. Bakken. 2006. Behaviour and percentage eye-white in cows waiting to be fed concentrate—A brief report. *Appl. Anim. Behav. Sci.* 97:145–151.

1679. Sandem, A. I., B. O. Braastad and K. E. Boe. 2002. Eye white may indicate emotional state on a frustration-contentedness axis in dairy cows. *Appl. Anim. Behav. Sci.* 79:1–10.

1680. Sandem, A. I., A. M. Janczak, R. Salte and B. O. Braastad. 2006. The use of diazepam as a pharmacological validation of eye white as an indicator of emotional state in dairy cows. *Appl. Anim. Behav. Sci.* 96:177–183.

1681. Sandler, B. E., G. A. Van Gelder, W. B. Buck and G. G. Karas. 1968. Effect of dieldrin exposure on detour behavior in sheep. *Psychol. Rep.* 23:451–455.

1682. Sandler, B. E., G. A. Van Gelder, D. D. Elsberg, G. G. Karas and W. B. Buck. 1969. Dieldrin exposure and vigilance behavior in sheep. *Psychonom. Sci.* 15:261–262.

1683. Sandler, B. E., G. A. Van Gelder, G. G. Karas and W. B. Buck. 1971. An operant feeding device for sheep. *J. Exp. Anal. Behav.* 15:95–96.

1684. Sapolsky, R. M. 1997. The importance of a well-groomed child. *Science* 277:1620–1621.

1685. Sappington, B. F. and L. Goldman. 1994. Discrimination learning and concept formation in the Arabian horse. *J. Anim. Sci.* 72:3080–3087.

1686. Sato, S. 1982. Leadership during actual grazing in a small herd of cattle. *Appl. Anim. Ethol.* 8:53–65.

1687. Sato, S. S. S. and A. Maeda. 1991. Social licking patterns in cattle (*Bos taurus*): Influence of environmental and social factors. *Appl. Anim. Behav. Sci.* 32:3–12.

1688. Sato, S., K. Tarumizu and K. Hatae. 1993. The influence of social factors on allogrooming in cows. *Appl. Anim. Behav. Sci.* 38:235–244.

1689. Say, L. and D. Pontier. 2004. Spacing pattern in a social group of stray cats: Effects on male reproductive success. *Anim. Behav.* 68:175–180.

1690. Scarlett, J. M., S. Donoghue, J. Saidla and J. Wills. 1994. Overweight cats: Prevalence and risk factors. *Int. J. Obes. Relat. Metab. Disord.* 18(Suppl 1): S22–S28.

1691. Schafer, M. 1975. *The language of the horse*. New York, NY: Arco Publishing Co.

1692. Schaffer, C. B. and J. Phillips. (Directors). 1993. *The tuskagee behaviour test for selecting therapy dogs*. [Video/DVD] Tuskagee: Tuskegee University School of Veterinary Medicine.

1693. Schake, L. M. and J. K. Riggs. 1969. Activities of lactating beef cows in confinement. *J. Anim. Sci.* 28:568–572.

1694. Schalke, E., J. Stichnoth, S. Ott and R. Jones-Baade. 2007. Clinical signs caused by the use of electric training collars on dogs in everyday life situations. *Appl. Anim. Behav. Sci.* 105:369–380.

1695. Scheepens, C. J. M., M. J. C. Hessing, E. Laarakker, W. G. P. Schouten and M. J. M. Tielen. 1991. Influence of intermittent daily draught on the behaviour of weaned pigs. *Appl. Anim. Behav. Sci.* 31:69–82.

1696. Schein, M. W. and M. H. Fohrman. 1955. Social dominance relationships in a herd of dairy cattle. *Br. J. Anim. Behav.* 3:45–55.

1697. Schichowski, C., E. Moors and M. Gauly. 2008. Effects of weaning lambs in two stages or by abrupt separation on their behavior and growth rate. *J. Anim. Sci.* 86:220–225.

1698. Schino, G. 1998. Reconciliation in domestic goats. *Behaviour* 135:343–356.

1699. Schloeth, R. 1961. Das sozialleben des camargue-rindes. Qualitative und quantitative untersuchungen uber die sozialen beziehungen-insbesondere die soziale rangordnung–des halbwilden franzosischen SP–kampfrindes. *Z. Tierpsychol.* 18:574–627.

1700. Schneirla, T. C., J. S. Rosenblatt and E. Tobach. 1963. Maternal behavior in the cat. In H. L. Rheingold (Ed.), *Maternal behavior in mammals*, pp. 122–168. New York, NY: John Wiley & Sons.

1701. Schoen, A. M. S., E. M. Banks and S. E. Curtis. 1976. Behavior of young Shetland and Welsh ponies (Equus caballus). *Biol. Behav.* 1:199–216.

1702. Schoen, A. M. S., S. E. Curtis, E. M. Banks and H. W. Norton. 1974. Behavior and performance of swine subjected to preweaning handling. *J. Anim. Sci.* 39:136–137.

1703. Schofield, W. L. and J. P. Mulville. 1998. Assessment of the modified Forssell's procedure for the treatment of oral stereotypies in 10 horses. *Vet. Rec.* 142:572–575.

1704. Schryver, H. F., M. T. Parker, P. D. Daniluk, K. I. Pagan, J. Williams, L. V. Soderholm and H. F. Hintz. 1987. Salt consumption and the effect of salt on mineral metabolism in horses. *Cornell Vet.* 77:122–131.

1705. Schryver, H. F., S. VanWie, P. Daniluk and H. F. Hintz. 1978. The voluntary intake of calcium by horses and ponies fed a calcium deficient diet. *J. Eq. Med. Surg.* 2:337–340.

1706. Schutz, K., D. Davison and L. Matthews. 2006. Do different levels of moderate feed deprivation in dairy cows affect feeding motivation? *Appl. Anim. Behav. Sci.* 101:253–263.

1707. Scott, D. W., R. W. Kirk and J. Bentinck-Smith. 1979. Some effects of short-term methylprednisolone therapy in normal cats. *Cornell Vet.* 69:104–115.

1708. Scott, J. P. 1962. Critical periods in behavioral development. *Science* 138:949–958.

1709. Scott, J. P. 1958. *Aggression*. Chicago, IL: University of Chicago Press.

1710. Scott, J. P. 1958. *Animal behavior*. Chicago, IL: University of Chicago Press.

1711. Scott, J. P. 1948. Dominance and the frustration-aggression hypothesis. *Physiol. Zool.* 21:31–39.

1712. Scott, J. P. 1946. Dominance reaction in a small flock of goats. *Anat. Rec.* 94:38–381.

1713. Scott, J. P. 1945. Social behavior, organization and leadership in a small flock of domestic sheep. *Comp. Psychol. Monogr.* 18:1–29.

1714. Scott, J. P. and J. L. Fuller. 1974. *Dog behavior. The genetic basis*. Chicago, IL: University of Chicago Press.

1715. Scott, J. P. and M. V. Marston. 1950. Critical periods affecting the development of normal and maladjustive social behavior of puppies. *J. Genet. Psychol.* 77:25–60.

1716. Scott, L. L. and F. D. Provenza. 2000. Lambs fed protein or energy imbalanced diets forage in locations and on foods that rectify imbalances. *Appl. Anim. Behav. Sci.* 68:293–305.

1717. Scott, M. D. and K. Causey. 1973. Ecology of feral dogs in Alabama. *J. Wildl. Manag.* 37:253–265.

1718. Scott, P. P. 1970. Cats. In E. S. E. Hafez (Ed.), *Reproduction and breeding techniques for laboratory animals*, pp. 192–208. Philadelphia, PA: Lea & Febiger.

1719. Seabrook, M. F. 1972. A study to determine the influence of the herdsman's personality on milk yield. *J. Agric. Labour Sci.* 1:45–59.

1720. Seath, D. M. and G. D. Miller. 1946. Effect of warm weather on grazing performance of milking cows. *J. Dairy Sci.* 29:199–206.

1721. Sechzer, J. A. and J. L. Brown. 1964. Color discrimination in the cat. *Science* 144:427–429.

1722. Segerstad, C. H. and G. Hellekant. 1989. The sweet taste in the calf. I. Chorda tympani proper nerve responses to taste stimulation of the tongue. *Physiol. Behav.* 45:633–638.

1723. Seguin, M. J., R. M. Friendship, R. N. Kirkwood, A. J. Zanella and T. M. Widowski. 2006. Effects of boar presence on agonistic behavior, shoulder scratches, and stress response of bred sows at mixing. *J. Anim. Sci.* 84:1227–1237.

1724. Seidel, W. F., T. Roth, T. Roehrs, F. Zorick and W. C. Dement. 1984. Treatment of a 12-hour shift of sleep schedule with benzodiazepines. *Science* 224:1262–1264.

1725. Seitz, P. F. D. 1959. Infantile experiences and adult behavior in animal subjects. II. Age of separation from the mother and adult behavior in the cat. *Psychosom. Med.* 21:353–378.

1726. Seksel, K., E. J. Mazurski and A. Taylor. 1999. Puppy socialisation programs: Short and long term behavioural effects. *Appl. Anim. Behav. Sci.* 62:335–349.

1727. Selman, I. E., A. D. McEwan and E. W. Fisher. 1970. Studies on natural suckling in cattle during the first eight hours post partum. I. Behavioural studies (dams). *Anim. Behav.* 18:276–283.

1728. Selman, I. E., A. D. McEwan and E. W. Fisher. 1970. Studies on natural suckling in cattle during the first eight hours post partum. II. Behavioural studies (calves). *Anim. Behav.* 18:284–289.

1729. Senn, C. L. and J. D. Lewin. 1975. Barking dogs as an environmental problem. *J. Am. Vet. Med. Assoc.* 166:1065–1068.

1730. Seoane, J. R. and C. A. Baile. 1973. Feeding behavior in sheep as related to the hypnotic activities of barbiturates injected into the third ventricle. *Pharmacol. Biochem. Behav.* 1:47–53.

1731. Seoane, J. R. and C. A. Baile. 1973. Feeding elicited by injections of ca++ and mg++ into the third ventricle of sheep. *Experientia* 29:61–62.

1732. Seoane, J. R., C. A. Baile and R. H. Martin. 1972. Humoral factors modifying feeding behavior of sheep. *Physiol. Behav.* 8:993–995.

1733. Serpell, J. and J. A. Jagoe. 1995. Early experience and the development of behaviour. In J. Serpell (Ed.), *The domestic dog: Its evolution, behaviour and interactions with people*, pp. 79–102. Cambridge, UK: Cambridge University Press.

1734. Serpell, J. A. and Y. Hsu. 2001. Development and validation of a novel method for evaluating behavior and temperament in guide dogs. *Appl. Anim. Behav. Sci.* 72:347–364.

1735. Setchell, B. P. 1978. *The mammalian testis.* Ithaca, NY: Cornell University Press.

1736. Settle, R. H., B. A. Sommerville, J. McCormick and D. M. Broom. 1994. Human scent matching using specially trained dogs. *Anim. Behav.* 48:1443–1448.

1737. Shackleton, D. M. and C. C. Shank. 1984. A review of the social behavior of feral and wild sheep and goats. *J. Anim. Sci.* 58:500–509.

1738. Shank, C. C. 1972. Some aspects of social behaviour in a population of feral goats (Capra hircus L.). *Z. Tierpsychol.* 30:488–528.

1739. Share, I., E. Martyniuk and M. I. Grossman. 1952. Effect of prolonged intragastric feeding on oral food intake in dogs. *Am. J. Physiol.* 169:229–235.

1740. Shaw, E. and K. A. Houpt. 1985. Pre- and post-partum behaviour in mules impregnated by embryo transfer. *Equine Vet. J.* 17:73.

1741. Shaw, E. B., K. A. Houpt and D. F. Holmes. 1988. Body temperature and behaviour of mares during the last two weeks of pregnancy. *Equine Vet. J.* 20:199–202.

1742. Shaw, R. A. 1978. A time-controlled feeding system for cattle. *Anim. Prod.* 27:277–284.

1743. Shearer, M. K. and L. S. Katz. 2006. Female-female mounting among goats stimulates sexual performance in males. *Horm. Behav.* 50:33–37.

1744. Sheppard, A. J., R. E. Blaser and C. M. Kincaid. 1957. The grazing habits of beef cattle on pasture. *J. Anim. Sci.* 16:681–687.

1745. Sheppard, G. and D. S. Mills. 2003. Evaluation of dog-appeasing pheromone as a potential treatment for dogs fearful of fireworks. *Vet. Rec.* 152:432–436.

1746. Sherry, C. J., T. J. Walters, G. G. Rodney Jr. and P. J. Henry. 1994. Behavioral chaining in the goat (*Capra hircus*). *Appl. Anim. Behav. Sci.* 40:241–251.

1747. Shi, J. and R. I. M. Dunbar. 2006. Feeding competition within a feral goat population on the Isle of Rum, NW Scotland. *J. Ethol.* 24:117–124.

1748. Shi, J., R. I. M. Dunbar, D. Buckland and D. Miller. 2003. Daytime activity budgets of feral goats (*Capra hircus*) on the Isle of Rum: Influence of season, age, and sex. *Can. J. Zool.* 81:803–815.

1749. Walser, E. S. and P. Hague. 1981. Field observations on a flock of ewes and lambs made of Clun Forest, Dalesbred and Jacob sheep. *Appl. Anim. Ethol.* 7:175–178.

1750. Walser, E. S. and P. Hague. 1980. Variations in the structure of bleats from sheep of four different breeds. *Behaviour* 75:22–35.

1751. Walser, E. S., E. Walters and P. Hague. 1981. A statistical analysis of the structure of bleats from sheep of four different breeds. *Behaviour* 77:67–76.

1752. Walser, E. S., S. Willadsen and P. Hague. 1982. Maternal vocal recognition in lambs born to Jacob and Dalesbred ewes after embryo transplantation between breeds. *Appl. Anim. Ethol.* 8:479–486.

1753. Walser, E. E. S. 1986. Recognition of the sow's voice by neonatal piglets. *Behaviour* 99:177–187.

1754. Shillito, E. and G. Alexander. 1975. Mutual recognition amongst ewes and lambs of four breeds of sheep (*Ovis aries*). *Appl. Anim. Ethol.* 1:151–165.

1755. Shillito, E. E. 1975. A comparison of the role of vision and hearing in lambs finding their own dams. *Appl. Anim. Ethol.* 1:369–377.

1756. Shillito, E. E. and V. J. Hoyland. 1971. Observations on parturition and maternal care in Soay sheep. *J. Zool.* 165:509–512.

1757. Shipka, M. P. and L. C. Ellic. 1998. No effect of bull exposure on expression of estrous behavior in high-producing dairy cows. *Appl. Anim. Behav. Sci.* 57:1–7.

1758. Shipka, M. P. and S. P. Ford. 1991. Relationship of circulating estrogen and progesterone concentrations during late pregnancy and the onset phase of maternal behavior in the ewe. *Appl. Anim. Behav. Sci.* 31:91–99.

1759. Shreffler, C. and W. D. Hohenboken. 1974. Dominance and mating behavior in ram lambs. *J. Anim. Sci.* 39:725–731.

1760. Shuleikina, K. V. 1976. Sensory mechanisms of learning in the behaviour of newborn kittens. *Act. Nerv. Super. (Praha)* 18:48–50.

1761. Sibbald, A. M. 1997. The effect of body condition on the feeding behaviour of sheep with different times of access to food. *Anim. Sci.* 64:239–246.

1762. Sibbald, A. M., H. W. Erhard, R. J. Hooper, B. Dumont and A. Boissy. 2006. A test for measuring individual variation in how far grazing animals will move away from a social group to feed. *Appl. Anim. Behav. Sci.* 98:89–99.

1763. Sibbald, A. M., S. P. Oom, R. J. Hooper and R. M. Anderson. 2008. Effects of social behaviour on the spatial distribution of sheep grazing a complex vegetation mosaic. *Appl. Anim. Behav. Sci.* 115:149–159.

1764. Sibbald, A. M., L. J. Shellard and T. S. Smart. 2000. Effects of space allowance on the grazing behaviour and spacing of sheep. *Appl. Anim. Behav. Sci.* 70:49–62.

1765. Signoret, J.-P. 1975. Influence of the sexual receptivity of a teaser ewe on the mating preference in the ram. *Appl. Anim. Ethol.* 1:229–232.

1766. Signoret, J.-P. 1970. Sexual behaviour patterns in female domestic pigs (*Sus scrofa* L.) reared in isolation from males. *Anim. Behav.* 18:165–168.

1767. Signoret, J.-P. 1967. Duree du cycle oestrien et de l'oestrus che la truie. action du benzoate d'oestradiol chez la femelle ovariectomisee. *Ann. Biol. Anim. Biochem. Biophys.* 7:407–421.

1768. Signoret, J.-P., B. A. Baldwin, D. Fraser and E. S. E. Hafez. 1975. The behaviour of swine. In E. S. E. Hafez (Ed.), *The behaviour of domestic animals*, pp. 295–329. Baltimore, MD: Williams & Wilkins.

1769. Signoret, J.-P. and P. Mauleon. 1962. Action de l'ablation des bulbes olfactifs sur les mecanismes de la reproductin chez la truie. *Ann. Biol. Anim. Biochem. Biophys.* 2:167–174.

1770. Simitzis, P. E., M. A. Charismiadou, B. Kotsampasi, G. Papadomichelakis, E. P. Christopoulou, E. K. Papavlasopoulou and S. G. Deligeorgis. 2009. Influence of maternal undernutrition on the behaviour of juvenile lambs. *Appl. Anim. Behav. Sci.* 116:191–197.

1771. Simpson, B. S. 2002. Neonatal foal handling. *Appl. Anim. Behav. Sci.* 78:303–317.

1772. Simpson, C. W., C. A. Baile and L. F. Krabill. 1975. Neurochemical coding for feeding in sheep and steers. *J. Comp. Physiol. Psychol.* 88:176–182.

1773. Sivak, J. and B. D. Allen. 1975. An evaluation of the "ramp" retina of the horse eye. *Vision Res.* 15:1353–1356.

1774. Siwak, C. T., H. L. Murphey, B. A. Muggenburg and N. W. Milgram. 2002. Age-dependent decline in locomotor activity in dogs is environment specific. *Physiol. Behav.* 75:65–70.

1775. Skinner, B. F. 1938. *The behavior of organisms.* New York, NY: Appleton-Century Co.

1776. Slabbert, J. M. and J. S. J. Odendaal. 1999. Early prediction of adult police dog efficiency–a longitudinal study. *Appl. Anim. Behav. Sci.* 64:269–288.

1777. Slabbert, J. M. and O. A. E. Rasa. 1997. Observational learning of an acquired maternal behaviour pattern by working dog pups: An alternative training method? *Appl. Anim. Behav. Sci.* 53:309–316.

1778. Sly, J. and F. R. Bell. 1979. Experimental analysis of the seeking behaviour observed in ruminants when they are sodium deficient. *Physiol. Behav.* 22:499–505.

1779. Smith, B. L., J. H. Jones, G. P. Carlson and J. R. Pascoe. 1994. Body position and direction preferences in horses during road transport. *Equine Vet. J.* 26:374–377.

1780. Smith, F. V. 1965. Instinct and learning in the attachment of lamb and ewe. *Anim. Behav.* 13:84–86.

1781. Smith, F. V., C. Van-Toller and T. Boyes. 1966. The "critical period" in the attachment of lambs and ewes. *Anim. Behav.* 14:120–125.

1782. Smith, S. and L. Goldman. 1999. Color discrimination in horses. *Appl. Anim. Behav. Sci.* 62:13–25.

1783. Snowder, G. D. and A. D. Knight. 1995. Breed effects of foster lamb and foster dam on lamb viability and growth. *J. Anim. Sci.* 73:1559–1566.

1784. Sobocinska, J. 1978. Gastric distention and thirst: Relevance to the osmotic thirst threshold and metering of water intake. *Physiol. Behav.* 20:497–501.

1785. Soffie, M., G. Thines and G. De Marneffe. 1976. Relation between milking order and dominance value in a group of dairy cows. *Appl. Anim. Behav. Sci.* 2:271–276.

1786. Solomon, R. L. and L. C. Wynne. 1953. Traumatic avoidance learning: Acquisition in normal dogs. *Psychol. Monogr.* 67:1–19.

1787. Soltysik, S. and B. A. Baldwin. 1972. The performance of goats in triple choice delayed response tasks. *Acta Neurobiol. Exp. (Wars)* 32:73–86.

1788. Somerville, S. H. and B. G. Lowman. 1979. Observations on the nursing behaviour of beef cows suckling Charolais cross calves. *Appl. Anim. Ethol.* 5:369–373.

1789. Sorrells, A. D., S. D. Eicher, K. A. Scott, M. J. Harris, E. A. Pajor, D. C. Lay Jr and B. T. Richert. 2006. Postnatal behavioral and physiological responses of piglets from gilts housed individually or in groups during gestation. *J. Anim. Sci.* 84:757–766.

1790. Souza, A. S. and A. J. Zanella. 2008. Social isolation elicits deficits in the ability of newly weaned female piglets to recognise conspecifics. *Appl. Anim. Behav. Sci.* 110:182–188.

1791. Spain, C. V., J. M. Scarlett and K. A. Houpt. 2004. Long-term risks and benefits of early-age gonadectomy in cats. *J. Am. Vet. Med. Assoc.* 224:372–379.

1792. Spangenberg, E. M. F., L. Björklund and K. Dahlborn. 2006. Outdoor housing of laboratory dogs: Effects on activity, behaviour and physiology. *Appl. Anim. Behav. Sci.* 98:260–276.

1793. Spencer, G. S. 1992. Immunization against cholecystokinin decreases appetite in lambs. *J. Anim. Sci.* 70:3820–3824.

1794. Spinka, M. and B. Algers. 1995. Functional view on udde massage after milk let-down in pigs. *Appl. Anim. Behav. Sci.* 43:197–212.

1795. Spinka, M., I. J. H. Duncan and T. M. Widowski. 1998. Do domestic pigs prefer short-term to medium-term confinement? *Appl. Anim. Behav. Sci.* 58:221–232.

1796. Spinka, M., G. Illmann, F. de Jonge, M. Andersson, T. Schuurman and P. Jensen. 2000. Dimensions of maternal behaviour characteristics in domestic and wildxdomestic crossbred sows. *Appl. Anim. Behav. Sci.* 70:99–114.

1797. Sprague, R. H. and J. J. Anisko. 1973. Elimination patterns in the laboratory beagle. *Behaviour* 47:257–267.

1798. Sprott, R. L. 1967. Barometric pressure fluctuations: Effects on the activity of laboratory mice. *Science* 157:1206–1207.

1799. Squires, V. R. and G. T. Daws. 1975. Leadership and dominance relationships in Merino and Border Leicester sheep. *Appl. Anim. Ethol.* 1:263–274.

1800. St. Hoy and J. Bauer. 2005. Dominance relationships between sows dependent on the time interval between separation and reunion. *Appl. Anim. Behav. Sci.* 90:21–30.

1801. Stahlbaum, C. C. and K. A. Houpt. 1989. The role of the Flehmen response in the behavioral repertoire of the stallion. *Physiol. Behav.* 45:1207–1214.

1802. Stangel, G. and P. Jensen. 1991. Behaviour of semi-naturally kept sows and piglets (except suckling) during 10 days postpartum. *Appl. Anim. Behav. Sci.* 31:211–227.

1803. Stanley, W. C., W. E. Bacon and C. Fehr. 1970. Discriminated instrumental learning in neonatal dogs. *J. Comp. Physiol. Psychol.* 70:335–343.

1804. Stanley, W. C., J. E. Barrett and W. E. Bacon. 1974. Conditioning and extinction of avoidance and escape behavior in neonatal dogs. *J. Comp. Physiol. Psychol.* 87:163–172.

1805. Stanley, W. C. and O. Elliot. 1962. Differential human handling as reinforcing events and as treatments influencing later social behavior in Basenji puppies. *Psychol. Rep.* 10:775–788.

1806. Steigerwald, E. S., M. Sarter, P. March and M. Podell. 1999. Effects of feline immunodeficiency virus on cognition and behavioral function in cats. *J. Acquir. Immune Defic. Syndr. Hum. Retrovirol.* 20:411–419.

1807. Stellflug, J. N., N. E. Cockett and G. S. Lewis. 1989. Relationship between sexual behavior classifications of rams and lambs sired in a competitive breeding environment. *Horm. Behav.* 23:290–303.

1808. Stephen, J. and R. Ledger. 2007. Relinquishing dog owners' ability to predict behavioural problems in shelter dogs post adoption. *Appl. Anim. Behav. Sci.* 107:88–99.

1809. Stephens, D. B. 1980. The effects of 2-deoxy-D-glucose given via the jugular or hepatic-portal vein on food intake and plasma glucose levels in pigs. *Physiol. Behav.* 25:691–697.

1810. Stephens, D. B. 1975. Effects of gastric loading on the sucking response and voluntary milk intake in neonatal piglets. *J. Comp. Physiol. Psychol.* 88:796–805.

1811. Stephens, D. B. 1974. Studies on the effect of social environment on the behaviour and growth rates of artificially reared British Friesian male calves. *Anim. Prod.* 18:23–24.

1812. Stephens, D. B. and B. A. Baldwin. 1971. Observations on the behaviour of groups of artificially reared lambs. *Res. Vet. Sci.* 12:219–224.

1813. Stephens, D. B., D. L. Ingram and D. F. Sharman. 1983. An investigation into some cerebral mechanisms involved in schedule-induced drinking in the pig. *Q. J. Exp. Physiol.* 68:653–660.

1814. Stephens, D. B. and J. L. Linzell. 1974. The development of sucking behaviour in the newborn goat. *Anim. Behav.* 22:628–633.

1815. Sterman, M. B., T. Knauss, D. Lehmann and C. D. Clemente. 1965. Circadian sleep and waking patterns in the laboratory cat. *Electroencephalogr. Clin. Neurophysiol.* 19:509–517.

1816. Stewart, J. C. and J. P. Scott. 1947. Lack of correlation between leadership and dominance relationships in a herd of goats. *J. Comp. Physiol. Psychol.* 40:255–264.

1817. Stone, C. C., M. S. Brown and G. H. Waring. 1974. An ethological means to improve swine production. *J. Anim. Sci.* 39:137.

1818. Stookey, J. M. and H. W. Gonyou. 1998. Recognition in swine: Recognition through familiarity or genetic relatedness? *Appl. Anim. Behav. Sci.* 55:291–305.

1819. Stookey, J. M. and H. W. Gonyou. 1994. The effects of regrouping on behavioral and production parameters in finishing swine. *J. Anim. Sci.* 72:2804–2811.

1820. Strain, G. M., B. M. Olcott, R. M. Archer and B. K. McClintock. 1984. Narcolepsy in a Brahman bull. *J. Am. Vet. Med. Assoc.* 185:538–541.

1821. Strasia, C. A., M. Thorn, R. W. Rice and D. R. Smith. 1970. Grazing habits, diet and performance of sheep on Alpine ranges. *J. Range Manag.* 23:201–208.

1822. Stricklin, W. R. and H. W. Gonyou. 1981. Dominance and eating behavior of beef cattle fed from a single stall. *Appl. Anim. Behav. Sci.* 7:135–140.

1823. Stricklin, W. R., C. C. Kautz-Scanavy and D. L. Greger. 1985. Determination of dominance-subordinance relationships among beef Heifers in a dominance tube. *Appl. Anim. Behav. Sci.* 14:111–116.

1824. Stroup, W. W., M. K. Nielsen and J. A. Gosey. 1987. Cyclic variation in cattle feed intake data: Characterization and implications for experimental design. *J. Anim. Sci.* 64:1638–1647.

1825. Studnitz, M. and K. H. Jensen. 2002. Expression of rooting motivation in gilts following different lengths of deprivation. *Appl. Anim. Behav. Sci.* 76:203–213.

1826. Studnitz, M., M. K. Jensen and L. J. Pedersen. 2007. Why do pigs root and in what will they root?: A review on the exploratory behaviour of pigs in relation to environmental enrichment. *Appl. Anim. Behav. Sci.* 107:183–197.

1827. Sturgeon, R. D., P. D. Brophy and R. A. Levitt. 1973. Drinking elicited by intracranial microinjection of angiotensin in the cat. *Pharmacol. Biochem. Behav.* 1:353–355.

1828. Sueda, K. L. C., B. L. Hart and K. D. Cliff. 2008. Characterisation of plant eating in dogs. *Appl. Anim. Behav. Sci.* 111:120–132.

1829. Sufit, E., K. A. Houpt and M. Sweeting. 1985. Physiological stimuli of thirst and drinking patterns in ponies. *Equine Vet. J.* 17:12–16.

1830. Sung, W. and S. L. Crowell-Davis. 2006. Elimination behavior patterns of domestic cats (Felis catus) with and without elimination behavior problems. *Am. J. Vet. Res.* 67:1500–1504.

1831. Sutherland, G. F. 1939. Salivary conditioned reflexes in swine. *Am. J. Physiol.* 126:P640–P641.

1832. Svartberg, K. 2006. Breed-typical behaviour in dogs—Historical remnants or recent constructs? *Appl. Anim. Behav. Sci.* 96:293–313.

1833. Svartberg, K. 2002. Shyness-boldness predicts performance in working dogs. *Appl. Anim. Behav. Sci.* 79:157–174.

1834. Svartberg, K. and B. Forkman. 2002. Personality traits in the domestic dog (*Canis familiaris*). *Appl. Anim. Behav. Sci.* 79:133–155.

1835. Svobodova, I., P. Vapenik, L. Pinc and L. Bartos. 2008. Testing German shepherd puppies to assess their chances of certification. *Appl. Anim. Behav. Sci.* 113:139–149.

1836. Sweeting, M. P., C. E. Houpt and K. A. Houpt. 1985. Social facilitation of feeding and time budgets in stabled ponies. *J. Anim. Sci.* 60:369–374.

1837. Sweetwood, H. L., D. F. Kripke, I. Grant, J. Yager and M. S. Gerst. 1976. Sleep disorder and psychobiological symptomatology in male psychiatric outpatients and male nonpatients. *Psychosom. Med.* 38:373–378.

1838. Swenson, R. M. and W. Randall. 1977. Grooming behavior in cats with pontile lesions and cats with tectal lesions. *J. Comp. Physiol. Psychol.* 91:313–326.

1839. Syme, G. J., L. A. Syme and T. P. Jefferson. 1974. A note on variations in the level of aggression within a herd of goats. *Anim. Prod.* 18:309–312.

1840. Syme, L. A., G. J. Syme, T. G. Waite and A. J. Pearson. 1975. Spatial distribution and social status in a small herd of dairy cows. *Anim. Behav.* 23:609–614.

1841. Symoens, J. and M. Van Den Brande. 1969. Prevention and cure of aggressiveness in pigs using the sedative azaperone. *Vet. Rec.* 85:64–67.

1842. Takeda, K., S. Sato and K. Sugawara. 2000. The number of farm mates influences social and maintenance behaviours of Japanese black cows in a communal pasture. *Appl. Anim. Behav. Sci.* 67:181–192.

1843. Takeuchi, Y., C. Hashizume, S. Arata, M. Inoue-Murayama, T. Maki, B. L. Hart and Y. Mori. 2009. An approach to canine behavioural genetics employing guide dogs for the blind. *Anim. Genet.* 40:217–224.

1844. Takeuchi, Y., C. Hashizume, E. M. Chon, Y. Momozawa, K. Masuda, T. Kikusui and Y. Mori. 2005. Canine tyrosine hydroxylase (TH) gene and dopamine beta-hydroxylase (DBH) gene: Their sequences, genetic polymorphisms, and diversities among five different dog breeds. *J. Vet. Med. Sci.* 67:861–867.

1845. Takeuchi, Y., K. A. Houpt and J. M. Scarlett. 2000. Evaluation of treatments for separation anxiety in dogs. *J. Am. Vet. Med. Assoc.* 217:342–345.

1846. Takeuchi, Y., F. Kaneko, C. Hashizume, K. Masuda, N. Ogata, T. Maki, M. Inoue-Murayama, B. L. Hart and Y. Mori. 2009. Association analysis between canine behavioural traits and genetic polymorphisms in the Shiba Inu breed. *Anim. Genet.* 40:616–622.

1847. Tallet, C., I. Veissier and X. Boivin. 2009. How does the method used to feed lambs modulate their affinity to their human caregiver? *Appl. Anim. Behav. Sci.* 119:56–65.

1848. Tallet, C., I. Veissier and X. Boivin. 2006. A note on the consistency and specificity of lambs' responses to a stockperson and to their photograph in an arena test. *Appl. Anim. Behav. Sci.* 98:308–314.

1849. Talling, J. C., N. K. Waran, C. M. Wathes and J. A. Lines. 1998. Sound avoidance by domestic pigs depends upon characteristics of the signal. *Appl. Anim. Behav. Sci.* 58:255–266.

1850. Tan, S. S. L. and D. M. Shackleton. 1990. Effects of mixing unfamiliar individuals and of azapaerone on the social behaviour of finishing pigs. *Appl. Anim. Behav. Sci.* 26:157–168.

1851. Tanida, H., A. Miura, T. Tanaka and T. Yoshimoto. 1995. Behavioral response to humans to individually handled weanling pigs. *Appl. Anim. Behav. Sci.* 42:249–259.

1852. Tanida, H., N. Miyazaki, T. Tanaka and T. Yoshimoto. 1991. Selection of mating partners in boars and sows under multi-sire mating. *Appl. Anim. Behav. Sci.* 32:13–21.

1853. Tapki, I., A. Sahin and A. G. Onal. 2006. Effect of space allowance on behaviour of newborn milk-fed dairy calves. *Appl. Anim. Behav. Sci.* 99:12–20.

1854. Taylor, N., N. Prescott, G. Perry, M. Potter, C. Le Sueur and C. Wathes. 2006. Preference of growing pigs for illuminance. *Appl. Anim. Behav. Sci.* 96:19–31.

1855. Taylor, A. A. and D. M. Weary. 2000. Vocal responses of piglets to castration: Identifying procedural sources of pain. *Appl. Anim. Behav. Sci.* 70:17–26.

1856. Taylor, K. and D. S. Mills. 2007. A placebo-controlled study to investigate the effect of dog appeasing pheromone and other environmental and management factors on the reports of disturbance and house soiling during the night in recently adopted puppies. *Appl. Anim. Behav. Sci.* 105:358–368.

1857. Teixeira, D. L., M. J. Hötzel and L. C. P. M. Filho. 2006. Designing better water troughs: 2. Surface area and height, but not depth, influence dairy cows' preference. *Appl. Anim. Behav. Sci.* 96:169–175.

1858. Telezhenko, E. and C. Bergsten. 2005. Influence of floor type on the locomotion of dairy cows. *Appl. Anim. Behav. Sci.* 93:183–197.

1859. Tellington-Jones, L. and U. Bruns. 1988. *An introduction to the Tellington-Jones equine awareness method.* Millwood, NY: Breakthrough Publications, Inc.

1860. Tennessen, T., M. A. Price and R. T. Berg. 1985. The social interactions of young bulls and steers after regrouping. *Appl. Anim. Behav. Sci.* 14:37–47.

1861. Terlouw, E. M., C. A. B. Lawrence and A. W. Illius. 1991. Influences of feeding level and physical restriction on development of stereotypies in sows. *Anim. Behav.* 42:981–991.

1862. Terlouw, E. M. C., A. Wiersma, A. B. Lawrence and H. A. MacLeod. 1993. Ingestion of food facilitates the performance of stereotypies in sows. *Anim. Behav.* 46:939–950.

1863. Ternouth, J. H. and A. W. Beattie. 1970. A note on the voluntary food consumption and the sodium-potassium ratio of sheep after shearing. *Anim. Prod.* 12:343–346.

1864. Thiery, J. A. and J.-P. Signoret. 1978. Effect of changing the teaser ewe on the sexual activity of the ram. *Appl. Anim. Ethol.* 4:87–90.

1865. Thinus-Blanc, C., B. Poucet and N. Chapuis. 1982. Object permanence in cats: Analysis in locomotor space. *Behav. Proc.* 7:81–86.

1866. Thomas, D. T., A. J. Rintoul and D. G. Masters. 2007. Sheep select combinations of high and low sodium chloride, energy and crude protein feed that improve their diet. *Appl. Anim. Behav. Sci.* 105:140–153.

1867. Thompson, L. H. and J. S. Savage. 1978. Age at puberty and ovulation rate in gilts in confinement as influenced by exposure to a boar. *J. Anim. Sci.* 47:1141–1144.

1868. Thompson, W. R. and W. Heron. 1954. The effects of early restriction on activity in dogs. *J. Comp. Physiol. Psychol.* 47:77–82.

1869. Thompson, W. R. and W. Heron. 1954. The effects of restricting early experience on the problem-solving capacity of dogs. *Can. J. Psychol.* 8:17–31.

1870. Thorhallsdotir, A. G., F. D. Provenza and D. F. Balph. 1990. The role of the mother in the intake of harmful foods by lambs. *Appl. Anim. Behav. Sci.* 25:35–44.

1871. Thorndike, E. L. 1911. *Animal intelligence: Experimental studies*. New York, NY: Macmillan.

1872. Thorpe, W. H. 1963. *Learning and instinct in animals*. Cambridge, MA: Harvard University Press.

1873. Thrasher, T. N., C. J. Brown, L. C. Keil and D. J. Ramsay. 1980. Thirst and vasopressin release in the dog: An osmoreceptor or sodium receptor mechanism? *Am. J. Physiol.* 238:R333–R339.

1874. Tilbrook, A. J. 1987. Physical and behavioural factors affecting the sexual "attractiveness" of the ewe. *Appl. Anim. Behav. Sci.* 17:109–115.

1875. Tilbrook, A. J., P. H. Hemsworth, J. S. Topp and A. W. N. Cameron. 1990. Parallel changes in the proceptive and receptive behaviour of the ewe. *Appl. Anim. Behav. Sci.* 27:73–92.

1876. Timney, B. and K. Keil. 1992. Visual acuity in the horse. *Vision Res.* 32:2289–2293.

1877. Tischner, M. 1982. Patterns of stallion sexual behaviour in the absence of mares. *J. Reprod. Fertil. Suppl.* 32:65–70.

1878. Tischner, M., K. Kosiniak and W. Bielanski. 1974. Analysis of the pattern of ejaculation in stallions. *J. Reprod. Fertil.* 41:329–335.

1879. Titterington, R. W. and D. Fraser. 1975. The lying behaviour of sows and piglets during early lactation in relation to the position of the creep heater. *Appl. Anim. Ethol.* 2:47–53.

1880. Tobach, E., L. R. Aronson and E. Shaw. 1971. *The biopsychology of development*. New York, NY: Academic Press.

1881. Tod, E., D. Brander and N. Waran. 2005. Efficacy of dog appeasing pheromone in reducing stress and fear related behaviour in shelter dogs. *Appl. Anim. Behav. Sci.* 93:295–308.

1882. Todd, N. B. 1963. *The catnip response*. Cambridge, MA: Harvard University Press.

1883. Toerien, C. A., T. Sahlu and W. W. Wong. 1999. Energy expenditure of Angora bucks in peak breeding season estimated with the doubly-labeled water technique. *J. Anim. Sci.* 77:3096–3105.

1884. Tolu, C. and T. Savas. 2007. A brief report on intra-species aggressive biting in a goat herd. *Appl. Anim. Behav. Sci.* 102:124–129.

1885. Tomkins, T. and M. J. Bryant. 1974. Oestrous behaviour of the ewe and the influence of treatment with progestagen. *J. Reprod. Fert.* 41:121–132.

1886. Tomlinson, K. A., E. O. Price and D. T. Torell. 1982. Responses of tranquilized post-partum ewes to alien lambs. *Appl. Anim. Ethol.* 8:109–117.

1887. Tonokura, M., K. Fujita, M. Morozumi, Y. Yoshida, T. Kanbayashi and S. Nishino. 2003. Narcolepsy in a hypocretin/orexin-deficient chihuahua. *Vet. Rec.* 152:776–779.

1888. Topal, J., A. Miklosi and V. Csanyi. 1997. Dog-human relationship affects problem solving behavior in the dog. *Anthrozoos* 10:214.

1889. Topel, D. G., G. M. Weiss, D. G. Siers and J. H. Magilton. 1973. Comparison of blood source and diurnal variation on blood hydrocortisone, growth hormone, lactate, glucose and electrolytes in swine. *J. Anim. Sci.* 36:531–534.

1890. Torrey, S., E. L. Toth Tamminga and T. M. Widowski. 2008. Effect of drinker type on water intake and waste in newly weaned piglets. *J. Anim. Sci.* 86:1439–1445.

1891. Torrey, S. and T. M. Widowski. 2007. Relationship between growth and non-nutritive massage in suckling pigs. *Appl. Anim. Behav. Sci.* 107:32–44.

1892. Torrey, S. and T. M. Widowski. 2006. Is belly nosing redirected suckling behaviour? *Appl. Anim. Behav. Sci.* 101:288–304.

1893. Tortora, D. F. 1980. Animal behavior therapy: The behavioral diagnosis and treatment of dominance-motivated aggression in canines: Part I. *Canine Pract.* 7:10–19.

1894. Tortora, D. F. 1980. Animal behavior therapy: The behavioral diagnosis and treatment of dominance-motivated aggression in canines: Part II. *Canine Pract.* 8:13–28.

1895. Toscano, M. J. and D. C. Lay Jr. 2005. Parsing the characteristics of a simulated udder to determine relative attractiveness to piglets in the 72 h following parturition. *Appl. Anim. Behav. Sci.* 92:283–291.

1896. Toth, L., M. Gacsi, J. Topal and A. Miklosi. 2008. Playing styles and possible causative factors in dogs' behaviour when playing with humans. *Appl. Anim. Behav. Sci.* 114:473–484.

1897. Toutain, P. L., C. Toutain, A. J. Webster and J. D. McDonald. 1977. Sleep and activity, age and fatness, and the energy expenditure of confined sheep. *Br. J. Nutr.* 38:445–454.

1898. Towbin, E. J. 1949. Gastric distention as a factor in the satiation of thirst in esophagostomized dogs. *Am. J. Physiol.* 159:533–541.

1899. Tribe, D. E. 1949. The importance of sense of smell to the grazing sheep. *J. Agric. Sci. (Camb.)* 39:309–312.

1900. Trivers, R. L. 1974. Parent offspring conflict. *Am. Zool.* 14:249–264.

1901. Trout, W. E., J. C. Pekas and B. D. Schanbacher. 1989. Immune, growth and carcass responses of ram lambs to active immunization against desulfated cholecystokinin (CCK-8). *J. Anim. Sci.* 67:2709–2714.

1902. Trumler, E. 1959. Das "rossigkeitgesicht" und ahnliches ausdrucks verhalten bei einhufern. *Z. Tierpsychol.* 16:478–488.

1903. Tuchscherer, M., B. Puppe, A. Tuchscherer and E. Kanitz. 1998. Effects of social status after mixing on immune, metabolic, and endocrine responses in pigs. *Physiol. Behav.* 64:353–360.

1904. Tucker, C. B., A. R. Rogers, G. A. Verkerk, P. E. Kendall, J. R. Webster and L. R. Matthews. 2007. Effects of shelter and body condition on the behaviour and physiology of dairy cattle in winter. *Appl. Anim. Behav. Sci.* 105:1–13.

1905. Turek, F. W. and S. Losee-Olson. 1986. A benzodiazepine used in the treatment of insomnia phase-shifts the mammalian circadian clock. *Nature* 321:167–168.

1906. Turner, A. S., N. White 2nd and J. Ismay. 1984. Modified Forssell's operation for crib biting in the horse. *J. Am. Vet. Med. Assoc.* 184:309–312.

1907. Turner, D. C. and P. Bateson. 1988. *The domestic cat: The biology of its behaviour.* New York, NY: Cambridge University Press.

1908. Turner, D. C., J. Feaver, M. Mendl and P. Bateson. 1986. Variation in domestic cat behaviour towards humans: A paternal effect. *Anim. Behav.* 34:1890–1892.

1909. Tyler, S. J. 1972. The behaviour and social organization of the new forest ponies. *Anim. Behav. Monogr.* 5:85–196.

1910. Ungerfeld, R., M. A. Ramos and R. Möller. 2006. Role of the vomeronasal organ on ram's courtship and mating behaviour, and on mate choice among oestrous ewes. *Appl. Anim. Behav. Sci.* 99:248–252.

1911. Ungerfeld, R. and L. Silva. 2005. The presence of normal vaginal flora is necessary for normal sexual attractiveness of estrous ewes. *Appl. Anim. Behav. Sci.* 93:245–250.

1912. Ursin, R. 1970. Sleep stage relations within the sleep cycles of the cat. *Brain Res.* 20:91–97.

1913. Ursin, R. 1968. The two stages of slow wave sleep in the cat and their relation to REM sleep. *Brain Res.* 11:347–356.

1914. Ursin, R., H. Cohen, S. Henriksen, G. Mitchell and W. Dement. 1976. Effects of sleep of restricted sleep. A cat case study. *Electroencephalogr. Clin. Neurophysiol.* 41:96–101.

1915. Vaarst, M., M. B. Jensen and A. Sandager. 2001. Behaviour of calves at introduction to nurse cows after the colostrum period. *Appl. Anim. Behav. Sci.* 73:27–33.

1916. Vailes, L. D. and J. H. Britt. 1990. Influence of footing surface on mounting and other sexual behaviors of estrual Holstein cows. *J. Anim. Sci.* 68:2333–2339.

1917. Val-Laillet, D., V. Guesdon, M. A. G. von Keyserlingk, A. M. De Passille and J. Rushen. 2009. Allogrooming in cattle: Relationships between social preferences, feeding displacements and social dominance. *Appl. Anim. Behav. Sci.* 116:141–149.

1918. Valros, A. E., M. Rundgren, M. Spinka, H. Saloniemi, L. Rydhmer and B. Algers. 2002. Nursing behaviour of sows during 5 weeks lactation and effects on piglet growth. *Appl. Anim. Behav. Sci.* 76:93–104.

1919. Van Den Berg, L., M. B. Schilder, H. de Vries, P. A. Leegwater and B. A. van Oost. 2006. Phenotyping of aggressive behavior in golden retriever dogs with a questionnaire. *Behav. Genet.* 36:882–902.

1920. Van Den Bos, R. 1998. Post-conflict stress-response in confined group-living cats (*Felis silvestris catus*). *Appl. Anim. Behav. Sci.* 59:323–330.

1921. Van Den Bos, R., M. K. Meijer and B. M. Spruijt. 2000. Taste reactivity patterns in domestic cats (*Felis silvestris catus*). *Appl. Anim. Behav. Sci.* 69:149–168.

1922. Van Der Borg, J. A. M., W. J. Netto and D. J. U. Planta. 1991. Behavioural testing of dogs in animal shelters to predict problem behaviour. *Appl. Anim. Behav. Sci.* 32:237–251.

1923. Van Der Staay, F. J., J. de Groot, T. Schuurman and S. M. Korte. 2008. Repeated social defeat in female pigs does not induce neuroendocrine symptoms of depression, but behavioral adaptation. *Physiol. Behav.* 93:453–460.

1924. van Miert, A. S., F. Kaya and C. T. van Duin. 1992. Changes in food intake and forestomach motility of dwarf goats by recombinant bovine cytokines (IL-1 beta, IL-2) and IFN-gamma. *Physiol. Behav.* 52:859–864.

1925. van Putten, G. 1969. An investigation into tail-biting among fattening pigs. *Br. Vet. J.* 125:511–517.

1926. Van Putten, G. and R. G. Bure. 1997. Preparing gilts for group housing by increasing their social skills. *Appl. Anim. Behav. Sci.* 54:173–183.

1927. Van Putten, G. and J. Dammers. 1976. A comparative study of the well-being of piglets reared conventionally and in cages. *Appl. Anim. Ethol.* 2:339–356.

1928. Vandenheede, M. and M.-F. Bouissou. 1993. Sex differences in fear reactions in sheep. *Appl. Anim. Behav. Sci.* 37:39–55.

1929. VanDierendonck, M. C., H. de Vries, B. H. Schilder, B. Colenbrander, A. G. Porhallsdottir and H. Sigurjonsdottir. 2009. Interventions in social behaviour in a herd of mares and geldings. *Appl. Anim. Behav. Sci.* 116:67–73.

1930. Van-Laillet, D. and R. Nowak. 2006. Socio-spatial criteria are important for the establishment of maternal preference in lambs. *Appl. Anim. Behav. Sci.* 96:269–280.

1931. VanWagoner, H. C., D. W. Bailey, D. D. Kress, D. C. Anderson and K. C. Davis. 2006. Differences among beef sire breeds and relationships between terrain use and performance when daughters graze foothill rangelands as cows. *Appl. Anim. Behav. Sci.* 97:105–121.

1932. Vas, J., J. Topal, B. Gyori and A. Miklosi. 2008. Consistency of dogs' reactions to threatening cues of an unfamiliar person. *Appl. Anim. Behav. Sci.* 112:331–344.

1933. Vecchiotti, G. G. and R. Galanti. 1987. Evidence of heredity of cribbing, weaving and stall walking. *Livestock Prod. Sci.* 14:91–95.

1934. Veeckman, J. and F. O. Odberg. 1978. Preliminary studies on the behavioural detection of oestrus in Belgian "Warm-Blood" mares with acoustic and tactile stimuli. *Appl. Anim. Ethol.* 4:109–118.

1935. Veissier, I. 1993. Observational learning in cattle. *Appl. Anim. Behav. Sci.* 33:235–243.

1936. Veissier, I., S. Andanson, H. Dubroeucq and D. Pomies. 2008. The motivation of cows to walk as thwarted by tethering. *J. Anim. Sci.* 86:2723–2729.

1937. Veissier, I., A. M. de Passille, G. Despres, J. Rushen, I. Charpentier, A. R. Ramirez de la Fe and P. Pradel. 2002. Does nutritive and non-nutritive sucking reduce other oral behaviors and stimulate rest in calves? *J. Anim. Sci.* 80:2574–2587.

1938. Veissier, I., D. Lamy and P. Le Neindre. 1990. Social behaviour in domestic beef cattle when yearling calves are left with the cows for the next calving. *Appl. Anim. Behav. Sci.* 27:193–200.

1939. Veissier, I. and P. Le Neindre. 1989. Weaning of calves: Its effect on social organization. 24:43–54.

1940. Verberne, G. and J. de Boer. 1976. Chemocommunication among domestic cats, mediated by the olfactory and vomeronasal senses. I. Chemocommunication. *Z. Tierpsychol.* 42:86–109.

1941. Vervaecke, H., J. M. G. Stevens, H. Vandemoortele, H. Sigurjonsdottir and H. De Vries. 2007. Aggression and dominance in matched groups of subadult Icelandic horses (*Equus caballus*). *J. Ethol.* 25:239–248.

1942. Vichova, J. and L. Bartos. 2005. Allosuckling in cattle: Gain or compensation? *Appl. Anim. Behav. Sci.* 94:223–235.

1943. Vierin, M. and M.-F. Bouissou. 2002. Influence of maternal experience on fear reactions in ewes. *Appl. Anim. Behav. Sci.* 75:307–315.

1944. Villablanca, J. R. and C. E. Olmstead. 1979. Neurological development of kittens. *Dev. Psychobiol.* 12:101–127.

1945. Villalba, J. J., F. D. Provenza and J. O. Hall. 2008. Learned appetites for calcium, phosphorus, and sodium in sheep. *J. Anim. Sci.* 86:738–747.

1946. Villalba, J. J., F. D. Provenza, J. O. Hall and C. Peterson. 2006. Phosphorus appetite in sheep: Dissociating taste from postingestive effects. *J. Anim. Sci.* 84:2213–2223.

1947. Villalba, J. J., F. D. Provenza and K. C. Olson. 2006. Terpenes and carbohydrate source influence rumen fermentation, digestibility, intake, and preference in sheep. *J. Anim. Sci.* 84:2463–2473.

1948. Vince, M. A. 1984. Teat seeking and presucking behaviour in newly born lambs: Possible effects of maternal skin temperatures. *Anim. Behav.* 32:249–254.

1949. Vince, M. A. and M. W. Stanier. 1991. The effect of food intake on young Soay and Clun Forest lambs' response to touch on the face. *Appl. Anim. Behav. Sci.* 30:37–96.

1950. Vince, M. A. and T. M. Ward. 1984. The responses of newly born Clun Forest lambs to odour sources in the ewe. *Behaviour* 89:117–121.

1951. Vince, M. A., T. M. Ward and M. Reader. 1984. Tactile stimulation and teat seeking behaviour in newly born lambs. *Anim. Behav.* 32:1179–1184.

1952. Viranyi, Z., J. Topal, M. Gacsi, A. Miklosi and V. Csanyi. 2004. Dogs respond appropriately to cues of humans' attentional focus. *Behav. Processes* 66:161–172.

1953. Virga, V., K. A. Houpt and J. M. Scarlett. 2001. Efficacy of amitriptyline as a pharmacological adjunct to behavioral modification in the management of aggressive behaviors in dogs. *J. Am. Anim. Hosp. Assoc.* 37:325–330.

1954. Visser, E. K., A. D. Ellis and C. G. Van Reenen. 2008. The effect of two different housing conditions on the welfare of young horses stabled for the first time. *Appl. Anim. Behav. Sci.* 114:521–533.

1955. Visser, E. K., C. G. Van Reenen, M. Rundgren, M. Zetterqvist, K. Morgan and H. J. Blokhuis. 2003.

Responses of horses in behavioural tests correlate with temperament assessed by riders. *Equine Vet. J.* 35:176–183.

1956. Visser, E. K., C. G. van Reenen, M. B. H. Schilder, A. Barneveld and H. J. Blokhuis. 2003. Learning performances in young horses using two different learning tests. *Appl. Anim. Behav. Sci.* 80:311–326.

1957. Vitale, A. F., M. Tenucci, M. Papini and S. Lovari. 1986. Social behaviour of the calves of semi-wild Maremma cattle, *Bos primigenius taurus*. *Appl. Anim. Behav. Sci.* 16:217–231.

1958. Vogel, H. H. Jr., J. P. Scott and M.-V. Marston. 1950. Social facilitation and allelomimetic behavior in dogs. I. Social facilitation in a non-competitive situation. *Behaviour* 2:121–134.

1959. Voith, V. L. and P. L. Borchelt. 1985. Elimination behavior and related problems in dogs. *Comp. Contin. Ed.* 7:537–546.

1960. von Borstel, U. U., I. J. H. Duncan, A. K. Shoveller, K. Merkies, L. J. Keeling and S. T. Millman. 2009. Impact of riding in a coercively obtained rollkur posture on welfare and fear of performance horses. *Appl. Anim. Behav. Sci.* 116:228–236.

1961. von Keyserlingk, M. A. and D. M. Weary. 2007. Maternal behavior in cattle. *Horm. Behav.* 52:106–113.

1962. Wagnon, K. A., R. G. Loy, W. C. Rollins and F. D. Carroll. 1966. Social dominance in a herd of Angus, Hereford, and Shorthorn cows. *Anim. Behav.* 14:474–479.

1963. Walker, D. B., J. C. Walker, P. J. Cavnar, J. L. Taylor, D. H. Pickel, S. B. Hall and J. C. Suarez. 2006. Naturalistic quantification of canine olfactory sensitivity. *Appl. Anim. Behav. Sci.* 97:241–254.

1964. Walker, D. E. 1962. Suckling and grazing behaviour of beef heifers and calves. *N. Z. J. Agric. Res.* 5:331–338.

1965. Walker, S. L., R. F. Smith, D. N. Jones, J. E. Routly and H. Dobson. 2008. Chronic stress, hormone profiles and estrus intensity in dairy cattle. *Horm. Behav.* 53:493–501.

1966. Wallace, L. R. 1949. Observations of lambing behaviour in ewes. *Proc. N. Z. Soc. Anim. Prod.* 9:85–96.

1967. Waller, G. R., G. H. Price and E. D. Mitchell. 1969. Feline attractant, cis,trans-nepetalactone: Metabolism in the domestic cat. *Science* 164:1281–1282.

1968. Waltl, B., M. C. Appleby and J. Solkner. 1995. Effects of relatedness on the suckling behaviour of calves in a herd of beef cattle rearing twins. *Appl. Anim. Behav. Sci.* 45:1–9.

1969. Wangsness, P. J., L. E. Chase, A. D. Peterson, T. G. Hartsock, D. J. Kellmel and B. R. Baumgardt. 1976. System of monitoring feeding behavior of sheep. *J. Anim. Sci.* 42:1544–1549.

1970. Waran, N. K. and D. Cuddeford. 1995. Effects of loading and transport on the heart rate and behaviour of horses. *Appl. Anim. Behav. Sci.* 43:71–81.

1971. Ward, C. and B. B. Smuts. 2007. Quantity-based judgments in the domestic dog (*Canis lupus familiaris*). *Anim. Cogn.* 10:71–80.

1972. Waring, G. H. 1983. *Horse behavior: The behavioral traits and adaptations of domestic and wild horses, including ponies*. Park Ridge, NJ: Noyes Publications.

1973. Waring, G. H. 1982. Onset of behavior patterns in the newborn foal. *Eq. Pract.* 4:28–34.

1974. Waring, G. H., S. Wierzbowski and E. S. E. Hafez. 1975. The behaviour of horses. In E. S. E. Hafez (Ed.), *The behaviour of domestic animals*, pp. 330–369. Baltimore, MD: Williams & Wilkins.

1975. Warren, J. M. and A. Baron. 1956. The formation of learning sets by cats. *J. Comp. Physiol. Psychol.* 49:227–231.

1976. Warren, J. T. and I. Mysterud. 1993. Extensive ranging by sheep released onto an unfamiliar range. *Appl. Anim. Behav. Sci.* 38:67–73.

1977. Waters, A. J., C. J. Nicol and N. P. French. 2002. Factors influencing the development of stereotypic and redirected behaviours in young horses: Findings of a four year prospective epidemiological study. *Equine Vet. J.* 34:572–579.

1978. Wattanakul, W., C. A. Bulman, H. L. Edge and S. A. Edwards. 2005. The effect of creep feed presentation method on feeding behaviour, intake and performance of suckling piglets. *Appl. Anim. Behav. Sci.* 92:27–36.

1979. Weary, D. M., M. C. Appleby and D. Fraser. 1999. Responses of piglets to early separation from the sow. *Appl. Anim. Behav. Sci.* 63:289–300.

1980. Weary, D. M. and B. Chua. 2000. Effects of early separation on the dairy cow and calf: 1. Separation at 6 h, 1 day and 4 days after birth. *Appl. Anim. Behav. Sci.* 69:177–188.

1981. Weary, D. M. and D. Fraser. 1995. Calling by domestic piglets: Reliable signals of need? *Anim. Behav.* 50:1047–1055.

1982. Weary, D. M., E. A. Pajor, M. Bonenfant, D. Fraser and D. L. Kramer. 2002. Alternative housing of sows and litters. Part 4. Effects of sow-controlled housing combined with a communal piglet area on pre- and post-weaning behaviour and performance. *Appl. Anim. Behav. Sci.* 76:279–290.

1983. Weary, D. M., E. A. Pajor, M. Bonenfant, S. K. Ross, D. Fraser and D. L. Kramer. 1999. Alternative housing for sows and litters. Part 2. Effects of communal piglet area on pre- and post-weaning behaviour and performance. *Appl. Anim. Behav. Sci.* 65:123–135.

1984. Weaver, S. A., F. X. Aherne, M. J. Meaney, A. L. Schaefer and W. T. Dixon. 2000. Neonatal handling permanently alters hypothalamic-pituitary-adrenal axis function, behaviour, and body weight in boars. *J. Endocrinol.* 164:349–359.

1985. Webb, F. M., V. N. Colenbrander, T. H. Blosser and D. E. Waldern. 1963. Eating habits of dairy cows under drylot conditions. *J. Dairy Sci.* 46:1433–1435.

1986. Weeks, J. W., S. L. Crowell-Davis, A. B. Caudle and G. L. Heusner. 2000. Aggression and social spacing in light horse (Equus caballus) mares and foals. *Appl. Anim. Behav. Sci.* 68:319–337.

1987. Wehrend, A., E. Hofmann, K. Failing and H. Bostedt. 2006. Behaviour during the first stage of labour in cattle: Influence of parity and dystocia. *Appl. Anim. Behav. Sci.* 100:164–170.

1988. Weiguo, L. and C. J. C. Phillips. 1991. The effects of supplementary light on the behaviour and performance of calves. *Appl. Anim. Behav. Sci.* 30:27–34.

1989. Weir, W. C. and D. T. Torell. 1959. Selective grazing by sheep as shown by a comparison of the chemical composition of range and pasture forage obtained by hand clipping and that collected by esophageal-fistulated sheep. *J. Anim. Sci.* 18:641–649.

1990. Weiss, E. and G. Greenberg. 1997. Service dog selection tests: Effectiveness of dogs from animal shelters. *Appl. Anim. Behav. Sci.* 53:297–308.

1991. Welch, A. R. and M. R. Baxter. 1986. Responses of newborn piglets to thermal and tactile properties of their environment. *Appl. Anim. Behav. Sci.* 15:203–215.

1992. Welch, R. A. S. and R. Kilgour. 1970. Mis-mothering among Romneys. *N. Z. J. Agric.* 121:26–27.

1993. Weldon, W. C., A. J. Lewis, G. F. Louis, J. L. Kovar, M. A. Giesemann and P. S. Miller. 1994. Postpartum hypophagia in primiparous sows: I. Effects of gestation feeding level on feed intake, feeding behavior, and plasma metabolite concentrations during lactation. *J. Anim. Sci.* 72:387–394.

1994. Weller, R. F. and R. H. Phipps. 1985. The effect of silage preference on the performance of dairy cows. *Anim. Prod.* 42:435.

1995. Wells, D. L. 2006. Aromatherapy for travel-induced excitement in dogs. *J. Am. Vet. Med. Assoc.* 229:964–967.

1996. Wells, D. L. 2003. Lateralised behaviour in the domestic dog, *Canis familiaris*. *Behav. Processes* 61:27–35.

1997. Wells, D. L. 2001. The effectiveness of a citronella spray collar in reducing certain forms of barking in dogs. *Appl. Anim. Behav. Sci.* 73:299–309.

1998. Wells, D. L., L. Graham and P. G. Hepper. 2002. The influence of auditory stimulation on the behaviour of dogs housed in a rescue shelter. *Anim. Welfare* 11:385–393.

1999. Wells, D. L. and P. G. Hepper. 1998. A note on the influence of visual conspecific contact on the behaviour of sheltered dogs. *Appl. Anim. Behav. Sci.* 60:83–88.

2000. Wells, S. M. and B. von Goldschmidt-Rothschild. 1979. Social behaviour and relationships in a herd of camargue horses. *Z. Tierpsychol.* 49:363–380.

2001. Wemelsfelder, F., M. Haskell, M. T. Mendl, S. Calvert and A. B. Lawrence. 2000. Diversity of behaviour during novel object tests is reduced in pigs housed in substrate-impoverished conditions. *Anim. Behav.* 60:385–394.

2002. Wesley, F. and F. D. Klopfer. 1962. Visual discrimination learning in swine. *Z. Tierpsychol.* 19:93–104.

2003. West, M. 1974. Social play in the domestic cat. *Am. Zool.* 14:427–436.

2004. West, M. J. 1977. Exploration and play with objects in domestic kittens. *Dev. Psychobiol.* 10:53–57.

2005. West, R. E. and R. J. Young. 2002. Do domestic dogs show any evidence of being able to count? *Anim. Cogn.* 5:183–186.

2006. Whalen, R. E. 1963. The initiation of mating in naive female cats. *Anim. Behav.* 11:463.

2007. Whatson, T. S. 1985. Development of eliminative behaviour in piglets. *Appl. Anim. Behav. Sci.* 14:365–377.

2008. Whipp, S. C., R. L. Wood and N. C. Lyon. 1970. Diurnal variation in concentrations of hydrocortisone in plasma of swine. *Am. J. Vet. Res.* 31:2105–2107.

2009. Whistance, L. K., D. R. Arney, L. A. Sinclair and C. J. C. Phillips. 2007. Defaecation behaviour of dairy cows housed in straw yards or cubicle systems. *Appl. Anim. Behav. Sci.* 105:14–25.

2010. Whistance, L. K., L. A. Sinclair, D. R. Arney and C. J. C. Phillips. 2009. Trainability of eliminative behaviour in dairy heifers using a secondary reinforcer. *Appl. Anim. Behav. Sci.* 117:128–136.

2011. White, W., G. J. Schwartz and T. H. Moran. 1999. Meal-synchronized CEA in rats: Effects of meal size, intragastric feeding, and subdiaphragmatic vagotomy. *Am. J. Physiol.* 276:R1276–R1288.

2012. Whittlestone, W. G. and L. R. Cate. 1973. An animal activated feeding device for cattle. *J. Dairy Sci.* 56:1352–1353.

2013. Whittlestone, W. G., R. Kilgour, H. de Langen and G. Duirs. 1970. Behavioral stress and the cell count of bovine milk. *J. Milk Food Technol.* 33:217–220.

2014. Whittlestone, W. G., M. M. Mullord, R. Kilgour and L. R. Cate. 1975. Electric shocks during machine milking. *N. Z. Vet. J.* 23:105–108.

2015. Widdowson, E. M. 1971. Food intake and growth in the newly-born. *Proc. Nutr. Soc.* 30:127–135.

2016. Widowski, T. M. and S. W. Curtis. 1990. The influence of straw, cloth tassel, or both on the prepartum behavior of sows. *Appl. Anim. Behav. Sci.* 27:53–71.

2017. Wieckert, D. A. 1971. Social behavior in farm animals. *J. Anim. Sci.* 32:1274–1277.

2018. Wieckert, D. A. and G. R. Barr. 1966. Studies on learning ability in young pigs. *J. Anim. Sci.* 25:1280.

2019. Wieckert, D. A., L. P. Johnson, K. P. Offord and G. R. Barr. 1966. Measuring learning ability in dairy cows. *J. Dairy Sci.* 49:729.

2020. Wiepkema, P. R., K. K. Van Hellemond, P. Roessingh and H. Romberg. 1987. Behaviour and abomasal damage in individual veal calves. *Appl. Anim. Behav. Sci.* 18:257–268.

2021. Wierbowski, S. 1978. The sexual behaviour of experimentally underfed bulls. *Appl. Anim. Ethol.* 4:55–60.

2022. Wierbowski, S. 1959. Odruchy plciowe ogierow. *Roczn. Nauk Rolnicz.* 73:753–788.

2023. Wierenga, H. K. 1990. Social dominance in dairy cattle and the influences of housing and management. *Appl. Anim. Behav. Sci.* 27:201–229.

2024. Wikmar, G. and J. M. Warren. 1972. Delayed response learning by cage-reared normal and prefrontal cats. *Psychonom. Sci.* 26:243–245.

2025. Wilcox, S., K. Dusza and K. A. Houpt. 1991. The relationship between recumbent rest and masturbation in stallions. *Eq. Vet. Sci.* 11:23–26.

2026. Willham, R. L., D. F. Cox and G. G. Karas. 1963. Genetic variation in a measure of avoidance learning in swine. *J. Comp. Physiol. Psychol.* 56:294–297.

2027. Willham, R. L., G. G. Karas and D. C. Henderson. 1964. Partial acquisition and extinction of an avoidance response in two breeds of swine. *J. Comp. Physiol. Psychol.* 57:117–122.

2028. Williams, J. L., T. H. Friend, C. H. Nevill and G. Archer. 2004. The efficacy of a secondary reinforcer (clicker) during acquisition and extinction of an operant task in horses. *Appl. Anim. Behav. Sci.* 88:331–341.

2029. Williams, J. L., T. H. Friend, M. J. Toscano, M. N. Collins, A. Sisto-Burt and C. H. Nevill. 2002. The effects of early training sessions on the reactions of foals at 1, 2, and 3 months of age. *Appl. Anim. Behav. Sci.* 77:105–114.

2030. Williams, M. and J. M. Johnston. 2002. Training and maintaining the performance of dogs (*Canis familiaris*) on an increasing number of odor discriminations in a controlled setting. *Appl. Anim. Behav. Sci.* 78:55–65.

2031. Williamson, N. B., R. S. Morris, D. C. Blood and C. M. Cannon. 1972. A study of oestrous behaviour and oestrus detection methods in a large commercial dairy herd. I. The relative efficiency of methods of oestrus detection. *Vet. Rec.* 91:50–58.

2032. Wilson, E. O. 1975. *Sociobiology. the new synthesis.* Cambridge, MA: The Belknap Press of Harvard University Press.

2033. Wilson, M., J. M. Warren and L. Abbott. 1965. Infantile stimulation, activity, and learning by cats. *Child Dev.* 36:843–853.

2034. Wilson, S. C., F. M. Mitlohner, J. Morrow-Tesch, J. W. Dailey and J. J. McGlone. 2002. An assessment of several potential enrichment devices for feedlot cattle. *Appl. Anim. Behav. Sci.* 76:259–265.

2035. Wilsson, E. 1984. The social interaction between mother and offspring during weaning in German Shepherd dogs: Individual differences between mothers and their effects on offspring. *Appl. Anim. Behav. Sci.* 13:101–112.

2036. Wilsson, E. and P.-E. Sundgren. 1998. Effects of weight, litter size and parity of mother on the behaviour of the puppy and the adult dog. *Appl. Anim. Behav. Sci.* 56:245–254.

2037. Wilsson, E. and P.-E. Sundgren. 1997. The use of a behaviour test for the selection of dogs for service and breeding, I: Method of testing and evaluating test results in the adult dog, demands on different kinds of service dogs, sex and breed differences. *Appl. Anim. Behav. Sci.* 53:279–295.

2038. Wilsson, E. and P.-E. Sundgren. 1997. The use of a behaviour test for the selection of dogs for service and breeding. II. Heritability for tested parameters and effect of selection based on service dog characteristics. *Appl. Anim. Behav. Sci.* 54:235–241.

2039. Winchester, C. F. 1943. The energy cost of standing in horses. *Science* 97:24.

2040. Winfield, C. G., P. H. Hemsworth, M. R. Taverner and P. D. Mullaney. 1974. Observations on the sucking behaviour of piglets in litters of varying size. *Proc. Aust. Soc. Anim. Prod.* 10:307–310.

2041. Winfield, C. G. and R. Kilgour. 1976. A study of following behaviour in young lambs. *Appl. Anim. Ethol.* 2:235–243.

2042. Winfield, C. G. and A. W. Makin. 1978. A note on the effect of continuous contact with ewes showing regular oestrus and post-weaning growth rate on the sexual activity of corriedale rams. *Anim. Prod.* 27:361–364.

2043. Winfield, C. G. and P. D. Mullaney. 1973. A note on the social behaviour of a flock of Merino and Wiltshire Horn sheep. *Anim. Prod.* 17:93–95.

2044. Winfield, C. G., G. J. Syme and A. J. Pearson. 1981. Effect of familiarity with each and breed on the spatial behaviour of sheep in an open field. *Appl. Anim. Ethol.* 7:67–75.

2045. Winkler, W. G. 1977. Human deaths induced by dog bites, United States, 1974–75. *Public Health Rep.* 92:425–429.

2046. Winskill, L. C., N. K. Waran and R. J. Young. 1996. The effect of a foraging device (a modified "Edinburgh Foodball") on the behaviour of a stabled horse. *Appl. Anim. Behav. Sci.* 48:25–35.

2047. Winslow, C. N. 1944. The social behavior of cats. II. Competitive, aggressive, and food-sharing behavior when both competitors have access to the goal. *J. Comp. Psychol.* 37:315–326.

2048. Winter, A. and J. E. Hillerton. 1995. Behaviour associated with feeding and milking of early lactation cows housed in an experimental automatic milking system. *Appl. Anim. Behav. Sci.* 46:1–15.

2049. Wirant, S. C., K. T. Halvorsen and B. McGuire. 2007. Preliminary observations on the urinary behaviour of female Jack Russell Terriers in relation to stage of the oestrous cycle, location, and age. *Appl. Anim. Behav. Sci.* 106:161–166.

2050. Wise, R. A. and V. Dawson. 1974. Diazepam-induced eating and lever pressing for food in sated rats. *J. Comp. Physiol. Psychol.* 86:930–941.

2051. Wolf, A. V. 1950. Osmometric analysis of thirst in man and dog. *Am. J. Physiol.* 161:75–86.

2052. Wolf, B. T., S. D. McBride, R. M. Lewis, M. H. Davies and W. Haresign. 2008. Estimates of the genetic parameters and repeatability of behavioural traits of sheep in an arena test. *Appl. Anim. Behav. Sci.* 112:68–80.

2053. Wolff, A. and M. Hausberger. 1996. Learning and memorisation of two different tasks in horses: The effects of age, sex and sire. *Appl. Anim. Behav. Sci.* 46:137–143.

2054. Wolski, T. R. 1982. Social behavior of the cat. *Vet. Clin. North Am. Small Anim. Pract.* 12:693–706.

2055. Wolski, T. R., K. A. Houpt and R. Aronson. 1980. The role of the senses in mare-foal recognition. *Appl. Anim. Ethol.* 6:121–138.

2056. Wood, M. T. 1977. Social grooming patterns in two herds of monozygotic twin dairy cows. *Anim. Behav.* 25:635–642.

2057. Wood, P. D., G. F. Smith and M. F. Lisle. 1967. A survey of intersucking in dairy herds in England and Wales. *Vet. Rec.* 81:396–398.

2058. Wood, R. J., B. J. Rolls and D. J. Ramsay. 1977. Drinking following intracarotid infusions of hypertonic solutions in dogs. *Am. J. Physiol.* 232:R88–R92.

2059. Wood, T., S. Stanley and T. Tobin. 1989. Operant conditioning and its applications in equine pharmacology. *J. Eq. Vet. Sci.* 9:124–130.

2060. Wood-Gush, D. G. M. 1983. *Elements of ethology.* London, UK: Chapman and Hall.

2061. Wood-Gush, D. G. M. and K. Vestergaard. 1991. The seeking of novelty and its relation to play. *Anim. Behav.* 42:599–606.

2062. Woods, G. L. and K. A. Houpt. 1986. An abnormal facial gesture in an estrous mare. *Appl. Anim. Behav. Sci.* 16:199–202.

2063. Worobec, E. K., I. J. H. Dundan and T. M. Widowski. 1999. The effects of weaning at 7, 14, and 28 days on piglet behaviour. *Appl. Anim. Behav. Sci.* 62:173–182.

2064. Wright, J. C. 1980. Early development of exploratory and dominance in three litters of German Shepherds. In *Early experiences and early behavior*, pp. 181–206. New York, NY: Academic Press.

2065. Wright, J. C. and M. S. Nesselrote. 1987. Classification of behavior problems in dogs: Distributions of age, breed, sex and reproductive status. *Appl. Anim. Behav. Sci.* 19:169–178.

2066. Yamane, A., J. Emoto and N. Ota. 1996. Factors affecting feeding order and social tolerance to kittens in the group-living feral cat (Felis catus). *Appl. Anim. Behav. Sci.* 52:119–127.

2067. Yang, T. S., B. Howard and W. V. Macfarlane. 1981. Effects of food on drinking behaviour of growing pigs. *Appl. Anim. Ethol.* 7:259–270.

2068. Yang, T. S., M. A. Price and F. X. Aherne. 1984. The effect of level of feeding on water turnover in growing pigs. *Appl. Anim. Behav. Sci.* 12:103–109.

2069. Yaniz, J., P. Santolaria and F. Lopez-Gatius. 2003. Relationship between fertility and the walking activity of cows at oestrus. *Vet. Rec.* 152:239–240.

2070. Yarney, T. A., G. W. Rahnefeld, R. J. Parker and W. M. Palmer. 1982. Hourly distribution of time of parturition in beef cows. *Can. J. Anim. Sci.* 62:597–605.

2071. Yeon, S. C., G. Golden, W. Sung, H. N. Erb, A. J. Reynolds and K. A. Houpt. 2001. A comparison of tethering and pen confinement of dogs. *J. Appl. Anim. Welfare Sci.* 4:257–260.

2072. Yerkes, R. M. 1916. The mental life of monkeys and apes: A study of ideational behavior. *Behav. Monogr.* 3:145.

2073. Yerkes, R. M. and C. A. Coburn. 1915. A study of the behavior of the pig (*Sus scrofa*) by the multiple choice method. *J. Anim. Behav.* 5:185–225.

2074. Young, C. A. 1991. Verbal commands as discriminative stimuli in domestic dogs (*Canis familiaris*). *Appl. Anim. Behav. Sci.* 32:75–89.

2075. Young, R. J., J. Carruthers and A. B. Lawrence. 1994. The effect of a foraging device (the "Edinburgh Foodball") on the behaviour of pigs. *Appl. Anim. Behav. Sci.* 39:237–247.

2076. Zablocka, T. 1975. Go-no go differentiation to visual stimuli in cats with different early visual experiences. *Acta Neurobiol. Exp. (Wars)* 35:399–402.

2077. Zablocka, T., J. Konorski and B. Zernicki. 1975. Visual discrimination learning in cats with different early visual experiences. *Acta Neurobiol. Exp. (Wars)* 35:389–398.

2078. Zahorik, D. M. and K. A. Houpt. 1981. Species differences in feed strategies, food hazards, and the ability to learn food aversions. In A. C. Kamil and T. D. Sargent (Eds.), *Foraging behavior*, pp. 289–310. New York, NY: Garland STPM Press.

2079. Zahorik, D. M. and K. A. Houpt. 1977. The concept of nutritional wisdom: Applicability of laboratory learning models to large herbivores. In L. M. Barker, M. R. Best and M. Domjan (Eds.), *Learning mechanisms in food selection*, pp. 45–67. Waco, TX: Baylor University Press.

2080. Zahorik, D. M., K. A. Houpt and J. Swartzman-Ander. 1990. Taste-aversion learning in three species of ruminants. *Appl. Anim. Behav. Sci.* 26:27–39.

2081. Zapelin, H. 1989. Mammalian sleep. In K. H. Kryger, T. Roth and W. C. Dement (Eds.), *Principles and practice of sleep medication*, pp. 30–49. Philadelphia, PA: W.B. Saunders Company.

2082. Zenchak, J. J. and G. C. Anderson. 1980. Sexual performance levels of rams (Ovis aries) as affected by social experiences during rearing. *J. Anim. Sci.* 50:167–174.

2083. Zenchak, J. J. and G. C. Anderson. 1973. Discrimination learning in sheep. *J. Anim. Sci.* 37:227.

2084. Zimmerman, M. B., E. M. Stricker and E. H. Blaine. 1978. Water and NaCl intake after furosemide treatment in sheep (Ovis aires). *J. Comp. Physiol. Psychol.* 92:501–510.

2085. Zonderland, J. J., L. Cornelissen, M. Wolthuis-Fillerup and H. A. M. Spoolder. 2008. Visual acuity of pigs at different light intensities. *Appl. Anim. Behav. Sci.* 111:28–37.

2086. Salter, R. E. and R. J. Hudson. 1979. Feeding ecology of feral horses in Western Alberta. *J. Range Manag.* 32:221–225.

2087. Keiper, R. R. and M. A. Keenan. 1980. Nocturnal activity patterns of feral horses. *J. Mammal.* 61:116–118.

2088. Rubenstein, D. I. 1981. Behavioural ecology of island feral horses. *Equine Vet.* 13:27–34.

2089. Willard, J. G., J. C. Willard, S. A. Wolfram and J. P. Baker. 1977. Effect of diet on cecal pH and feeding behavior of horses. *J. Anim. Sci.* 45:87–93.

2090. Ralston, S. L., G. Van den Broek and C. A. Baile. 1979. Feed intake patterns and associated blood glucose, free fatty acid and insulin changes in ponies. *J. Anim. Sci.* 49:838–845.

2091. Flannigan, G. and J. M. Stookey. 2001. Day-time time budgets of pregnant mares housed in tie stalls: A comparison of draft versus light mares. *Appl. Anim. Behav. Sci.* 78:125–144.

2092. McDonnell, S. M., D. A. Freeman, N. F. Cymbaluk, H. C. Schott, 2nd, K. Hinchcliff and B. Kyle. 1999. Behavior of stabled horses provided continuous or intermittent access to drinking water. *Am. J. Vet. Res.* 60(11):1451–1456.

2093. Ogilvie-Graham, T. S. 1994. *Time Budget Studies in Stalled Horses*. Edinburgh, Scotland: The University of Edinburgh.

2094. Boyd, L. E., D. A. Carbonaro and K. A. Houpt. 1988. The 24-hour time budget of Przewalski horses. *Appl. Anim. Behav. Sci.* 21:5–17.

2095. Boyd, L. E. 1988. Time budgets of adult Przewalski horses: Effects of sex, reproductive status and enclosure. *Appl. Anim. Behav. Sci.* 21:19–39.

2096. Bailey, P. J., A. H. Bishop and C. T. Boord. 1974. Grazing behaviour of steers. *Proc. Aust. Soc. Anim. Prod.* 10:303–306.

2097. Castle, M. E. and R. J. Halley. 1953. The grazing behaviour of dairy cattle at the national institute of research in dairying. *Br. J. Anim. Behav.* 1:139–143.

2098. Culley, M. J. 1938. Grazing habits of range cattle. *J. Forestry.* 36:715–717.

2099. Hardison, W. A., H. L. Fisher, G. G. Graf and N. R. Thompson. 1956. Some observations on the behavior of grazing lactating cows. *J. Dairy Sci.* 39:1735–1741.

2100. Hein, M. A. 1935. Grazing time of beef steers on permanent pastures. *J. Am. Soc. Agron.* 27:675–679.

2101. Holder, J. M. 1960. Observations on the grazing behaviour of lactaging dairy cattle in a subtropical environment. *J. Agric. Sci.* 55:261–267.

2102. Kropp, J. R., J. W. Holloway, D. F. Stephens, L. Knori, R. D. Morrison and R. Totusek. 1973. Range behavior of Hereford, Hereford X Holstein and Holstein non-lactating heifers. *J. Anim. Sci.* 36(4):797–802.

2103. Lampkin, G. H., J. Quarterman and M. Kidner. 1958. Observations on the grazing habits of grade and zebu steers in a high altitude temperature climate. *J. Agric. Sci.* 50:211–218.

2104. Larsen, H. J. 1963. Feeding habits of grazing and green feeding cows. *J. Anim. Sci.* 22:1134.

2105. Lofgreen, G. P., J. H. Meyer and J. L. Hull. 1957. Behavior patterns of sheep and cattle being fed pasture of Silage. *J. Anim. Sci.* 16:773–780.

2106. Moorefield, J. G. and H. H. Hopkins. 1951. Grazing habits of cattle in a mixed-prairie pasture. *J. Range Manag.* 4:151–157.

2107. O'Donnell, T. G. and G. A. Walton. 1969. Some observations on the behaviour and hill-pasture utilization of Irish cattle. *J. Br. Grassland Soc.* 24:128–133.

2108. Sneva, F. A. 1970. Behavior of yearling cattle on eastern Oregon range. *J. Range Manag.* 23:155–158.

2109. Wardrop, J. C. 1953. Studies in the behaviour of dairy cows at pasture. *Br. J. Anim. Behav.* 1:23–31.

2110. Zemo, T. and J. O. Klemmedson. 1970. Behavior of fistulated steers on a desert grassland. *J. Range Manag.* 23:158–163.

2111. Friend, T. H. and C. E. Polan. 1974. Social rank, feeding behavior, and free stall utilization by dairy cattle. *J. Dairy Sci.* 57:1214–1220.

2112. Lewis, R. C. and J. D. Johnson. 1954. Observations of dairy cow activities in loose-housing. *J. Dairy Sci.* 37:269–275.

2113. Schmisseur, W. E., J. L. Albright, W. M. Dillon, E. W. Kehrberg and W. H. Morris. 1966. Animal behavior responses to loose and free stall housing. *J. Dairy Sci.* 49(1):102–104.

2114. Turner, R. R. 1961. Silage self-feeding. *Vet. Rec.* 73:1432–1436.

2115. Squires, V. R. 1974. Grazing distribution and activity patterns of Merino sheep on a saltbush community in south-east Australia. *Appl. Anim. Behav. Sci.* 1:17–30.

2116. Wertz-Lutz, A. E., T. J. Knight, R. H. Pritchard, J. A. Daniel, J. A. Clapper, A. J. Smart, A. Trenkle and D. C. Beitz. 2006. Circulating ghrelin concentrations fluctuate relative to nutritional status and influence feeding behavior in cattle. *J. Anim. Sci.* 84: 3285–3300.

Index

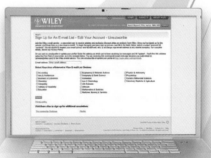
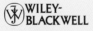